Recent Progress in Osteoporosis Research

Recent Progress in Osteoporosis Research

Edited by Reed Spears

hayle
medical

New York

Hayle Medical,
750 Third Avenue, 9th Floor,
New York, NY 10017, USA

Visit us on the World Wide Web at:
www.haylemedical.com

ISBN: 978-1-63241-723-7

The publisher's policy is to use permanent paper from mills that operate a sustainable forestry policy. Furthermore, the publisher ensures that the text paper and cover boards used have met acceptable environmental accreditation standards.

Printed in China.

Cataloging-in-Publication Data

Recent progress in osteoporosis research / edited by Reed Spears.
p. cm.
Includes bibliographical references and index.
ISBN 978-1-63241-723-7
1. Osteoporosis. 2. Osteoporosis--Research. 3. Bones--Diseases. I. Spears, Reed.
RC931.O73 R43 2019
616.716--dc23

Table of Contents

Preface

Osteoporosis is a disease associated with bone weakness. In osteoporosis, the weakness in bones often increases the risk of a broken bone. The hip bone, the bones of the forearm and the vertebrae in the spine are some of the common bones which usually break due to osteoporosis. It is usually caused in the elderly. Fractures occur commonly in osteoporosis and can potentially result in disability. Osteoporotic fractures generally occur in the shoulder, hip, spine and wrist. Multiple vertebral fractures lead to loss of height, a stooped posture and chronic pain. A dual-energy X-ray absorptiometry is primarily used to diagnose osteoporosis. Some of the common medications include bisphosphonates and teriparatide. This book will provide interesting topics for research, which interested readers can take up. It aims to shed light on some of the unexplored aspects of osteoporosis and the recent researches related to it. The extensive content of this book provides the readers with a thorough understanding of the subject.

This book is a result of research of several months to collate the most relevant data in the field.

When I was approached with the idea of this book and the proposal to edit it, I was overwhelmed. It gave me an opportunity to reach out to all those who share a common interest with me in this field. I had 3 main parameters for editing this text:

1. Accuracy - The data and information provided in this book should be up-to-date and valuable to the readers.

2. Structure - The data must be presented in a structured format for easy understanding and better grasping of the readers.

3. Universal Approach - This book not only targets students but also experts and innovators in the field, thus my aim was to present topics which are of use to all.

Thus, it took me a couple of months to finish the editing of this book.

I would like to make a special mention of my publisher who considered me worthy of this opportunity and also supported me throughout the editing process. I would also like to thank the editing team at the back-end who extended their help whenever required.

Editor

1

Isolation of Antiosteoporotic Compounds from Seeds of *Sophora japonica*

Hossam M. Abdallah[1,2], Ahmed M. Al-Abd[3,4], Gihan F. Asaad[3,5], Ashraf B. Abdel-Naim[4], Ali M. El-halawany[1,2]*

1 Department of Natural Products, Faculty of Pharmacy, King Abdulaziz University, Jeddah, Saudi Arabia, **2** Department of Pharmacognosy, Faculty of Pharmacy, Cairo University, Cairo, Egypt, **3** Pharmacology Department, Medical Division, National Research Center, Giza, Egypt, **4** Department of Pharmacology and Toxicology, Faculty of Pharmacy, King Abdulaziz University, Jeddah, Saudi Arabia, **5** Pharmacology Department, Faculty of Pharmacy, Jazan University, Jazan, Saudia Arabia

Abstract

Chemical investigation of *Sophora japonica* seeds resulted in the isolation of seven metabolites identified as: genistin (**1**), sophoricoside (**2**), sophorabioside (**3**), sophoraflavonoloside (**4**), genistein 7,4′-di-*O*-β-D-glucopyransoide (**5**), kaempferol 3-*O*-α–L-rhamnopyranosyl(1→6)β-D-glucopyranosyl(1→2)β-D-glucopyranoside (**6**) and rutin (**7**). Compounds **1**, **2** and **5** showed significant estrogenic proliferative effect in MCF-7 cell in sub-cytotoxic concentration range. Compounds **1** and **2** showed minimal cell membrane damaging effect using LDH leakage assay. Accordingly, compound **2** (sophoricoside, (SPH)) was selected for further *in-vivo* studies as a potential anti-osteoporosis agent. The anti-osteoporotic effect of SPH was assessed in ovarectomized (OVX) rats after oral administration (15 mg/kg and 30 mg/kg) for 45 days compared to estradiol (10 µg/kg) as a positive control. Only in a dose of 30 mg/kg, SPH regained the original mechanical bone hardness compared to normal non-osteoporotic group. However, SPH (15 mg/kg) significantly increased the level of alkaline phosphatase (ALP) to normal level. Treatment with SPH (30 mg/kg) increased the level of ALP to be higher than normal group. SPH (15 mg/kg) did not significantly increase the serum level of osteocalcin (OC) compared to OVX group. On the other hand, treatment with SPH (30 mg/kg) significantly increased the level of OC to 78% higher than normal non-ovarectomized animals group. In addition, SPH (15 mg/kg) decreased the bone resorption marker, acid phosphatase (ACP) to normal level and SPH (30 mg/kg) further diminished the level of serum ACP. Histopathologically, sophoricoside ameliorated the ovarectomy induced osteoporosis in a dose dependent manner. The drug showed thicker bony trabeculae, more osteoid, and more osteoblastic rimming compared to OVX group.

Editor: Jean-Marc A. Lobaccaro, Clermont Université, France

Funding: This project was funded by the Deanship of Scientific Research (DSR), King Abdulaziz University, Jeddah, under grant no. 208/166/1433. The authors, therefore, acknowledge with thanks DSR technical and financial support. The funders had no role in study design, data collection and analysis, decision to publish, or preparation of the manuscript.

* E-mail: ali.elhalawany@pharma.cu.edu.eg

Introduction

According to the World Health Organization "Osteoporosis is a disease characterized by low bone mass and micro-architectural deterioration of bone tissues, leading to enhanced fragility and consequent increase in fracture risk that results in fractures with minimal trauma". Osteoporosis, a silent epidemic has become a chief health hazard in recent years, afflicting over 2000 million people worldwide [1]. Osteoporosis is associated with deficiency of ovarian hormone following menopause. A sharp decrease in ovarian estrogen production is the predominant cause of rapid, hormone-related bone loss after menopause [2] as a result of higher bone turnover, an imbalance between bone formation and bone resorption & net bone loss [3]. The common sites of fracture among postmenopausal women include the vertebrae, forearm and hip. The incidence of hip fractures & cost for treatment will rise in the future, unless successful prophylactic actions are taken [4].

In Saudi Arabia, the incidence of osteoporosis is common among postmenopausal women; it is often associated with early or late onset of menopause. It was found that osteoporosis is familiar (60%) among postmenopausal Saudi Arabian women [5,6].

Hormone replacement therapy (HRT) effectively ameliorates postmenopausal symptoms and lowers the risk for coronary heart disease and osteoporosis. However, HRT increases the risk of breast cancer and cardiovascular diseases. To overcome the wide range of side effects produced by HRT, there is an increasing demand for "backing to nature" which is considered to be healthier and safer for the treatment of osteoporosis. Phytoestrogens are plant-derived compounds that structurally or functionally mimic mammalian estrogens, and therefore are considered to play an important role in the prevention of cancers, heart disease, menopausal symptoms, and osteoporosis.

Recent reports indicate that phytoestrogens exert their effects in selective estrogen receptor modulators (SERMs) -like manner [7]. The plant food sources high in phytoestrogens are numerous and include soybeans, flaxseeds, and certain other fruits and vegetables rich in polyphenolic compounds.

Sophora japonica L. family Fabaceae, is a tree native to China and Korea. It is also named Japanese pagoda tree (Enju) or Chinese scholar tree. It has been used in Chinese traditional medicine as a haemostatic agent. Flavones from the buds and pericarp were discovered as haemostatic constituents [8,9]. Triterpenes, phospholipids, alkaloids, amino acids and fatty acids have been reported as the main chemical constituents of the seeds of this plant [10,11].

The naringinase-digested methanol extract of *S. japonica* seeds showed potent estrogen agonist activity due to its genistein and kaempferol contents [12]. Genistein from *S. japonica* was also reported to prevent osteoporosis [13]. Moreover, *in-vivo* studies have shown that *S. japonica* extracts prevented bone loss, partly by inhibiting osteoclastic activity [14]. Dichloromethane (DCM) of *S. japonica* fruit extract stimulated alkaline phosphatase activity and matrix mineralization. The DCM fraction also induced expression of osteoblast markers such as alkaline phosphatase, osterix, and osteocalcin in C3H10T1/2 cells and primary bone marrow cells [15].

In the present study the major phenolic compounds from *S. japonica* seed were isolated and their estrogenic activity was determined in MCF-7 cells. Compound that proved highest estrogenic proliferative activity was tested *in-vivo* for its osteoprotective effect in ovarectomized rats.

Results

The methanol extract of *S. japonica* seeds was partitioned with chloroform and the remaining water soluble portion was fractionated on a Diaion HP-20 column to afford 25%, 50%, and 100% methanol fractions. The 50% methanol fraction was purified on several silica gel, ODS and Sephadex LH-20 columns to produce seven compounds. The identification of isolated compounds was achieved systematically by trying the response of the isolated compounds to different spray reagents using thin layer chromatography (TLC) aiming to identify the nature of the compounds. ^{1}H NMR study was carried out for all compounds to, un-ambiguously, identify its structure. Compounds with more than one sugar moiety such as compounds **3–6** were further subjected to ^{13}C NMR measurement to clearly identify site of sugar attachment (Figure S1–S5). The identity of compounds was confirmed by comparing NMR data with previously reported ones as (Figure S1–S5, Table S1), genistin (**1**) [16], sophoricoside (**2**) [17], sophorabioside (**3**), sophoraflavonoloside (**4**), genistein 7,4'-di-*O*-*β*-D-glucopyransoide (**5**) [18], kaempferol 3-*O*-*α*-L-rhamnopyranosyl(1→6)*β*-D-glucopyranosyl(1→2)*β*-D-glucopyranoside (**6**) [19], and rutin (**7**) (Fig. 1). Purity of all isolated compounds was confirmed through HPLC analysis. The purity of compounds **4–6** was over 92%, while that of the remaining compounds was over 95% as indicated by their HPLC chromatograms (Figure S6).

The estrogenic/proliferative properties of compounds isolated from *S. japonica* in MCF-7 cell line

The proliferative effect in estrogen dependent MCF-7 cell line of the isolated compounds was tested. Sub-cytotoxic dose range with potential estrogenic proliferative effect of compounds under investigation was determined using trypan blue exclusion assay and further confirmed using LDH leakage assay.

Trypan blue positive cells was less than 50% after exposure to all compounds under investigation indicative of negative cytotoxic effect until 100 µM concentration. Exposure to 1 mM of compounds **3**, **4**, **6**, and **7** induced trypan staining in more than 50% of cells. On the other hand, exposure to compounds **1**, **2**, and **5** showed trypan blue positive cells less than 1% until 100 µM concentration; and accordingly these compounds can be considered the safest to cell integrity (Table 1).

Effect of compounds under investigation on the cell membrane integrity was further confirmed using more sensitive technique (LDH leakage assay). Exposure to 1 µM of compounds **3**, **4** and **6** induced 2.2, 2.6 and 2.8 folds LDH leakage that in the control group, respectively. The concentration of LDH in media was about 5 folds control group after exposure to 100 µM of compounds **3**, **4** and **6**. On the other hand, the amount of LDH in media over cells treated with concentrations less than 10 µM of compounds **1**, **2**, **5**, and **7** did not exceed double the concentration of LDH leakage in control group. These indicate the harmless effect of these compounds on cell membrane (Figure 2-A).

With respect to the proliferative effect in MCF-7 cell, compounds **3**, **4**, and **6** did not show any significant proliferation enhancement after 72 h of exposure to concentration range of 0.01 to 100 µM. The proliferative effect of compounds **1**, **2**, and **5** was significant in MCF-7 starting from a concentration of 0.01 µM (1.4, 1.5, and 1.2 folds, respectively); and most prominent at concentration of 0.1 µM showing 1.5, 1.6, and 1.3 folds, respectively (Figure 2-B). Based on the cytotoxicity profile, effect on membrane integrity and estrogenic proliferative activity; compound **2** (sophoricoside) was selected for further studies as a potential anti-osteoporosis agent *in-vivo*.

Anti-osteoporosis effect of sophoricoside *in-vivo*

The anti-osteoporosis effect of sophoricoside was investigated mechanically and biochemically in ovarectomized rats after oral administration (15 mg/kg and 30 mg/kg) for 45 days compared to estradiol (10 µg/kg). Mechanical hardness of femur bones was determined after applying longitudinal and vertical forces to the bone shaft and identifying the breaking point pressure.

Mechanically, the forces required to break the femur bones longitudinally and vertically were significantly decreased in response to ovarectomy to be 34% and 56% of the normal bone hardness, respectively. Treatment with E_2 (10 µg/kg) and low dose SPH (15 mg/kg) did not affect the bone hardness in response to longitudinal force; however high dose SPH (30 mg/kg) improved the bone hardness by 43.3% compared to OVX group. In other words, treatment with SPH (30 mg/kg) regained the original longitudinal bone hardness (Figure 3-A). On the other hand, treatment with E_2 (10 µg/kg), SPH (15 mg/g) and SPH (30 mg/kg) significantly improved bone hardness to vertical force by 89.3% and 97.4%, respectively compared to OVX group (Figure 3-B).

Osteoporosis was assessed biochemically by measuring the serum concentration of alkaline phosphatase (ALP) and osteocalcin (OC) as markers for bone formation. In addition, acid phosphatase (ACP) was measured as an indicator for bone resorption. Serum level of ALP was significantly decreased in OVX group indicative of osteoporosis. Treatment with E_2 significantly increased the level of ALP to above normal level. Treatment with sophoricoside (15 mg/kg) significantly increased the level of ALP and brought it to normal level. However, treatment with sophoricoside (30 mg/kg) increased the level of ALP to be higher than normal group (Figure 3- C).

Similar to ALP, Serum level of OC was significantly decreased to about half its original value in response to ovarectomy confirming the incidence of osteoporosis. Treatment with E_2 significantly increased the level of OC back to its normal level. Treatment with sophoricoside (15 mg/kg) did not significantly increase the serum level of OC compared to OVX group. However, treatment with sophoricoside (30 mg/kg) significantly increased the level of OC to 78% higher than normal group non-ovarectomized animals (Figure 3- D).

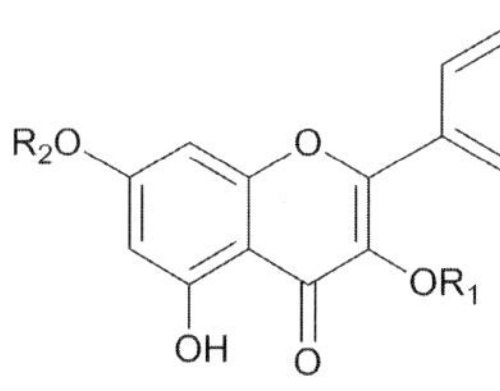

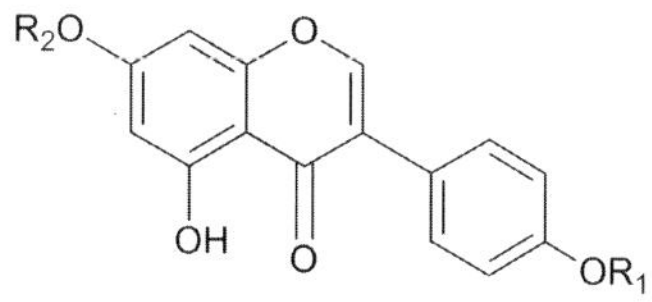

4 R_1= glc (2-1) glc R_2=H

6 R_1= glc (2-1) glc (6-1) rha R_2=H

1 R_1= H R_2=glc
2 R_1= glc R_2=H
3 R_1= glc (2-1) rha R_2=H
5 R_1= glc R_2=glc

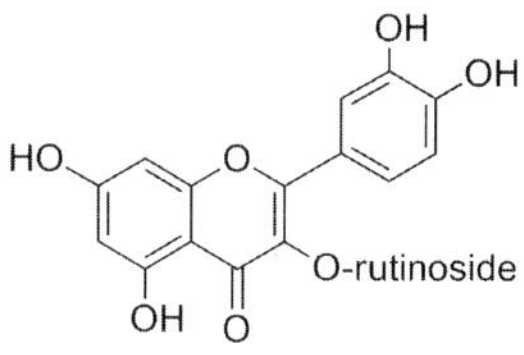

7

Figure 1. Chemical structure for compounds isolated from *Sophora japonica* seeds.

Serum level of ACP was significantly increased (60% compared to control group) in response to OVX indicating prominent hormone dependent bone resorption. ACP level was significantly depressed by E_2 treatment to reach 17.2% of OVX group level. Treatment with sophoricoside (15 mg/kg) significantly decreased the level of ACP and brought it to normal level. Surprisingly, treatment with sophoricoside (30 mg/kg) extensively decreased the level of ACP to be only 4.5% of OVX group level (Figure 3- E).

Histopathological assessment of the anti-osteoporosis effect of sophoricoside

The anti-osteoporotic effect of sophoricoside was confirmed pathologically. Histological pictures of femurs of normal animals showed intact, well-formed, dense bony trabeculae with osteoblastic rimming and average intervening bone marrow (Fig. 4-A). Ovarectomy resulted in prominent osteoporosis in OVX group manifested as thin and widely separated trabeculae with notched and eroded surfaces (Fig. 4-B). Estradiol partly reversed the osteoporosis status showing thicker bony trabeculae and more osteoid and osteoblastic rimming compared to OVX group (Fig. 4-C). Sophoricoside ameliorated the ovarectomy induced osteoporosis in a dose dependent manner. Femurs of animals treated with SPH (15 mg/kg) showed thicker bony trabeculae, more osteoid, and more osteoblastic rimming compared to OVX group (Fig. 4-D). Femurs of animals treated with higher dose of SPH (30 mg/kg) showed thicker bony trabeculae, higher osteoid activity with narrow bone marrow spaces compared to OVX group (Fig. 4-E).

Discussion

Osteoporosis is a major health problem particularly for post-menopause women due to hormonal deficiency [15]. The osteoprotective use of natural compounds with estrogenic activity enabled the avoidance of estrogen replacement therapy and its debilitating side effects [15]. Natural products with inherit nutritional value on top of estrogenic activity such as *S. japonica* represent an interesting nutraceutical alternative for osteoporosis [20–22]. In the current study, we examined the estrogenic proliferative activity of seven compounds isolated from *S. Japonica*

Table 1. Cytotoxicity assessment of compounds isolated from *S. Japonica* using trypan blue exclusion assay.

Cpd	Compound name	Percent dead cells				
		0.1 μM	1 μM	10 μM	100 μM	1 mM
1	Genistin	<1%	<1%	<1%	<1%	42.5±3.6%
2	Sophoricoside	<1%	<1%	<1%	<1%	39.2±2.8%
3	Sophorabicoside	<1%	<1%	2.4±0.2%	15.7±2.7%	63.9±5.1%
4	Sophoraflavonoloside	<1%	1.5±0.3%	8.3±2.6%	17.5±3.1%	74.2±7.4%
5	genistein glucoside	<1%	<1%	<1%	<1%	41.7±3.7%
6	kaempferol glucoside	2.6±0.8%	8.6±1.5%	14.8±3.6%	21.7±4.2%	87.3±5.1%
7	Rutin	<1%	<1%	6.8±2.15	14.3±3.1%	68.5±4.9%

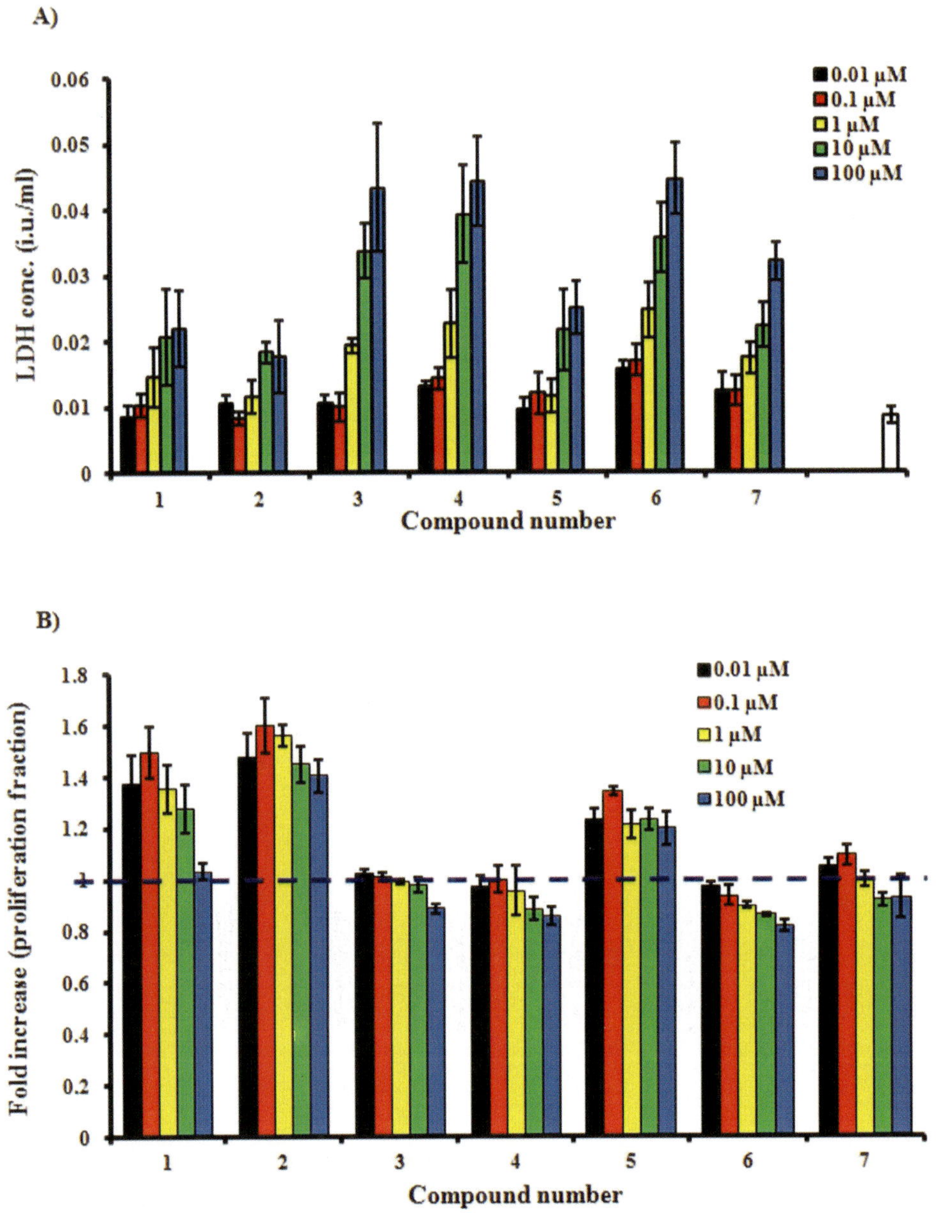

Figure 2. Assessing the estrogenic properties of compounds isolated from *S. japonica* in estrogen dependent MCF-7 cell line. Sub-cytotoxic concentrations of the isolated compounds were determined using LDH leakage assay (A); and proliferative effect was determined using SRB assay (B).

in the estrogen dependent MCF-7 cell line. The best candidate estrogenic compound (Sophoricoside) was further tested for potential osteo-protective activity using ovarectomized rat model.

In the current study, genistin, sophoricoside and genistein 7,4'-di-*O*-*β*-D-glucopyransoide showed significant proliferative activity in estrogen dependent MCF-7 cell line in a subcytotoxic concentration range. Sophoricoside which is highly abundant phytoestrogen in the methanolic extract of *S. Japonica* seeds [12] did not induce any tangible cell membrane damage up to 100 µM concentration. In a previous report, prominent anti-osteoporosis effect of dichloromethane extract of *S. Japonica* fruits was attributed to the high content of the genistein aglycone as evidenced by LC-MS analysis [15]. Sophoricoside which is another genistein glycoside, possess potent estrogenic activity as assessed in our previous work using yeast hybrid assay [12].

Herein, sophoricoside (15 mg/kg and 30 mg/kg) showed promising and dose dependent osteo-protective effect against ovarectomy induced osteoporosis rat model compared to estradiol. Sophoricoside improved the mechanical bone hardness in ovarectomized rats after treatment for 6 weeks. Sophoricoside (4–16 mg/kg for 4 weeks) improved the pathological picture of trabecular bones in ovarectomized rats in previous report [20]; however, herein both mechanical as well as pathological evidences are presented for the osteo-protective effect of sophoricoside. In addition, it was observed that sophoricoside induced significant elevation in the osteogenic biochemical markers such as serum alkaline phosphate and osteocalcin.

Osteo-protective effect of sophoricoside might be attributed to the resulting genistein after hydrolysis in GIT flora or directly to the parent compound *per se*. Therefore, the use of the total

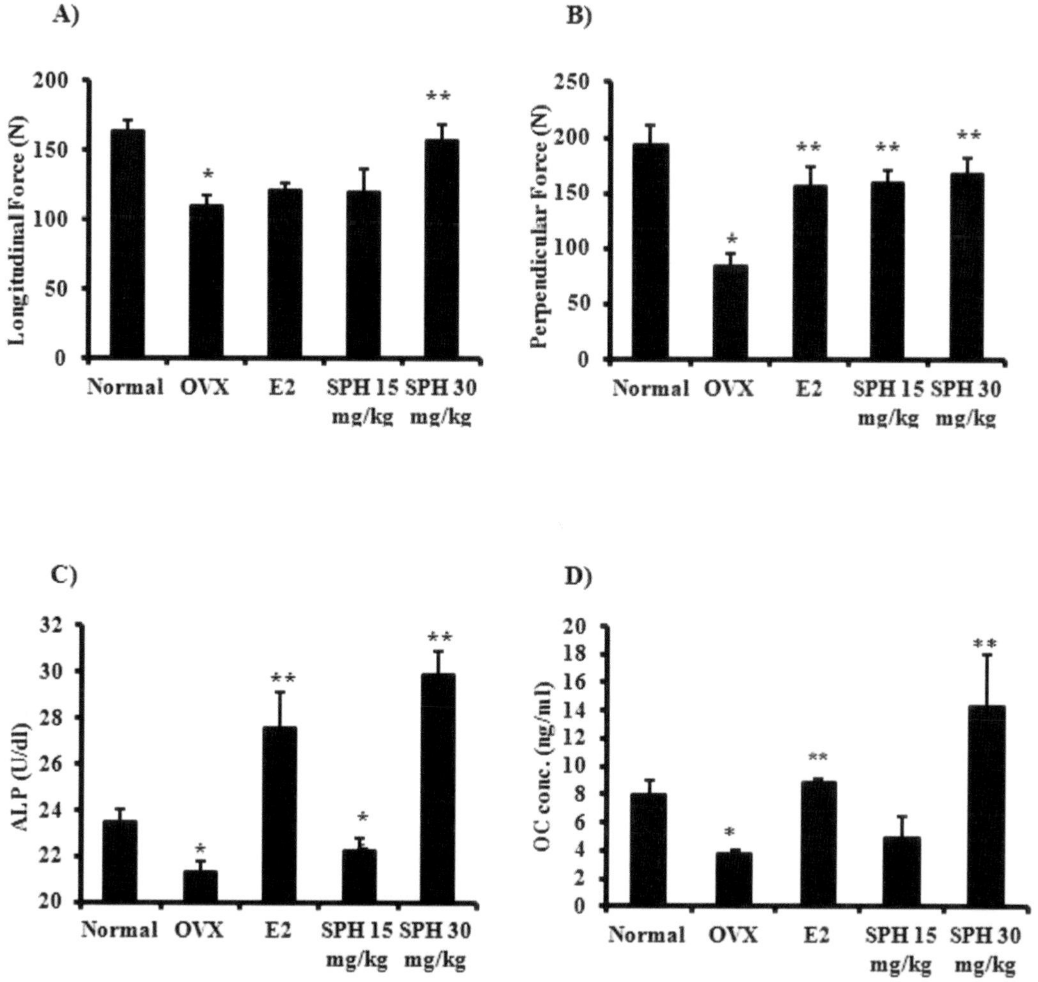

Figure 3. Mechanical and biochemical assessment for anti-osteoporosis effect of sophoricoside *in-vivo*. Ovariectomized rats were treated with SPH (15 mg/kg and 30 mg/kg) for 6 weeks and compared to E_2 treated animals (10 µg/kg) and sham-operation group. Mechanical hardness was evaluated using hardness tester along (A) and perpendicular (B) to femur bone shaft. Biochemical assessment of osteoporosis was evaluated by measuring serum alkaline phosphatase (C) and osteocalcin (D) at the end of treatment period.

alcoholic extract of *S. japonica* seeds could be as effective as sophoricoside due to its high content of geniestein-derived glycosides which will be transformed to genistein upon hydrolysis by GIT flora.

Materials and Methods

General

TLC was carried out on precoated Silica gel 60 F_{254} (0.25 mm, Merck) and RP-18 $F_{254}S$ (0.25 mm, Merck Co., Dermstadt) and spots were detected under UV light or after spraying with anisaldehyde-H_2SO_4 reagent followed by heating. Column chromatography (CC) was carried out on (BW-820MH silica gel), Wakosil C-300 (40–64 µm) (Wako, Osaka, Japan), ODS DM 1020T (ODS, Fuji Silysia, Nagoya, Japan), Diaion HP-20 (Mitsubishi Kasei, Tokyo, Japan) and Sephadex LH-20 (Pharmacia Co.). Medium pressure liquid chromatography (MPLC) was performed on LiChroprep RP-18 and LiChroprep Si 60 (size A and B, Merck Co.). HPLC analysis was conducted on Agilent 1200 liquid chromatography equipped a photodiode array detector. A C18 reversed-phase packing column (4.5 mm×15 cm, 5 µm) were used for separation throughout this study.

Plant material

Seeds of *S. japonica* were collected from the ripe fruits cultivated in the Medicinal Plant Station of Faculty of Pharmacy, Cairo University during December 2012. Authentication of the plant was established by Ass. Prof. Dr. Sherif El-Khanagry, Agriculture Museum, El-Dokki, Cairo, Egypt. A Herbarium specimen (SJ-1023) was prepared and kept at the Herbarium of the Department of Natural Products and Alternative Medicine, Faculty of Pharmacy, King Abdulaziz University.

Extraction and isolation

The pulverized seeds of *S. japonica* (1300 g) were extracted with MeOH (1L x 3) at room temperature and the combined extract was evaporated in *vacuo*. The methanol extract (104 g) was suspended in MeOH and water and successively partitioned with hexane and chloroform to produce hexane (31 g) and chloroform (4 g) soluble fractions. The remaining aqueous layer was fractionated on a Diaion HP-20 column (60 cm×6 cm) stepwisely eluted with H_2O, 25%, 50% and 100% MeOH. The eluates were evaporated under vacuum to afford H_2O fraction (26 g), 25% MeOH fraction (8.5 g), 50% MeOH fraction (14 g) and 100% MeOH fraction 5.8 g. The 50% MeOH (12 g) was applied to a

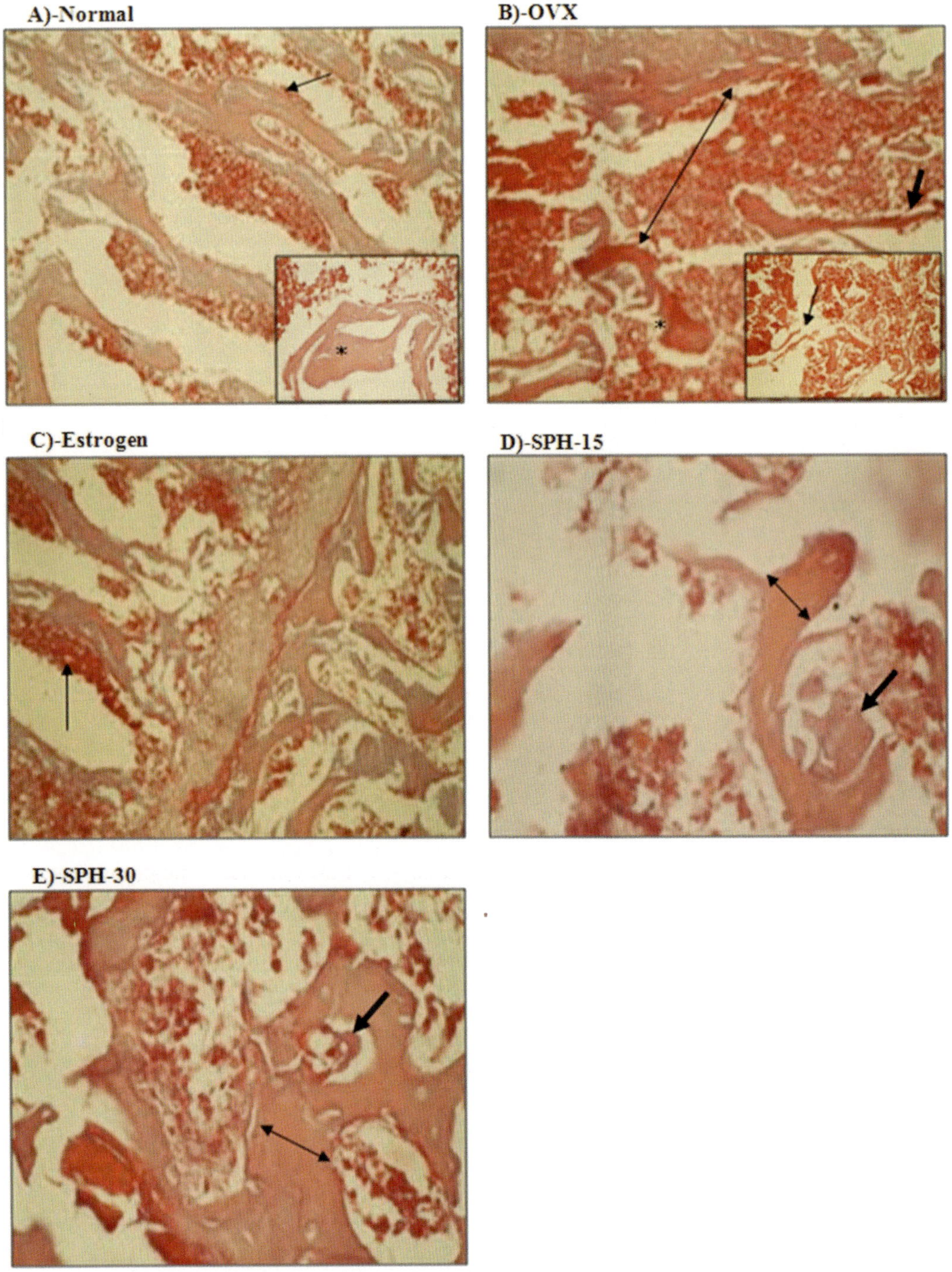

Figure 4. Histopathological assessment of the anti-osteoporosis effect of sophoricoside. Normal group (A) shows normal bony tissue with intact well-formed dense trabeculae (star in the inner panel) with osteoblastic rimming (arrow) and average intervening bone marrow. OVX group (B) showed scant, disconnected (arrow in inner panel), thin (arrow in the outer panel), and widely separated trabeculae (double-headed arrow in the outer panel) with eroded surface (star in the outer panel). Estrogen treated group (C) showed widely distributed osteoid and osteoblastic rimming (arrow). SPH-15 group (D) showed thick trabeculae (double-headed arrow), more osteoid, and osteoblastic activity (arrow). SPH-30 group (E) showed thick trabeculae (double-headed arrow), more osteoid and osteoblastic activity (arrow).

silica gel column (300 g silica) and gradienltly eluted with $CHCl_3$-MeOH-H_2O (9:1:0.1 v/v/v) to obtain 8 fractions. Fraction 3 (2 g) gave a yellow precipitate upon concentration, that was washed several times by chloroform-methanol to obtain compound **3** (193 mg). The supernatant of this fraction was purified on an MPLC RP-18 column (size A) using MeOH-H_2O (4:6 v/v) to afford compounds **1** (120 mg), and **2** (500 mg). Fraction 4 gave compound **4** (358 mg) upon crystallization from MeOH and the remaining supernatant was applied to an MPLC RP-18 column (size A) eluted with MeOH-H_2O (3:7 v/v) to get **7** (5 mg). Fraction 5 gave compound **5** (180 mg) by crystallization from MeOH-$CHCl_3$.Fraction 6 (1.5 g) was purified on a Sephadex LH-

20 column (30 cm×3 cm) eluted with MeOH-H_2O (1:1 v/v). Subfractions 17–30 of this column was combined together and applied to an MPLC RP-18 column (size A) eluted with MeOH-H_2O (3:7 v/v) to get compound **6** (37.4 mg). Purity of all compounds were analyzed using HPLC using a gradient elution (water – TFA, 0.1% v/v) to solvent B (acetonitrile), with a flow rate of 1.0 ml min

Chemicals and drugs

Sulfarhodamine B (SRB) and 17β-hydroxyesradiol were purchased from Sigma-Aldrich Chemical Company (St. Louis, MO, USA), RPMI-1640 media, fetal bovine serum and other cell culture materials were purchased from Euroclone (Milano, Italy). Urethane was purchased from Biobasic Inc. (Toronto, Canada). All other chemicals were of the highest available analytical grade.

Cell culture

Human estrogen dependent breast adenocarcinoma cells (MCF-7 cell line) were obtained from the Vacsera (Giza, Egypt). Cells were maintained in RPMI-1640 supplemented with 100 μg/mL streptomycin, 100 units/mL penicillin and 10% heat-inactivated fetal bovine serum in a humidified, 5% (v/v) CO_2 atmosphere at 37°C.

Cytotoxicity assessment

Cytotoxicity of compounds isolated from *S. Japonica* was tested in MCF-7 cells by trypan-blue exclusion assay. Briefly, exponentially growing cells were plated in 96-well plates. Cells were exposed to serial dilutions of isolated compounds for 2, 4, 7 and 10 days and the percent of trypan blue positive cells was determined in live culture [1,23].

Cell membrane integrity assessment

The influence of compounds isolated from *S. Japonica* against the cell membrane integrity was assessed in MCF-7 cells by LDH leakage assay [24]. Briefly, exponentially growing cells were plated in 6-well plates. Cells were exposed to serial concentrations of isolated compounds for 24 h and the LDH was determined in the culture media using colorimetric assay (Biosystems, Barcelona, Spain).

Proliferation assay

The proliferative effect of compounds isolated from *S. Japonica* was tested in MCF-7 cells by SRB assay as well. Briefly, exponentially growing cells were exposed to sub-cytotoxic concentrations of the isolated compounds for 72 h and subsequently stained with SRB solution for quantification [25,26].

Animals and animal treatment

Animal handling and treatment was approved by the bioethical and research committee of The National Research Center. Female Sprague Drawly rats (300 g weight) were acclimatized in the animal house facility of The National Research Center, Cairo, Egypt, for at least one week prior to experimentation. Animals were kept at 20±2°C and 65±10% relative humidity during the whole experiment. Standard food pellets and water were supplied *ad labium*. All experiments were performed between 8–10 A.M.

Osteoporosis was induced in rats by ovarectomy as previously described with minor modification [3]. Briefly, rats in the same menstrual phase were selected and confirmed by vaginal smear and underwent experimental ovarectomy. Animals were anesthetized by i.p. injection of urethane (1 g/kg). Surgical incision of about 5 mm was made in each of the hind dorsal flank regions of rats exposing the ovary and surrounding periovarian fat bed. Both fallopian tubes were suture-closed at the most distal end and both ovaries were surgically excised carefully. The incision was sutured and dressed with sterile povidone iodine solution. Sham operations were performed to animals of control groups. Animal were let for two weeks to recover from the surgical trauma. Then, animals were divided into 5 groups (n = 10 per group). Control group which was subjected to sham operation; OVX group was surgically ovarectomized and received saline vehicle daily. Estrogen group (E_2) was subjected to surgical ovarectomy and received 17β-estradiol (10 μg/kg) via i.p. injection daily; sophoricoside low dose group (SPH-15) was subjected to surgical ovarectomy and received sophoricoside (15 mg/kg) p.o. daily. Sophoricoside high dose group (SPH-30) was subjected to surgical ovarectomy and received sophoricoside (30 mg/kg) p.o. daily. All animals were allowed free access for food and water throughout the whole experiment (45 day). Blood samples were withdrawn by retro-orbital plexus puncture; and the serum was collected then animals were sacrificed by cervical dislocation. Both right and left femur bones were dissected immediately *post mortem*; left femurs were used to measure hardness; and the right femurs were fixed in buffered formalin solution (4%) for histological assessment.

Bone hardness assessment

To quantify the degree of osteoporosis, hardness of left femurs was measured using hardness tester (Erweka GmbH, Heusenstamm, Germany) as previously described with minor modification [27]. Briefly, left femurs were placed in the clamp assembly of the hardness tester in a vertical (n = 5) and horizontal (n = 5) positions to the force direction. Minimum force required to induce bone shaft fracture was recorded.

Serological evaluation of osteoporosis in-vivo

To assess the ossification process in response to treatment with sophoricoside, serum level of alkaline phosphatase (ALP), acid phophatase (ACP) and osteocalcin (OC) were measured. ALP and tartarate-resistant ACP were determined by direct HTS-ready colorimetric assay (Abcam, Cambridge, UK) [28]. Osteocalcin was determined using Uscan immunoassay ELISA Kit (Life Science Inc. Wuhan, China) according to the manufacturer's instructions [29]

Histological examination for rat lamellar bone tissue

Histological assessment for lamellar bone was performed according the lab routine protocol. Briefly, paraformaldhyde fixed tissues were decalcified by EDTA and embedded in paraffin wax. Cross vertical sections (5 μm) were obtained and after dewaxing and rehydration sections were stained with H&E.

Statistical analysis

Data are presented as mean ± SEM. Analysis of variance (ANOVA) with LSD post hoc test was used for testing the significance using SPSS for windows, version 17.0.0. $p<0.05$ was taken as a cut off value for significance.

Supporting Information

Figure S1 ^{1}H-NMR charts of compounds 1, 2 and 7. (A) Compound 1; (B) Compound 2; (C) Compound 7.

Figure S2 ^{1}H-NMR and ^{13}C-NMR charts of compound 3.

Figure S3 ^{1}H-NMR and ^{13}C-NMR charts of compound 4.

Figure S4 ^{1}H-NMR and ^{13}C-NMR charts of compound 5.

Figure S5 ^{1}H-NMR and ^{13}C-NMR charts of compound 6.

Figure S6 HPLC chromatograms of isolated compounds.

Table S1 ^{13}C NMR data of compounds 3-6.

Author Contributions

Conceived and designed the experiments: HMA AMA ABA AME. Performed the experiments: HMA AMA GFA AME. Analyzed the data: AMA AME. Contributed reagents/materials/analysis tools: HMA AMA. Wrote the paper: HMA AMA GFA AME.

References

1. Cowan JD, Von Hoff DD, Neueneflldt B, Mills LS GM, Clark GM (1984) Predictive value of trypan blue exclusion viability measurements for colony formation in a human tumor cloning assay. Canc Drug Del 1: 95–100.
2. Gruber HE, Ivey JL, Baylink DJ, Matthews M, Nelp WB, et al. (1984) Long-term calcitonin therapy in postmenopausal osteoporosis. Metabolism 33: 295–303.
3. Reddy NP, Lakshmana M (2005) Assessment of experimental osteoporosis using CT-scanning, quantitative X-ray analysis and impact test in calcium deficient ovariectomized rats. J Pharmacol Toxicol 52: 350–355.
4. Obrant KJ, Bengner U, Johnell O, Nilsson BE, Sernbo I (1989) Increasing age-adjusted risk of fragility fractures: a sign of increasing osteoporosis in successive generations? Calcif Tissue Int 44: 157–167.
5. Addar M, El Desouki M, Babay Z (2004) Correlates of age at menopause and osteoporosis in Saudi women. Clin Exp Obstet Gyn 32: 135–137.
6. Sadat-Ali M, Al-Habdan IM, Al-Mulhim FA, El-Hassan AY (2004) Bone mineral density among postmenopausal Saudi women. Saudi Med J 25: 1623–1625.
7. Brzezinski A, Debi A (1999) Phytoestrogens: the "natural" selective estrogen receptor modulators? Eur J Obstet Gyn R B 85: 47–51.
8. Ishida H, Umino T, Tsuji K, Kosuge T (1989) Studies on the anti-hemorrhagic substances in herbs classified as hemostatics in Chinese medicine. X. On hemostatic activities of the parched herbs for hemostatics]. Yakugaku zasshi 109: 179.
9. Tang Y, Lou F, Wang J, Zhuang S (2001) Four New Isoflavone Triglycosides from *Sophora japonica*. J Nat Prod 64: 1107–1110.
10. Grishkovets V, Gorbacheva L (1995) Triterpene glycosides of*Sophora japonica* seeds. Chem Nat Comp 31: 596–599.
11. Mukhamedova KS, Glushenkova A (1997) Phospholipids of ripeSophora japonica seeds. Chem Nat Comp 33: 445–448.
12. El-Halawany AM, Chung MH, Abdallah HM, Nishihara T, Hattori M (2010) Estrogenic activity of a naringinase-treated extract of *Sophora japonica* cultivated in Egypt. Pharm Biol 48: 177–181.
13. Wang Z, Sun J, Wang D, Xie Y, Wang S, et al. (2006) Pharmacological studies of the large-scaled purified genistein from Huaijiao *Sophora japonica* – Leguminosae) on anti-osteoporosis. Phytomedicine 13: 718–723.
14. Shim JG, Yeom SH, Kim HJ, Choi YW, Song KY, et al. (2005) Bone loss preventing effect of Sophorae Fructus on ovariectomized rats. Arch Pharm Res 28: 106–110.
15. Yoon H-J, Seo C-R, Kim M, Kim Y-J, Song N-J, et al. (2013) Dichloromethane extracts of *Sophora japonica* L. stimulate osteoblast differentiation in mesenchymal stem cells. Nutr Res 33: 1035–1062.
16. Mostafa K, Ahmed A, Ali A (2003) Chemical constituents and antidiabetic activity of *Trifolium alexandrinum* L. Bull Fac Pharm 41: 253–263.
17. Min B, Oh SR, Lee H-K, Takatsu K, Chang I-M, et al. (1999) Sophoricoside analogs as the IL-5 inhibitors from *Sophora japonica*. Planta Med 65: 408–412.
18. Watanabe K, Kinjo J, Nohara T (1993) Three new isoflavonoid glycosides from *Lupinus luteus* L.and *polyphyllus arboreus*. Chem Pharm Bull 41: 394–396.
19. Tang Y-P, Li Y-F, Hu J, Lou F-C (2002) Isolation and identification of antioxidants from *Sophora japonica*. J Asian Nat Prod Res 4: 123–128.
20. Du N, Xu Y, Chen WZ, Zhang FH (2003) [Effect of Sophoricoside on histomorphology of bone in ovariectomized rats]. Zhong Xi Yi Jie He Xue Bao 1: 44–46.
21. Jia TL, Wang HZ, Xie LP, Wang XY, Zhang RQ (2003) Daidzein enhances osteoblast growth that may be mediated by increased bone morphogenetic protein (BMP) production. Biochem Pharmacol 65: 709–715.
22. Shim JG, Yeom SH, Kim HJ, Choi YW, Lee DI, et al. (2005) Bone loss preventing effect of Sophorae Fructus on ovariectomized rats. Arch Pharm Res 28: 106–110.
23. Mahmoud AM, Al-Abd AM, Lightfoot DA, El-Shemy HA (2012) Anti-cancer characteristics of mevinolin against three different solid tumor cell lines was not solely p53-dependent. J Enzyme Inhib Med Chem 27: 673–679.
24. Phillips CA, Hughes DR, Huja SS (2009) Modifications of the lactate dehydrogenase assay, a histochemical determinant of osteocyte viability–A qualitative study. Acta Histochem 111: 166–171.
25. Skehan P, Storeng R, Scudiero D, Monks A, McMahon J, et al. (1990) New colorimetric cytotoxicity assay for anticancer-drug screening. J Natl Cancer I 82: 1107–1112.
26. Mosli HA, Tolba MF, Al-Abd AM, Abdel-Naim AB (2013) Catechol estrogens induce proliferation and malignant transformation in prostate epithelial cells. Toxicol Lett 220: 247–258.
27. Ko Y-J, Wu J-B, Ho H-Y, Lin W-C (2012) Antiosteoporotic activity of *Davallia formosana*. J Ethnopharmacol 139: 558–565.
28. Gerhardt W, Nielsen ML, Nielsen OV, Olsen J, Statland B (1974) Clinical evaluation of routine measurement of liver and bone alkaline phosphatases in human serum: Differential inhibition by l-phenylalanine and carbamide (urea) on the LKB 8600 reaction rate analyzer. Clin Chim Acta 53: 291–297.
29. Fu J, Muller D (1999) Simple, rapid enzyme-linked immunosorbent assay (ELISA) for the determination of rat osteocalcin. Calcif Tissue Int 64: 229–233.

2

Mitigation of Oxidative Damage by Green Tea Polyphenols and Tai Chi Exercise in Postmenopausal Women with Osteopenia

Guoqing Qian[1], Kathy Xue[1], Lili Tang[1], Franklin Wang[1], Xiao Song[2], Ming-Chien Chyu[3], Barbara C. Pence[4], Chwan-Li Shen[4,5,6], Jia-Sheng Wang[1]*

1 Department of Environmental Health Science, University of Georgia, Athens, Georgia, United States of America, **2** Department of Epidemiology and Biostatistics, University of Georgia, Athens, Georgia, United States of America, **3** Department of Mechanical Engineering, Texas Tech University, Lubbock, Texas, United States of America, **4** Laboratory Science and Primary Care, Texas Tech University Health Sciences Center, Lubbock, Texas, United States of America, **5** Department of Pathology, Texas Tech University Health Sciences Center, Lubbock, Texas, United States of America, **6** Laura W. Bush Institute for Women's Health, Texas Tech University Health Sciences Center, Lubbock, Texas, United States of America

Abstract

Background: Osteoporosis is a degenerative bone disease predominantly in postmenopausal women. Green tea polyphenols (GTP) and Tai Chi (TC) have been shown to be beneficial on human bone health. This study examined the efficacy of GTP and TC on mitigation of oxidative damage in postmenopausal women with osteopenia.

Methods: A 6-month randomized and placebo-controlled clinical trial was conducted in 171 postmenopausal women with osteopenia, who were recruited from Lubbock County, Texas. These participants were treated with placebo, GTP (500 mg daily), placebo + TC (60-minute group exercise, 3 times/week), or GTP (500 mg daily) + TC (60-minute group exercise, 3 times/week), respectively. Their blood and urine samples were collected at the baseline, 1-, 3- and 6-months during intervention for assessing levels of 8-hydroxy-2′-deoxyguanosine (8-OHdG), an oxidative DNA damage biomarker, and concentrations of serum and urine GTP components.

Results: The elevated concentrations of serum and urinary GTP components demonstrated a good adherence for the trial. A significant reduction of urinary 8-OHdG concentrations was found in all three treated groups during 3-month ($P<0.001$) and 6-month ($P<0.001$) intervention, as compared to the placebo group. The significant time- and dose-effects on mitigation of the oxidative damage biomarker were also found for GTP, TC, and GTP+TC intervened groups.

Conclusion: Our study demonstrated that GTP and TC interventions were effective strategies of reducing the levels of oxidative stress, a putative mechanism for osteoporosis in postmenopausal women, and more importantly, working in an additive manner, which holds the potential as alternative tools to improve bone health in this population.

Trial Registration: ClinicalTrials.gov NCT00625391

Editor: D William Cameron, University of Ottawa, Canada

Funding: This work was supported by the National Center for Complementary and Alternative Medicine (R21AT003735)(nccam.nih.gov/) and National Cancer Institute, National Institutes of Health (RO1CA90997)(www.cancer.gov). The funders had no role in study design, data collection and analysis, decision to publish, or preparation of the manuscript.

Competing Interests: The authors have declared that no competing interests exist.

* E-mail: jswang@uga.edu

Introduction

Osteoporosis is a degenerative bone disease characterized by low bone mass and structural deterioration of bone tissue. Bone fragility and increased susceptibilities to bone fracture especially in the hip, spine and wrist are common outcomes [1]. Worldwide, osteoporosis is a huge health and social concern as approximately 200 million women suffer from this chronic disease [2]. In the United States, it is estimated that about 44 million people at age of 50 and older suffer from osteoporosis or low bone mass [3]. Postmenopausal women have four times the risk to develop osteoporosis than men due to decreased estrogen levels after menopause and represent the highest risk population [4]. Etiological risk factors associated with osteoporosis include poor nutrition, imbalanced cytokines and hormones, and the aging process [5,6]. It has been noticed that reactive oxygen species (ROS) plays a key role in the aging process, and contributes greatly to osteoporosis [7–9]. Roles of ROS in the pathology of osteoporosis have been reviewed in detail by Manolagas [10], including influences of the generation and survival of osteoclasts, osteoblasts, and osteocytes, disturbance of FoxOs in early mesenchymal progenitors and Wnt signaling pathway, which led to decreased osteoblastogenesis. Excess ROS can damage DNA to form 8-hydroxy-2′-deoxyguanosine (8-OHdG), an oxidative biomarker that has been widely used in human studies to indicate the oxidative stress status [11,12].

Green tea polyphenols (GTP, extract of green tea) have shown its osteo-protective effects via decreasing oxidative stress, increasing activity of antioxidant enzymes, and decreasing expression of proinflammatory mediators in rodent models [13], and the beneficial effects of GTP on bone health has been reviewed recently [14]. Biomarkers of green tea consumption using green tea components have been validated in human studies [15], and the GTP supplementation has demonstrated chemopreventive effects on cancer [16], cardiovascular diseases [17], and neurodegenerative diseases [18]. However, limited information is available about the beneficial effect of consumption of tea or its bioactive components (i.e., GTP) on bone health in postmenopausal women. On the other hand, Tai Chi (TC) exercise, a form of low to moderate intensity mind-body exercise with aerobic and muscular fitness activity, has been demonstrated to potentially benefit bone health in several human studies [19–21]. The potential mechanisms include slowing the decrease of bone mineral density (BMD) [22], reducing the oxidative damage, and enhancing the enzyme activity of superoxide dismutase (SOD) [23]. Nevertheless, the information on effects of GTP and TC, especially their combined effects, on oxidative stress status of postmenopausal women is lacking.

In this study, a 6-month placebo-controlled randomized trial was conducted to examine the pharmacokinetics of GTP and effects of GTP and TC on mitigation of the oxidative damage biomarker in 171 study participants, who were recruited from a large community pool including 1,065 postmenopausal women. As for the whole project of this clinical trial, the detailed study protocol [24], the data on the safety issues and life quality of study participants [25], and clinical outcomes on bone health [26] have been published previously.

Methods

The protocol for this trial and supporting CONSORT checklist are available as supporting information; see Checklist S1 and Protocol S1.

1. Study Participants and Design

The detailed flow of the trial is described in Figure 1. The study participants were screened and enrolled in 2007 from Lubbock, Texas and the surrounding area. The trial was conducted in 2007–2008. The study followed the randomized and placebo-controlled clinical trial guidelines from National Institute of Health (NIH). Briefly, a total of 171 community-dwelling postmenopausal women were recruited to participate in this 6-month trial. The recruited participants were randomized in a stratified method based on age (≥65 or <65 years old), history of green tea consumption, and history of mind-body exercise and assigned to one of the four treatment groups: Placebo group (age: 57.6 (7.5), mean (SD)): medicinal starch 500 mg daily; GTP group (age: 56.5 (5.5), mean (SD)): GTP 500 mg daily; Placebo+TC group (age: 58.3 (7.7), mean (SD)): medicinal starch 500 mg daily and 24-move simplified Yang-style TC training (60 minutes per session, 3 sessions per week), and GTP+TC group (age: 57.6 (6.7), mean (SD)): GTP 500 mg daily and 24-move simplified Yang-style TC training (60 minutes per session, 3 sessions per week). A daily dose of GTP or placebo material was administered as two capsules (250 mg each). Daily consumption of such a GTP dose (500 mg) was equivalent to 4 cups of green tea (about 500 mL). During intervention, all participants were provided with 500 mg elemental calcium and 200 IU vitamin D (as cholecalciferol) daily. The complete study protocol has been reported in detail previously [24]. Inclusion criteria in this study included: postmenopausal women (at least 2 years after menopause) with osteopenia (mean lumbar spine and/or hip BMD T-score between 1 and 2.5 standard deviation (SD) below the normal sex-matched areal BMD of the reference database; normal function of thyroid, liver, and kidney; and serum 25-hydroxy vitamin D (25-OH-D, ≥20 ng/mL)). Women were excluded if they had a disease condition or were taking medication known to affect bone metabolism; history of cancer except for treated superficial basal or squamous cell carcinoma of the skin; uncontrolled intercurrent illness or physical condition that would be a contraindication to exercise; depression; cognitive impairment; and if unwilling to accept randomization. Written informed consent was obtained from all the participants before enrollment and the study was approved by the Texas Tech University Health Sciences Center Institutional Review Board.

2. Randomization and Blinding

A central allocation schedule for randomization was prepared through a computer-generated random sequence of the four treatment allocations. Treatment assignments were then made from separate randomization sequences created for each stratum. Placebo or GTP capsules dispersion was conducted by the site research pharmacist according to the patient's randomization assignment. Research staff and medical staff were unaware of the treatment assignment. Sample analysis, data collection and statistical analysis were blinded to the technical personnel.

3. Sample Size

Data from previous studies were used for calculation of sample size. The effect size of 0.75 was assumed based on the baseline mean and standard deviation (SD) values for the primary outcome of urinary 8-OHdG (7.5±2.5 pmol/mL) [27]. Equal sample size for each group was assumed. The main comparisons are expected to be made as follows: placebo vs. GTP; placebo vs. placebo+TC; and placebo vs. GTP+TC. The sample size was calculated based on detecting a 25% change in urinary 8-OHdG, as compared to placebo group, with a power of 0.8 at $\alpha = 0.05$. An assumed correlation coefficient of 0.80 between baseline and follow-up measurements within a treatment group was used. The sample size for each group was estimated to be 32 for urinary 8-OHdG based on a previously reported method [28]. Therefore, a total sample size of 128 participants is needed which requires 151 participants at an attrition rate of 15%.

4. Chemicals and Instruments

GTP capsules and placebo agents were supplied by Zhejiang Yixin Pharmaceutical Co., Ltd. China (GTP IND no. 77,470 by FDA of USA). The main GTP components were 46.5% of epigallocatechin-3-gallate (EGCG), 21.25% of epigallocatechin (ECG), 10% of epicatechin (EC), 7.5% of epicatechin-3-gallate (EGC), 9.5% of gallocatechingallate (GCG), and 4.5% of catechin with the purity higher than 98.5%. Authentic standards of EC, ECG, EGC, and EGCG, beta-glucuronidase, sulfatase, and tetrahydroxyfuran (THF) were purchased from Sigma Chemical Co. (St. Louis, MO). Acetonitrile (ACN) was purchased from Burdick & Jackson (Muskegon, MI). Ethyl acetate, methylene chloride, and sodium dihydrophosphate (NaH_2PO4) were products of Fisher Scientific (Pittsburgh, PA). An ESA HPLC-CoulArray system (Chelmsford, MA) was used for detection of GTP components and metabolites as well as urinary 8-OHdG.

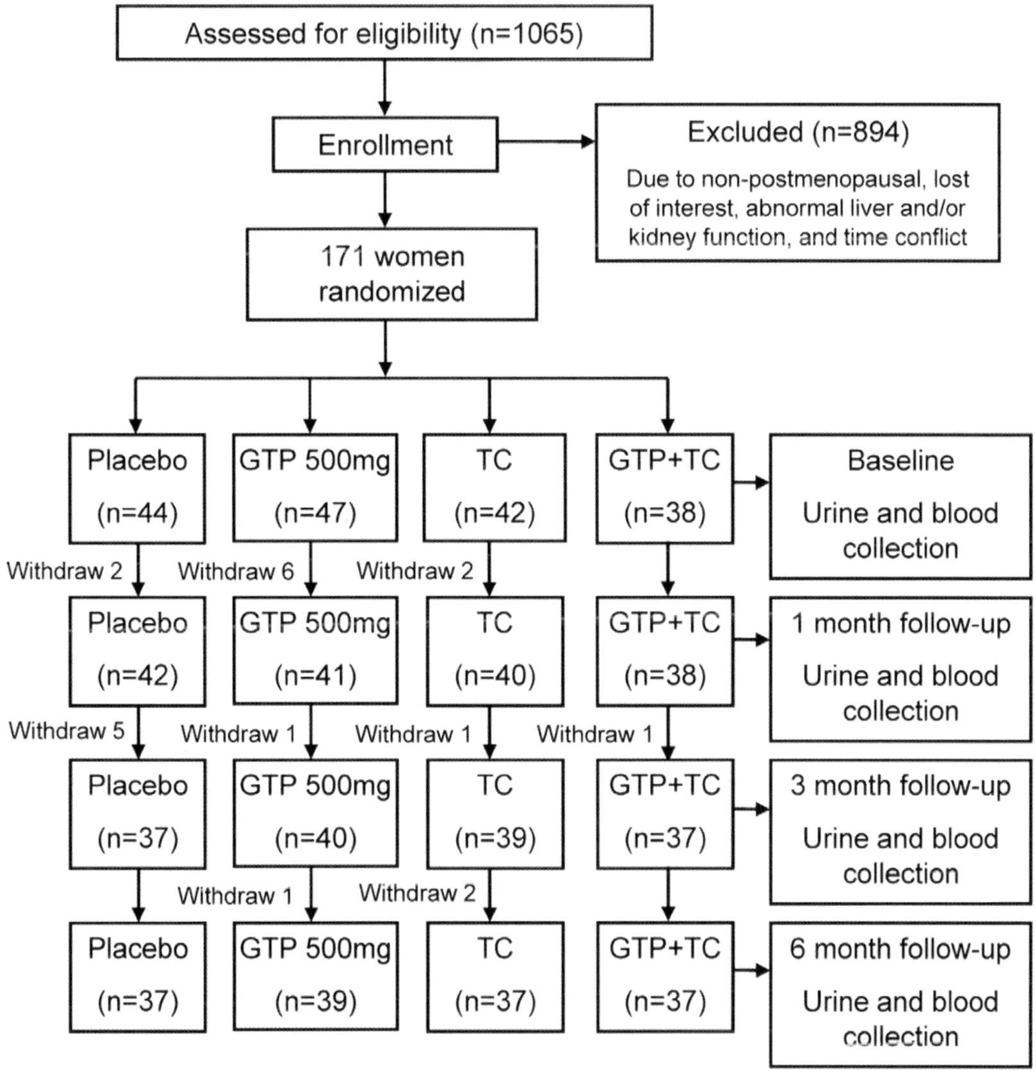

Figure 1. Flow chart of the trial.

5. Blood and Urine Sample Collection and Processing

All participants reported to Clinical Research Center at Texas Tech University Medical Center for blood/urine collection. The blood samples were collected between 7:00 and 10:00 a.m. after an overnight fast with abstinence of food, drink, nicotine, and caffeine. Blood was drawn from a superficial arm vein with a syringe, transferred to a vacutainer, allowed to clot at room temperature, and then centrifuged at 1500 g for 10 min within 2 hours of collection to separate plasma or serum. Urine samples were also collected in acid-washed polyethylene containers. After the total volume of the urine sample was measured to an accuracy of 0.1 ml and recorded, urine was aliquoted. All plasma and urine samples were stored at −80°C before analyses.

6. Extraction of Serum and Urinary GTP

The protocol for serum GTP extraction was previously published [15]. Briefly, 200 μL serum samples were incubated with beta-glucuronidase (500 units) and sulfatase (20 units) at 37°C for 45 min to release the conjugated GTP components before repeated extraction with 400 μL methylene chloride to remove proteins and lipids. The aqueous phases were pooled for twice extraction with 700 μL ethyl acetate, and the organic phase was vacuum-dried with a Labconco Centrivap concentrator (Kansas City, MO) and reconstituted for HPLC-ECD analysis.

Urinary GTP extraction followed a previously established protocol [27]. Briefly, thawed urine samples were centrifuged and 1 mL supernatant was taken for 60 min incubation with beta-glucuronidase (500 units) and sulfatase (2 units) at 37°C to release conjugated GTP, then directly extracted twice with ethyl acetate. Organic phases were pooled, dried *in vacuo*, and reconstituted in 15% acetonitrile before analysis.

7. HPLC-ECD Analysis of Serum and Urinary GTP Components

The method for analyzing serum and urinary GTP conjugates was modified from previously established protocols [27]. GTP analysis was conducted in the ESA HPLC-CoulArray system (Chelmsford, MA). The mobile phases consisted of buffer A (30 mM NaH_2PO_4:ACN:THF at 98%: 1.8%: 0.2%, v/v, pH 3.35) and buffer B (15 mM NaH_2PO_4:ACN:THF at 30%: 63%: 7%, v/v, pH 3.45). The Zorbax Eclipse XDB-C18 (5 micron, 4.6×250 mm) was used and maintained at 35°C during separation. Flow rate was set at 1 mL/min and a gradient was generated to separate the GTP components within 60 min. The 8 channels of the CoulArray detector were sequentially set at −90, −10, 70, 150, 230, 310, 380 and 450 mV potentials for the detection of GTP components. The main peaks appeared at −10 mV (EGC), 70 mV (EC, EGCG), and 150 mV (ECG). Calibration curves for individual standard GTP component were generated separately, and EGC, EC, EGCG, and ECG were eluted at around 14, 21, 24, and 29 min, respectively. Quality assurance and quality control procedures included analysis of one authentic standard for every set of five samples and simultaneous analysis of a quality control sample daily. The limits of detection were 1.0 ng/mL urine for EC and EGC and 0.5 ng/mL serum for EGCG and ECG, respectively. Urinary GTP components were adjusted by creatinine level to eliminate the variation in urine volume. Urinary creatinine concentration was determined colorimetrically with a Diagnostics Creatinine Kit (Sigma Co).

8. Measurement of Urinary 8-OHdG

The procedure for 8-OHdG analysis was modified from established protocols [27]. Urinary 8-OHdG was extracted from 1 mL urine with the Oasis® HLB 3 cc (60 mg) cartridge. The eluents were dried under ultra-pure N_2 stream and reconstituted in buffer (10 mM ammonium acetate in 2% MeOH, pH 4.3) for analysis with the ESA HPLC-CoulArray system. The HPLC column for 8-OHdG analysis was Waters YMC basicTM column (S3 µm, 4.6×150 mm). The mobile phases consisted of buffer A (10 mM ammonium acetate, pH 4.3) and buffer B (100% methanol). Flow rate was kept at 0.8 mL/min and a linear gradient (0–40% MeOH in 15 min) was applied for chromatographic separation with the peak of 8-OHdG eluted at around 9.5 min. The CoulArray Detector was set at 270, 300, 330, and 360 mv, with the highest peak appeared at 330 mv channel. Authentic standard 8-OHdG was used for qualification by retention times and response patterns, and quantification by calibration curves. Quality assurance and quality control procedures included analysis of one authentic standard for every set of five samples and simultaneous analysis of a spiked urine sample daily. The limit of detection for 8-OHdG was 1 ng/mL urine. The amount of 8-OHdG was adjusted by urinary creatinine concentrations, which was also determined with a Diagnostics Creatinine Kit (Sigma Co).

9. Statistical Analysis

All of the data generated were stored in an Excel database and analyzed with SAS software version 9.3 (SAS Institute Inc., Cary, NC). Median, mean, standard deviations (SD) and range were calculated for concentrations of 8-OHdG, EC and EGC in urine, and EGCG and ECG in serum. The values were expressed as median and mean ± SD unless otherwise stated. To assess the efficacy of GTP, TC, or GTP+TC intervention arms, the statistical evaluation focused on the comparisons among different treatment arms and different time points. For the parameters that were normally distributed (serum EGCG and ECG), repeated measures ANOVA and Bonferroni correction were used to compare differences among means of different times separately for serum EGCG and ECG. For the parameters that were not normally distributed (urinary EC, EGC and 8-OHdG), the Kruskal-Wallis test of one-way ANOVA followed by Wilcoxon rank sum test with Bonferroni correction was used to compare the differences among different treatment groups; and the Friedman's test followed by Wilcoxon signed rank test with Bonferroni correction was used to compare the differences among different time points (urinary EC, EGC and 8-OHdG) given the dependence of measurements. For urinary EC and EGC, the test of difference between GTP and GTP+TC groups at the same time point was done by Wilcoxon rank sum test with Bonferroni correction. To evaluate the effect of dose and time interactions on treatment arms, a nonparametric model for analysis of repeated measurements was applied as previously described [29]. A *P*-value of less than 0.05 (two-tailed) was considered statistically significant.

Results

1. Overall Study Outcome

A total of 88% (150/171) participants completed for this 6-month clinical trial with complete data. Seven (16%) participants in the Placebo arm, 5 (12%) in the Placebo+TC arm, 8 (17%) in the GTP arm, and 1 (3%) in the GTP+TC arm withdrew before the end of the study due to accidental fall at home (1 participant), relocation (2 participants), time conflicts (6 participants), lost to follow-up (5 participants) and lost interest (7 participants). The compliance rate was 89% for both GTP and placebo capsules and the adherence rate for TC classes was 83%.

2. Serum GTP in Study Participants

To examine the adherence and compliance of study participants in this intervention trial, serum and urinary GTP concentrations were measured at different intervention intervals, 0, 1-, 3- and 6-month. There were no detectable GTP components in the placebo group and TC group over 4 collection times of serum samples. There were no GTP components in the baseline of all 4 treatment groups, which was consistent with the questionnaire data, i.e., no green tea drinking habits in these study participants. Among GTP-intervention groups (GTP and GTP+TC), only EGCG and ECG were constantly detectable in serum samples of the study participants after intervention. Serum EGCG concentrations in both GTP and GTP+TC groups were elevated in study participants at 1-month after intervention and kept at the similar levels at 3- and 6-months (Figure 2A). No significant time effect on serum EGCG concentrations was found in GTP+TC Group $P=0.413$) while significant time effect were found in GTP group ($P=0.019$) and between 3- and 6-months ($P<0.050$). Serum ECG concentrations in both GTP and GTP+TC groups were also elevated in study participants at 1-month after the intervention and kept at similar concentrations at 3- and 6-months (Figure 2B.). No statistically significant time effect on serum ECG concentrations was found ($P=0.321$ in GTP group and $P=0.438$ in GTP+TC group), though there were some fluctuations in data between 3-month and 6-month time points.

3. Urinary GTP in Study Participants

There were no detectable green tea polyphenol components in the placebo group and TC group participants over 4 time-points collected urine samples. Among GTP intervention groups (GTP and GTP+TC), only EC and EGC were constantly detectable in urinary samples of the study participants. As shown in Figure 3A, urinary EC concentrations in both GTP and GTP+TC groups were elevated in study participants at 1-month after the intervention and kept at higher concentrations at 3- and 6-months. No significant time effect on urinary EC concentrations was found ($P=0.201$ in GTP group and $P=0.575$ in GTP+TC group). Urinary EGC concentrations in GTP-intervened group were elevated in study participants at 1-month after the intervention and kept at constantly higher concentrations at 3- and 6-months (Figure 3B), whereas urinary EGC concentrations in GTP+TC group were kept elevated linearly in study participants in 1-, 3-, and 6-months. No significant time effect on urinary EGC

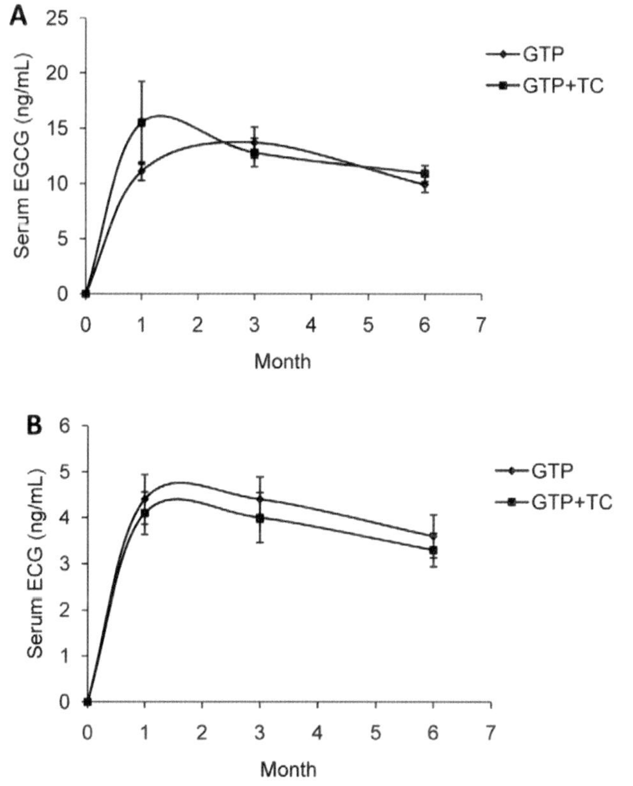

Figure 2. Mean (±SEM) serum GTP concentrations in study participants in the clinical trial. A: serum EGCG concentrations; B: serum ECG concentrations. Starting from first month, serum EGCG and ECG kept constant with minor fluctuations in the GTP and GTP+TC groups. The differences among different time points (1-, 3-, or 6-months) within each group and between groups were tested with repeated measures ANOVA followed by Bonferroni correction for multiple comparisons for each outcome and the significant difference was found in EGCG concentrations in the GTP group between 3- and 6-months ($P<0.050$). No significant differences were found between these two groups at each time point ($P>0.050$).

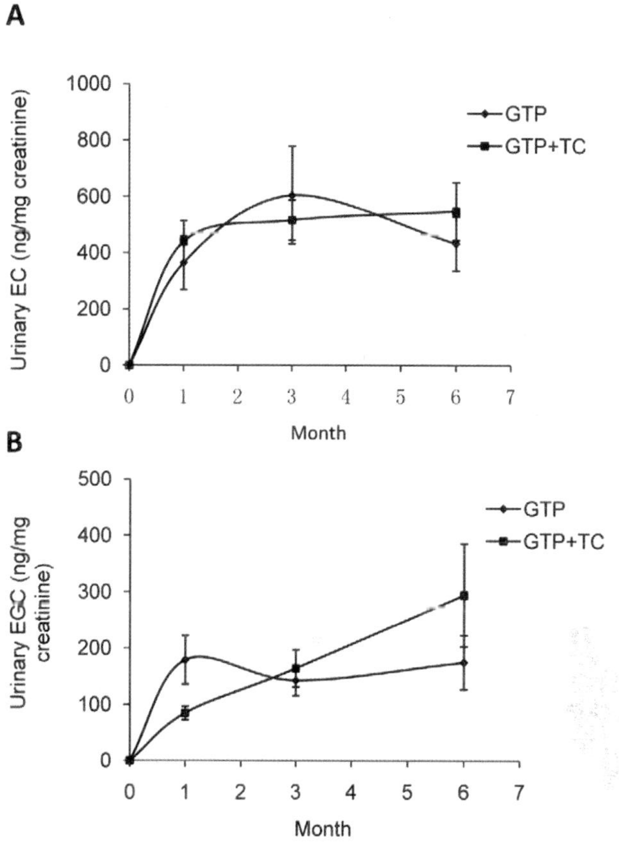

Figure 3. Mean (±SEM) urinary GTP concentrations in study participants in intervention groups. A: urinary EC concentrations; B: urinary EGC concentrations. Starting from first month, urinary EC and EGC concentrations kept constant with minor fluctuations in GTP and GTP+TC groups. No significant differences were found between these two groups at same time points ($P>0.050$, tested with Wilcoxon rank sum test). The differences among differnt time points within each group were tested with Friedman's test followed by Wilcoxon signed rank test with Bonferroni correction for multiple comparisons for each outcome and the significant difference only existed in the EGC concentrations in GTP+TC group between 1- and 3-months ($P<0.050$).

concentrations was found in GTP group ($P=0.689$), while significant difference occurred in GTP+TC group ($P=0.035$) with difference found between 1- and 3-months.

4. Urinary 8-OHdG Concentrations in Study Participants

Urinary concentrations of 8-OHdG in study participants from each treatment group at the baseline, 1-, 3-, and 6-months of the intervention trial were summarized in Table 1, Figures 4 and 5. Data in Table 1 included the mean concentration of 8-OHdG with standard deviation, median, and detectable range. Detailed distribution of the whole dataset was shown in Figures 4 and 5. As shown in Figure 4A, the mean baseline concentrations among 4 treatment groups, although varied, were comparable ($P=0.299$). After 1-month intervention, though no statistical significance was found among groups, the median concentration of 8-OHdG decreased by 27.4%, 43.9%, and 40.1% in TC, GTP, and GTP+TC treated groups, respectively (Figure 4B). After 3-months intervention, the median concentration of 8-OHdG decreased by 44.1%, 62.4%, and 64.8% in TC, GTP, and GTP+TC treated groups, respectively (Figure 4C), which showed statistical significance among treatment groups ($P<0.001$). After 6-months intervention, the median concentration of 8-OHdG decreased by 40.1%, 60.1%, and 73.3% in TC, GTP, and GTP+TC treated groups, respectively (Figure 4D), which also showed statistical significance among treatment groups ($P<0.001$).

Over the 6-month period, urinary 8-OHdG concentrations in the placebo group showed minimal changes as compared with the baseline level and no significant time effect was found ($P=0.133$, Figure 5A). As shown in Figure 5B, urinary 8-OHdG concentrations in TC group significantly decreased over intervention time ($P<0.001$). The time effect was even more striking in GTP group ($P<0.001$, Figure 5C) and GTP+TC group ($P<0.001$, Figure 5D), suggesting that treatment with TC, GTP, or GTP+TC significantly decreased 8-OHdG concentrations in study participants.

5. Non-parametric Model Analysis of Treatment and Time on Concentrations of Urinary 8-OHdG

The effects of treatment and time interactions on urinary 8-OHdG concentrations were analyzed in a non-parametric model for repeated measures, which were summarized in Table 2. Statistical significances in the main effect of treatment and time and their interaction were found by this model analysis ($P\leq0.001$). The treatment of TC, GTP and GTP+TC all had significant effects on urinary 8-OHdG concentrations, as compared with the

Table 1. Urinary 8-OHdG concentrations in study participants in the intervention trial.

Groups	No. of participants	Urinary 8-OHdG (ng/mg creatinine)				P-values (Time)[2]
		Baseline	1-month	3-month	6-month	
Placebo	n = 37	64.5±42.7	65.8±48.5	68.3±48.1	73.5±51.0	0.133
		58.0 (3.5–197.4)	55.4 (3.0–241.6)	66.5 (2.6–256.2)	62.6 (4.9–258.2)	
Placebo + TC	n = 37	64.1±23.6	45.6±25.4[3,4]	40.6±20.2[3,4]	37.8±17.7[3,4]	<0.001
		65.1 (23.5–154.9)	40.2 (9.6–132.6)	37.2 (4.0–104.8)	37.5 (8.9–93.6)	
GTP	n = 39	84.6±74.3	48.2±44.6[3,4]	38.7±37.8[3,4]	33.5±33.1[3,4]	<0.001
		65.4 (7.6–290.6)	31.1 (2.5–175.1)	25.0 (1.1–154.4)	25.0 (0.5–164.5)	
GTP + TC	n = 37	75.8±61.0	45.7±43.5[3,4]	32.8±34.7[3,4]	20.7±19.8[3,4]	<0.001
		65.9 (4.2–249.8)	33.2 (1.2–194.5)	23.4 (0.5–167.2)	16.7 (0.5–76.8)	
P-values (Treatment)[1]		0.299	0.110	<0.001	<0.001	

Urinary 8-OHdG values are expressed as Mean±SD, median (range).
[1]P-values (Treatment) were from Kruskal-Wallis test of one-way ANOVA.
[2]P-values (Time) were from Friedman's test.
[3]Significantly different from Placebo at the same time point, tested by Wilcoxon rank sum test with Bonferroni correction for multiple comparisons, $P<0.050$.
[4]Significantly different from baseline in the same group, tested by Wilcoxon signed rank test with Bonferroni correction for multiple comparisons, $P<0.001$.

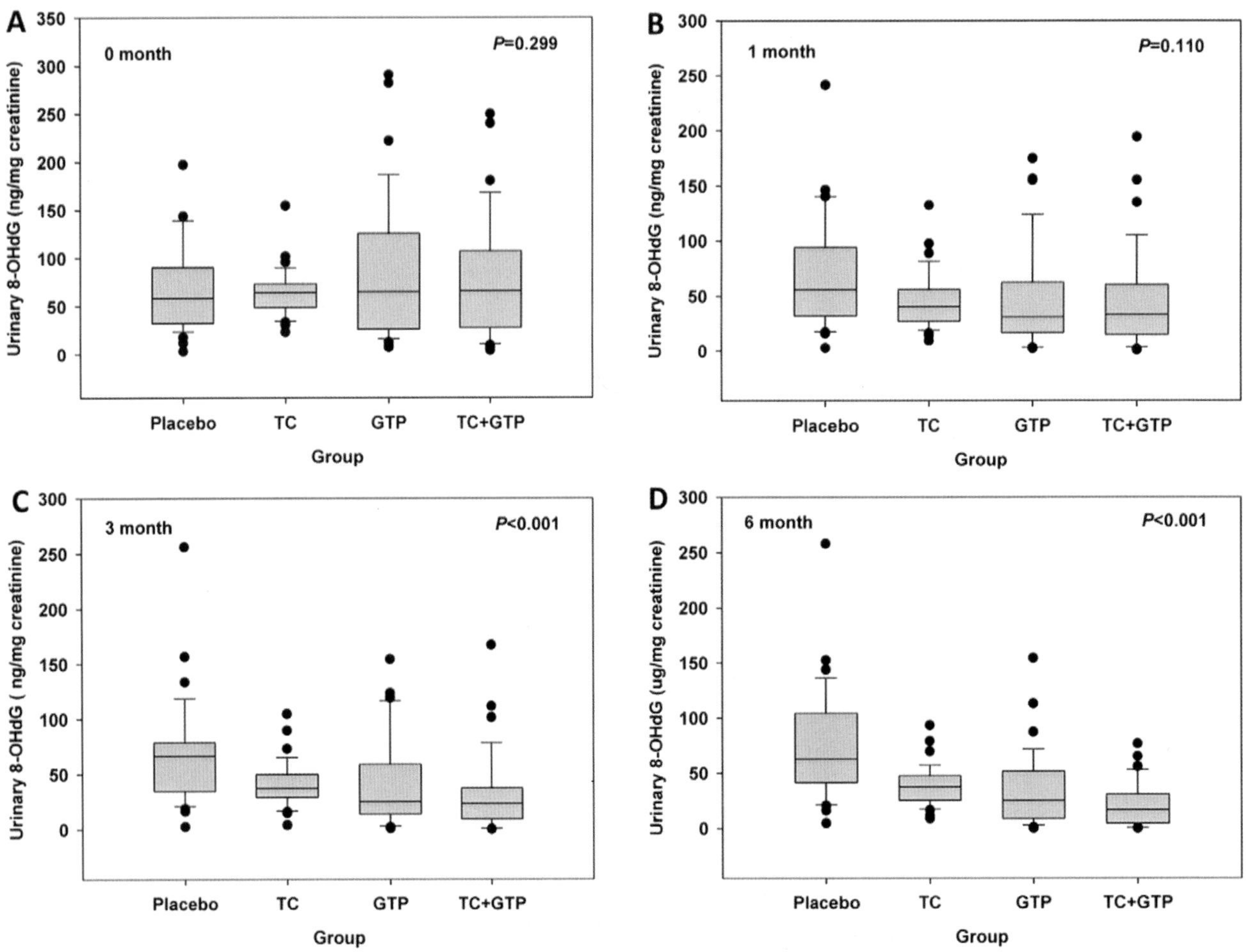

Figure 4. Urinary 8-OHdG concentrations in study participants in different groups. A: baseline, no significant differences in urinary 8-OHdG were found ($P=0.299$); B: 1 month, urinary 8-OHdG concentrations were reduced by all treatments, but no significant differences were observed ($P=0.110$); C: 3 month, urinary 8-OHdG concentrations were significantly reduced in all treatment groups ($P<0.001$); D: 6 month, urinary 8-OHdG concentrations were significantly reduced in all treatment groups ($P<0.001$).

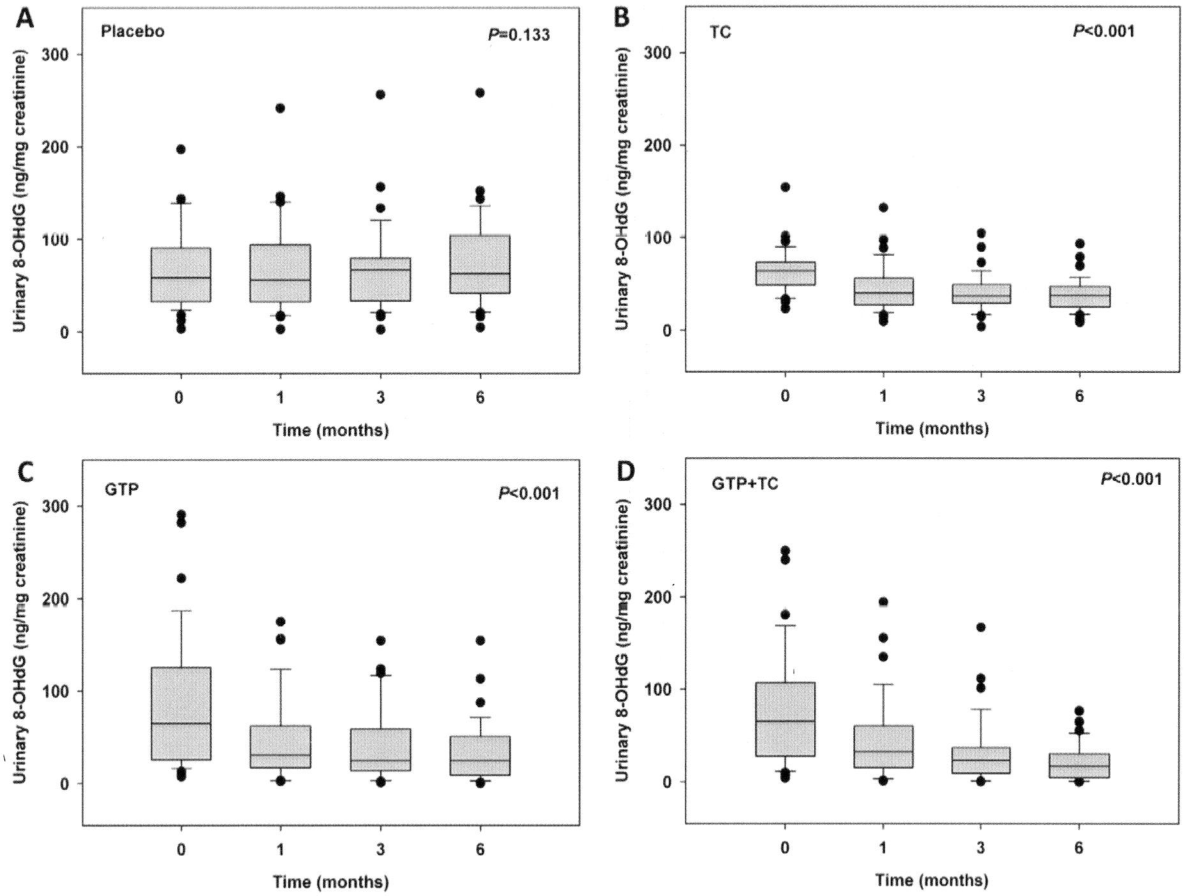

Figure 5. Temporal patterns of urinary 8-OHdG concentrations in study participants. A: Placebo, no significant differences was observed in different treatment periods ($P = 0.133$); B: TC, compared to baseline, urinary 8-OHdG concentrations were significantly reduced at 1-, 3-, and 6-months treatment ($P < 0.001$); C: GTP, compared to baseline, urinary 8-OHdG concentrations were all significantly reduced at 1-, 3-, and 6-months treatment ($P < 0.001$); and D: GTP+TC, compared to baseline, urinary 8-OHdG concentrations were all significantly reduced at 1-, 3- and 6-months treatment ($P < 0.001$).

placebo group ($P < 0.050$); the urinary concentrations of 8-OHdG were also significantly modified by time for each of the treatment group ($P < 0.050$). For each group, the duration of treatment proved to have cumulative effects on urinary 8-OHdG in the six month period. These results demonstrated the efficacy of treatment and time on lowering urinary 8-OHdG concentrations in study participants in this trial.

Discussion

In this study, we assessed the adherence and compliance of the 6-month clinical trial by measuring GTP components in blood and urine of the participants. Our previous studies have validated that measurement of blood and urinary GTP components are good biomarkers for determining green tea consumption and GTP intervention in human population studies [15,27]. Among the four major GTP components, all EGCG, EGC, EC, and ECG, were detectable in blood and urine samples [16], but only EGCG and ECG in serum and EC and EGC in urine showed dose-response correlations [27]. Results of serum concentrations of EGCG and ECG and urinary excretion of EC and EGC in this study showed significant elevation after GTP intervention and no detectable concentrations in the baseline and the placebo participants over the study period, which further confirmed the excellent adherence and compliance of the overall trial. In addition, these results were

Table 2. Non-paramatric model analysis of treatment and time on concentrations of urinary 8-OHdG.

Effect	Test statistic (*P*-value)
Treatment	5.58 ($P = 0.001$)
Time	97.92 ($P < 0.001$)
Treatment*Time	17.15 ($P < 0.001$)
TC v.s. Placebo	10.62 ($P = 0.001$)
GTP v.s. Placebo	3.76 ($P = 0.037$)
(GTP+TC) v.s. Placebo	4.80 ($P = 0.029$)
TC*Time (time effect in TC group)	13.38 ($P < 0.001$)
GTP*Time (time effect in GTP group)	67.20 ($P < 0.001$)
(GTP+TC)*Time (time effect in (GTP+TC) group)	3.24 ($P = 0.043$)

The test statistics and *P*-values shown here were generated from a non-parametric model designed for repeated measurements using SAS macro F1_LD_F1, the more detailed information on model assumption and hypothesis is referred to reference #30, chapter 8.

consistent with our previous findings, i.e., blood and urinary GTP components are practical and reliable biomarkers for green tea consumption [27].

In this study, we further assessed the efficacy of GTP supplement and TC exercise for their individual and combined effects on the oxidative DNA damage biomarker, 8-OHdG, in postmenopausal women with osteopenia in the 6-month clinical trial. Results from this study showed that individual GTP supplement, TC exercise, or the combination significantly decreased urinary excretion of 8-OHdG after 1-, 3-, and 6-months intervention in postmenopausal women, as compared with the placebo group, which demonstrated the efficacy of this trial in reducing the oxidative stress biomarker levels.

Several lines of evidence have indicated the role of ROS in induction of osteoporosis [10,14]: ROS are capable of influencing the generation and survival of osteoclasts, osteoblasts, and osteocytes; ROS-activated FoxOs in early mesenchymal progenitors also leads to decreased osteoblastogenesis through disruption of Wnt signaling pathway [10]; ROS also increases serum osteopontin and transforming growth factor-β levels in iron overloaded rats, suggesting osteoclast-mediated bone resorption through the receptor activator of nuclear factor-κB/RANK ligand (RANK/RANKL) mediated signaling pathway [30]. In postmenopausal women, the reduced estrogen level might be a key factor in boosting the ROS level because estrogen has been reported to be able to diminish production of ROS and stimulate the activity of glutathione reductase [31]. The ability of green tea and GTP as potent ROS scavengers has been well recognized as the basis for its biological activity [16,32]. Previous studies by others and ours showed strong evidence of protective effects of GTP on the capacity of bone formation due to its anti-oxidative stress potentials [33,34]. An animal study shows that urinary excretion of 8-OHdG is a reliable indicator of oxidative stress in postmenopausal rats [9]. More importantly, urinary 8-OHdG concentration has also been widely used as a DNA oxidative damage biomarker in many human studies [11,35]. In this study we observed a significant decrease in urinary 8-OHdG concentrations in postmenopausal women appearing at 1- to 6-months after the GTP intervention as compared to the placebo control group, which further suggests evidence of oxidative stress in the study participants. The result of this study is consistent with the previous finding in HBsAg carrier groups, which also showed statistically significant reduced urinary 8-OHdG after 3-months GTP intervention at 500 mg or 1,000 mg/day [27].

TC exercise has been characterized as a moderate intensity mind-body exercise, coupling muscular activity with an internally directed focus, producing a temporary self-contemplative mental state [36]. In this study, the TC exercise significantly decreased urinary 8-OHdG concentrations after 3-months intervention as compared with the control group. The effect of exercise on oxidative stress has been reviewed [37]. It was reported that high-intensity exercise increased oxidative stress biomarkers, including 8-OHdG and malondialdehyde (MDA)-modified low-density lipoprotein in humans, whereas moderate exercise tended to decrease both indices of oxidative stress [38]. A recent study has also demonstrated that TC exercise stimulated endogenous antioxidant enzymes (superoxide dismutase, SOD) and reduced oxidative damage markers (MDA) in middle-aged adults [23]. These reports support our observation that TC, a moderate exercise, reduced oxidative stress in postmenopausal women.

This is the first study to investigate the combined effects of GTP and TC on oxidative DNA damage in postmenopausal women with osteopenia. An additive effect of GTP supplementation and TC exercise on suppression of oxidative stress was found, as evidenced by a 40% reduction of urinary 8-OHdG in the TC group and 60% reduction in the GTP group alone and a 73% reduction was observed in the GTP+TC group. Results of this study further suggest that a combinative intervention strategy, including dietary supplementation and moderate exercise, may be more effective in promoting bone health in postmenopausal women with osteopenia.

The strength of our study was in its design as a randomized and placebo controlled clinical trial that could limit the biases usually introduced through the design and data acquisition. Limitations to this study included a relatively small sample size that might limit the statistical power, such as parameters after 1-month of intervention. A wide inter-individual variation found in concentration of biomarkers measured may be due to the individual variations in GTP metabolism enzymes, endogenous susceptibility factors, and/or DNA repair capacity; the large variation in urinary 8-OHdG levels (43.9±42.1 ng/mg creatinine) has also been reported previously in females [35], which supports this finding in our study. The stratified randomization and non-parametric analysis used could limit potential biases (randomization) and increase the power of detecting the differences (non-parametric model analysis). The intent to treat (ITT) analysis could benefit the comparison; however, considering the comparable compliance and adherence rates for the treatment groups, the effect of dropouts might be minimal. On the other hand, the exclusion of dropouts into statistical analysis may not severely affect the statistical power as an originally estimated 140 participants (34 participants for each group) would be sufficient for a power of about 0.90 for the outcome of urinary 8-OHdG level.

In conclusion, this study provides evidence that 500 mg GTP supplement, Tai Chi exercise, either alone or together, can effectively reduce an oxidative stress biomarker in postmenopausal women with osteopenia. Based on the putative role of oxidative stress in osteoporosis and the observed beneficial effects on bone health as published previously, these intervention strategies hold the potential as an alternative tool to benefit the bone health in postmenopausal women which deserves further long-term human studies.

Supporting Information

Checklist S1 CONSORT Checklist.

Protocol S1 Trial Protocol.

Safety and clinical outcomes S1.

Acknowledgments

Authors acknowledge all participants in this study, Dr. Jay Magaziner (University of Maryland, MD) for his advice, and the assistance of Mary J. Flores, Raul Y. Dagda, and Marisela Dagda in the clinical data collection. We also thank Dr. Li Xu for her input in the statistical analysis.

Author Contributions

Conceived and designed the experiments: JSW CLS MCC BCP. Performed the experiments: GQ KX LT FW. Analyzed the data: XS LT GQ. Contributed reagents/materials/analysis tools: JSW. Wrote the paper: GQ. Read and approved the final manuscript: GQ KX LT FW XS MCC BCP CLS JSW.

References

1. NIH (2001) Osteoporosis prevention, diagnosis, and therapy. JAMA 285: 785–795.
2. Lane NE (2006) Epidemiology, etiology, and diagnosis of osteoporosis. Am J Obstet Gynecol 194: S3–11.
3. Boonen S, Dejaeger E, Vanderschueren D, Venken K, Bogaerts A, et al. (2008) Osteoporosis and osteoporotic fracture occurrence and prevention in the elderly: a geriatric perspective. Best Pract Res Clin Endocrinol Metab 22: 765–785.
4. Looker AC, Johnston CC, Jr., Wahner HW, Dunn WL, Calvo MS, et al. (1995) Prevalence of low femoral bone density in older U.S. women from NHANES III. J Bone Miner Res 10: 796–802.
5. Inada M, Miyaura C (2010) [Cytokines in bone diseases. Cytokine and postmenopausal osteoporosis]. Clin Calcium 20: 1467–1472.
6. Clarke BL, Khosla S (2010) Female reproductive system and bone. Arch Biochem Biophys 503: 118–128.
7. Syed FA, Ng AC (2010) The pathophysiology of the aging skeleton. Curr Osteoporos Rep 8: 235–240.
8. Basu S, Michaelsson K, Olofsson H, Johansson S, Melhus H (2001) Association between oxidative stress and bone mineral density. Biochem Biophys Res Commun 288: 275–279.
9. Isomura H, Fujie K, Shibata K, Inoue N, Iizuka T, et al. (2004) Bone metabolism and oxidative stress in postmenopausal rats with iron overload. Toxicology 197: 93–100.
10. Manolagas SC (2010) From estrogen-centric to aging and oxidative stress: a revised perspective of the pathogenesis of osteoporosis. Endocr Rev 31: 266–300.
11. Valavanidis A, Vlachogianni T, Fiotakis C (2009) 8-hydroxy-2′ -deoxyguanosine (8-OHdG): A critical biomarker of oxidative stress and carcinogenesis. J Environ Sci Health C Environ Carcinog Ecotoxicol Rev 27: 120–139.
12. Pilger A, Rudiger HW (2006) 8-Hydroxy-2′-deoxyguanosine as a marker of oxidative DNA damage related to occupational and environmental exposures. Int Arch Occup Environ Health 80: 1–15.
13. Shen CL, Yeh JK, Samathanam C, Cao JJ, Stoecker BJ, et al. (2011) Green tea polyphenols attenuate deterioration of bone microarchitecture in female rats with systemic chronic inflammation. Osteoporos Int 22: 327–337.
14. Shen CL, Yeh JK, Cao JJ, Wang JS (2009) Green tea and bone metabolism. Nutr Res 29: 437–456.
15. Wang JS, Luo H, Wang P, Tang L, Yu J, et al. (2008) Validation of green tea polyphenol biomarkers in a phase II human intervention trial. Food Chem Toxicol 46: 232–240.
16. Yang CS, Lambert JD, Ju J, Lu G, Sang S (2007) Tea and cancer prevention: molecular mechanisms and human relevance. Toxicol Appl Pharmacol 224: 265–273.
17. Jochmann N, Baumann G, Stangl V (2008) Green tea and cardiovascular disease: from molecular targets towards human health. Curr Opin Clin Nutr Metab Care 11: 758–765.
18. Li Q, Li Y (2010) [Review on the neuroprotective effects of green tea polyphenols for the treatment of neurodegenerative diseases]. Wei Sheng Yan Jiu 39: 123–126.
19. Woo J, Hong A, Lau E, Lynn H (2007) A randomised controlled trial of Tai Chi and resistance exercise on bone health, muscle strength and balance in community-living elderly people. Age Ageing 36: 262–268.
20. Lui PP, Qin L, Chan KM (2008) Tai Chi Chuan exercises in enhancing bone mineral density in active seniors. Clin Sports Med 27: 75–86.
21. Qin L, Choy W, Leung K, Leung PC, Au S, et al. (2005) Beneficial effects of regular Tai Chi exercise on musculoskeletal system. J Bone Miner Metab 23: 186–190.
22. Lee MS, Pittler MH, Shin BC, Ernst E (2008) Tai chi for osteoporosis: a systematic review. Osteoporos Int 19: 139–146.
23. Goon JA, Aini AH, Musalmah M, Anum MY, Nazaimoon WM, et al. (2009) Effect of Tai Chi exercise on DNA damage, antioxidant enzymes, and oxidative stress in middle-age adults. J Phys Act Health 6: 43–51.
24. Shen CL, Chyu MC, Yeh JK, Felton CK, Xu KT, et al. (2009) Green tea polyphenols and Tai Chi for bone health: designing a placebo-controlled randomized trial. BMC Musculoskelet Disord 10: 110.
25. Shen CL, Chyu MC, Pence BC, Yeh JK, Zhang Y, et al. (2010) Green tea polyphenols supplementation and Tai Chi exercise for postmenopausal osteopenic women: safety and quality of life report. BMC Complement Altern Med 10: 76.
26. Shen CL, Chyu MC, Yeh JK, Zhang Y, Pence BC, et al. (2012) Effect of green tea and Tai Chi on bone health in postmenopausal osteopenic women: a 6-month randomized placebo-controlled trial. Osteoporos Int 23: 1541–1552.
27. Luo H, Tang L, Tang M, Billam M, Huang T, et al. (2006) Phase IIa chemoprevention trial of green tea polyphenols in high-risk individuals of liver cancer: modulation of urinary excretion of green tea polyphenols and 8-hydroxydeoxyguanosine. Carcinogenesis 27: 262–268.
28. Hedeker D, Gibbons RD, Waternaux C (1999) Sample size estimation for longitudinal designs with attrition: Comparing time-related contrasts between two groups. Journal of Educational and Behavioral Statistics 24: 70–93.
29. Brunner E DS, Langer F. (2002) Nonparametric analysis of longitudinal data in factorial experiments. New York, NY:Wiley.
30. Yamamoto N, Sakai F, Kon S, Morimoto J, Kimura C, et al. (2003) Essential role of the cryptic epitope SLAYGLR within osteopontin in a murine model of rheumatoid arthritis. J Clin Invest 112: 181–188.
31. Almeida M, Martin-Millan M, Ambrogini E, Bradsher R, Han L, et al. (2010) Estrogens attenuate oxidative stress and the differentiation and apoptosis of osteoblasts by DNA-binding-independent actions of the ERalpha. J Bone Miner Res 25: 769–781.
32. Chan K, Qin L, Lau M, Woo J, Au S, et al. (2004) A randomized, prospective study of the effects of Tai Chi Chun exercise on bone mineral density in postmenopausal women. Arch Phys Med Rehabil 85: 717–722.
33. Salah N, Miller NJ, Paganga G, Tijburg L, Bolwell GP, et al. (1995) Polyphenolic flavanols as scavengers of aqueous phase radicals and as chain-breaking antioxidants. Arch Biochem Biophys 322: 339–346.
34. Rice-Evans C (1999) Implications of the mechanisms of action of tea polyphenols as antioxidants in vitro for chemoprevention in humans. Proc Soc Exp Biol Med 220: 262–266.
35. Wu LL, Chiou CC, Chang PY, Wu JT (2004) Urinary 8-OHdG: a marker of oxidative stress to DNA and a risk factor for cancer, atherosclerosis and diabetics. Clin Chim Acta 339: 1–9.
36. Lan C, Chen SY, Lai JS (2004) Relative exercise intensity of Tai Chi Chuan is similar in different ages and gender. Am J Chin Med 32: 151–160.
37. Finaud J, Lac G, Filaire E (2006) Oxidative stress : relationship with exercise and training. Sports Med 36: 327–358.
38. Goto C, Higashi Y, Kimura M, Noma K, Hara K, et al. (2003) Effect of different intensities of exercise on endothelium-dependent vasodilation in humans: role of endothelium-dependent nitric oxide and oxidative stress. Circulation 108: 530–535.

c-Fms Signaling Mediates Neurofibromatosis Type-1 Osteoclast Gain-In-Functions

Yongzheng He[1], Steven D. Rhodes[2], Shi Chen[1], Xiaohua Wu[1], Jin Yuan[1], Xianlin Yang[1], Li Jiang[1], Xianqi Li[3], Naoyuki Takahashi[3], Mingjiang Xu[1], Khalid S. Mohammad[4], Theresa A. Guise[4], Feng-Chun Yang[1]*

1 Department of Pediatrics, Indiana University School of Medicine, Indianapolis, Indiana, United States of America, **2** Department of Anatomy and Cell Biology, Indiana University School of Medicine, Indianapolis, Indiana, United States of America, **3** Division of Hard Tissue Research, Matsumoto Dental University, Shiojiri, Nagano, Japan, **4** Department of Medicine, Indiana University School of Medicine, Indianapolis, Indiana, United States of America

Abstract

Skeletal abnormalities including osteoporosis and osteopenia occur frequently in both pediatric and adult neurofibromatosis type 1 (NF1) patients. *NF1* (*Nf1*) haploinsufficient osteoclasts and osteoclast progenitors derived from both NF1 patients and $Nf1^{+/-}$ mice exhibit increased differentiation, migration, and bone resorptive capacity *in vitro*, mediated by hyperactivation of $p21^{Ras}$ in response to limiting concentrations of macrophage-colony stimulating factor (M-CSF). Here, we show that M-CSF binding to its receptor, c-Fms, results in increased c-Fms activation in $Nf1^{+/-}$ osteoclast progenitors, mediating multiple gain-in-functions through the downstream effectors Erk1/2 and p90RSK. PLX3397, a potent and selective c-Fms inhibitor, attenuated M-CSF mediated $Nf1^{+/-}$ osteoclast migration by 50%, adhesion by 70%, and pit formation by 60%. *In vivo*, we administered PLX3397 to $Nf1^{+/-}$ osteoporotic mice induced by ovariectomy (OVX) and evaluated changes in bone mass and skeletal architecture. We found that PLX3397 prevented bone loss in $Nf1^{+/-}$-OVX mice by reducing osteoclast differentiation and bone resorptive activity *in vivo*. Collectively, these results implicate the M-CSF/c-Fms signaling axis as a critical pathway underlying the aberrant functioning of *Nf1* haploinsufficient osteoclasts and may provide a potential therapeutic target for treating NF1 associated osteoporosis and osteopenia.

Editor: Michael Glogauer, University of Toronto, Canada

Funding: This work was supported in part by the Department of Defense NF043032 (FCY), NF073112 (FCY) and National Institutes of Health/National Cancer Institute/5R01CA074177 (FCY and DWC), Indiana Clinical and Translational Sciences Institute Career Development Award PHS NCCR Grant No: 5TL1RR025759-03 (SDR), and Children's Tumor Foundation Young Investigator Award 2011-01-010 (SDR). Plexxikon Inc. provided the PLX3397 compound. The funders had no role in study design, data collection and analysis, decision to publish, or preparation of the manuscript.

Competing Interests: The authors have declared that no competing interests exist.

* E-mail: fyang@iupui.edu

Introduction

Neurofibromatosis type 1 (NF1) is one of the most common genetic diseases with an incidence of 1 out of 3000 individuals [1]. NF1 is caused by mutations of the *NF1* tumor suppressor gene, which encodes neurofibromin, a GTPase activating protein for p21ras [2]. Individuals with NF1 have a high incidence of both malignant and non-malignant complications [3,4]. Clinical studies have reported that NF1 patients are at a significant risk for both generalized osteoporotic abnormalities [5,6,7] and focal skeletal abnormalities including dystrophic kyphoscoliosis and pseudarthrosis [8,9]. NF1 patients have an increased prevalence of osteoporosis beginning from childhood and adolescence [10,11,12], leading to greater risk of fracture later in life [13]. Given that osteoporosis occurs in a younger patient population and the predisposition to pseudarthrosis is 2–5% in individuals with NF1 [3,14,15], the ultimate health costs and sequelae of this condition in NF1 patients may be significantly greater. Although NF1 related osteopenia commonly presents in the childhood years, there is no efficient treatment so far. Despite evidence of low serum Vitamin D levels in some NF1 patients, clinical studies involving Vitamin D supplementation have yielded conflicting results on whether improvements in bone mineral density (BMD) can be achieved [10,16,17].

Osteoclasts are specialized bone resorbing cells which differentiate from the myeloid monocyte/macrophage lineage. Many skeletal diseases, in particular diseases with decreased bone mineral density (BMD), occur as a consequence of a skeletal imbalance that favors bone resorption. Although a significant number of skeletal diseases, including skeletal manifestations in NF1 patients, have been linked to abnormal osteoclast function(s) [18,19,20,21], the intracellular mechanisms by which osteoclasts normally function or contribute to disease states are poorly understood.

Ras signaling pathways are highly relevant to bone formation and the maintenance of skeletal homeostasis. Several Ras-activating growth factors, including M-CSF, are known to affect skeletal development and remodeling. Mitogen-activated protein kinase, a major downstream effector of Ras, is critical in the mitogenic response to extracellular stimuli including growth, podosome formation, and bone resorption of the osteoclast [22]. Previously, we reported that haploinsufficient *Nf1* ($^{+/-}$) myeloid progenitors are hypersensitive to M-CSF, leading to increased osteoclast formation and bone erosive activity *in vitro* [18].

Furthermore, we have shown that the phenotype of *Nf1*$^{+/-}$ osteoclasts appears to be associated with hyperactivation of the MAPK pathway [18].

Upstream of the Ras/MAPK pathway, M-CSF binding to its membrane receptor, c-Fms, stimulates phosphorylation of Y807 in the activation loop, resulting in a conformational shift that enhances intrinsic kinase activity and docking of adaptor proteins such as Grb2 and Sos with subsequent activation of the Ras/Raf/MEK/ERK cascade. Here we show that *Nf1* haploinsufficient osteoclast progenitors exhibit increased c-Fms activation in response to M-CSF, resulting in multiple osteoclast gain-in-functions including migration, adhesion, and bone resorptive capacity, which are correlated with hyperphosphorylation of the downstream effectors Erk1/2 and p90^{rsk}. Administration of PLX3397, a potent and selective small molecule inhibitor of c-Fms receptor tyrosine kinase activity, was sufficient to mitigate hyperfunctioning *Nf1*$^{+/-}$ osteoclast phenotypes *in vitro*. *In vivo*, ovariectomized (OVX) *Nf1*$^{+/-}$ mice exhibit accelerated bone loss as compared to WT controls in response to bone resorptive stress. In the present study, we found that treatment with PLX3397 was sufficient to correct this phenotype, normalizing bone mineral density and trabecular bone mass in *Nf1*$^{+/-}$ -OVX mice vs. vehicle treated controls. Collectively, these data implicate the M-CSF/c-Fms signaling axis as a critical pathway underlying the aberrant functioning of *Nf1* haploinsufficient osteoclasts and warrant further investigation of c-Fms as a potential therapeutic target for treating NF1 associated osteoporosis and osteopenia.

Materials and Methods

Ethics Statement

This study was carried out in strict accordance Indiana University's Institutional Animal Care and Use Committee (IACUC). Animals and records of their ovariectomy surgery were maintained in compliance with Indiana University's Institutional Animal Care and Use Committee with approval protocol ID #3401- A4. All surgery was performed under isoflurane anesthesia, and all efforts were made to minimize suffering.

Animal and material preparation

Nf1$^{+/-}$ mice were obtained from Tyler Jacks at the Massachusetts Institute of Technology (Cambridge, Massachusetts, USA) in a C57BL/6J.129 background and backcrossed for 13 generations into a C57BL/6J strain [23]. Studies were conducted with a protocol approved by the Indiana University Laboratory Animal Research Center. Chemicals were purchased from Sigma (St. Louis, MO) unless otherwise stated. All cytokines were purchased from PeproTech (Rocky Hills, NC). PLX3397 was provided by Plexxikon Inc. (Berkeley, CA).

Clonogenic progenitor assays

Colony-forming unit-macrophage/monocyte (CFU-M) of bone marrow mononuclear cells (BMMNCs) was assayed, as described previously [19]. BMMNCs were isolated from 6- to 8-week-old WT and *Nf1*$^{+/-}$ mice by flushing the bone marrow and using Ficoll density gradient centrifugation. 2.5×10^4 BMMNCs were seeded onto a 35-mm gridded dish containing methylcellulose supplemented with 30 ng/mL M-CSF and 20 ng/mL murine recombinant receptor activator of nuclear factor kappa-B ligand (RANKL) at 37°C in a 5% CO_2 incubator for 7 days. Colonies were counted using an inverted light microscope.

Generation of murine osteoclasts

Murine osteoclasts were obtained *in vitro* from BMMNCs, as described previously [18]. BMMNCs were cultured in alpha minimum essential medium (α-MEM) supplemented with 10% fetal bovine serum (FBS, Sigma) and M-CSF 30 ng/mL and RANKL 20 ng/mL for 3 days. Cell culture media was switched on day 4 to α-MEM supplemented with 10% FBS, M-CSF (30 ng/mL), and RANKL (60 ng/mL) for an additional 3 days of culture. Adherent cells were fixed and stained for tartrate resistant acid phosphatase (TRACP) to identify osteoclasts, as described previously [18]. Osteoclasts were visualized using a Nikon TE2000-S microscope (Nikon Inc., Melville, NY) and images were taken by a QImaging camera and QCapture-Pro software (Fryer Company Inc., Cincinnati, OH). Multinucleated TRACP$^+$ cells containing more than three nuclei were scored as mature osteoclasts. The numbers and areas of multinucleated, TRACP$^+$ osteoclasts were calculated using Image Pro Express (Media Cybernetics, In., MD).

Migration assay

Osteoclast migration was evaluated using a transwell assay, as described previously with minor modifications [18]. Briefly, equivalent numbers of pre-osteoclasts were loaded onto the upper chamber of an 8 μm polycarbonate transwell (Corning Incorporated, Corning, NY) coated with vitronectin (Takara, Japan). The lower chamber contained α-MEM supplemented with M-CSF (30 ng/mL) and 0.1% bovine serum albumin with phosphate buffered saline (PBS) vehicle or PLX3397 (200 nM). Cells that migrated to the bottom chamber were stained with crystal violet and counted. Six fields per experimental condition were counted.

Adhesion assay

A single-cell suspension of osteoclast precursors were pipetted into 96-well plates pre-coated with vitronectin at a density of 1×10^4 cells/well as previously described [19]. After 30 minutes of incubation in the presence of M-CSF (30 ng/mL) with PBS vehicle or PLX3397 (200 nM), nonattached cells were gently removed with PBS and adherent cells were stained with crystal violet and counted.

Bone resorption assay

Osteoclasts can form a specialized cell-extracellular matrix to initiate degradation of bone matrix by secreting proteinases. To directly assess the effect of PLX3397 on osteoclast bone resorption, independent of adhesion and differentiation, pit formation assay was performed using cells that were cultured for 3 days in media containing M-CSF and RANKL as described previously [18]. Briefly, preosteoclasts were detached from plates after 3 days culture in α-MEM supplemented with M-CSF (30 ng/mL) and RANKL (20 ng/mL) and replated at 1×10^5/well on dentine discs (ALPCO Diagnostic, Windham, NH) in a 96-well plate. The cells were incubated at 37°C, 5% CO_2 in the presence of 30 ng/mL M-CSF and 60 ng/mL RANKL and allowed to adhere overnight. On the following day, vehicle (PBS) or PLX3397 (200 nM) was added to the culture with media changed every three days. Wells containing media alone, without M-CSF, were used as negative controls (data not shown). Following 7 days of culture, the dentine discs were rinsed with PBS, immersed in 1 M ammonium hydroxide overnight, and stained with a 1% toluidine blue in 0.5% sodium tetraborate solution. The resorptive areas or "pits" were imaged using reflective light microscopy. Pit area (μm^2) per low power field was quantitated using Image Pro Express software. Six fields per experimental condition were evaluated.

High content image assay

As described above, murine preosteoclasts were obtained *in vitro* from BMMNCs isolated from 6- to 8-week-old WT and $Nf1^{+/-}$ mice. After being cultured in α-MEM supplemented with M-CSF (30 ng/mL) and RANKL (20 ng/mL), preosteoclasts were starved in 0.5%BSA in α-MEM for 6 hours, pretreated with or without PLX3397 in serial dilution for 2 hours and then stimulated with M-CSF (30 ng/mL) for 5 minutes. The cells were then fixed and incubated with anti-phospho-c-Fms antibody (Cell signaling) at 1:100 for immunofluorescence staining. Thereafter, the cells were incubated with Alexa Fluor® 488 goat anti-rabbit IgG (H+L) (Invitrogen) at 1:500 and Hoechst (Invitrogen) at 1:1000 in PBS at room temperature for 90 minutes and imaged on a BD AttoVision™ instrument. The mean fluorescence intensity of phospho-c-Fms was acquired and normalized to each cell based on the nuclear counts. Data readout was analyzed as phospho-c-Fms mean fluorescence intensity. The half maximal inhibition concentration (IC_{50}) of PLX3397 was calculated by Prism software.

Ovariectomy surgery

To determine if application of PLX3397 prevents bone loss in $Nf1^{+/-}$-OVX mice *in vivo*, two groups of 8 week-old WT or $Nf1^{+/-}$ female mice were subject to ovariectomy surgery (OVX) to induce low bone mass as previously reported [18]. Briefly, the mice were anesthetized via inhalation of 1.5% isoflurane (IsoFlo; Abbott Laboratories, North Chicago, IL) mixed with O_2 (1.5 liter/minute). Ovariectomy was preceded by a 2 cm midline dorsal skin incision. The peritoneal cavity was incised to access the ovaries, which were then excised with scissors. The success of OVX was verified by examining the uterine weight of the mice following sacrifice (Figure S1A–B).

Drug administration

After two weeks of recovery from the OVX surgery, the mice were treated with either the PBS vehicle or PLX3397 (80 mg/kg/day) by daily gavage as recommended by the Plexxikon Inc. for a period of twelve weeks. At the end of the treatment, the mice were euthanized for analysis. To ensure that these mice received sufficient amounts of PLX3397, blood was collected in heparin coated tubes by cardiac puncture and plasma was separated to determine the concentration of PLX3397 in the blood (Figure S1C).

Histomorphometric analysis

Utilizing our previously established methods [18,24,25], the femurs of syngeneic experimental mice were fixed with 4% buffered paraformaldehyde (PFA) and decalcified for paraffin embedding. Histological sections from the distal metaphysis were stained for the osteoclast enzyme TRACP. The area of TRACP positive ($TRACP^+$) osteoclasts per unit trabecular surface was counted under the microscope with a QImaging camera and QCapture-Pro software (Version 5.1, Fryer Company Inc., Cincinnati, OH).

Detection of C-terminal telopeptide of type I collagen (CTX) in plasma

To evaluate the impact of PLX3397 on osteoclast activity *in vivo*, the CTX levels in the plasma were measured. Briefly, blood was collected by heart puncture and transferred into ethylenediaminetetraacetic acid (EDTA) coated tubes. The tubes were immediately placed on ice, and centrifuged within 30 minutes for plasma separation. All samples were analyzed in the same assay. The concentration of CTX was determined by using a commercial enzyme immunoassay kit (Ratlaps™ EIA, Immunodiagnostic systems Inc., Fountain Hills, AZ).

Liquid chromatography/mass spectroscopy (LC/MS) analysis of mice plasma

Plasma was collected following centrifugation at 3,000 rpm at 4°C for 20 minutes and processed for liquid chromatography/mass spectroscopy (LC/MS) analysis. Briefly, murine plasma samples were prepared for LC/MS analysis by precipitating plasma with 3x volumes of ice cold acetonitrile. The precipitated samples were centrifuged and the clarified samples were diluted with 5×0.2% formic acid in water. Samples were analyzed by LC/MS in a formic acid, water, methanol chromatography system using an MDS SCIEX API 3000 spectrometer (Applied Biosystems, Carlsbad, California).

Measurement of BMD *in vivo*

Bone mineral density (BMD) of the femur was evaluated *in vivo* using peripheral dual energy x-ray absorptiometry (pDEXA) designed for analyzing mouse skeletons (GE-Lunar Corp., Madison, USA). The mice were anesthetized via inhalation of 1.5% isoflurane (IsoFlo; Abbott Laboratories, North Chicago, IL) mixed with O2 (1.5 liter/minute) and were placed in the prone position on a specimen tray for scanning. For this experiment, 8 week-old female mice were scanned for BMD once before surgery. Then, after 12 weeks of drug treatment, the mice were scanned for BMD again before euthanasia. The BMD of the left femoral metaphysis was measured by defining a region of interest of 11 pixels x 10 pixels proximal to the distal growth plate, which contains a high content of trabecular bone.

Micro (μ) computed tomography (CT)

After euthanasia, bone volume and microarchitecture of the femoral distal metaphysis were evaluated using a desktop μCT (μCT 20; Scanco Medical AG, Bassersdorf, Switzerland). Each specimen was scanned with a slice increment of 9 μm starting at 15% of the total femur length measured from the tip of femoral condyle and extending proximally for 200 slices. Microarchitecture parameters including bone volume (BV, mm^3) and bone volume fraction (BV/TV, %) were measured.

Western blotting analysis

The phosphorylation levels of c-Fms, Erk1/2 and p90RSK in preosteoclasts were determined by western blot using phospho-specific antibodies (Cell Signaling, Danvers, MA). Phosphorylation levels were quantitated with Image J and standardized by total β-actin expression levels (Cell Signaling). Briefly, preosteoclasts were deprived of growth factors for 12 hours in α-MEM supplemented with 0.5% bovine serum albumin (BSA) before being pretreated with PLX3397 at different concentrations as indicated, and were stimulated with M-CSF (30 ng/mL) for 5 minutes in the presence of PLX3397. The cells were then lysed in ProteoJET lysis buffer (Fermentas, Glen Burnie, MD) supplemented with Complete Mini protease inhibitor cocktail (Roche, Indianapolis, IN) for protein extraction. Protein separated by sodium dodecyl sulfate polyacrylamide gel electrophoresis (SDS-PAGE) were transferred to nitrocellulose filters and probed with specific antibodies.

Statistical analyses

The data are presented as mean ± standard error of the mean (SEM). Differences among experimental groups were analyzed by repeated measures of paired *t*-tests or analysis of variance (ANOVA) with appropriate post hoc *t*-tests. *P* values less than

0.05 were considered significant. Statistical analyses were performed with Prism 5.0 software (GraphPad, La Jolla, CA).

Results

Aberrant c-Fms activation mediates M-CSF hyperresponsiveness in *Nf1* haploinsufficient osteoclast progenitors

Although *Nf1*$^{+/-}$ osteoclasts and osteoclast progenitors are hyperresponsive to limiting doses of M-CSF, the molecular mechanisms mediating this phenotype remain unclear. We therefore sought to determine whether *Nf1* haploinsufficiency may result in aberrant M-CSF signaling via hyperactivation of its receptor, c-Fms. We first examined the phosphorylation level of c-Fms by immunofluorescence staining of WT and *Nf1*$^{+/-}$ preosteoclasts. *Nf1*$^{+/-}$ preosteoclasts exhibited increased phospho-c-Fms staining both at base line and after being stimulated with M-CSF (30 ng/mL) for 5 minutes as compared with WT preosteoclasts. The expression levels of phospho-c-Fms decreased markedly following treatment with a small molecule inhibitor of the c-Fms receptor tyrosine kinase, PLX3397, at 62.5 nM and reached the lowest level at 1 μM in WT cultures and 0.1 μM in *Nf1*$^{+/-}$ cultures, respectively (Figure 1A and 1B).

To further validate these findings and determine the impact of increased c-Fms activation with respect to the downstream MAPK pathway, the phosphorylation levels of c-Fms, p90RSK, and Erk were detected by western blotting. *Nf1*$^{+/-}$ preosteoclasts demonstrated increased phosphorylation levels of c-Fms, p90RSK and Erk as compared with WT preosteoclasts when stimulated by M-CSF. Pretreatment of PLX3397 blocked the phosphorylation of these proteins both in WT and *Nf1*$^{+/-}$ preosteoclasts (Figure 1C and Figure S2).

Pharmacologic c-Fms inhibition reduces osteoclast progenitor frequency and osteoclast differentiation *in vitro*. Given that *Nf1* haploinsufficiency leads to M-CSF induced hyperactivation of c-Fms and the downstream MAPK effector pathway, we sought to investigate the effect of pharmacologic c-Fms inhibition on *Nf1*$^{+/-}$ osteoclast differentiation *in vitro*. Since osteoclasts are derived from monocyte/macrophage progeny within the bone marrow, we quantified the number of colony forming unit-macrophage (CFU-M) per femur following culture in semisolid methylcellulose media. Consistent with our previous data [18], a significantly increased number of CFU-M was observed in *Nf1*$^{+/-}$ bone marrow mononuclear cells (BMMNCs) as compared to WT BMMNCs. Addition of PLX3397 significantly reduced the frequencies of CFU-M at

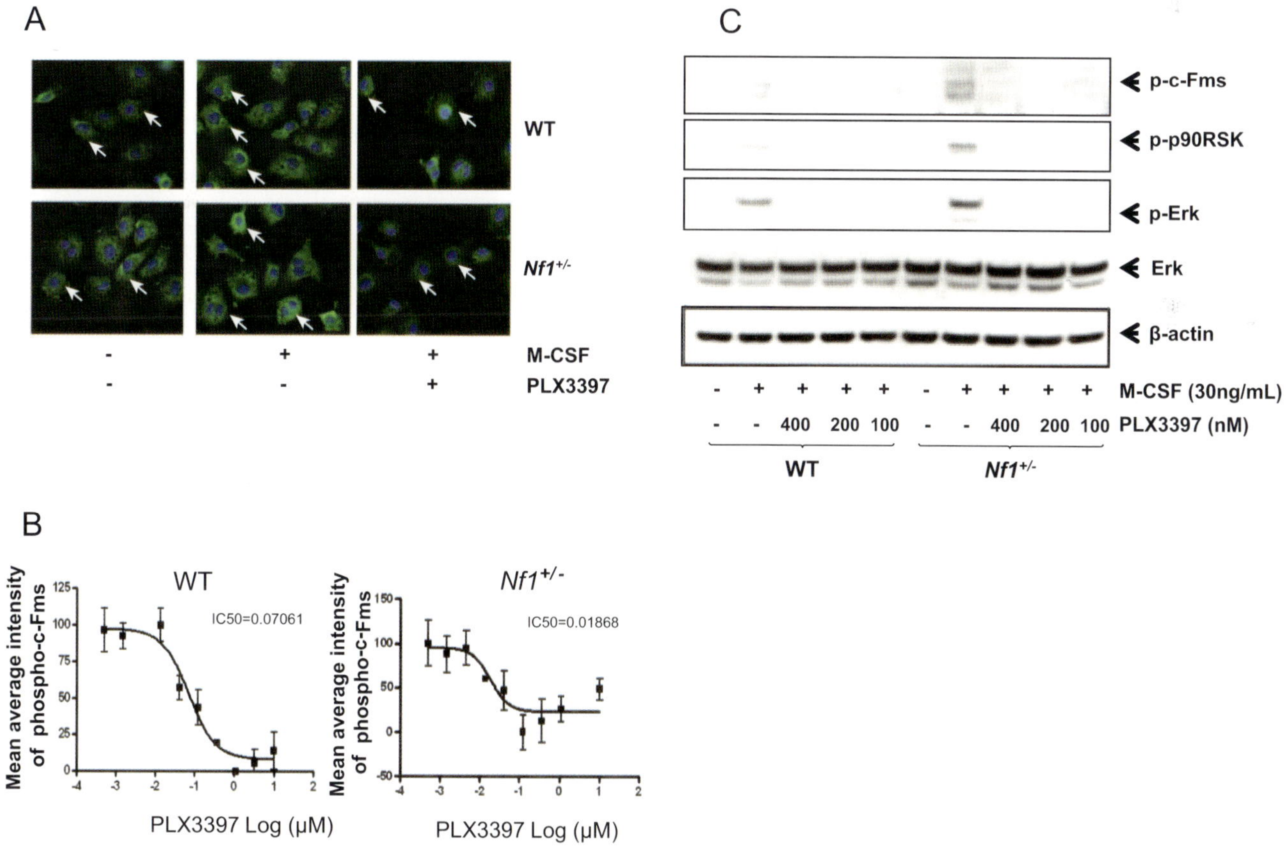

Figure 1. Increased c-Fms activation in *Nf1*$^{+/-}$ osteoclast progenitors. (**A**) Expression level of phospho-c-Fms in WT and *Nf1*$^{+/-}$ preosteoclasts was evaluated by immunofluorescence staining. Preosteoclasts were obtained by 3 days culture in the presence of M-CSF (30 ng/mL) and RANKL (20 ng/mL). After serum deprivation in 0.5% BSA in α-MEM for 6 hours, cells were pretreated with PLX3397 or PBS vehicle before stimulated with M-CSF (30 ng/mL). The cells were then fixed and stained for phospho-c-Fms (Arrows indicate the phospho-c-Fms positive cells). (**B**) *Nf1*$^{+/-}$ osteoclast progenitors show enhanced phosphorylation of c-Fms both at baseline and in the presence of M-CSF. Treatment with PLX3397 significantly reduced the activation of c-Fms both in the WT and *Nf1*$^{+/-}$ preosteoclasts. Maximal inhibitory concentration (IC_{50}) indicates the half maximal (50%) inhibitory concentration (IC) of a substance (50% IC, or IC_{50}). (**C**) After being stimulated with M-CSF (30 ng/mL) for 5 minutes, the phosphorylation levels of c-Fms, Erk, and P90RSK in both WT and *Nf1*$^{+/-}$ preosteoclasts were detected by western blot. Pretreatment of PLX3397 completely blocked the activation of Erk and p90RSK in those cells. These experiments were repeated on three independent occasions with similar results.

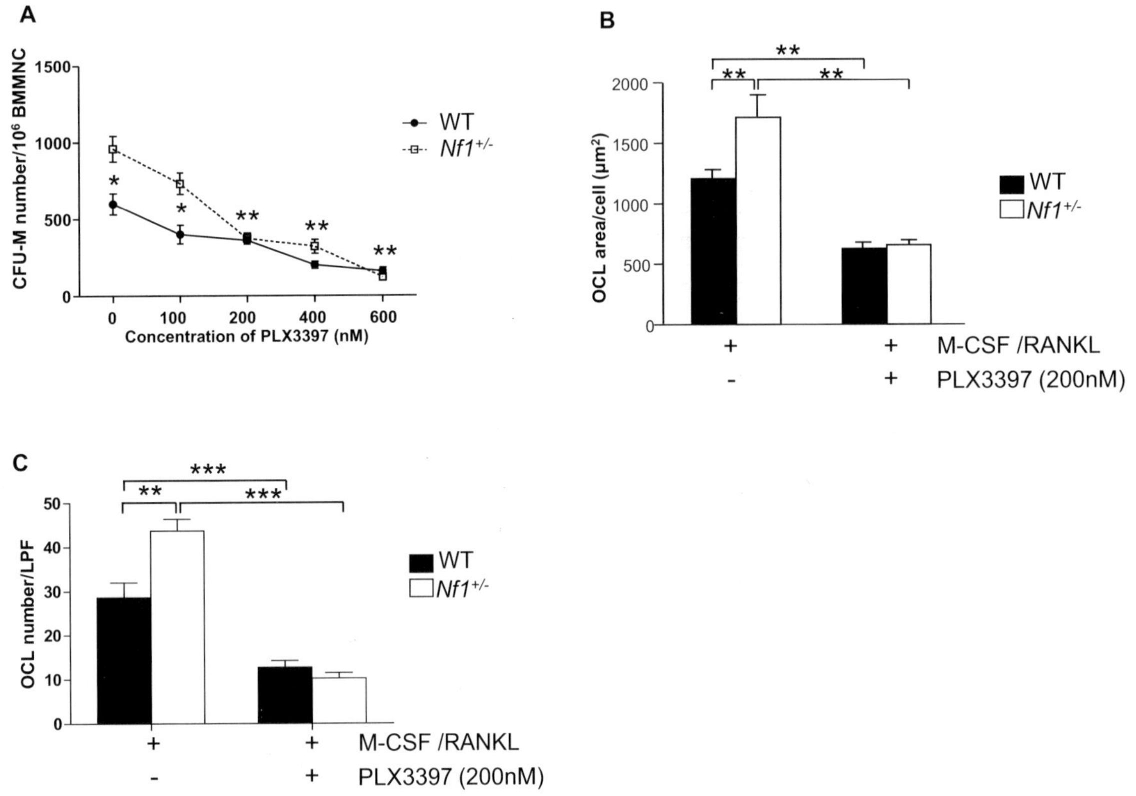

Figure 2. c-Fms hyperactivity mediates increased osteoclast progenitor frequency and differentiation capacity in bone marrow cells from *Nf1*$^{+/-}$ mice. (**A**) Clonogenic assays were performed to establish the number of osteoclast progenitors, CFU-M, per femur from WT and *Nf1*$^{+/-}$ mice. Addition of PLX3397 reduced CFU-M at a dose dependent manner. *$p<0.05$ and **$p<0.01$. (**B**) The ability of WT and *Nf1*$^{+/-}$ BMMNCs to form osteoclasts in response to M-CSF with PLX3397 or PBS vehicle was evaluated by TRACP staining. The y-axis shows the osteoclast area per cell. (**C**) The numbers of TRACP$^+$ osteoclasts in WT and *Nf1*$^{+/-}$ culture was evaluated by TRACP staining. Data are represented as mean ± SEM, with n = 3. **$p<0.01$ and ***$p<0.001$ compared with the control group. Three independent experiments were conducted with similar results.

concentrations of 200 nM both in WT and *Nf1*$^{+/-}$ cultures (Figure 2A).

To assess whether inhibition of M-CSF signaling affected osteoclast formation, we established osteoclast cultures in the presence of M-CSF/RANKL with PBS vehicle or PLX3397. Osteoclast differentiation was determined by calculating the TRACP$^+$ area per osteoclast (Figure 2B) and by counting the number of TRACP$^+$ osteoclasts per low power field (Figure 2C). *Nf1*$^{+/-}$ cultures contained significantly increased TRACP$^+$ area and osteoclast numbers as compared to WT cultures Addition of PLX3397 reduced osteoclast formation in both WT and *Nf1*$^{+/-}$ cultures.

M-CSF/c-Fms signaling mediates *Nf1*$^{+/-}$ preosteoclast migration and adhesion

The ability of osteoclasts to migrate across the bone surface is a key cellular function required for bone resorption. We have previously reported that haploinsufficiency of *Nf1* resulted in enhanced preosteoclast migration in response to M-CSF [18]. To assess the impact of c-Fms inhibition on preosteoclast motility mediated by M-CSF, preosteoclast migration was assessed by transwell assays. Bottom chambers containing media alone without M-CSF were used as negative controls (data not shown). After four hours of stimulation, M-CSF induced a significantly higher level of migration in *Nf1*$^{+/-}$ cultures than that of WT cultures (Figure 3A). Addition of PLX3397 reduced *Nf1*$^{+/-}$ preosteoclast migration to WT levels.

To determine the impact of M-CSF/c-Fms signaling on preosteoclast adhesion, a key process for initiation of bone resorption, adhesion assays were performed. Consistent with our previous findings [18], significantly increased *Nf1*$^{+/-}$ preosteoclasts were observed to adhere to vitronectin following M-CSF stimulation. Pretreatment with PLX3397 (200 nM) dramatically decreased the number of adherent cells in both WT and *Nf1*$^{+/-}$ preosteoclasts mediated by M-CSF (Figure 3B).

PLX3397 inhibits osteoclast bone resorption

To assess the impact of PLX3397 on osteoclast bone resorptive activity, pit formation assays were performed [18,19]. Consistent with our previous study [18], *Nf1*$^{+/-}$ osteoclasts induced a 2–3 fold increased pit forming area as compared to WT osteoclasts (Figure 3C). Importantly, PLX3397 reduced pit forming areas in both WT and *Nf1*$^{+/-}$ cultures. These data indicate that c-Fms inhibition not only inhibits osteoclast differentiation but also diminishes osteoclast bone resorptive activity.

Pharmacologic c-Fms inhibition prevents bone loss in ovariectomized *Nf1*$^{+/-}$ mice

Based on our findings that *Nf1*$^{+/-}$ osteoclasts exhibit increased bone lytic activity and that PLX3397 inhibits osteoclast formation and bone resorptive activity *in vitro*, we postulated that pharmacologic inhibition of c-Fms with PLX3397 may exert anti-catabolic effects on bone *in vivo*. To further test our hypothesis that PLX3397 may prevent bone loss *in vivo*, we gavage-fed PLX3397

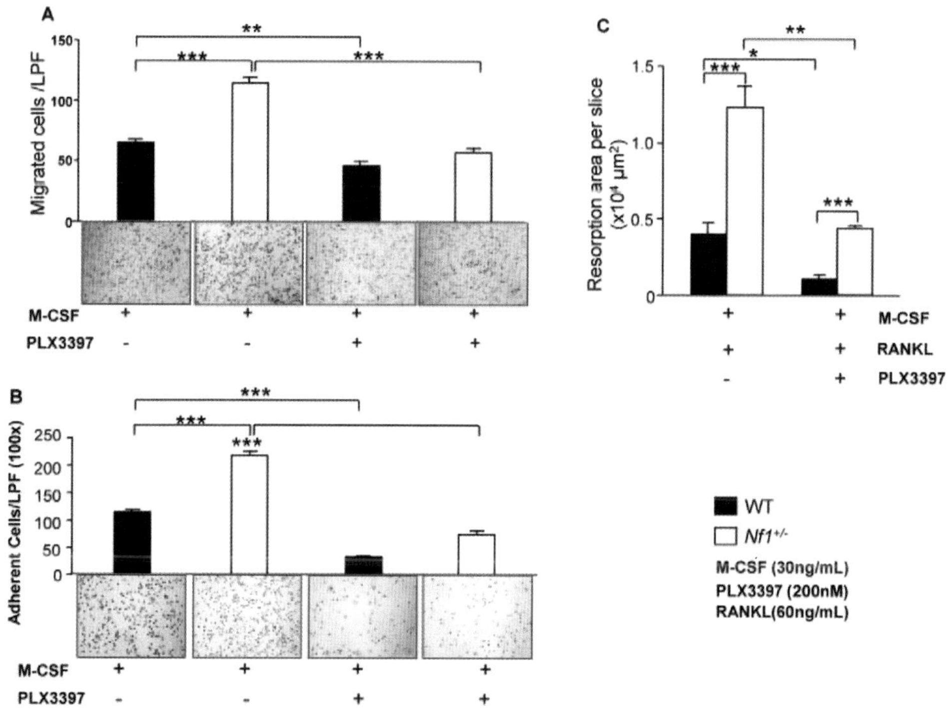

Figure 3. Pharmacologic c-Fms inhibition mitigates multiple *Nf1*$^{+/-}$ osteoclast gain in functions including migration, adhesion, and bone resorptive activity. (**A**) A transwell assay was used to investigate the effect of the c-Fms inhibitor PLX3397 on osteoclast migration. Experiments were conducted in triplicates per condition. Five fields were counted per well. Three independent experiments were performed with similar results. $^{**}p<0.01$;. (**B**) Adhesion assays were used to investigate the effect of the PLX3397 on osteoclast attachment to vitronectin. Experiments were conducted in triplicates per condition. Five fields were counted per well. Three independent experiments were performed with similar results. $^{***}p<0.001$. (**C**) Quantitative evaluation of bone resorption. Data represent the mean ± SEM of 6 fields per genotype. Each condition was carried out in triplicates and four independent experiments were performed. $^{*}p<0.05$; $^{**}p<0.01$; $^{***}p<0.001$.

to *Nf1*$^{+/-}$ mice undergoing ovariectomy (OVX), an established osteoporotic stress model [18]. 80 mg/kg/day of PLX3397 were administered to both WT-OVX and *Nf1*$^{+/-}$-OVX mice for a period of twelve weeks, and PBS was used as vehicle in control groups.

Similar to our previous study, the OVX surgery resulted in reduced BMD in both genotypes of mice [18]. Moreover, the *Nf1*$^{+/-}$ -OVX mice lost significantly more bone mass than the WT- OVX mice (Figure 4A), confirming that a pro-resorptive challenge induces a greater osteoclastic response in *Nf1* haploinsufficient mice. *Nf1*$^{+/-}$-OVX mice fed with PLX3397 showed a significantly increased BMD as compared to the vehicle control group.

To further investigate the role of PLX3397 on modulating trabecular bone, microcomputed tomography (μCT) was performed to examine the architecture of trabecular bone. Representative μCT 3D reconstructions are shown (Figure 4B). *Nf1*$^{+/-}$-OVX mice displayed significantly less trabecular bone, as determined by bone volume/tissue volume (BV/TV), and as compared to WT-OVX mice that received vehicle treatment. PLX3397 significantly increased the trabecular bone in *Nf1*$^{+/-}$-OVX mice (Figure 4C).

In addition, CTX, a sensitive marker of bone loss, was significantly increased in the plasma of both WT-OVX and *Nf1*$^{+/-}$-OVX mice as compared to controls ($^{*}p<0.05$ for *Nf1*$^{+/-}$-OVX vs. *Nf1*$^{+/-}$ sham) (Figure 4D). CTX was even higher in the plasma of *Nf1*$^{+/-}$-OVX mice than that of WT-OVX mice ($^{*}p<0.05$ for *Nf1*$^{+/-}$-OVX vs. WT-OVX). Importantly, administration of PLX3397 attenuated the plasma CTX levels in both WT-OVX mice and *Nf1*$^{+/-}$-OVX mice. Collectively, these data suggest that pharmacologic c-Fms inhibition is sufficient to prevent bone loss by abrogating osteoclast bone resorptive activity *in vivo*.

c-Fms hyperactivity mediates expansion of the osteoclast progenitor pool in *Nf1*$^{+/-}$ OVX mice *in vivo*

Since osteoclasts are considered to be the key lineage mediating bone loss in ovariectomy induced resorptive stress, we next investigated the effect of ovariectomy on the number of osteoclast progenitors in the bone marrow by performing CFU-M assays. Ovariectomy surgery significantly increased the frequency of CFU-M in both WT-OVX and *Nf1*$^{+/-}$-OVX groups as compared to the sham group. PLX3397, but not by vehicle gavage-feeding, suppressed the CFU-M formation to the level of sham groups in the *Nf1*$^{+/-}$ mice (Figure 5A).

To examine the impact of PLX3397 on osteoclastogenesis *in vivo*, the TRACP^{+} cell area/bone surface area of the femur was scored following TRACP staining. A significant increase in the TRACP^{+} area/bone surface area was observed in *Nf1*$^{+/-}$ Sham as compared to the WT Sham group. Furthermore, OVX surgery induced an even more dramatic increase in osteoclastogenesis in *Nf1*$^{+/-}$ mice as evidence by the increased TRACP^{+} cells compared to WT-OVX mice. Importantly, PLX3397 treatment reduced the number of TRACP^{+} osteoclasts in *Nf1*$^{+/-}$-OVX mice (Figure 5B and 5C). Collectively, these data indicate that elevated c-Fms signaling, following ovariectomy induced resorptive stress, results in increased numbers of osteoclast progenitors and mature osteoclasts in *Nf1*$^{+/-}$ mice, and consequently accelerated bone loss.

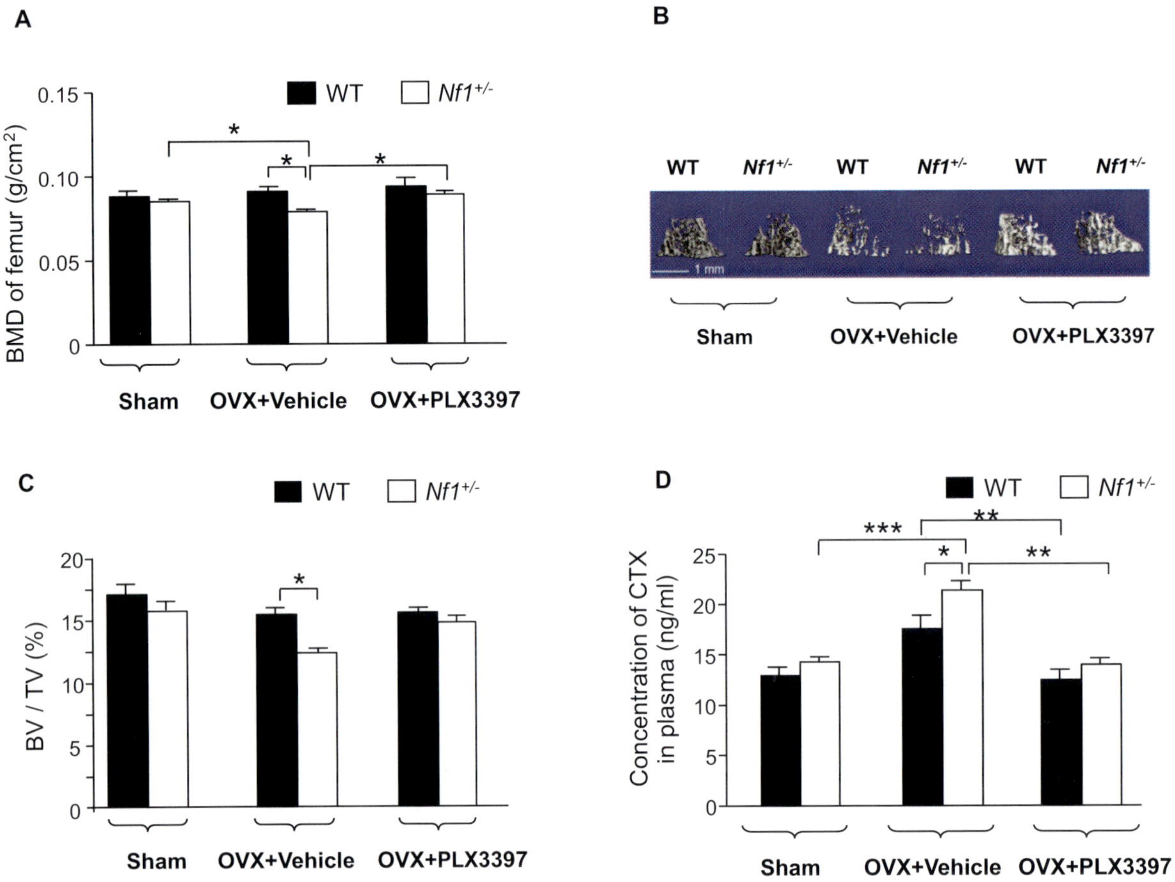

Figure 4. PLX3397 treatment restores bone mass in *Nf1*$^{+/-}$ OVX mice *in vivo*. (**A**) The BMD of femoral metaphysis was measured by pDEXA and analyzed with Lunar Piximus. **p*<0.05; ****p*<0.001 (**B**) Micro-CT (μCT) scans were performed on the distal femur of all groups of mice. Representative reconstructed 3D pictures are shown. The cortical portion of each femur has been removed to allow visualization of the metaphyseal architecture. (**C**) Bone volume fraction (BV/TV) was assessed by μCT. **p*<0.05. (**D**) The concentration of CTX in plasma in WT and *Nf1*$^{+/-}$ mice was measured after OVX. Data are represented as mean ± SEM, with n = 8. **p*<0.05, ***p*<0.01 and ****p*<0.001 compared with the control group.

Discussion

Osteoporosis and osteopenia affect both children and adults with NF1 [5,6,7,12,26,27]. As *Nf1*$^{+/-}$ mice have normal bone mass, ovariectomy is an established experimental model to induce low bone mass in Nf1+/− mice [18]. Previously, we reported an increased frequency of osteoclast progenitors in *Nf1*$^{+/-}$ bone marrow induced by M-CSF as assessed by the colony forming unit-macrophage (CFU-M) assay [18]. We also showed that haploinsufficiency of *Nf1* results in hypersensitivity of osteoclast progenitors to M-CSF correlated with hyperactivation of the Ras/MAPK pathway [18]. In the present study, we show that the M-CSF receptor, c-Fms, is hyperactivated in *Nf1* haploinsufficient osteoclasts and progenitors following M-CSF stimulation. Utilizing a small molecule c-Fms kinase inhibitor, PLX3397, we demonstrate that c-Fms overactivity mediates multiple *Nf1*$^{+/-}$ osteoclast gain-in-function phenotypes both *in vitro* and *in vivo* including expansion of osteoclast progenitors in the bone marrow, increased osteoclast migration, adhesion, and differentiation, and accelerated bone loss following ovariectomy induced resorptive stress.

M-CSF is a critical cytokine for the development of macrophages and their subsequent differentiation to the osteoclast cell lineage [28]. It has been reported recently that macrophage colony stimulating factor (M-CSF), together with signals from a family of biologically related tumor necrosis factor receptor like proteins (particularly RANKL), control the induction of osteoclast differentiation and are key to the physiologic and pathologic responses of osteoclasts [29,30]. Post-menopausal patients, as well as those with common chronic diseases such as arthritis, have a high incidence of osteoporosis, due to increased production of M-CSF and RANKL, which leads to increased osteoclast activation and consequent bone loss [31]. It has been shown that PI3K is a critical downstream effector of the M-CSF/c-Fms pathway [32]. Once activated by M-CSF, PI3K modulates osteoclast survival as well as actin remodeling [33,34]. Pharmacologic inhibitors of PI3K, including LY294002 and wortmannin, show a dramatic reduction of osteoclast formation in cultures treated with M-CSF and RANKL. Furthermore, treating osteoclasts with pharmacologic inhibitors of PI3K also impairs the resorptive activity of osteoclasts, which is associated with impaired membrane ruffling, deficient actin ring formation, and reduced pit formation [35]. Unfortunately, the clinical utility of commercially available PI3K inhibitors such as wortmannin and LY294002 is limited as these compounds target the ATP-binding site of all PI3K family members and interfere with other PI3K related kinases at therapeutic concentrations. As such, these inhibitors are broad spectrum, non-specific and are associated with significant toxicity *in vivo*. PLX3397 is a novel small molecule that potently and selectively inhibits c-Fms, Kit, and Flt3-ITD kinases [36,37]. Since osteoclasts cultured from *Nf1*$^{+/-}$ mice and human NF1 patients

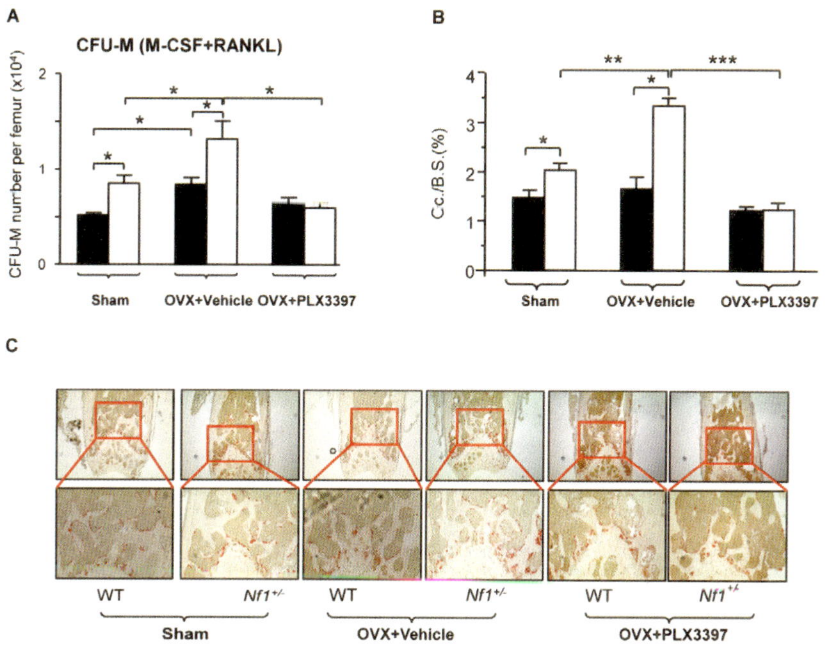

Figure 5. c-Fms inhibition attenuates osteoclast formation *in vivo*. (**A**) The CFU-M number of the BMMNC from WT and *Nf1*$^{+/-}$ mice after OVX with vehicle or PLX3397 treatment was counted. *$p<0.05$. (**B**) Quantitative analysis of the percentage of TRACP^{+} osteoclast area/bone surface area (Oc./BS). Data are represented as mean ± SEM, with n = 5. *$p<0.05$; **$p<0.01$; ***$p<0.001$. (**C**) Femur samples were processed for TRACP staining. Representative photographs (40x upper panels, 100x lower panels) of the trabecular bone following TRACP staining are shown. The red stained area indicates TRACP^{+} osteoclasts.

exhibit hyperactivation of the c-Fms receptor kinase in response to M-CSF, we reasoned that pharmacologic inhibition of c-Fms with PLX3397 may exert anti-catabolic effects on bone in the NF1 murine model.

M-CSF is critical for the proliferation of osteoclast precursors and addition of an M-CSF neutralizing antibody considerably reduced macrophage differentiation at the early precursor stage [38,39]. Consistent with these findings, our *in vivo* study indicates that administration of PLX3397 significantly reduced the frequency of osteoclast progenitors as shown by reduced numbers of CFU-M. In addition, M-CSF is also essential for osteoclast formation and maturation by contributing to proliferation and survival [1√8] [40]. In the present study, we show that pharmacologic c-Fms inhibition reduces osteoclast differentiation and bone resorption. In addition, our data demonstrates that PLX3397 inhibited M-CSF mediated MAPK signaling pathway by diminishing the activation of c-Fms, p90RSK and Erk, which are key to the hyperfunctioning of *Nf1*$^{+/-}$ osteoclasts in response to M-CSF.

Underscoring the critical role of c-Fms in mediating excessive osteoclast bone resorptive activity in NF1, administration of PLX3397 was sufficient to prevent bone loss in an established murine model of NF1 low bone mass. This normalization of bone mineral density and trabecular bone mass in response to pharmacologic c-Fms inhibition *in vivo* was associated with the attenuation of osteoclast development and cellular functions, including osteoclast differentiation, migration and bone resorption. Collectively, these data suggest that the M-CSF signaling through its receptor c-Fms may play a critical role in osteoclast-mediated osteoporotic manifestations in NF1. Biochemically, our data show that administration of PLX3397 can prevent the activation of the MAPK signaling cascade in response to M-CSF, thereby correcting aberrant osteoclast functions in the *Nf1*$^{+/-}$ murine model. As such, further studies are needed to assess whether targeting M-CSF/c-Fms signaling might provide a potential treatment for osteoporosis in NF1.

Supporting Information

Figure S1 (**A**) Uteri of WT or *Nf1*$^{+/-}$ mice undergoing OVX surgery were compared to sham operated controls. (**B**) Uterine weight of WT and *Nf1*$^{+/-}$ mice undergoing OVX surgery vs. sham controls. Data are represented as mean ± SEM, with n = 5. *$p<0.05$; **$p<0.01$; ***$p<0.001$. (**C**) The plasma concentration of PLX3397 in mice receiving treatment is shown.

Figure S2 The phosphorylation levels of c-Fms, Erk, and p90RSK in both WT and *Nf1*+/− preosteoclasts were detected by western blot (Figure 1C) and quantified by densitometry as shown below.

Acknowledgments

We thank Lisa Harris for administrative support. Plexxikon Inc. provided the PLX3397 compound.

Author Contributions

Conceived and designed the experiments: YH FCY TAG. Performed the experiments: YH SDR SC XW JY XY LJ XL NT. Analyzed the data: YH KSM TAG FCY MX. Contributed reagents/materials/analysis tools: NT XL. Wrote the paper: YH FCY MX.

References

1. Lammert M, Friedman JM, Kluwe L, Mautner VF (2005) Prevalence of neurofibromatosis 1 in German children at elementary school enrollment. Arch Dermatol 141: 71–74.
2. Hiatt KK, Ingram DA, Zhang Y, Bollag G, Clapp DW (2001) Neurofibromin GTPase-activating protein-related domains restore normal growth in Nf1−/− cells. J Biol Chem 276: 7240–7245.
3. Riccardi VM (1981) Von Recklinghausen neurofibromatosis. N Engl J Med 305: 1617–1627.
4. Friedman JM (2002) Neurofibromatosis 1: clinical manifestations and diagnostic criteria. J Child Neurol 17: 548–554; discussion 571–542, 646–551.
5. Kuorilehto T, Poyhonen M, Bloigu R, Heikkinen J, Vaananen K, et al. (2005) Decreased bone mineral density and content in neurofibromatosis type 1: lowest local values are located in the load-carrying parts of the body. Osteoporos Int 16: 928–936.
6. Lammert M, Kappler M, Mautner VF, Lammert K, Storkel S, et al. (2005) Decreased bone mineral density in patients with neurofibromatosis 1. Osteoporos Int 16: 1161–1166.
7. Illes T, Halmai V, de Jonge T, Dubousset J (2001) Decreased bone mineral density in neurofibromatosis-1 patients with spinal deformities. Osteoporos Int 12: 823–827.
8. Jacques C, Dietemann JL (2005) [Imaging features of neurofibromatosis type 1]. J Neuroradiol 32: 180–197.
9. Stevenson DA, Zhou H, Ashrafi S, Messiaen LM, Carey JC, et al. (2006) Double inactivation of NF1 in tibial pseudarthrosis. Am J Hum Genet 79: 143–148.
10. Brunetti-Pierri N, Doty SB, Hicks J, Phan K, Mendoza-Londono R, et al. (2008) Generalized metabolic bone disease in Neurofibromatosis type I. Mol Genet Metab 94: 105–111.
11. Seitz S, Schnabel C, Busse B, Schmidt HU, Beil FT, et al. (2010) High bone turnover and accumulation of osteoid in patients with neurofibromatosis 1. Osteoporos Int 21: 119–127.
12. Stevenson DA, Moyer-Mileur LJ, Murray M, Slater H, Sheng X, et al. (2007) Bone mineral density in children and adolescents with neurofibromatosis type 1. J Pediatr 150: 83–88.
13. Heervä E, Koffert A, Jokinen E, Kuorilehto T, Peltonen S, et al. (2012) A controlled register based study of 460 neurofibromatosis 1 (NF1) patients: Increased fracture risk in children and adults over 41 years. J Bone Miner Res.
14. Crawford AH, Jr., Bagamery N (1986) Osseous manifestations of neurofibromatosis in childhood. J Pediatr Orthop 6: 72–88.
15. Friedman JM, Birch PH (1997) Type 1 neurofibromatosis: a descriptive analysis of the disorder in 1,728 patients. Am J Med Genet 70: 138–143.
16. Elefteriou F, Kolanczyk M, Schindeler A, Viskochil DH, Hock JM, et al. (2009) Skeletal abnormalities in neurofibromatosis type 1: approaches to therapeutic options. Am J Med Genet A 149A: 2327–2338.
17. Mondal R, Nandi M, Chandra PK Neurofibromatosis, pathological fracture and hypervitaminosis-D. Indian Pediatr 47: 881–882.
18. Yang FC, Chen S, Robling AG, Yu X, Nebesio TD, et al. (2006) Hyperactivation of p21ras and PI3K cooperate to alter murine and human neurofibromatosis type 1-haploinsufficient osteoclast functions. J Clin Invest 116: 2880–2891.
19. Yan J, Chen S, Zhang Y, Li X, Li Y, et al. (2008) Rac1 mediates the osteoclast gains-in-function induced by haploinsufficiency of Nf1. Hum Mol Genet 17: 936–948.
20. Heervä E, Alanne MH, Peltonen S, Kuorilehto T, Hentunen T, et al. (2010) Osteoclasts in neurofibromatosis type 1 display enhanced resorption capacity, aberrant morphology, and resistance to serum deprivation. Bone 47: 583–590.
21. Alanne MH, Siljamaki E, Peltonen S, Vaananen K, Windle JJ, et al. (2012) Phenotypic characterization of transgenic mice harboring Nf1(+/−) or Nf1(−/−) osteoclasts in otherwise Nf1(+/+) background. J Cell Biochem.
22. He Y, Staser K, Rhodes SD, Liu Y, Wu X, et al. (2011) Erk1 positively regulates osteoclast differentiation and bone resorptive activity. PLoS One 6: e24780.
23. Jacks T, Shih TS, Schmitt EM, Bronson RT, Bernards A, et al. (1994) Tumour predisposition in mice heterozygous for a targeted mutation in Nf1. Nat Genet 7: 353–361.
24. Wu X, Chen S, He Y, Rhodes SD, Mohammad KS, et al. (2011) The haploinsufficient hematopoietic microenvironment is critical to the pathological fracture repair in murine models of neurofibromatosis type 1. PLoS One 6: e24917.
25. Zhang W, Rhodes SD, Zhao L, He Y, Zhang Y, et al. (2011) Primary osteopathy of vertebrae in a neurofibromatosis type 1 murine model. Bone 48: 1378–1387.
26. Yilmaz K, Ozmen M, Bora Goksan S, Eskiyurt N (2007) Bone mineral density in children with neurofibromatosis 1. Acta Paediatr 96: 1220–1222.
27. Dulai S, Briody J, Schindeler A, North KN, Cowell CT, et al. (2007) Decreased bone mineral density in neurofibromatosis type 1: results from a pediatric cohort. J Pediatr Orthop 27: 472–475.
28. Yoshida H, Hayashi S, Kunisada T, Ogawa M, Nishikawa S, et al. (1990) The murine mutation osteopetrosis is in the coding region of the macrophage colony stimulating factor gene. Nature 345: 442–444.
29. Lacey DL, Timms E, Tan HL, Kelley MJ, Dunstan CR, et al. (1998) Osteoprotegerin ligand is a cytokine that regulates osteoclast differentiation and activation. Cell 93: 165–176.
30. Yasuda H, Shima N, Nakagawa N, Yamaguchi K, Kinosaki M, et al. (1998) Osteoclast differentiation factor is a ligand for osteoprotegerin/osteoclastogenesis-inhibitory factor and is identical to TRANCE/RANKL. Proc Natl Acad Sci U S A 95: 3597–3602.
31. Raisz LG (2005) Pathogenesis of osteoporosis: concepts, conflicts, and prospects. J Clin Invest 115: 3318–3325.
32. Golden LH, Insogna KL (2004) The expanding role of PI3-kinase in bone. Bone 34: 3–12.
33. Pilkington MF, Sims SM, Dixon SJ (1998) Wortmannin inhibits spreading and chemotaxis of rat osteoclasts in vitro. J Bone Miner Res 13: 688–694.
34. Palacio S, Felix R (2001) The role of phosphoinositide 3-kinase in spreading osteoclasts induced by colony-stimulating factor-1. Eur J Endocrinol 144: 431–440.
35. Nakamura I, Takahashi N, Sasaki T, Tanaka S, Udagawa N, et al. (1995) Wortmannin, a specific inhibitor of phosphatidylinositol-3 kinase, blocks osteoclastic bone resorption. FEBS Lett 361: 79–84.
36. Anthony SP, Puzanov I, Lin PS, Nolop KB, West B, et al. (2011) Pharmacodynamic activity demonstrated in phase I for PLX3397, a selective inhibitor of FMS and Kit. J Clin Oncol (suppl; abstr 3093) 29.
37. DeNardo DG, Brennan DJ, Rexhepaj E, Ruffekk B, Shiao SL, et al. (2011) Leukocyte complexity predicts breast cancer survival and functionally regulates response to chemotherapy. Drug Discovery 1: 54–67.
38. Liggett W, Jr., Shevde N, Anklesaria P, Sohoni S, Greenberger J, et al. (1993) Effects of macrophage colony stimulating factor and granulocyte-macrophage colony stimulating factor on osteoclastic differentiation of hematopoietic progenitor cells. Stem Cells 11: 398–411.
39. Biskobing DM, Fan X, Rubin J (1995) Characterization of MCSF-induced proliferation and subsequent osteoclast formation in murine marrow culture. J Bone Miner Res 10: 1025–1032.
40. Otero K, Turnbull IR, Poliani PL, Vermi W, Cerutti E, et al. (2009) Macrophage colony-stimulating factor induces the proliferation and survival of macrophages via a pathway involving DAP12 and beta-catenin. Nat Immunol 10: 734–743.

4

MiR-133a in Human Circulating Monocytes: A Potential Biomarker Associated with Postmenopausal Osteoporosis

Yang Wang[1], Ling Li[1], Benjamin T. Moore[1], Xian-Hao Peng[1], Xiang Fang[2], Joan M. Lappe[1], Robert R. Recker[1], Peng Xiao[1]*

1 Osteoporosis Research Center, School of Medicine, Creighton University, Omaha, Nebraska, United States of America, **2** Biostatistical Core, Office of Research and Compliance, Creighton University, Omaha, Nebraska, United States of America

Abstract

Background: Osteoporosis mainly occurs in postmenopausal women, which is characterized by low bone mineral density (BMD) due to unbalanced bone resorption by osteoclasts and formation by osteoblasts. Circulating monocytes play important roles in osteoclastogenesis by acting as osteoclast precursors and secreting osteoclastogenic factors, such as IL-1, IL-6 and TNF-α. MicroRNAs (miRNAs) have been implicated as important biomarkers in various diseases. The present study aimed to find significant miRNA biomarkers in human circulating monocytes underlying postmenopausal osteoporosis.

Methodology/Principal Findings: We used ABI TaqMan® miRNA array followed by qRT-PCR validation in circulating monocytes to identify miRNA biomarkers in 10 high and 10 low BMD postmenopausal Caucasian women. MiR-133a was upregulated ($P = 0.007$) in the low compared with the high BMD groups in the array analyses, which was also validated by qRT-PCR ($P = 0.044$). We performed bioinformatic target gene analysis and found three potential osteoclast-related target genes, CXCL11, CXCR3 and SLC39A1. In addition, we performed Pearson correlation analyses between the expression levels of miR-133a and the three potential target genes in the 20 postmenopausal women. We did find negative correlations between miR-133a and all the three genes though not significant.

Conclusions/Significance: This is the first *in vivo* miRNA expression analysis in human circulating monocytes to identify novel miRNA biomarkers underlying postmenopausal osteoporosis. Our results suggest that miR-133a in circulating monocytes is a potential biomarker for postmenopausal osteoporosis.

Editor: Qingyang Huang, Central China Normal University, China

Funding: This study was supported by grants from the State of Nebraska (LB692 and LB595) and the NIH (R01AR04054496-02S1). The funders had no role in study design, data collection and analysis, decision to publish, or preparation of the manuscript.

Competing Interests: The authors have declared that no competing interests exist.

* E-mail: pxiao@creighton.edu

Introduction

Tissue-specific expressed microRNAs (miRNAs) are short non-coding RNA molecules that regulate gene expression, generally by destabilizing mRNAs or suppressing translation. MiRNAs have been identified as important biomarkers and regulators in various human diseases such as cancer [1,2], diabetes [3,4] and myocardial disease [5]. In the bone area, many miRNAs regulate osteoblastogenesis [6–16]. However, very few miRNAs have been related to osteoclastogenesis [17,18]. MiRNA miR-223 played an essential role in osteoclastogenesis in a mouse osteoclast precursor cell line [18]. MiR-146a inhibited osteoclastogenesis from human circulating mononuclear cells [17].

Circulating monocytes are important cells that participate in osteoclatogenesis by acting as osteoclast precursors [19–22] and secreting osteoclastogenesis-related factors, such as IL-1 (interleukin-1), IL-6 and TNF-α (tumor necrosis factor-alpha) [23–25]. In addition, human studies have found associations of gene expression levels in circulating monocytes and osteoporosis, such as ANXA2 (annexin A2) [26], STAT1 (signal transducer and activator of transcription 1) [27], CCR3 [chemokine (C-C motif) receptor 3], HDC (histidine decarboxylase), and GCR (glucocorticoid receptor) [28].

However, no study has been conducted to identify miRNA biomarkers in circulating monocytes associated with human osteoporosis *in vivo*. Our present study aimed to identify differentially expressed miRNAs in circulating monocytes isolated from postmenopausal Caucasian women with discordant bone mineral density (BMD) using ABI miRNA array technology followed by qRT-PCR (quantitative RT-PCR). We found the significance of miR-133a in human circulating monocytes associated with postmenopausal osteoporosis. Further bioinformatic analysis of miR-133a identified its potential target genes that may be important in osteoclastogenesis.

Materials and Methods

Human subjects and characteristics

The study was approved by the Institutional Review Board at Creighton University, and all the subjects signed informed-consent documents before entering the project. All the subjects were Caucasians of European origin recruited from the vicinity of Creighton University in Omaha, NE. The exclusion criteria were detailed in our previous mRNA expression profiling study on B cells isolated from postmenopausal Caucasians for different BMD status [29]. The information such as age, ethnicity, menstrual status, medication history, and disease history was obtained via questionnaire. We recruited 20 unrelated postmenopausal Caucasian women, 10 with high BMD (spine or hip Z-score>0.84) and 10 with low BMD (spine or hip Z-score<−0.84). The high and low BMD groups are the top and bottom 20% BMD distributions of the age-, sex- and ethnicity-matched population. BMD (g/cm^2) for the lumbar spine (L1-4) and total hip (femoral neck, trochanter, and intertrochanteric region) were measured by Hologic 4500A dual energy X-ray absorptiometry (DXA) scanners (Hologic Inc., Bedford, MA). The machine was calibrated daily. The measurement precision as reflected by the coefficient of variation (CV) was 0.9% and 1.4% for spine and hip BMD, respectively. Postmenopausal status was defined as the date of the last menses followed by at least 12 months of no menses. All the study subjects were aged 57–68. The detailed characteristics of the study subjects are summarized in Table 1.

As shown in Table 1, both hip and spine BMD were significantly different between the high and low BMD groups. For age, weight and height traits, only height showed marginal difference between the two BMD groups. However, height only demonstrated a very small effect on quantitative BMD variations [30]. Moreover, in this study, BMD was classified as a quality trait into two categories, the low and the high BMD. Therefore, the effect of height on BMD can be ignored in this study.

Monocyte isolation

Blood mononuclear cells (MNCs) from 70 ml peripheral blood from each study subject were separated by density gradients with UNI-SEP tubes containing a solution of 5.6% polysucrose and 9.6% sodium metrizoate with a density of 1.077 g/ml (Novamed, Jerusalem, Israel). Monocytes were isolated by a negative isolation kit, Dynabeads® Untouched™ Human Monocytes (Dynal Biotech, Lake Success, NY, USA), which contains a cocktail of CD2, CD7, CD16, CD19, CD56 and CD235a antibodies to deplete T cells, B cells, natural killer cells, erythrocytes and granulocytes, leaving monocytes naive and free of the surface-bound antibody and beads. The purity of isolated monocytes was assessed by flow cytometry with fluorescence labeled antibodies CD19-PE and CD45-FITC (BD Biosciences, San Jose, CA USA), and the average purity is about 85% with 3% deviation.

Table 1. Characteristics of the study subjects.

Traits	High BMD (n = 10)	Low BMD (n = 10)	*P* Value
Age (yrs)	63.6±3.2	61.6±2.6	0.15
Height (cm)	159.2±3.2	163.6±4.7	0.03
Weight (kg)	76.7±7.9	72.9±17.6	0.55
Spine BMD (g/cm^2)	1.128±0.058	0.826±0.069	<0.001
Spine Z-Score	2.24±0.59	−0.63±0.64	<0.001
Hip BMD (g/cm^2)	1.057±0.101	0.725±0.045	<0.001
Hip Z-Score	1.94±0.99	−1.04±0.45	<0.001

Note: The data are mean ±SD.

Total RNA extraction

The *mir*Vana miRNA Isolation Kit (Ambion, Austin, Texas, USA) was used to extract total RNA including miRNAs from each cell sample following the manufacturer's protocol. Total RNA concentration and integrity were evaluated by an Agilent 2100 Bioanalyzer (Agilent, Palo Alto, CA, USA). Each RNA sample has a high quality with an excellent integrity number >9.0.

MiRNA array procedures

We used TaqMan® Human MicroRNA Array v1.0 (Applied Biosystems, Foster City, CA, USA) to perform miRNA expression profiling for each RNA sample. Each array covers 365 human miRNAs and endogenous controls RNU48 and RNU44. First, TaqMan miRNA Multiplex Reverse Transcription Kit (Applied Biosystems) was used for the RT reaction. For each RNA sample, the RT reaction was performed in a 63 µl reaction system including 1.8 µl 100 mM dNTPs, 18 µl Reverse Transcriptase (50 U/ml), 9 µl 10× RT Buffer, 1.13 µl RNase Inhibitor (20 U/µl), 16 µl sample RNA, and 17.08 µl nuclease-free water. The reaction conditions were as follows: 30 min at 16°C, 30 min at 42°C, and 5 min at 85°C. After that, we mixed 450 µl diluted RT reaction product (diluted 62.5-fold) with 450 µl TaqMan Universal PCR Master Mix (ABI) and loaded 100 µl real-time PCR reaction mix into each port of the array card (8 ports/card). The real-time qRT-PCR for each array was carried out on an Applied BioSystems 7900HT Fast Real-time PCR System with the following reaction conditions: 2 min at 50°C, 10 min at 95°C, 40 cycles of 15 sec at 95°C plus 1 min at 60°C. For each array card, there was only one probe for each target miRNA.

In the miRNA array data analysis, the raw expression level was determined by the cycle number at which the reaction crossed a predetermined cycle threshold (CT) as identified for each miRNA probe. The relative quantity (RQ) of each miRNA for each sample is determined by $2^{-\Delta\Delta CT}$, where $\Delta CT = (CT_{\text{Target miRNA}} - CT_{\text{endogenous control RNU48}})$ and $\Delta\Delta CT = (\Delta CT - \text{average } \Delta CT$ of all the samples). The RQ data were used for student's t test to identify differentially expressed miRNAs between the high and the low BMD groups.

qRT-PCR for miRNAs

To correct for the multiple-testing comparison and eliminate false positive results in the miRNA array analysis, we conducted qRT-PCR among the same 20 RNA samples to further validate the identified significant miRNAs in the array analysis. Two-step qRT-PCR was used to confirm the differentially expressed miRNAs. The first step is RT of cDNA and the second step is real-time quantitative PCR. All the reagents are provided by Applied Biosystems. The RT reaction was performed in a 15 µl volume, containing 1.5 µl Taqman RT Buffer (10×), 0.15 µl 100 mM dNTPs (100 mM), 1.0 µl Reverse Transcriptase, 0.19 µl RNase inhibitor (20 U/µl), 3.0 µl specific miRNA primer, 100 ng total RNA, and nuclease-free water to make the final volume 15 µl. The real-time quantitative PCR was performed in a 20 µl reaction volume using standard protocols on the Applied Biosystems 7900HT System. Briefly, 2.5 µl cDNA was mixed with 10.0 µl TaqMan universal PCR master mix (2×), 1.0 µl TaqMan miRNA assay and 6.5 µl nuclease-free water. The reaction conditions were the same as the above real-time PCR in the array experiments. For each RNA sample, the target miRNA and RNU48 reactions were run as triplicates in the same plate. The RQ of each miRNA for each sample is determined by $2^{-\Delta\Delta CT}$, where ΔCT = (average of triplicate $CT_{Target\ miRNA}$ − average of triplicate $CT_{endogenous\ control\ RNU48}$) and $\Delta\Delta CT$ = (ΔCT − average ΔCT of all the samples). The RQ data were used for student's *t* test between the two groups.

Target gene prediction and verification

We conducted bioinformatic sequence analysis of each significant miRNA to identify potential target genes [31]. MiRNAs normally repress gene expression by base pairing at complementarity sites mainly but not exclusively in the 3′-untraslated region (3′-UTR) of the target mRNAs [32,33]. The currently available miRNA target gene databases are all limited in the 3′-UTR analyses. We used both miRDB (http://www.miRDB.org/) and TargetScan (http://www.targetscan.org/) databases to predict target genes by searching for the presence of conserved 8-mer and 7-mer sites in their 3′-UTRs that match the seed region of each significant miRNA [34]. In addition, we also conducted qRT-PCR for the potential target genes of the significant miRNA among the same 20 RNA samples. Similar to miRNA qRT-PCR, the mRNA qRT-PCR was also composed of RT and real-time qPCR. The first step is RT of cDNA and the second step is real-time quantitative PCR. The RT and qPCR were in 100 µl and 25 µl volumes, respectively, following the company's standard protocols (Applied Biosystems). For each RNA sample, the target mRNA and internal control β-actin were run as triplicates in the same plate. We used the same calculation for RQ $2^{-\Delta\Delta CT}$ as we did for miRNA qRT-PCR and performed student's *t* test between the two groups.

Results

MiRNA array analyses

Among the 365 miRNAs in the array, the expression of many miRNAs were missing among the 20 study samples, probably due to tissue-specific expression or extremely low expression. To obtain enough power, we selected miRNAs that were expressed in at least 5 samples in each BMD group for the analyses. According to this criterion, 156 qualified miRNAs (Table S1) were subject to the statistical analyses and two miRNAs, miR-133a and miR-382, showed significant upregulation in the low BMD group compared with the high BMD group (Figure 1). Specifically, miR-133a displayed a fold change of 6.48 between the low and high BMD groups as mean ± SD (4.21±2.15 vs. 0.65±0.75, P = 0.007), and miR-382 showed a fold change of 3.65 between the low and high BMD groups (2.74±2.18 vs. 0.75±0.63, P = 0.027).

qRT-PCR for miRNAs

We further performed qRT-PCR to validate the differential expression of miR-133a and miR-382. However, only the upregulation of miR-133a in monocytes in the low vs. the high BMD group (2.21±2.08 vs. 0.76±0.37) was validated by qRT-PCR (P = 0.044). The difference in expression of miR-382 in monocytes in the low vs. the high BMD group (6.56±2.84 vs. 7.93±9.73) was not significant (P = 0.67) (Figure 2).

Target gene prediction and verification

Our bioinformatic sequence analyses identified 226 potential target genes that are overlapped in both miRDB and TargetScan databases. By searching relevant references for all the 226 genes, we found that three of them are related to osteoclastogenesis, CXCL11 [chemokine (C-X-C motif) ligand 11], CXCR3 [chemokine (C-X-C motif) receptor 3], and SLC39A1 [solute carrier family (zinc transporter), member 1]. Table 2 demonstrates the specific putative binding sites of miR-133a in the 3′ UTRs of the three genes. We conducted qRT-PCR analyses for all the three genes among the same 20 study samples and did not find significant differential expression. In addition, we performed correlation analysis of the expression levels of miR-133a and each gene. All three genes did demonstrate negative correlation with miR-133a, although they were not significant (P>0.05) (Table 3).

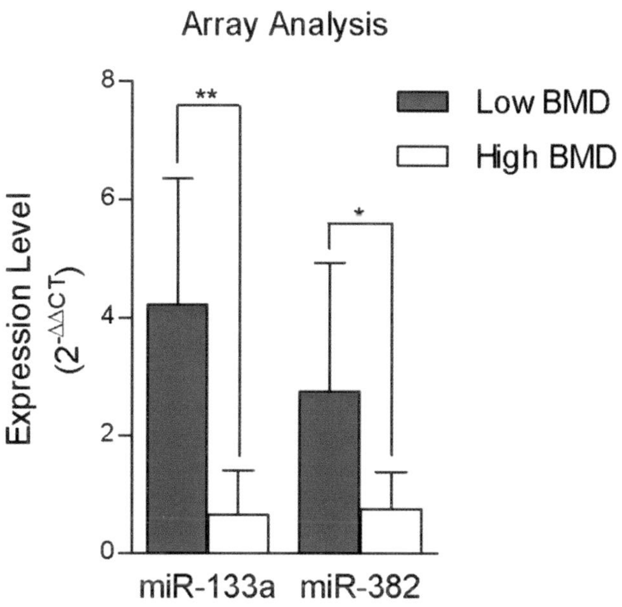

Figure 1. Expression levels ($2^{-\Delta\Delta CT}$) of significant miRNAs measured by array analysis in circulating monocytes in the low and high BMD groups (: P<0.01; *: P<0.05).**

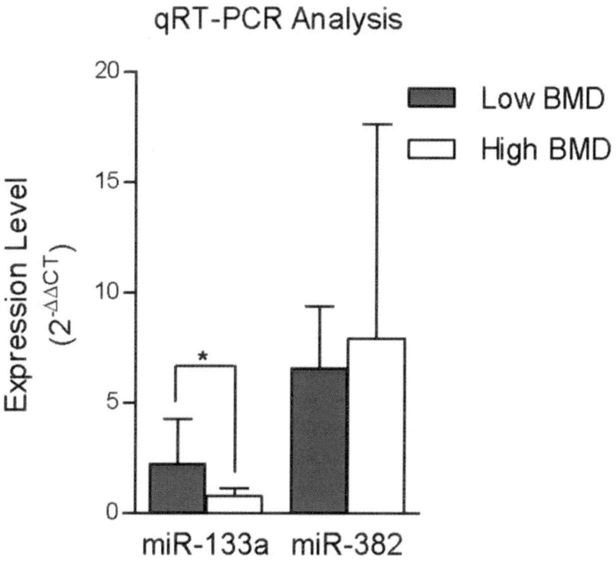

Figure 2. Expression levels ($2^{-\Delta\Delta CT}$) of miR-133a and miR-382 measured by qRT-PCR analysis in circulating monocytes in the low and high BMD groups (*: P<0.05).

Table 2. Putative binding sites of miR-133a in predicted target genes in humans.

Target Gene	3′ UTR Position	Consequential Pairing Target gene binding region (top) and miR-133a sequence (bottom)
CXCL11	171–177	5′...AAAGGUGGGUGAAA**GGACCAA**A... ||||||| 3′ GUCGACCAACUUCC**CCUGGUU**U
CXCR3	444–450	5′...AAACAAGAUCGUCA**GGACCAA**A... ||||||| 3′ GUCGACCAACUUCC**CCUGGUU**U
SLC39A1	107–113	5′...AAGGGAAAUACUGA**GGACCAA**A... ||||||| 3′ GUCGACCAACUUCC**CCUGGUU**U

Discussion

In this study, we aimed to identify important miRNAs in human circulating monocytes associated with discordant BMD status in postmenopausal Caucasian women. We found significant upregulation of miR-133a in the low BMD group in both the array and the qRT-PCR analyses.

Human mature miR-133a is encoded by two genes: MIR133A1 for miR-133a1 at 18q11.2 (194,036,59–194,077,46 bp) and MIR133A2 for miR-133a2 at 20q13.33 (611,601,19–611,642,20 bp). Both genes encode different pre-mature miRNAs but generate the same mature miR-133a sequence. Interestingly, human genetic studies also found the association of 18q11.2 to osteoporosis-related traits [35] and linkage of 20q13 to bone phenotypes [36–38]. In humans, there are two types of miR-133 miRNA isoforms, miR-133a and miR-133b, with one base difference (g-a) in the last nucleotide at the 3′ end (miRBase: http://www.mirbase.org/). The ABI miRNA array used in this study includes both miR-133a and miR-133b probes. Interestingly, miR-133b is marginally unregulated in the low vs. the high BMD groups (1.51 ± 0.67 vs. 0.95 ± 0.63, $P=0.08$). In addition, we detected miR-133a expression levels in circulating B cells from the same 20 high or low BMD postmenopausal women. Circulating B cells were isolated by Dynabeads® CD19 (Pan B) (Dynal Biotech). However, miR-133a was not differentially expressed in B cells between the high and the low BMD groups ($P=0.49$). Therefore, miR-133a is most likely to be a monocyte specific biomarker underlying postmenopausal osteoporosis.

Many studies demonstrated that miR-133 and 133a are important in the development of muscle, such as skeletal muscle [39–43], and heart/cardiovascular muscle [44–47]. In bone, particularly, miR-133 and 133a have been found to regulate osteoblastogenesis by targeting and regulating Runx2 expression [6,48]. A recent study also demonstrated that miR-133a was upregulated in osteoblast-like periodontal ligament stem cells treated with ibandronate, a nitrogen-containing bisphosphonate that inhibits bone resorption and is widely used to treat osteoporosis [49]. However, our study for the first time showed the association of miR-133a expression levels in circulating monocytes, the osteoclast precursors, with postmenopausal osteoporosis.

To further predict what genes are targeted and regulated by miR-133a in monocytes in bone metabolism, we used two miRNA target gene predicting databases (miRDB and TargetScan) [50–55]. Our bioinformatic sequence analyses and reference searching identified three potential target genes of miR-133a related to the inhibition of osteoclastogenesis, which are CXCL11, CXCR3, and SLC39A1 (Table 2). CXCL11 is a small cytokine of the CXC chemokine family. CXCL11 has been shown to inhibit osteoclast differentiation of CD14+ monocytes [56]. CXCR3 is a $G\alpha_i$ protein-coupled receptor in the CXC chemokine receptor family. CXCR3 expression significantly decreased during osteoclast differentiation [57]. The SLC39A1 gene encodes zinc transporter 1 (ZIP1). Zinc deficiency has been correlated with reduction of bone growth and development of osteoporosis [58,59]. SLC39A1 has been detected in osteoclasts and inhibited osteoclastogenesis and osteoclast function through zinc uptake [60].

All three genes did show negative correlation with miR-133a, though not significant (Table 3). Since one single miRNA normally regulates the expression of hundreds of genes, the regulatory effect of each gene may be small. Osteoporosis is a complex disease and regulated by multiple genes [61]. To investigate the combined effects, we also utilized a principle component analysis (PCA) to analyze the qRT-PCR observations from all three potential target genes. The PCA was performed using the correlation matrix. The analysis reduced the original data into two principle components (PC) that account for 58.17% and 32.78% of the total variance, respectively. A plot of the second PC against the first PC in the 10 high and 10 low BMD subjects is shown in Figure 3. We can see that both PCs are above the average levels in 6 out of 10 high BMD subjects and below the average levels in 7 out of 10 low BMD subjects, which means that the three genes are systematically upregulated in the high vs. low BMD groups. This result is

Table 3. Correlation of expression levels ($2^{-\Delta\Delta CT}$) of miR-133a with those of three potential target genes and the ratio of expression levels of each gene in the high and low BMD groups, as measured by qRT-PCR.

Gene	Fold Change (H/L)	Correlation Coefficient	P Value
CXCL11	2.70	−0.04	0.88
CXCR3	3.02	−0.22	0.36
SLC39A1	1.33	−0.02	0.94

Note: H/L: high/low BMD groups.

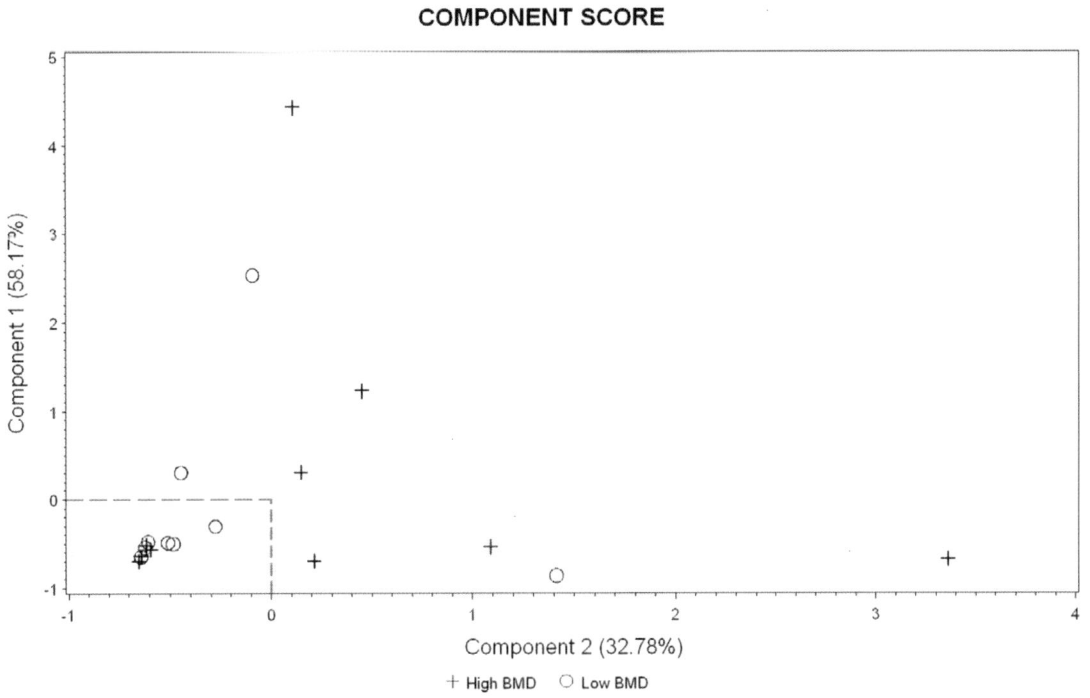

Figure 3. PCA of the expression levels of the three potential target genes measured by qRT-PCR in the 10 high and 10 low BMD subjects. In each axis, "0" represents the average level of each principle component.

consistently correlated with the downregulation of miR-133a in the high vs. low BMD groups.

There are some limitations for this study. In the miRNA array data, we performed the statistical tests for the 156 miRNAs according to expression data available in at least five samples in each group, and used raw *P* values but not adjusted *P* values for multiple tests. Actually, we did not find significant miRNAs after multiple testing adjustments by Bonferroni. However, the significant qRT-PCR *P* value confirmed the differential expression of miR-133a in the array analyses. The qRT-PCR validation largely solved the multiple testing problem. The sample size of 20 is relatively small. However, it is enough for an initial biomarker screening according to our previous [29,62] and other [63,64] gene expression profiling studies. Moreover, we are also planning to validate the miR-133a biomarker in a larger independent population. We did not find significant correlations of miR-133a and selected potential target genes. First, it may be due to the limited sample size to get enough power to detect the significant correlation. Second, many miRNAs inhibit gene expression by only suppressing protein translation instead of mRNA degradation [32,33]. Third, there may be other unknown target genes of miR-133a in circulating monocytes that affect osteoclastogenesis. Therefore, we will test the current and potential novel target gene expression and correlation with miR-133a in a bigger population at both mRNA and protein levels in the future.

In summary, this is an initial miRNA expression study to indentify miRNA biomarkers in human circulating monocytes underlying postmenopausal osteoporosis. Our study suggested that miR-133a is a potential miRNA biomarker and/or regulatory element in circulating monocytes for postmenopausal osteoporosis.

Supporting Information

Table S1 MiRNA array results of 156 miRNAs that were expressed in at least 5 samples in each BMD group. *: the ratio of the mean expression values between the low and high BMD groups.

Acknowledgments

We thank Dr. Xiang-Ding Chen for his help with the miRNA array experiments.

Author Contributions

Conceived and designed the experiments: YW LL BTM XHP XF JML RRR PX. Performed the experiments: YW LL BTM XHP PX. Analyzed the data: YW LL BTM XF PX. Contributed reagents/materials/analysis tools: PX. Wrote the paper: YW LL BTM XHP XF JML RRR PX.

References

1. Li Y, Vandenboom TG, Wang Z, Kong D, Ali S, et al. (2010) miR-146a suppresses invasion of pancreatic cancer cells. Cancer Res 70: 1486–1495.
2. Ma L, Teruya-Feldstein J, Weinberg RA (2007) Tumour invasion and metastasis initiated by microRNA-10b in breast cancer. Nature 449: 682–688.
3. Balasubramanyam M, Aravind S, Gokulakrishnan K, Prabu P, Sathishkumar C, et al. (2011) Impaired miR-146a expression links subclinical inflammation and insulin resistance in Type 2 diabetes. Mol Cell Biochem 351: 197–205.
4. Poy MN, Eliasson L, Krutzfeldt J, Kuwajima S, Ma X, et al. (2004) A pancreatic islet-specific microRNA regulates insulin secretion. Nature 432: 226–230.
5. Thum T, Gross C, Fiedler J, Fischer T, Kissler S, et al. (2008) MicroRNA-21 contributes to myocardial disease by stimulating MAP kinase signalling in fibroblasts. Nature 456: 980–984.
6. Li Z, Hassan MQ, Volinia S, van Wijnen AJ, Stein JL, et al. (2008) A microRNA signature for a BMP2-induced osteoblast lineage commitment program. Proc Natl Acad Sci U S A 105: 13906–13911.
7. Eskildsen T, Taipaleenmaki H, Stenvang J, Abdallah BM, Ditzel N, et al. (2011) MicroRNA-138 regulates osteogenic differentiation of human stromal (mesenchymal) stem cells in vivo. Proc Natl Acad Sci U S A 108: 6139–6144.

8. Zhang J, Tu Q, Bonewald LF, He X, Stein G, et al. (2011) Effects of miR-335-5p in modulating osteogenic differentiation by specifically downregulating Wnt antagonist DKK1. J Bone Miner Res 26: 1953–1963.
9. Hassan MQ, Gordon JA, Beloti MM, Croce CM, van Wijnen AJ, et al. (2010) A network connecting Runx2, SATB2, and the miR-23a~27a~24-2 cluster regulates the osteoblast differentiation program. Proc Natl Acad Sci U S A 107: 19879–19884.
10. Kapinas K, Kessler C, Ricks T, Gronowicz G, Delany AM (2010) miR-29 modulates Wnt signaling in human osteoblasts through a positive feedback loop. J Biol Chem 285: 25221–25231.
11. Huang J, Zhao L, Xing L, Chen D (2010) MicroRNA-204 regulates Runx2 protein expression and mesenchymal progenitor cell differentiation. Stem Cells 28: 357–364.
12. Mizuno Y, Yagi K, Tokuzawa Y, Kanesaki-Yatsuka Y, Suda T, et al. (2008) miR-125b inhibits osteoblastic differentiation by down-regulation of cell proliferation. Biochem Biophys Res Commun 368: 267–272.
13. Luzi E, Marini F, Sala SC, Tognarini I, Galli G, et al. (2008) Osteogenic differentiation of human adipose tissue-derived stem cells is modulated by the miR-26a targeting of the SMAD1 transcription factor. J Bone Miner Res 23: 287–295.
14. Inose H, Ochi H, Kimura A, Fujita K, Xu R, et al. (2009) A microRNA regulatory mechanism of osteoblast differentiation. Proc Natl Acad Sci U S A 106: 20794–20799.
15. Kim YJ, Bae SW, Yu SS, Bae YC, Jung JS (2009) miR-196a regulates proliferation and osteogenic differentiation in mesenchymal stem cells derived from human adipose tissue. J Bone Miner Res 24: 816–825.
16. Li H, Xie H, Liu W, Hu R, Huang B, et al. (2009) A novel microRNA targeting HDAC5 regulates osteoblast differentiation in mice and contributes to primary osteoporosis in humans. J Clin Invest 119: 3666–3677.
17. Nakasa T, Shibuya H, Nagata Y, Niimoto T, Ochi M (2011) The inhibitory effect of microRNA-146a expression on bone destruction in collagen-induced arthritis. Arthritis Rheum 63: 1582–1590.
18. Sugatani T, Hruska KA (2007) MicroRNA-223 is a key factor in osteoclast differentiation. J Cell Biochem 101: 996–999.
19. Fujikawa Y, Quinn JM, Sabokbar A, McGee JO, Athanasou NA (1996) The human osteoclast precursor circulates in the monocyte fraction. Endocrinology 137: 4058–4060.
20. Higuchi S, Tabata N, Tajima M, Ito M, Tsurudome M, et al. (1998) Induction of human osteoclast-like cells by treatment of blood monocytes with anti-fusion regulatory protein-1/CD98 monoclonal antibodies. J Bone Miner Res 13: 44–49.
21. Matayoshi A, Brown C, DiPersio JF, Haug J, Abu-Amer Y, et al. (1996) Human blood-mobilized hematopoietic precursors differentiate into osteoclasts in the absence of stromal cells. Proc Natl Acad Sci U S A 93: 10785–10790.
22. Purton LE, Lee MY, Torok-Storb B (1996) Normal human peripheral blood mononuclear cells mobilized with granulocyte colony-stimulating factor have increased osteoclastogenic potential compared to nonmobilized blood. Blood 87: 1802–1808.
23. Cohen-Solal ME, Graulet AM, Denne MA, Gueris J, Baylink D, et al. (1993) Peripheral monocyte culture supernatants of menopausal women can induce bone resorption: involvement of cytokines. J Clin Endocrinol Metab 77: 1648–1653.
24. Cohen-Solal ME, Boitte F, Bernard-Poenaru O, Denne MA, Graulet AM, et al. (1998) Increased bone resorbing activity of peripheral monocyte culture supernatants in elderly women. J Clin Endocrinol Metab 83: 1687–1690.
25. Pacifici R (1996) Estrogen, cytokines, and pathogenesis of postmenopausal osteoporosis. J Bone Miner Res 11: 1043–1051.
26. Deng FY, Lei SF, Zhang Y, Zhang YL, Zheng YP, et al. (2011) Peripheral blood monocyte-expressed ANXA2 gene is involved in pathogenesis of osteoporosis in humans. Mol Cell Proteomics 10: M111.
27. Chen XD, Xiao P, Lei SF, Liu YZ, Guo YF, et al. (2010) Gene expression profiling in monocytes and SNP association suggest the importance of the STAT1 gene for osteoporosis in both Chinese and Caucasians. J Bone Miner Res 25: 339–355.
28. Liu YZ, Dvornyk V, Lu Y, Shen H, Lappe JM, et al. (2005) A novel pathophysiological mechanism for osteoporosis suggested by an in vivo gene expression study of circulating monocytes. J Biol Chem 280: 29011–29016.
29. Xiao P, Chen Y, Jiang H, Liu YZ, Pan F, et al. (2008) In vivo genome-wide expression study on human circulating B cells suggests a novel ESR1 and MAPK3 network for postmenopausal osteoporosis. J Bone Miner Res 23: 644–654.
30. Zerbini CA, Latorre MR, Jaime PC, Tanaka T, Pippa MG (2000) Bone mineral density in Brazilian men 50 years and older. Braz J Med Biol Res 33: 1429–1435.
31. Rajewsky N (2006) microRNA target predictions in animals. Nat Genet 38 Suppl: S8–13.
32. He L, Hannon GJ (2004) MicroRNAs: small RNAs with a big role in gene regulation. Nat Rev Genet 5: 522–531.
33. Bartel DP (2004) MicroRNAs: genomics, biogenesis, mechanism, and function. Cell 116: 281–297.
34. Grimson A, Farh KK, Johnston WK, Garrett-Engele P, Lim LP, et al. (2007) MicroRNA targeting specificity in mammals: determinants beyond seed pairing. Mol Cell 27: 91–105.
35. Hsu YH, Zillikens MC, Wilson SG, Farber CR, Demissie S, et al. (2010) An integration of genome-wide association study and gene expression profiling to prioritize the discovery of novel susceptibility Loci for osteoporosis-related traits. PLoS Genet 6: e1000977.
36. Ralston SH, Galwey N, MacKay I, Albagha OM, Cardon L, et al. (2005) Loci for regulation of bone mineral density in men and women identified by genome wide linkage scan: the FAMOS study. Hum Mol Genet 14: 943–951.
37. Deng FY, Xiao P, Lei SF, Zhang L, Yang F, et al. (2007) Bivariate whole genome linkage analysis for femoral neck geometric parameters and total body lean mass. J Bone Miner Res 22: 808–816.
38. Mitchell BD, Cole SA, Bauer RL, Iturria SJ, Rodriguez EA, et al. (2000) Genes influencing variation in serum osteocalcin concentrations are linked to markers on chromosomes 16q and 20q. J Clin Endocrinol Metab 85: 1362–1366.
39. Deng Z, Chen JF, Wang DZ (2011) Transgenic overexpression of miR-133a in skeletal muscle. BMC Musculoskelet Disord 12: 115.
40. McCarthy JJ, Esser KA (2007) MicroRNA-1 and microRNA-133a expression are decreased during skeletal muscle hypertrophy. J Appl Physiol 102: 306–313.
41. Rao PK, Kumar RM, Farkhondeh M, Baskerville S, Lodish HF (2006) Myogenic factors that regulate expression of muscle-specific microRNAs. Proc Natl Acad Sci U S A 103: 8721–8726.
42. Huang MB, Xu H, Xie SJ, Zhou H, Qu LH (2011) Insulin-like growth factor-1 receptor is regulated by microRNA-133 during skeletal myogenesis. PLoS One 6: e29173.
43. Chen JF, Mandel EM, Thomson JM, Wu Q, Callis TE, et al. (2006) The role of microRNA-1 and microRNA-133 in skeletal muscle proliferation and differentiation. Nat Genet 38: 228–233.
44. Bostjancic E, Zidar N, Stajer D, Glavac D (2010) MicroRNAs miR-1, miR-133a, miR-133b and miR-208 are dysregulated in human myocardial infarction. Cardiology 115: 163–169.
45. Villar AV, Merino D, Wenner M, Llano M, Cobo M, et al. (2011) Myocardial gene expression of microRNA-133a and myosin heavy and light chains, in conjunction with clinical parameters, predict regression of left ventricular hypertrophy after valve replacement in patients with aortic stenosis. Heart 97: 1132–1137.
46. Torella D, Iaconetti C, Catalucci D, Ellison GM, Leone A, et al. (2011) MicroRNA-133 controls vascular smooth muscle cell phenotypic switch in vitro and vascular remodeling in vivo. Circ Res 109: 880–893.
47. Liu N, Williams AH, Kim Y, McAnally J, Bezprozvannaya S, et al. (2007) An intragenic MEF2-dependent enhancer directs muscle-specific expression of microRNAs 1 and 133. Proc Natl Acad Sci U S A 104: 20844–20849.
48. Zhang Y, Xie RL, Croce CM, Stein JL, Lian JB, et al. (2011) A program of microRNAs controls osteogenic lineage progression by targeting transcription factor Runx2. Proc Natl Acad Sci U S A 108: 9863–9868.
49. Zhou Q, Zhao ZN, Cheng JT, Zhang B, Xu J, et al. (2011) Ibandronate promotes osteogenic differentiation of periodontal ligament stem cells by regulating the expression of microRNAs. Biochem Biophys Res Commun 404: 127–132.
50. Wang X (2008) miRDB: a microRNA target prediction and functional annotation database with a wiki interface. RNA 14: 1012–1017.
51. Wang X, El Naqa IM (2008) Prediction of both conserved and nonconserved microRNA targets in animals. Bioinformatics 24: 325–332.
52. Lewis BP, Burge CB, Bartel DP (2005) Conserved seed pairing, often flanked by adenosines, indicates that thousands of human genes are microRNA targets. Cell 120: 15–20.
53. Grimson A, Farh KK, Johnston WK, Garrett-Engele P, Lim LP, et al. (2007) MicroRNA targeting specificity in mammals: determinants beyond seed pairing. Mol Cell 27: 91–105.
54. Garcia DM, Baek D, Shin C, Bell GW, Grimson A, et al. (2011) Weak seed-pairing stability and high target-site abundance decrease the proficiency of lsy-6 and other microRNAs. Nat Struct Mol Biol 18: 1139–1146.
55. Friedman RC, Farh KK, Burge CB, Bartel DP (2009) Most mammalian mRNAs are conserved targets of microRNAs. Genome Res 19: 92–105.
56. Coelho LF, Magno de Freitas AG, Mennechet FJ, Blangy A, Uze G (2005) Interferon-alpha and -beta differentially regulate osteoclastogenesis: role of differential induction of chemokine CXCL11 expression. Proc Natl Acad Sci U S A 102: 11917–11922.
57. Grassi F, Piacentini A, Cristino S, Toneguzzi S, Cavallo C, et al. (2003) Human osteoclasts express different CXC chemokines depending on cell culture substrate: molecular and immunocytochemical evidence of high levels of CXCL10 and CXCL12. Histochem Cell Biol 120: 391–400.
58. Eberle J, Schmidmayer S, Erben RG, Stangassinger M, Roth HP (1999) Skeletal effects of zinc deficiency in growing rats. J Trace Elem Med Biol 13: 21–26.
59. Nishi Y (1996) Zinc and growth. J Am Coll Nutr 15: 340–344.
60. Khadeer MA, Sahu SN, Bai G, Abdulla S, Gupta A (2005) Expression of the zinc transporter ZIP1 in osteoclasts. Bone 37: 296–304.
61. Liu YJ, Shen H, Xiao P, Xiong DH, Li LH, et al. (2006) Molecular genetic studies of gene identification for osteoporosis: a 2004 update. J Bone Miner Res 21: 1511–1535.
62. Chen XD, Xiao P, Lei SF, Liu YZ, Guo YF, et al. (2010) Gene expression profiling in monocytes and SNP association suggest the importance of the STAT1 gene for osteoporosis in both Chinese and Caucasians. J Bone Miner Res 25: 339–355.

63. Atzmon G, Yang XM, Muzumdar R, Ma XH, Gabriely I, et al. (2002) Differential gene expression between visceral and subcutaneous fat depots. Horm Metab Res 34: 622–628.

64. Linder K, Arner P, Flores-Morales A, Tollet-Egnell P, Norstedt G (2004) Differentially expressed genes in visceral or subcutaneous adipose tissue of obese men and women. J Lipid Res 45: 148–154.

5

High Serum Carotenoids Associated with Lower Risk for Bone Loss and Osteoporosis in Post-Menopausal Japanese Female Subjects: Prospective Cohort Study

Minoru Sugiura[1]*, Mieko Nakamura[2], Kazunori Ogawa[1], Yoshinori Ikoma[1], Masamichi Yano[1]

1 Citrus Research Division, National Institute of Fruit Tree Science, Shizuoka City, Shizuoka, Japan, 2 Department of Community Health and Preventive Medicine, Hamamatsu University School of Medicine, Hamamatsu City, Shizuoka, Japan

Abstract

Introduction: Recent epidemiological studies show that high intakes of carotenoids might be useful to maintain bone health, but little is known about the association of serum carotenoids with change of bone mineral density (BMD). The objective of this study was to investigate longitudinally whether serum carotenoids are associated with bone loss.

Methods: We conducted a follow-up on 146 male and 99 pre- and 212 post-menopausal female subjects from the Mikkabi study. Those who participated in previous BMD surveys and completed four years of follow-up were examined longitudinally.

Results: During a 4-year follow-up, 15 of the post-menopausal female subjects developed new-onset osteoporosis. In contrast, none of the male and pre-menopausal female subjects did. In male and pre-menopausal female subjects, the six serum carotenoids at the baseline were not associated with bone loss. On the other hand, in post-menopausal female subjects, the 4-year bone loss of radius was inversely associated with the serum carotenoid concentrations, especially in β-carotene. After adjustments for confounders, the odds ratios (OR) for osteoporosis in the highest tertiles of serum β-carotene and β-cryptoxanthin against the lowest tertiles were 0.24 (95% confidence interval 0.05–1.21) and 0.07 (CI: 0.01–0.88), respectively. Serum β-cryptoxanthin was also inversely associated with the risk for osteopenia and/or osteoporosis (*P* for trend, 0.037). In addition, our retrospective analysis revealed that subjects who developed osteoporosis and/or osteopenia during the survey period had significantly lower serum concentrations of β-cryptoxanthin and β-carotene at the baseline than those in the normal group.

Conclusions: Antioxidant carotenoids, especially β-cryptoxanthin and β-carotene, are inversely associated with the change of radial BMD in post-menopausal female subjects.

Editor: Brenda Smith, Oklahoma State University, United States of America

Funding: This work was supported by a grant from the Ministry of Agriculture, Forestry, and Fisheries (MAFF) for a food research project titled "Integrated Research on Safety and Physiological Function of Food" and a grant from the Council for advancement of Fruit Tree Science. The funders had a role in data collection and analysis.

Competing Interests: The authors have declared that no competing interests exist.

* E-mail: msugiura@affrc.go.jp

Introduction

Osteoporosis and related fractures are a major public health problem [1]. Osteoporosis is a chronic disease characterized by low bone density and microarchitectural disruption, leading to bone fragility and an increased susceptibility to fractures [2]. Nutrition is an important modifiable factor in the development and maintenance of bone health, and numerous studies on nutrition and bone health have been conducted [3,4]. With regard to nutritional approaches to bone metabolism, calcium and vitamin D have been identified as important nutritional factors to maintain normal bone metabolism. Other nutrients, such as potassium, magnesium, zinc, copper, iron, vitamin C, and vitamin K, may also have beneficial effects. Fruit and vegetables are rich sources of these nutrients for bone metabolism. Therefore, the intake of these types of food might affect bone health. In fact, recent epidemiological studies have shown an association between fruit and vegetable intakes with the bone mineral density (BMD) in both young and elderly subjects [5,6,7,8,9,10].

On the other hand, fruits and vegetables are also rich sources of antioxidant carotenoids, which have been shown to contribute to the body's defense against reactive oxygen species [11,12]. Recent animal experiments and *in vitro* studies have shown that reactive oxygen species and free radicals are involved in osteoclastogenesis, in apoptosis of osteoblasts and osteocytes, and, therefore, in bone resorption [13,14,15]. Furthermore, recent epidemiological studies have shown a relationship between oxidative stress and BMD or osteoporosis [16,17,18]. These previous findings in epidemiological and experimental studies suggest that antioxidant carotenoids may provide benefits to bone metabolism against oxidative stress. In fact, several recent epidemiological reports have shown inverse associations of antioxidant micronutrient intake or serum level with low BMD, risk of fracture, and/or risk of osteoporosis [19,20,21,22,23,24,25]. However, to the best of our knowledge, a thorough longitudinal cohort study about the association of serum carotenoid levels with the change of BMD and/or incidence of osteoporosis has not been conducted.

Previously, we found that the serum concentrations of β-cryptoxanthin and β-carotene were weakly but positively associated with the radial BMD in post-menopausal female subjects [26,27]. These associations suggest that β-cryptoxanthin and β carotene might provide benefits to bone health in post-menopausal women. However, this data consisted of cross-sectional analyses. Therefore, only limited inferences can be made regarding temporality and causation. To determine whether antioxidant carotenoids are beneficial micronutrients on bone health, further cohort study will be required.

The objective of this study was to investigate longitudinally whether the change of BMD and/or the risk of development of osteoporosis is associated with serum carotenoid concentrations. The associations of six serum carotenoid concentrations, i.e., lutein, lycopene, α-carotene, β-carotene, β-cryptoxanthin, and zeaxanthin, with BMD were evaluated longitudinally.

Materials and Methods

Ethics Statement

This study was carried out in accordance with the Declaration of Helsinki and approved by the ethics committee of the National Institute of Fruit Tree Science. We obtained written informed consent from all participants involved in our study.

Study Population

This was a prospective survey involving participants in the Mikkabi cohort study conducted in the town of Mikkabi, Shizuoka Prefecture, Japan. In a baseline survey, study subjects were recruited from participants in an annual health check-up program conducted by the local government of Mikkabi in April 2005 [26]. Mikkabi is located in western Shizuoka, and about 40% of its residents work in agriculture. Fruit trees are the key industry in Mikkabi, which is an important producer of mandarin oranges in Japan. A total of 1,891 males and females were subjects for the annual health check-up program in 2005. As a result, 1,369 males and females (72.4% of total subjects), ranging in age from 30 to 70 years, had received the health check-up program. Study participants were recruited from baseline surveys, and written informed consent was obtained from 699 subjects (222 males and 477 females). The response rate was 51.1%. After four years of a baseline survey, subjects were invited to participate in a follow-up survey in April 2009. As a result, 457 subjects (146 males and 311 females) took part in the follow-up survey. The follow-up rate was 65.4%.

For the baseline survey, participants completed a self-administered questionnaire about a subject's history of osteoporosis, hormone use, and lifestyle, including tobacco use (current smoker, ex-smoker, or non-smoker), exercise (1+ times weekly), regular alcohol intake (1+ times weekly), dietary supplement use (non-user, occasional user, current user), and dietary habits. Diet was assessed with a modified validated simple food-frequency questionnaire (FFQ) developed especially for the Japanese [28,29]. Information about alcohol consumption and the daily intake of 18 nutrients was estimated from the monthly food intake frequencies with either standard portion size (for most types of food) or subject-specified typical portion size (for rice, bread, and alcoholic and non-alcoholic beverages) using the FFQ analysis software package for Windows (Food Frequency Questionnaire System, System Supply Co., Ltd., Kanagawa, Japan). This FFQ analysis software computes individual food and nutrient intake form FFQ data based on standard tables for food composition in Japan [30,31]. The intakes of total energy, calcium, potassium, magnesium, and vitamins C, D, and E of each subject were used in this report.

The concentrations of six serum carotenoids at the baseline survey, lutein, lycopene, α-carotene, β-carotene, β-cryptoxanthin, and zeaxanthin, were analyzed by reverse-phase high-performance liquid chromatography (HPLC) using β-apo-8′-carotenal as an internal standard at the Laboratory of Public Health and Environmental Chemistry, Kyoto Biseibutsu Kenkyusho (Kyoto, Japan), as described previously [32].

The radial BMD at the baseline and follow-up survey was measured using dual-energy X-ray absorptiometry (DXA) of each participant's nondominant forearm with an osteometer (model DCS-600EX-III, ALOKA Co., Ltd., Tokyo, Japan), as described previously [26]. The measurement of the radial BMD of each participant was performed by a well-trained clinical technologist of the Seirei Preventive Health Care Center (Shizuoka, Japan).

Statistical Analysis

All subjects were categorized into three groups stratified by sex and menopausal status at the baseline survey. Serum carotenoid concentrations and intakes of vitamins C, D, and E were skewed toward the higher concentrations. These values were $\log_e$ (natural)-transformed to improve the normality of their distribution. The paired *t*-test was used to test differences among the baseline and follow-up survey. All variables were presented as an original scale. The data are expressed as the means (standard deviation), geometric mean (95% confidence interval), range, or percent.

The multivariate adjusted mean of the 4-year change of the radial BMD by the tertiles of the serum carotenoid concentrations at the baseline survey was calculated after adjusting for age, weight, height, years since menopause, current tobacco use, regular alcohol intake, exercise habits, supplement use, and total energy intake at the baseline using the general linear model procedure. Differences in the multivariate adjusted mean of the change of the radial BMD among each tertile of serum carotenoid concentration at the baseline were tested by Bonferroni multiple comparison. In the test for linear trends, the associations among the change of the radial BMD across three categories assigned by means of the serum carotenoid concentrations in each tertile were carried out by linear regression.

Osteoporosis was defined as a person whose T-score (which shows how a subject's BMD compares with young adult mean) is less than 70% according to the guidelines on the management of osteoporosis by the Japan Osteoporosis Society [33]. A person whose T-score exceeds 70% and is less than 80% is defined as having osteopenia. To assess the relationship between the serum carotenoid concentrations at the baseline and the development of osteopenia and osteoporosis after four years, logistic regression analyses were performed after adjusting for age, weight, height, years since menopause, current tobacco use, regular alcohol intake, exercise habits, supplement use, and total energy intake at the baseline. Multivariable adjustment for the intakes of calcium, magnesium, potassium, and vitamins D, C, and E was further conducted as sensitivity analysis. In data analyses of the relationship between the serum carotenoid concentrations at the baseline and the development of osteoporosis, we used the data from 187 post-menopausal female subjects whose T-score at the baseline survey exceeded 70%. In a similar way, we analyzed the relationship between the serum carotenoid concentrations at the baseline and the development of osteopenia and/or osteoporosis using the data from 140 post-menopausal female subjects whose T-score at the baseline survey exceeded 80%. In the test for linear trends, the associations among the risk of osteoporosis and/or osteopenia across three categories assigned by means of the serum carotenoid concentrations in each tertile were carried out by logistic regression analysis.

We did not adjust each carotenoid concentration in the multivariate models because Pearson's correlation analyses of serum carotenoid concentrations revealed significant positive correlations among all combinations of the six carotenoids. All statistical analyses were performed using statistical software package for Windows (SPSS ver. 12.0J, SPSS Inc., Chicago, IL, USA) on personal computers.

Results

Baseline Characteristics and Radial BMD Status at the Baseline and Follow-up Survey in Study Subjects

Table 1 shows the characteristics of the study subjects at the baseline survey stratified by sex and menopausal status at the baseline. Among pre-menopausal female subjects at the baseline survey, 35 subjects had reached menopause.

Table 2 shows the radial BMD at the baseline survey and follow-up surveys stratified by sex and menopausal status at the baseline. The radial BMD at the follow-up survey in male and pre- and post-menopausal female subjects was significantly lower than that in each group at the baseline survey. Osteopenia, as newly diagnosed for male and pre-menopausal female subjects in our study, was identified in only two males and one female. None of the males or pre-menopausal females developed osteoporosis. On the other hand, in post-menopausal female subjects, two subjects in the normal group at the baseline and fifteen subjects in the osteopenia group at the baseline developed osteoporosis after four years. Furthermore, twenty-five subjects in the normal group at the baseline developed osteopenia. In our survey, two subjects identified as having osteoporosis at the baseline were identified as having osteopenia during the follow-up survey. Three subjects with osteopenia were diagnosed as normal during the follow-up survey. The radial BMD in these five subjects seemed to increase over the four-year follow-up.

In our follow-up survey, the baseline radial BMD in male and pre-menopausal female subjects was no different among fallout and follow-up subjects (data not shown). On the other hand, in post-menopausal female subjects, the mean of the baseline radial BMD in fallout subjects was significantly higher than that in subjects who participated in the follow-up survey ($P = 0.019$).

Table 1. Caracteristics of the study subject at baseline survey[a].

	Male		Pre-menopausal female		Post-menopausal female	
N	146		99		212	
Age (y)	57.1	(8.9)	44.8	(5.3)	60.5	(5.8)
Body height (cm)	165.8	(6.5)	155.4	(4.9)	151.9	(5.7)
Body weight (kg)	64.9	(8.7)	54.9	(9.7)	50.9	(7.4)
Body mass index (kg/m^2)	23.6	(2.7)	22.7	(3.9)	22.0	(2.8)
Total energy intake (kcal/day)						
Including ethanol	2157.4	(473.8)	1913.7	(437.5)	1940.5	(443.2)
Excluding ethanol	2017.7	(452.2)	1898.2	(441.6)	1928.0	(443.1)
Calcium intake (mg/day)	521.3	(219.3)	584.6	(190.8)	642.1	(232.2)
Potassium intake (mg/day)	2481.0	(824.5)	2512.2	(774.2)	2871.1	(860.7)
Magnesium intake (mg/day)	270.3	(72.5)	244.5	(66.1)	278.4	(72.6)
Vitamin C intake (mg/day)[b]	126.3	(115.3–138.4)	115.4	(104.7–127.2)	170.6	(161.0–180.8)
Vitamin D intake (μg/day)[b]	4.9	(4.4–5.5)	5.1	(4.5–5.7)	6.3	(5.8–6.8)
Vitamin E intake (mg/day)[b]	7.4	(7.0–7.9)	7.6	(7.2–8.1)	8.0	(7.7–8.3)
Serum carotenoid concentrations (μmol/L)[b]						
Lutein	0.45	(0.43–0.47)	0.47	(0.44–0.50)	0.56	(0.53–0.58)
Lycopene	0.31	(0.28–0.33)	0.46	(0.42–0.50)	0.38	(0.35–0.40)
α-Carotene	0.13	(0.12–0.14)	0.20	(0.18–0.22)	0.22	(0.20–0.24)
β-Carotene	0.58	(0.53–0.65)	0.90	(0.81–1.01)	1.16	(1.09–1.24)
β-Cryptoxanthn	1.26	(1.09–1.45)	1.05	(0.91–1.22)	1.80	(1.64–1.98)
Zeaxanthin	0.19	(0.18–0.20)	0.20	(0.19–0.21)	0.21	(0.20–0.21)
Current tobacco use (%)	25.3		2.0		1.9	
Exercise habits (%)[c]	21.2		14.1		17.9	
Regular alcohol intake (%)[c]	58.9		16.2		13.2	
Current supplement use (%)	3.4		14.1		9.0	

[a]Data are mean (standard deviation), geometric mean (95% confidence interval), range, or percent.
[b]These variables were represented as original scale after analysis by log (natural) transformed values.
[c]>=1 times/wk.

Table 2. Bone mineral density and T-score at baseline and follow-up survey[a].

	Male		Pre-menopausal female[b]		Post-menopausal female	
n	146		99		212	
Baseline survey in 2005						
Bone mineral density (g/cm^2)	0.770	(0.064)	0.680	(0.056)	0.554	(0.085)
Range		0.593–0.906		0.521–0.817		0.380–0.820
T-Score (%)	99.8	(8.2)	105.2	(8.7)	85.8	(13.2)
Normal [n, (%)]	144	(98.6)	99	(100.0)	140	(66.0)
Osteopenia [n, (%)]	2	(1.4)	0	(0.0)	47	(22.2)
Osteoporosis [n, (%)]	0	(0.0)	0	(0.0)	25	(11.8)
Follow-up survey in 2009						
Bone mineral density (g/cm^2)	0.765	(0.069)[c]	0.669	(0.062)[c]	0.527	(0.084)[c]
Range		0.565–0.913		0.482–0.803		0.330–0.725
T-Score (%)	99.1	(8.8)[c]	103.6	(9.6)[c]	81.7	(13.0)[c]
Normal [n, (%)]	142	(97.3)	98	(99.0)	116	(54.7)
Osteopenia [n, (%)]	4	(2.7)	1	(1.0)	56	(26.4)
Osteoporosis [n, (%)]	0	(0.0)	0	(0.0)	40	(18.9)

[a]Data are mean (standard deviation), range, or percent.
[b]Newly thirty five female subjects reached menopause four years later.
[c]$P<0.001$ vs baseline by paired *t*-test.

Multivariate Adjusted Means of the Change of Radial BMD for Four Years by Stratified Tertiles of each Serum Carotenoid Concentration

Figure 1 shows the multivariate-adjusted means of the change of the radial BMD for four years by the tertiles of the baseline serum carotenoid concentrations among post-menopausal female subjects. The change of the radial BMD in the highest tertile of serum β-carotene was significantly lower than that in the lowest one. This significant difference was also observed after further adjusting for intakes of calcium, magnesium, potassium, and vitamins D, C, and E (P for linear tend: 0.002). In contrast, in male and pre-menopausal female subjects, no significant associations were observed in any of the six serum carotenoids (data not shown).

Although newly thirty-five female subjects reached menopause four years later, significant associations between the changes of the radial BMD and baseline serum carotenoid concentration were not observed in either pre-menopausal female subjects or newly post-menopausal female subjects who were pre-menopausal at the baseline (data not shown).

Risk of Osteoporosis According to Tertiles of Baseline Serum Carotenoid Concentrations

The odds ratios of osteoporosis associated with the tertiles of six serum carotenoid concentrations at the baseline survey after adjusting for confounding factors are shown in Table 3. After excluding subjects whose T-scores were under 70% at the baseline survey, the odds ratios of osteoporosis in the middle (T2) and highest (T3) groups against the lowest tertile (T1) used for the reference group were calculated. After adjusting for age, weight, height, years since menopause, current tobacco use, regular alcohol intake, exercise habits, supplement use, and total energy intake, a significant lower odds ratio for osteoporosis among post-menopausal female subjects was observed in the highest group (T3) of serum β-cryptoxanthin. This inverse association between baseline serum β-cryptoxanthin and the development of osteoporosis was also observed after further adjusting for the intakes of calcium, magnesium, potassium, and vitamins C, D, and E. On the other hand, significantly lower odds ratios were not observed in other carotenoids. In this study population, although four post-menopausal female subjects were currently using female hormones, such as estrogen, the associations of the radial BMD with serum carotenoid concentrations did not change after excluding these four subjects.

Risk of Osteopenia and/or Osteoporosis According to Tertiles of Baseline Serum Carotenoid Concentrations

The odds ratios of osteopenia and/or osteoporosis associated with the tertiles of six serum carotenoid concentrations at the baseline survey after adjusting for confounding factors are shown in Table 4. After excluding subjects whose T-scores were under 80% at the baseline survey, the odds ratios of osteopenia and/or osteoporosis in the middle (T2) and highest (T3) groups against the lowest tertile (T1) used for the reference group were calculated. After adjusting for age, weight, height, years since menopause, current tobacco use, regular alcohol intake, exercise habits, supplement use, and total energy intake, significant lower odds ratios for osteopenia and/or osteoporosis among post-menopausal female subjects were observed in the middle (T2) and highest group (T3) with high serum β-cryptoxanthin. These significant lower odds ratios were also observed after multivariate adjustment. On the other hand, significant lower risks for osteopenia and/or osteoporosis were not observed in other carotenoids.

Baseline Serum Carotenoid Concentrations among Continuously Normal Subjects, Newly Diagnosed Osteopenia, and Newly Diagnosed Osteoporosis

Table 5 shows the baseline serum carotenoid concentrations of post-menopausal female subjects stratified by continuously normal subjects, newly diagnosed osteopenia, and newly diagnosed osteoporosis defined by T-score levels at the follow-up survey. In our survey, in post-menopausal female subjects, newly seventeen subjects developed osteoporosis and newly twenty-five subjects

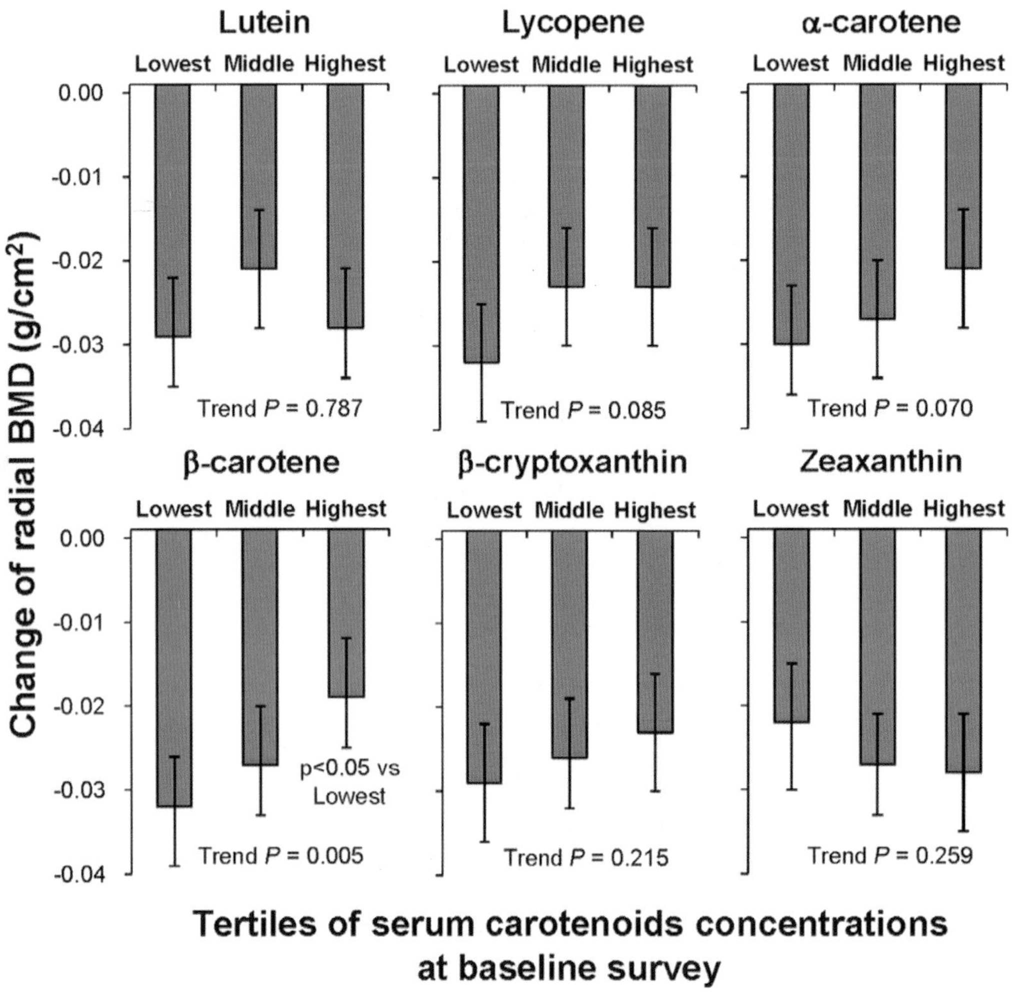

Figure 1. Change of radial bone mineral density by tertiles of serum carotenoids in post-menopausal female subjects. Multivariate-adjusted means of radial bone mineral density were calculated after adjusting for age, weight, height, years since menopause, current tobacco use, regular alcohol intake, exercise habits, supplement use, and total energy intake. *P*-values over the quartiles of serum carotenoids were assessed with a test for linear trends using linear regression.

developed osteopenia over the course of four years. A total of 113 subjects were diagnosed as continuously normal at the baseline and throughout the follow-up surveys. After multivariate adjustment, the baseline serum β-cryptoxanthin of subjects who were newly diagnosed osteoporosis was significantly lower than that of continuously normal subjects. Furthermore, the baseline serum β-carotene also tended to be low; however, it was not statistically significant.

Discussion

The objective of this study was to investigate longitudinally whether the change of BMD is associated with serum carotenoid concentration. The results indicated that higher serum β-carotene at the baseline in post-menopausal female subjects was significantly associated with less bone loss of the radius four years later. Furthermore, high serum β-cryptoxanthin was associated with a lower risk of osteoporosis and/or osteopenia. In addition, our retrospective analysis revealed that subjects who developed osteoporosis and/or osteopenia during the survey period had significantly lower serum concentrations of β-cryptoxanthin and β-carotene at the baseline compared to the continuously normal group. In other words, subjects who had had higher serum concentrations of β-cryptoxanthin and β-carotene at the baseline were less likely to develop osteoporosis and/or osteopenia in later years. Numerous antioxidant vitamins and carotenoids are contained in fruits and vegetables, and several recent epidemiological reports have shown inverse associations of antioxidant vitamin and carotenoid intake or serum level with low BMD, risk of fracture, and/or risk of osteoporosis [19,20,21,22,23,24,25]. Previously, we found that the serum concentrations of β-cryptoxanthin and β-carotene were weakly but positively associated with the radial BMD in post-menopausal female subjects from the cross-sectional analyses [26,27]. However, to the best of our knowledge, thorough longitudinal cohort studies about the association of bone loss with serum carotenoid concentration have not been conducted. This is the first longitudinal cohort study to examine the association of the serum carotenoid concentration with the change of BMD. Our findings further support the hypothesis that high intakes of fruit and vegetables rich in antioxidant carotenoids, especially β-cryptoxanthin and β-carotene, might provide benefits to bone health in post-menopausal female subjects.

Table 3. Odds ratios (and 95% confidence intervals) of tertiles of baseline serum carotenoid concentration on osteoporosis in post-menopausal Japanese female subjects.

Serum carotenoids		N	Mean and range of serum carotenoid (μmol/L)		Case	Model 1			Model 2		
						OR	95% CI	*P* for trend	OR	95% CI	*P* for trend
Lutein	Lowest (T1)	60	0.38	(0.23–0.47)	6	1.00			1.00		
	Middle (T2)	66	0.56	(0.49–0.63)	6	0.69	(0.19–2.51)		0.47	(0.10–2.13)	
	Highest (T3)	61	0.78	(0.65–2.11)	5	0.53	(0.14–2.05)	0.356	0.54	(0.11–2.60)	0.433
Lycopene	Lowest (T1)	59	0.23	(0.07–0.32)	7	1.00			1.00		
	Middle (T2)	61	0.38	(0.34–0.45)	4	0.71	(0.17–2.97)		0.57	(0.11–2.81)	
	Highest (T3)	67	0.62	(0.47–1.06)	6	0.91	(0.25–3.37)	0.890	0.58	(0.14–2.51)	0.481
α-Carotene	Lowest (T1)	67	0.13	(0.07–0.17)	7	1.00			1.00		
	Middle (T2)	56	0.21	(0.19–0.22)	5	0.80	(0.22–2.94)		0.64	(0.13–3.09)	
	Highest (T3)	64	0.38	(0.24–2.74)	5	0.76	(0.20–2.94)	0.694	0.71	(0.14–3.68)	0.733
β-Carotene	Lowest (T1)	61	0.69	(0.35–0.91)	9	1.00			1.00		
	Middle (T2)	64	1.17	(0.95–1.42)	4	0.32	(0.08–1.28)		0.26	(0.05–1.24)	
	Highest (T3)	62	1.91	(1.43–3.37)	4	0.30	(0.08–1.13)	0.071	0.24	(0.05–1.21)	0.082
β-Cryptoxanthin	Lowest (T1)	62	0.81	(0.24–1.41)	9	1.00			1.00		
	Middle (T2)	63	1.87	(1.43–2.39)	7	0.83	(0.24–2.90)		0.63	(0.16–2.42)	
	Highest (T3)	62	3.60	(2.41–10.53)	1	0.08	(0.01–0.75)	0.021	0.07	(0.01–0.88)	0.034
Zeaxanthin	Lowest (T1)	56	0.15	(0.09–0.18)	8	1.00			1.00		
	Middle (T2)	64	0.20	(0.19–0.21)	5	0.50	(0.14–1.84)		0.50	(0.12–2.04)	
	Highest (T3)	67	0.26	(0.23–0.37)	4	0.36	(0.09–1.38)	0.130	0.35	(0.08–1.52)	0.149

Model 1: Age, weight, height, years since menopause, current tobacco use, regular alcohol intake, exercise habits, supplement use, and total energy intake were adjusted.
Model 2: Intakes of calcium, magnesium, potassium, and vitamins D, C, and E were further adjusted.

Recent studies have also implicated the possible involvement of oxidative stress in BMD loss and increased risk of fractures. In fact, experimental evidence shows that smokers have increased risk of fractures [18,19], that osteoporosis patients have lower concentrations of serum vitamin C and vitamin E and exhibit elevated serum oxidative stress marker levels [16,17,19,20], and that NF-κB proteins that play an important role in bone resorption become activated when exposed to oxidative stress [34,35,36,37]. Although all types of carotenoids are known to have potent antioxidative properties, no association was found among carotenoids other than β-cryptoxanthin and β-carotene and BMD in our study. This finding suggests that mechanisms other than antioxidant activity might be involved in the effect of carotenoids on bone metabolism. Further research is needed.

Our observation is consistent with experimental results previously reported. Recently, Yamaguchi et al. reported the beneficial effects of β-cryptoxanthin on bone metabolism in *in vitro* and *in vivo* studies [38,39,40]. They found [38] that β-cryptoxanthin enhanced the calcium content and alkaline phosphatase activity in the femoral-diaphyseal and femoral-metaphyseal tissues of young rats at physiological low concentrations *in vitro*, while lycopene and lutein had no effects at the same dose. Furthermore, they found [39] a stimulatory effect on bone formation and an inhibitory effect on bone resorption in a tissue culture. In an *in vivo* study, they found [40] that the oral administration of β-cryptoxanthin caused a significant increase in the calcium content and alkaline phosphatase activity in the femoral-diaphyseal and femoral-metaphyseal tissues. These previous results support our findings that β-cryptoxanthin may have a direct stimulatory effect on bone formation and an inhibitory effect on bone resorption. The development of osteoporosis may be reduced by a dietary intake of β-cryptoxanthin.

Several epidemiological research teams are currently examining longitudinally the possible association of carotenoids with osteoporosis, changes in BMD, or risks of fractures. In the past, most epidemiological studies on the association between carotenoids and bone health have been carried out using either cross-sectional, case-control, and/or nested case-control designs to examine carotenoid intake and how it might affect BMD or bone health. A few studies assessing this association using the serum carotenoid levels were based on cross-sectional or case-control studies. According to these studies, lycopene, β-carotene, and β-cryptoxanthin have all been reported to be associated with bone health [21,22,23,24].

It is important to consider that dietary habits in populations vary across studies. Thus, studies conducted in Europe or the U.S., where lycopene intake is relatively high, tend to implicate lycopene as the type of carotenoid affecting bone metabolism. On the other hand, a few studies [22,23] targeting Italian and/or American populations have reported on the efficacy of β-cryptoxanthin. In recent years, the Framingham research group [24] published results from a longitudinal analysis of the association between carotenoid intake and BMD. This group analyzed the effects of carotenoid intake and associated changes in BMD over four years and concluded that a high intake of lycopene has inhibitory effects on BMD loss. Nonetheless, they found no association between β-cryptoxanthin and bone health.

Table 4. Odds ratios (and 95% confidence intervals) of tertiles of baseline serum carotenoid concentration on osteopenia and/or osteoprosis in post-menopausal Japanese female subjects.

Serum carotenoids		n	Mean and range of serum carotenoid (μmol/L)		Case	Model 1			Model 2		
						OR	95% CI	*P* for trend	OR	95% CI	*P* for trend
Lutein	Lowest (T1)	47	0.39	(0.28–0.47)	8	1.00			1.00		
	Middle (T2)	45	0.55	(0.49–0.62)	9	1.48	(0.46–4.68)		1.50	(0.45–5.01)	
	Highest (T3)	48	0.74	(0.63–1.14)	10	1.29	(0.41–4.08)	0.676	1.62	(0.47–5.56)	0.445
Lycopene	Lowest (T1)	48	0.24	(0.07–0.34)	7	1.00			1.00		
	Middle (T2)	46	0.40	(0.35–0.46)	10	1.61	(0.52–5.00)		2.04	(0.61–6.83)	
	Highest (T3)	46	0.66	(0.50–1.06)	10	1.54	(0.46–5.13)	0.481	1.57	(0.42–5.90)	0.480
α-Carotene	Lowest (T1)	46	0.13	(0.07–0.17)	8	1.00			1.00		
	Middle (T2)	46	0.21	(0.19–0.24)	9	1.18	(0.39–3.54)		1.55	(0.46–5.18)	
	Highest (T3)	48	0.39	(0.26–2.75)	10	0.89	(0.29–2.73)	0.806	0.97	(0.28–3.31)	0.889
β-Carotene	Lowest (T1)	47	0.70	(0.35–0.97)	9	1.00			1.00		
	Middle (T2)	47	1.23	(0.99–1.45)	10	0.78	(0.26–2.36)		0.87	(0.28–2.73)	
	Highest (T3)	46	1.94	(1.50–3.36)	8	0.56	(0.18–1.76)	0.324	0.58	(0.18–1.91)	0.378
β-Cryptoxanthin	Lowest (T1)	46	0.85	(0.24–1.45)	14	1.00			1.00		
	Middle (T2)	47	1.95	(1.50–2.44)	6	0.22	(0.07–0.76)		0.18	(0.05–0.67)	
	Highest (T3)	47	3.78	(2.47–10.51)	7	0.29	(0.09–0.96)	0.037	0.28	(0.08–0.99)	0.035
Zeaxanthin	Lowest (T1)	41	0.15	(0.11–0.18)	7	1.00			1.00		
	Middle (T2)	50	0.20	(0.19–0.21)	11	1.40	(0.44–4.42)		1.52	(0.46–4.99)	
	Highest (T3)	49	0.26	(0.23–0.37)	9	1.28	(0.40–4.14)	0.697	1.42	(0.41–4.91)	0.593

Model 1: Age, weight, height, years since menopause, current tobacco use, regular alcohol intake, exercise habits, supplement use, and total energy intake were adjusted.
Model 2: Intakes of calcium, magnesium, potassium, and vitamins D, C, and E were further adjusted.

In general, there is little available epidemiological research on the association between carotenoids and bone health. No studies have, in fact, been conducted to date to longitudinally analyze the association between serum carotenoid levels and bone health. In this respect, ours is the first study including a longitudinal analysis of the association between serum carotenoid levels and BMD and demonstrating the possible inhibitory effects of β-cryptoxanthin and β-carotene on BMD loss. In general, when the carotenoid intake of each subject is estimated on the basis of data collected from a diet survey, the estimated intake levels may not necessarily reflect the actual amount of carotenoid ingested or absorbed into the body. On the other hand, data on serum carotenoid levels are a relatively accurate measure of the actual amount of carotenoids present in the body, which therefore gives a more detailed account of the association between carotenoid levels and BMD.

In contrast to findings collected in Europe and the U.S., no significant association has been observed between lycopene and bone health in the subjects who participated in our study. This

Table 5. Baseline serum carotenoid concentrations of post-menopausal Japanese female subjects stratified by T-Score levels in 2009.

	Mean and range of serum carotenoid concentrations (μmol/L)						
	Continuously normal		Newly diagnosed osteopenia		Newly diagnosed osteoporosis		P for trend
N	113		25		17		
Lutein	0.54	(0.51–0.57)	0.56	(0.50–0.63)	0.52	(0.44–0.61)	0.660
Lycopene	0.39	(0.36–0.43)	0.41	(0.34–0.49)	0.38	(0.30–0.48)	0.969
α-Carotene	0.23	(0.20–0.25)	0.21	(0.17–0.27)	0.21	(0.16–0.28)	0.370
β-Carotene	1.22	(1.13–1.33)	1.06	(0.89–1.27)	0.97	(0.78–1.21)	0.025
β-Cryptoxanthin	1.94	(1.72–2.19)	1.59	(1.22–2.07)	1.16	(0.85–1.58)*	<0.001
Zeaxanthin	0.20	(0.19–0.21)	0.21	(0.19–0.23)	0.18	(0.16–0.21)	0.388

Age, weight, height, years since menopause, current tobacco use, regular alcohol intake, exercise habits, supplement use, and total energy intake were adjusted.
*p<0.01 vs Normal group by Bonferroni multiple comparison test.

may be partly due to the fact that the groups of subjects in the Mikkabi study have much lower dietary intake and serum levels of lycopene than individuals living in other parts of the world. Similarly, although a higher serum concentration of α-carotene has contributed to some extent to a decreasing rate of BMD loss, the association has not been found to be significant. A more extended follow-up may reveal a significant association. On the other hand, our analyses failed to show any association of lutein and zeaxanthin with BMD. In a previous study, lutein was found to be consumed in the highest amount by the subjects in the Mikkabi study, and the serum concentration of lutein was also found to be higher than those of α-carotene or lycopene [41]. However, no association was found between lutein and bone health. This finding suggests that none of these carotenoids is involved in the maintenance of bone health.

This study had some limitations. First, we could not evaluate the association of blood levels of vitamins C and E with the radial BMD. Some studies have shown an association of antioxidant vitamins with the risk of hip fracture in current smokers and aged osteoporotic women [19,20]. It would be necessary to measure blood levels of vitamins C and E in order to examine the associations of these antioxidant vitamin concentrations with the radial BMD. Second, in this report, we evaluated the radial BMD at 1/3 of the forearm length measured from the styloid process on the ulna. Therefore, an analysis of the association of serum carotenoids with BMD in cancellous bone, such as the femoral neck or lumbar spine, will be required. Last, in our study, sample size in post-menopausal female subjects was not so large and it had less statistical power. Further study in large scale will be required.

Our findings lead us to conclude that β-cryptoxanthin and β-carotene are probably the two types of carotenoids that are involved in the prevention of BMD loss in post-menopausal Japanese women. However, further evidence from epidemiological research is needed before a definitive conclusion on this issue can be drawn.

Acknowledgments

We are grateful to the participants in our survey and to the staff of the health examination program for residents of the town of Mikkabi, Shizuoka, Japan. We are also grateful to the staff of the Seirei Preventive Health Care Center (Shizuoka, Japan).

Author Contributions

Conceived and designed the experiments: MS MN. Performed the experiments: MS MN KO YI MY. Analyzed the data: MS MN KO. Contributed reagents/materials/analysis tools: MS MN KO. Wrote the paper: MS MN.

References

1. Ministry of Health, Labor and Welfare. Comprehensive survey of living conditions of the people on Health and Welfare. Section3 2004. Internet: http://www.mhlw.go.jp/toukei/saikin/hw/k-tyosa/k-tyosa04/4-2.html (accessed 11 July 2012).
2. Christodoulou C, Cooper C (2003) What is osteoporosis? Postgrad Med J 79: 133–138.
3. Gennari C (2001) Calcium and vitamin D nutrition and bone disease of the elderly. Public Health Nutr 4: 547–559.
4. Prentice A (2004) Diet, nutrition and the prevention of osteoporosis. Public Health Nutr 7: 227–243.
5. Macdonald HM, New SA, Golden MH, Campbell MK, Reid DM (2004) Nutritional associations with bone loss during the menopausal transition: evidence of a beneficial effect of calcium, alcohol, and fruit and vegetable nutrients and of a detrimental effect of fatty acids. Am J Clin Nutr 79: 155–165.
6. New SA, Bolton-Smith C, Grubb DA, Reid DM (1997) Nutritional influences on bone mineral density: a cross-sectional study in premenopausal women. Am J Clin Nutr 65: 1831–1839.
7. Prynne CJ, Mishra GD, O'Connell MA, Muniz G, Laskey MA, et al. (2006) Fruit and vegetable intakes and bone mineral status: a cross sectional study in 5 age and sex cohorts. Am J Clin Nutr 83: 1420–1428.
8. Okubo H, Sasaki S, Horiguchi H, Oguma E, Miyamoto K, et al. (2006) Dietary patterns associated with bone mineral density in premenopausal Japanese farmwomen. Am J Clin Nutr 83: 1185–1192.
9. McGartland CP, Robson PJ, Murray LJ, Cran GW, Savage MJ, et al. (2004) Fruit and vegetable consumption and bone mineral density: the Northern Ireland Young Hearts Project. Am J Clin Nutr 80: 1019–1023.
10. Tucker KL, Chen H, Hanna MT, Couples LA, Wilson PW, et al. (2002) Bone mineral density and dietary patterns in older adults: the Framingham Osteoporosis Study. Am J Clin Nutr 76: 245–252.
11. Gutteridge JM (1994) Biological origin of free radicals, and mechanisms of antioxidant protection. Chem Biol Interact 91: 133–140.
12. Rock CL, Jacob RA, Bowen PE (1996) Update on the biological characteristics of the antioxidant micronutrients: vitamin C, vitamin E, and the carotenoids. J Am Diet Assoc 96: 693–702.
13. Almeida M, Han L, Martin-Millan M, O'Brien CA, Manolagas SC (2007) Oxidative stress antagonizes Wnt signaling in osteoblast precursors by diverting beta-catenin from T cell factor- to forkhead box O-mediated transcription. J Biol Chem 282: 27298–27305.
14. Jilka RL, Weinstein RS, Parfitt AM, Manolagas SC (2007) Quantifying osteoblast and osteocyte apoptosis: challenges and rewards. J Bone Miner Res 22: 1492–1501.
15. Garrett IR, Boyce BF, Oreffo RO, Bonewald L, Poser J, et al. (1990) Oxygen-derived free radicals stimulate osteoclastic bone resorption in rodent bone in vitro and in vivo. J Clin Invest 85: 632–639.
16. Basu S, Michaelsson K, Olofsson H, Johansson S, Melhus H (2001) Association between oxidative stress and bone mineral density. Biochem Biophys Res Commun 288: 275–279.
17. Yalin S, Bagis S, Polat G (2005) Is there a role of free oxygen radicals in primary male osteoporosis? Clin Exp Rheumatol. 23: 689–692.
18. Law MR, Hackshaw AK (1997) A meta-analysis of cigarette smoking, bone mineral density and risk of hip fracture: recognition of a major effect. BMJ 315: 841–846.
19. Melhus H, Michaelsson K, Holmberg L, Wolk A, Ljunghall S (1999) Smoking, antioxidant vitamins, and the risk of hip fracture. J Bone Miner Res 14: 129–135.
20. Maggio D, Barabani M, Pierandrei M (2003) Marked decrease in plasma antioxidants in aged osteoporotic women: results of a cross-sectional study. J Clin Endocrinol Metab 88: 1523–1527.
21. Wattanapenpaiboon N, Lukito W, Wahlqvist ML, Strauss BJ (2003) Dietary carotenoid intake as a predictor of bone mineral density. Asia Pac J Clin Nutr 12: 467–473.
22. Maggio D, Polidori MC, Barabani M, Tufi A, Ruggiero C, et al. (2006) Low levels of carotenoids and retinol in involutional osteoporosis. Bone 38: 244–248.
23. Yang Z, Zhang Z, Penniston KL, Binkley N, Tanumihardjo SA (2008) Serum carotenoid concentrations in postmenopausal women from the United States with and without osteoporosis. Int J Vitam Nutr Res 78: 105–111.
24. Sahni S, Hannan MT, Blumberg J, Cupples LA, Kiel DP, et al. (2009) Inverse association of carotenoid intakes with 4-y change in bone mineral density in elderly men and women: the Framingham Osteoporosis Study. Am J Clin Nutr 89: 416–424.
25. Sahni S, Hannan MT, Gagnon D, Blumberg J, Cupples LA, et al. (2009) Protective effect of total and supplemental vitamin C intake on the risk of hip fracture–a 17-year follow-up from the Framingham Osteoporosis Study. Osteoporos Int 20: 1853–1861.
26. Sugiura M, Nakamura M, Ogawa K, Ikoma Y, Ando F, et al. (2008) Bone mineral density in post-menopausal female subjects is associated with serum antioxidant carotenoids. Osteoporos Int 19: 211–219.
27. Sugiura M, Nakamura M, Ogawa K, Ikoma Y, Ando F, et al. (2011) Dietary patterns of antioxidant vitamin and carotenoid intake associated with bone mineral density: Findings from post-menopausal Japanese female subjects. Osteoporos Int 22: 143–152.
28. Wakai K, Egami I, Kato K, Lin Y, Kawamura T, et al. (1999) A simple food frequency questionnaire for Japanese diet–Part I. Development of the questionnaire, and reproducibility and validity for food groups. J Epidemiol 9: 216–226.
29. Egami I, Wakai K, Kato K, Lin Y, Kawamura T, et al. (1999) A simple food frequency questionnaire for Japanese diet–Part II. Reproducibility and validity for nutrient intakes. J Epidemiol 9: 227–234.
30. Science and Technology Agency (1983) Standard tables of food composition in Japan. 4th ed. Tokyo, Japan: Printing Bureau, Ministry of Finance. (in Japanese).
31. Science and Technology Agency (1997) Standard tables of food composition in Japan. 5th ed. (for new foods) Tokyo, Japan: Printing Bureau, Ministry of Finance. (in Japanese).
32. Sugiura M, Nakamura M, Ikoma Y, Yano M, Ogawa K, et al. (2005) High serum carotenoids are inversely associated with serum gamma-glutamyltransferase in alcohol drinkers within normal liver function. J Epidemiol 15: 180–186.

33. Orimo H, Hayashi Y, Fukunaga M, Sone T, Fujiwara S, et al. (2001) Diagnostic criteria for primary osteoporosis: year 2000 revision. J Bone Miner Metab 19: 331–337.
34. Iotsova V, Caamaño J, Loy J, Yang Y, Lewin A, et al. (1997) Osteopetrosis in mice lacking NF-kappaB1 and NF-kappaB2. Nat Med 3: 1285–1289.
35. Baeuerle PA, Rupec RA, Pahl HL (1996) Reactive oxygen intermediates as second messengers of a general pathogen response. Pathol Biol (Paris) 44: 29–35.
36. Garrett IR, Boyce BF, Oreffo RO, Bonewald L, Poser J, et al. (1990) Oxygen-derived free radicals stimulate osteoclastic bone resorption in rodent bone in vitro and in vivo. J Clin Invest 85: 632–639.
37. Bax BE, Alam AS, Banerji B, Bax CM, Bevis PJ, et al. (1992) Stimulation of osteoclastic bone resorption by hydrogen peroxide. Biochem Biophys Res Commun 183: 1153–1158.
38. Yamaguchi M, Uchiyama S (2003) Effect of carotenoid on calcium content and alkaline phosphatase activity in rat femoral tissues in vitro: the unique anabolic effect of beta-cryptoxanthin. Biol Pharm Bull 26: 1188–1191.
39. Yamaguchi M, Uchiyama S (2004) beta-Cryptoxanthin stimulates bone formation and inhibits bone resorption in tissue culture in vitro. Mol Cell Biochem 258: 137–144.
40. Uchiyama S, Yamaguchi M (2004) Oral administration of beta-cryptoxanthin induces anabolic effects on bone components in the femoral tissues of rats in vivo. Biol Pharm Bull 27: 232–235.
41. Sugiura M, Nakamura M, Ogawa K, Ikoma Y, Matsumoto H, et al. (2009) Synergistic interaction of cigarette smoking and alcohol drinking with serum carotenoid concentrations: findings from the middle-Japanese population. Br J Nutr 102: 1211–1219.

6

Time of Progression to Osteopenia/Osteoporosis in Chronically HIV-Infected Patients: Screening DXA Scan

Eugenia Negredo[1]*, Anna Bonjoch[1], Moisés Gómez-Mateu[2], Carla Estany[1], Jordi Puig[1], Nuria Perez-Alvarez[1,2], Joaquin Rosales[3], Silvana di Gregorio[3], Luis del Rio[3], Guadalupe Gómez[2], Bonaventura Clotet[1,4]

1 Lluita contra la SIDA Foundation, Hospital Universitari Germans Trias i Pujol, Universitat Autònoma de Barcelona, Barcelona, Spain, **2** Statistics and Operations Research Department, Universitat Politècnica de Catalunya, Barcelona, Spain, **3** CETIR Centre Mèdic, Barcelona, Spain, **4** Irsicaixa Foundation, Barcelona, Spain

Abstract

Background: Algorithms for bone mineral density (BMD) management in HIV-infected patients are lacking. Our objective was to assess how often a dual-energy x-ray absorptiometry (DXA) scan should be performed by assessing time of progression to osteopenia/osteoporosis.

Methods: All DXA scans performed between 2000 and 2009 from HIV-infected patients with at least two DXA were included. Time to an event (osteopenia and osteoporosis) was assessed using the Kaplan–Meier method. Strata (tertiles) were defined using baseline minimum T scores. Differences between strata in time to an event were compared with the log-rank test.

Results: Of 391 patients (1,639 DXAs), 49.6% had osteopenia and 21.7% osteoporosis at their first DXA scan. Of the 112 (28.6%) with normal BMD, 35.7% progressed to osteopenia; median progression time was 6.7 years. These patients were stratified: "low-risk" (baseline minimum T score >-0.2 SD), "middle-risk" (between -0.2 and -0.6 SD), and "high-risk" (from -0.6 to -1 SD); median progression time to osteopenia was 8.7, >7.2, and 1.7 years, respectively ($p<0.0001$). Of patients with osteopenia, 23.7% progressed to osteoporosis; median progression time was >8.5 years. Progression time was >8.2 years in "low-risk" tertile (T score between -1.1 and -1.6 SD), >8.5 years in "middle-risk" (between -1.6 and -2), and 3.2 years in "high-risk" (from -2 to -2.4) ($p<0.0001$).

Conclusions: Our results may help to define the BMD testing interval. The lowest T score tertiles would suggest recommending a subsequent DXA in 1–2 years; in the highest tertiles, ≥6 years. Early intervention in patients with bone demineralization could reduce fracture-related morbidity/mortality.

Editor: Songtao Shi, University of Southern California, United States of America

Funding: This work was supported in part by a grant from the Spanish Ministry of Education and Science [Grant number MTM2008-06747-C02-00]. The funders had no role in study design, data collection and analysis, decision to publish, or preparation of the manuscript. No additional external funding was received for this study.

Competing Interests: The authors have declared that no competing interests exist.

* E-mail: enegredo@flsida.org

Introduction

Bone strength is the result of bone mineral density (BMD) and bone microarchitecture. A decrease in BMD leads to deterioration of microarchitecture, and is determined by the intensity of bone remodeling. These changes lead to critical damage and porosity that weaken bone and increase the probability of fractures.[1]

Many factors lead to accelerated bone loss, and HIV infection is one of the most recently identified [2,3,4]. The results of several studies confirm a higher incidence of osteopenia and osteoporosis in HIV-infected patients than in HIV-negative individuals. In fact, up to 25% of infected patients fulfill the criteria for osteoporosis and up to 50% fulfill those of osteopenia [2,3,4,5]. Accelerated bone demineralization in this population is due to an additional number of factors such as the HIV infection itself and the chronic inflammatory status, by increasing apoptosis of osteoblast cells and promotion of osteoclastic activity [6,7,8,9,10,11,12,13,14,15], the exposure to specific antiretroviral agents [2,13,16,17,18] and the immune reconstitution [14,19,20], together with traditional risk factors, such as vitamin D insufficiency, a secondary cause of osteoporosis that is very prevalent among HIV-infected patients.[21]

In addition, the first available longitudinal studies revealed that HIV-infected patients experience more rapid bone loss [5,19,20] and more frequent fractures than HIV-negative individuals.[20,22,23,24]

The high associated morbidity and mortality of bone fractures [25] means that optimal monitoring of bone mineralization should be offered to patients at high risk of low BMD, such as the HIV-infected population.

Dual-energy X-ray absorptiometry (DXA) is the method of choice for the assessment of BMD. Most clinicians attending HIV-infected patients agree that this group should undergo DXA screening, especially those patients with traditional risk factors for bone loss. [26,27] However, the optimal BMD testing intervals remains undetermined.

This study aims to determine how often a DXA scan should be performed in chronically HIV-infected patients by assessing the time of progression to osteopenia or osteoporosis in a large cohort.

Methods

Study design, population, and objective

We performed a retrospective longitudinal observational study of all DXA scans from HIV-infected patients who attended our HIV Unit between January 2000 and December 2009.

Of a total of 671 patients with at least one DXA scan, 391 had at least two DXA scans performed during the study period. These scans were included in the present analysis. The study was performed according to the stipulations of the Declaration of Helsinki, and all patients gave their written informed consent for their medical information to be used for purposes of scientific research in accordance with the ethical committee of the participating site. A more detailed description of the methodology applied has been described elsewhere. [2]

The objective of the study was to determine the time of progression to bone loss defined as time from normal BMD to osteopenia and from osteopenia to osteoporosis.

Osteopenia and osteoporosis were defined following the World Health Organization (WHO) criteria, as follows: normal, when the T score by DXA was higher than −1.0 SD, osteopenia when the T score was between −1.0 SD and −2.5 SD, and osteoporosis when the T score was less than −2.5 SD. [28]

Assessments

A total of 1,639 DXA scans from 391 patients were included in the present analysis.

The mean BMD and T score (comparison with normal reference values for young adults expressed as standard deviation units) for the lumbar spine and femoral neck were measured using the same DXA device (Lunar Prodigy, GE Healthcare, Belgium) at an external center (CETIR Grup Mèdic, Barcelona, Spain).

Epidemiological and HIV-related data (time since diagnosis of HIV infection, time on antiretroviral treatment, viral load, CD4 T-cell count, nadir CD4 T-cell count, total time on treatment, total time on protease inhibitors, total time on tenofovir, baseline antiretroviral treatment, time with viral suppression, and hepatitis B or C coinfection) were collected from the database of our HIV Unit at time of the first DXA scan.

Statistical analysis

A descriptive analysis of the main quantitative and categorical variables was performed.

We calculated time of progression in weeks from normal BMD to osteopenia. The calculation was based on those individuals whose BMD was considered normal according to a first DXA scan and who fulfilled the criteria for osteopenia in a subsequent scan. The same procedure was followed to compute time from osteopenia to osteoporosis (ie, patients with osteopenia in a first DXA scan who progressed to osteoporosis).

Patients with normal BMD at baseline and at least 3 DXA scans who progressed from normal BMD status to osteopenia and later to osteoporosis were considered for both time from normal BMD status to osteopenia and time from osteopenia to osteoporosis.

The time to an event, namely, change of category (normal to osteopenia, osteopenia to osteoporosis), was known only for those patients who presented the event before the last DXA scan. For the remaining patients, the only known data were that the time to the event was greater than the observation time. This approach is known as administrative censoring, and the incomplete data are termed right-censored. [29]

Additionally, data were stratified by tertiles of the baseline T score. These distinct groups represent the BMD baseline status. The initial value is related to the time to an event, assuming that the T score is a monotone and decreases over time.

Survival was analyzed using the Kaplan-Meier estimator; the log-rank test was used to compare strata. If the last time of observation is not censored, then the curve fall to zero and an exact value of time is provided while, if the last observed time is censored, the survival remains constant from the last time value and result is provided as ">than" this value.

All analyses were performed using the R software, and all reported *p* values are two-tailed.

Results

Epidemiological and clinical data are summarized in Table 1.

At the first DXA scan, 112 patients of 391 (28.6%) had normal BMD, 194 (49.6%) fulfilled the criteria for osteopenia, and 85 (21.7%) fulfilled the criteria for osteoporosis.

The mean (SD) number of DXA scans per patient (DXA scans/patient) was 4 (2); 100% of patients had 2 DXA scans, 67% had 3 DXA scans, 48% had 4 DXA scans, and 35% had 5 or more. No differences were observed in mean (SD) DXA scans/patient after stratification taking the first DXA as normal (5 (3) DXA/patient), osteopenia (4 (3) DXA/patient), and osteoporosis (4 (2) DXA/patient) ($p = 0.111$).

Table 1. Epidemiological and clinical data at first DXA scan.

Gender, male, n (%)	284 (73%)
Menopause, n (%)	10 (9.5%)
Age, years	39.4 (34.9; 44.2)
BMI, kg/m^2	22.5 (20.9; 24.6)
Calcium intake, g/d	16 (4%)
Hepatitis B/C coinfection, n (%)	93 (29%)
Concomitant therapy, n (%)	
Hormone treatment, n (%)	3 (1%)
Alendronate, n (%)	7 (2%)
Time since HIV diagnosis, years	7.9 (3.7; 12.1)
Current CD4+, absolute value, cells/μL	514 (348.5; 746.5)
Nadir CD4+, cells/μL	219.5 (106.8; 318.3)
Suppressed viral load, n (%)	268 (68.5%)
Proportion of time with suppressed viral load, n (%)	30.6 (11.7; 49.3)
Naïve, n (%)	48 (12%)
Time on antiretroviral therapy, years	4.8 (1.5; 8.5)
Current use of protease inhibitors, n (%)	171 (50%)
Time on protease inhibitors, years	2.4 (1.2; 4.1)
Current use of tenofovir, n (%)	173 (51%)
Time on tenofovir, years	1 (0.3; 2.3)
Creatinine, μmol/L	87 (76; 97.5)

Values are expressed as median (IQR) or number (%).

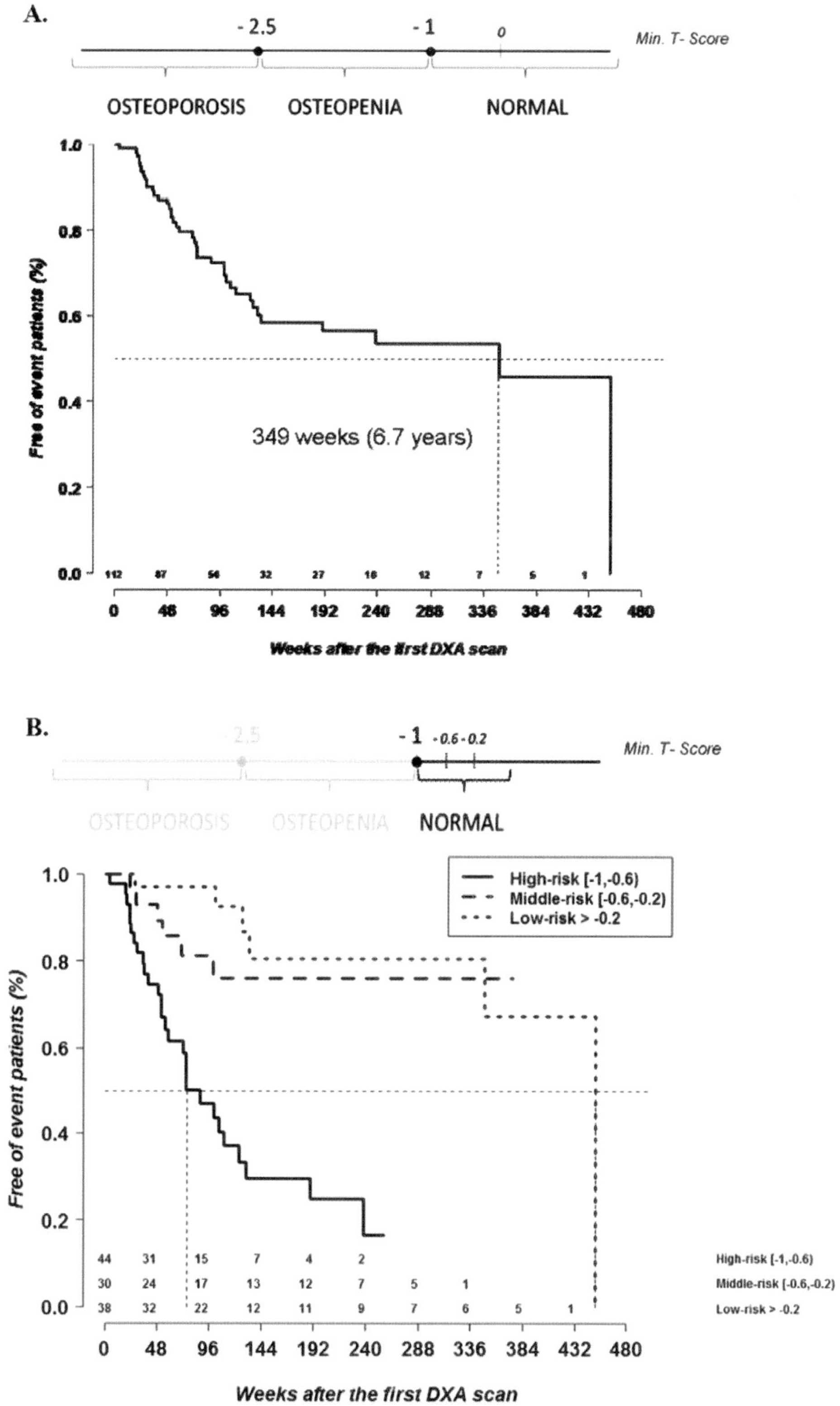

HIGH-RISK [–1, –0.6)	88 weeks
MIDDLE-RISK [–0.6,–0.2)	>375 weeks
LOW-RISK ≥–0.2	451 weeks

Figure 1. Time of progression. Time of progression from normal bone mineral density to osteopenia overall (n = 112 patients) (A) and after stratification according to minimum baseline T score ("low-risk", "middle-risk", and "high-risk") (B).

Table 2. Patients (n = 112) who progressed from normal bone mineral density to osteopenia/osteoporosis.

Follow-up (weeks)	HIGH-RISK	MIDDLE-RISK	LOW-RISK
48	25%	11%	3%
96	53%	19%	3%
144	70%	24%	20%
192	75%	24%	20%
240	84%	24%	20%
288		24%	20%
336		24%	20%
384			33%
432			33%
480			100%

Median (IQR) time between DXA scans was 33.71 weeks (25.1; 56) (0.65 years); median (IQR) time between the first and the last DXA scans was 133.1 weeks (62.7; 276.4) (2.6 years). No differences were detected in median (IQR) time between the first and the last DXA scans after stratification according to the first DXA scan (data not shown).

Change from normal BMD at baseline to osteopenia

Median follow-up for the 112 patients from this group was 152 weeks (59.1; 258) (2.9 years). Forty of these 112 patients (35.7%) progressed to osteopenia/osteoporosis.

The survival analysis showed a median (IQR) time of progression to osteopenia of 349 weeks (74; 451) (6.7 years) (Figure 1.A).

Patients with normal BMD at baseline were stratified in tertiles according to the minimum T score of their first DXA, as follows: "low-risk" tertile when the minimum T score was >−0.2 SD (38 patients, 33.9%), "middle-risk" tertile when the minimum T score was between −0.2 and −0.6 SD (30 patients, 26.8%) and "high-risk" tertile when the minimum T score was between −0.6 and −1 SD (44 patients, 39.3%) (Figure 1.B).

The three groups were similar with respect to age (p = 0.95), gender (p = 0.72), time with infection (p = 0.064), percentage of patients with viral suppression (p = 0.81), and CD4 T-cell count (p = 0.359).

The survival analysis revealed significant differences in time of progression after stratification by tertiles. Median (IQR) time of progression overall was 451 weeks (349; 451) (8.7 years) in patients from the "low-risk" tertile, >375 weeks (>375; >375) (>7.2 years) in those who were in the "middle-risk" tertile, and 88 weeks (39; 190) (1.7 years) in those who were in the "high-risk" tertile (p<0.0001) (Figure 1.B).

Table 2 shows those of the 112 patients whose status progressed from normal to osteopenia/osteoporosis after stratification by baseline minimum T score ("low-risk", "middle-risk", and "high-risk").

When patients were stratified by age tertiles in the same group, differences in time of progression were observed when we applied the following tertiles: those aged <30 years (20 patients, 17.9%), those aged 30–50 years (85 patients, 75.9%), and those aged >50 years (7 patients, 6.3%) (p = 0.016), but not when we applied the tertiles <33, 33–39, and >39 years (p = 0.418) (Figure 2.A and 2.B).

When patients were stratified by both the minimum T score of baseline DXA scan and by age, the median time of progression was significantly shorter in tertiles with a T score <−0.4, independently of age, than in those with a T score ≥−0.4 (p = 0.0003) (Figure 2.C).

No statistically significant differences were observed when patients were classified according to gender: time of progression was >392 weeks (130; >392) (>7.5 years) in women (n = 35) and 238 weeks (72; 451) (4.6 years) in men (n = 77) (p = 0.136).

Change from osteopenia at baseline to osteoporosis

A total of 211 patients had osteopenia at baseline; of these, 194 presented osteopenia at their first DXA scan and the remaining 17 had a normal DXA result at baseline, progressed to osteopenia in a subsequent DXA, and underwent additional DXA scans.

Median follow-up for the 211 patients from this group was 128 weeks (60.4; 279) (2.7 years). Fifty of these 211 patients (23.7%) progressed to osteoporosis.

Survival analysis showed a median (IQR) time of progression to osteoporosis of >443 weeks (186; >443) (>8.5 years) (Figure 3.A).

When the 211 patients were stratified according to the minimum T score of the first DXA scan, 73 (34.6%) were classed as "low-risk" (between −1.6 and −1.1 SD), 63 (29.9%) as "middle-risk" (between −2 and −1.6 SD and 75 (35.5%) as "high-risk" (between −2.4 and −2 SD) (Figure 3).

The 3 groups were similar with respect to age (p = 0.106), gender (p = 0.103), percentage of patients with viral suppression (p = 0.602), and CD4 T-cell count (p = 0.739), but not by time with infection, which was higher in patients from the "high-risk" tertile with respect to the "low-risk" tertile (9.4 years vs 7.8 years, p = 0.043).

The survival analysis showed significant differences in time of progression to osteoporosis between the 3 groups, as follows: median (IQR) time of progression of >425 weeks (359; >425), (>8.2 years) in the "low-risk" tertile, >443 weeks (347; >443) (>8.5 years) in the "middle-risk" tertile, and 164 weeks (53; 364) (3.2 years) in the "high-risk" tertile (p<0.0001) (Figure 3.B)

Table 3 shows those of the 211 patients who progressed from osteopenia to osteoporosis stratified by minimum T score ("low-risk", "middle-risk", and "high-risk").

When patients were stratified by age tertiles, no significant differences were seen for <37 years (74 patients, 35%), 37–43 years (74 patients, 35%), or >43 years of age (63 patients, 30%) (p = 0.214) (Figure 4.A).

When patients were stratified by both the minimum values of the T score of the DXA scan and age, median time of progression was significantly shorter in the group with a T score <−1.8 and age >40 years (p<0.0001) (Figure 4.B).

No differences were seen when patients were classified according to gender: median time of progression (IQR) was 359 (234; >443) weeks (6.9 years) in women (n = 60) and >428 weeks (179; >428) (>8.2 years) in men (n = 151) (p = 0.465).

As for patients with osteoporosis in the first DXA scan, 24.7% improved (osteoporosis to osteopenia or normal BMD), while 75.3% remained unchanged.

Discussion

Among our chronically HIV-infected patients, nearly one-third of those whose first DXA scan showed normal BMD progressed to osteopenia. Median time of progression to osteopenia was almost 7 years, but in those patients with normal BMD but whose baseline

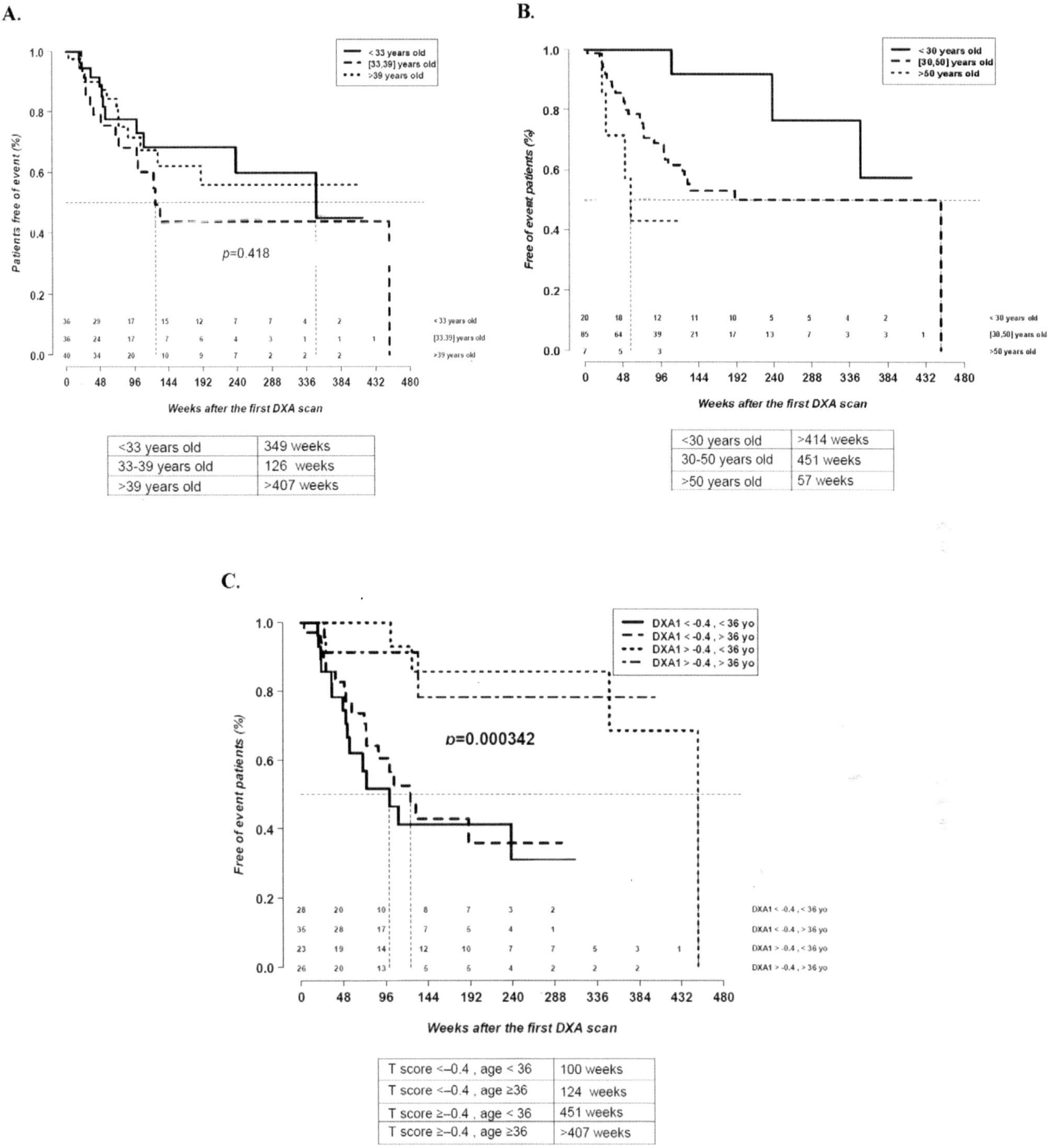

<33 years old	349 weeks
33-39 years old	126 weeks
>39 years old	>407 weeks

<30 years old	>414 weeks
30-50 years old	451 weeks
>50 years old	57 weeks

T score <–0.4 , age < 36	100 weeks
T score <–0.4 , age ≥36	124 weeks
T score ≥–0.4 , age < 36	451 weeks
T score ≥–0.4 , age ≥36	>407 weeks

Figure 2. Survival analysis by age. Survival analysis in patients with normal bone mineral density at baseline stratified by age (<33 years, 33–38 years and >38 years [A] and <30 years, 30–50 years, and >50 years [B]) and by both age and T score (less or higher than −0.4 and less or higher than 36 years [C]).

minimum T score was in the "high-risk" tertile, this progression was much faster (<2 years). Similarly, osteopenia progressed to osteoporosis in a quarter of patients. Although time of progression was more than 8 years, for patients with a minimum baseline T score <−2 SD (lower tertile) it was 3 years.

Alterations in bone strength predispose to fragility fractures, which are associated with increased morbidity and mortality in the HIV-negative population. [1,24,25,30]

Prevention of osteoporotic fractures, then, is of major interest from a public health perspective. In HIV-infected patients, osteoporosis is probably underdiagnosed. Adequate tools should be designed to identify patients at high risk for low BMD, who would be candidates for BMD screening by DXA. In the last few years, many efforts have been made to identify risk factors for bone loss—other than traditional factors—among HIV-infected patients. [2,27,31] Age (>50 years), the menopause, other secondary

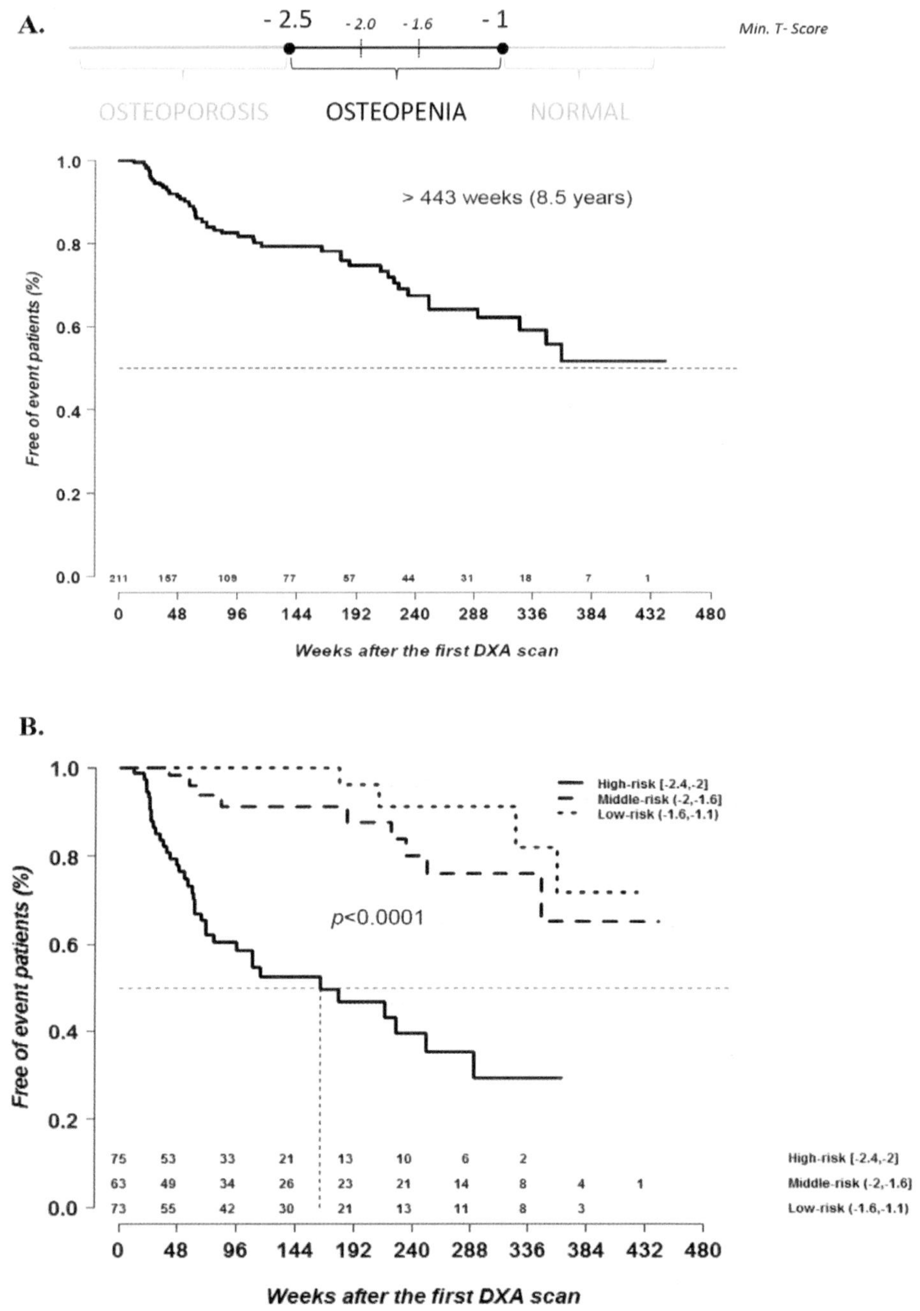

HIGH-RISK [–2.4, –2]	164 weeks
MIDDLE-RISK (–2, –1.6]	>443 weeks
LOW-RISK (–1.6, –1.1)	>425 weeks

Figure 3. Time of progression to osteoporosis. Time of progression from osteopenia to osteoporosis overall (n = 211 patients) (A) and after stratification by baseline minimum T score ("low-risk", "middle-risk", and "high-risk") (B).

causes of low BMD, and a personal or family (parents) history of fragility fractures, together with exposure to some antiretroviral drugs (tenofovir and boosted protease inhibitors), are relevant risk factors that speak in favor of screening with DXA. [31] The optimal BMD testing intervals using DXA scans, however, has not been established.

Data have been published on the rate of progression to bone loss [32,33,34], although our results are the first to show the time of progression to osteopenia/osteoporosis, information that is essential for monitoring. We observed that baseline T score, divided into tertiles, enabled us to establish time of progression of bone loss more accurately than the simple classification according to the WHO criteria (normal, osteopenia, and osteoporosis). According

Table 3. Patients (n = 211) who progressed from osteopenia to osteoporosis (B) after stratification according to minimum T score ("low-risk", "middle-risk" and "high-risk").

Follow-up (weeks)	HIGH-RISK	MIDDLE-RISK	LOW-RISK
48	22%	2%	0%
96	40%	9%	0%
144	60%	9%	0%
192	71%	13%	4%
240	71%	20%	9%
288	71%	24%	9%
336	71%	24%	18%
384		36%	28%
432		36%	
480			

to our results, time of progression to osteopenia in patients with normal BMD at the first DXA scan was enormously different depending on the tertile in which the patient was classified at baseline: from more than 8 years to less than 2 years according to whether the T score was in the low-risk tertile (>−0.2 SD) or if it was in the lowest tertile (from −0.6 to −1 SD), respectively. Similarly, the time of progression to osteoporosis varied widely among patients with osteopenia in the first DXA scan according to the tertile: 8 years for those whose minimum T score was in the higher tertile (between −1.1 and 1.6 SD), but only 3 years for those whose minimum T score was in the lowest tertile (from −2 to −2.4 SD). Ourt results are consistent with recent published data in older HIV-negative women. In this analysis of data from 4,957 women, baseline T score was the most determinant of a BMD testing interval; osteoporosis developed in 15 years for women with normal BMD or mild osteopenia (T score, greater than −1.5), 5 years for women with moderate osteopenia (T score from −1.5 to −1.99) and 1 year for women with advanced osteopenia (T score from −2.0 to −2.49) [35].

Current recommendations on the study of bone disease for HIV care providers mainly include information on candidates for BMD monitoring by DXA, [22,29] but provide very little information on the optimal frequency of subsequent DXA scans, based on the WHO categories of BMD. [31] According to our data, a reasonable proposal would be to set the frequency of DXA according to the tertile: patients in the lowest T score tertiles (defined as a T score from −0.6 to −1 in patients with normal BMD according to the WHO criteria, and from −2 to −2.4 among those with osteopenia) should undergo another DXA scan more frequently than those in the other 2 tertiles. A subsequent DXA scan should be recommended as soon as 1–2 years later for those in the lower tertiles, even when baseline BMD had been classified as normal; this frequency will help to diagnose early changes in BMD status (from normal BMD to osteopenia or from osteopenia to osteoporosis) and, in the case of progression, enable appropriate measures to be taken. Patients in the other 2 tertiles (T score from −0.6 to >−0.2 in patients with normal BMD and from −1.1 to −2 among those with osteopenia) could be assessed by a DXA scan after at least 6–7 years, even in those whose baseline BMD fulfilled the criteria for osteopenia. Since it is unlikely that a patient would progress in less than 7–8 years, more frequent DXA scanning would not affect management, although it would increase costs and inconvenience to patients.

Given our results, similar recommendations on the frequency of DXA scan should be implemented according to age, providing that the decision is based on the T score. Although age affected bone loss, when patients were classified according to their initial T score (tertiles), BMD status gave more information on the progression of bone loss. In clinical terms, however, the negative effect of age on risk of osteoporotic fracture, independently of BMD, has been reported, suggesting that both age and BMD should be taken into consideration [36] The lack of elderly patients prevents us from assessing this issue in greater depth.

As for gender, although no statistically significant differences were detected between men and women, variations in the time of progression to osteopenia/osteoporosis could be clinically relevant: those men with a normal baseline BMD, included in the high-risk tertile, progressed more rapidly to osteopenia than women (median of progression of 4.6 years in men and >7.5 years in women). This finding could suggest the need for special care and more rigorous monitoring of men from this group. These data are consistent with other published results showing the higher prevalence of low BMD and fragility fractures in men than in premenopausal women. [25]

As a retrospective observational study, our analysis presents some limitations. Variables were recorded using clinical documents as the source. Consequently, the first DXA scan for each patient did not correspond to a defined baseline; however, since at that time DXA scan was only performed when patients were seen for first time in our unit or in the context of clinical assays (metabolic studies, new antiretroviral strategies, antiretroviral-naive patients…), subjects included in the analysis seem to be a good representation of our population. Additionally, the time from normal BMD to osteopenia is only known to lie within the time interval between the first DXA with a value <−1 SD and the time immediately before this scan; the time from osteopenia to osteoporosis is only known to lie within the time interval between the first DXA with a value <−2.5 SD and the time immediately before this scan. Our analysis imputed the right end of this interval, that is the time with the first DXA <−1 SD as the time to osteopenia and <−2.5 SD as the time to osteoporosis. A statistical analysis taking into account the random nature of the intervals, where the change of status occurs, could diminish the bias due to this finding. [37] However, it is our belief that the effect of these limitations on the conclusions would be negligible. Finally, the retrospective nature of the analysis avoids knowing the presence of some clinical factors that may contribute to a different bone loss progression or bone recovery (steroid use, menopause, hypogonadism, bisphosphonate use, vitamin D or calcium supplementation, etc).

To conclude, in HIV-infected patients, the use of screening thresholds based on the minimum T scores (tertiles) provided by DXA is more efficient for predicting time of progression to osteopenia/osteoporosis and deciding on BMD testing intervals than the WHO criteria. The lowest minimum T-score tertiles indicate the recommendation of a subsequent DXA scan in 1–2 years, while in the highest tertiles, this interval could be 6 years or more. Since management algorithms are lacking, ours and other data are necessary to facilitate the design of suitable guidelines for this population. Early intervention in patients with bone demineralization could reduce the high morbidity and mortality associated with osteoporotic fractures.

A.

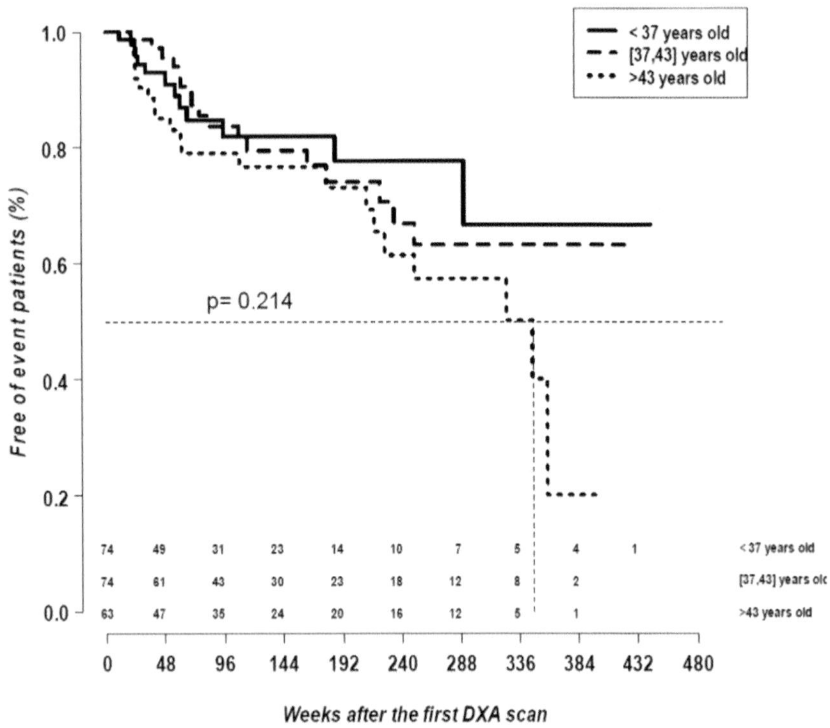

<37 years old	>443 weeks
37-43 years old	>428 weeks
>43 years old	347 weeks

B.

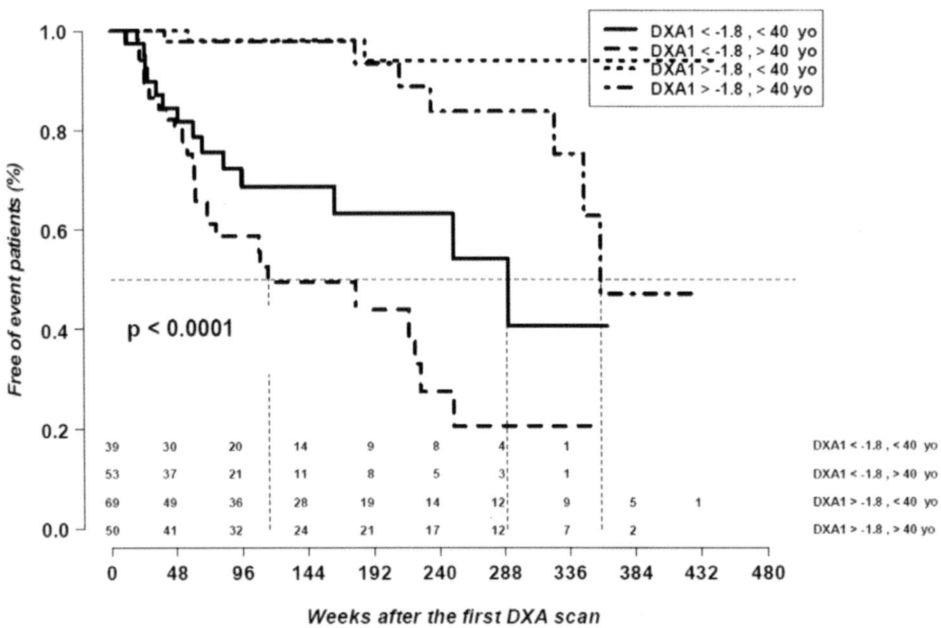

T score <-1.8, <40 years old	290 weeks
T score <-1.8, ≥40 years old	115 weeks
T score ≥-1.8, <40 years old	>443 weeks
T score ≥-1.8, ≥40 years old	359 weeks

Figure 4. Time of progression stratified by age and T score. Time of progression stratified by age: <37 years, 37–43 years and >43 years (A) and by both the minimum values of the T score and age (B).

Acknowledgments

We are grateful to Thomas O'Boyle for editorial assistance.

Author Contributions

Conceived and designed the experiments: EN AB BC. Performed the experiments: JP CE JR SdG LR. Analyzed the data: MG-M NP-A GG. Contributed reagents/materials/analysis tools: JP CE JR SdG LR. Wrote the paper: EN AB BC.

References

1. NIH Consensus Development Panel on Osteoporosis Prevention D, and Therapy, Conference CD (2001) Osteoporosis prevention, diagnosis, and therapy. JAMA 285: 785–795.
2. Bonjoch A, Figueras M, Estany C, Perez-Alvarez N, Rosales J, et al. (2010) High prevalence of and progression to low bone mineral density in HIV-infected patients: a longitudinal cohort study. AIDS 24: 2827–2833.
3. Brown TT, Qaqish RB (2006) Antiretroviral therapy and the prevalence of osteopenia and osteoporosis: a meta-analytic review. AIDS 20: 2165–2174.
4. Bruera D, Luna N, David DO, Bergoglio LM, Zamudio J (2003) Decreased bone mineral density in HIV-infected patients is independent of antiretroviral therapy. AIDS 17: 1917–1923.
5. Knobel H, Guelar A, Vallecillo G, Nogues X, Diez A (2001) Osteopenia in HIV-infected patients: is it the disease or is it the treatment? AIDS 15: 807–808.
6. Cotter EJ, Malizia AP, Chew N, Powderly WG, Doran PP (2007) HIV proteins regulate bone marker secretion and transcription factor activity in cultured human osteoblasts with consequent potential implications for osteoblast function and development. AIDS Res Hum Retroviruses 23: 1521–1530.
7. Fakruddin JM, Laurence J (2003) HIV envelope gp120-mediated regulation of osteoclastogenesis via receptor activator of nuclear factor kappa B ligand (RANKL) secretion and its modulation by certain HIV protease inhibitors through interferon-gamma/RANKL cross-talk. J Biol Chem 278: 48251–48258.
8. Gibellini D, De Crignis E, Ponti C, Borderi M, Clo A, et al. (2010) HIV-1 Tat protein enhances RANKL/M-CSF-mediated osteoclast differentiation. Biochem Biophys Res Commun 401: 429–434.
9. Gibellini D, De Crignis E, Ponti C, Cimatti L, Borderi M, et al. (2008) HIV-1 triggers apoptosis in primary osteoblasts and HOBIT cells through TNFalpha activation. J Med Virol 80: 1507–1514.
10. Grijsen ML, Vrouenraets SM, Steingrover R, Lips P, Reiss P, et al. (2010) High prevalence of reduced bone mineral density in primary HIV-1-infected men. AIDS 24: 2233–2238.
11. Gutierrez F, Masia M (2011) The role of HIV and antiretroviral therapy in bone disease. AIDS Rev 13: 109–118.
12. Hoy J (2011) Bone, fracture and frailty. Curr Opin HIV AIDS 6: 309–314.
13. Ofotokun I, Weitzmann MN (2010) HIV-1 infection and antiretroviral therapies: risk factors for osteoporosis and bone fracture. Curr Opin Endocrinol Diabetes Obes 17: 523–529.
14. Ofotokun I, Weitzmann MN (2011) HIV and bone metabolism. Discov Med 11: 385–393.
15. Wei S, Kitaura H, Zhou P, Ross FP, Teitelbaum SL (2005) IL-1 mediates TNF-induced osteoclastogenesis. J Clin Invest 115: 282–290.
16. Gallant JE, Staszewski S, Pozniak AL, DeJesus E, Suleiman JM, et al. (2004) Efficacy and safety of tenofovir DF vs stavudine in combination therapy in antiretroviral-naive patients: a 3-year randomized trial. JAMA 292: 191–201.
17. Gibellini D, Borderi M, de Crignis E, Clo A, Miserocchi A, et al. (2010) Analysis of the effects of specific protease inhibitors on OPG/RANKL regulation in an osteoblast-like cell line. New Microbiol 33: 109–115.
18. McComsey GA, Kitch D, Daar ES, Tierney C, Jahed NC, et al. (2011) Bone mineral density and fractures in antiretroviral-naive persons randomized to receive abacavir-lamivudine or tenofovir disoproxil fumarate-emtricitabine along with efavirenz or atazanavir-ritonavir: Aids Clinical Trials Group A5224s, a substudy of ACTG A5202. J Infect Dis 203: 1791–1801.
19. Ofotokun I WN, Vunnava A, Sheth A, Villinger F, Zhou J, Williams E, Sanford S, Rivas M, Lennox J, (2011) HAART-induced Immune Reconstitution: A Driving Force Behind Bone Resorption in HIV/AIDS CROI 2011.
20. Yong MK, Elliott JH, Woolley IJ, Hoy JF (2011) Low CD4 Count Is Associated With an Increased Risk of Fragility Fracture in HIV-Infected Patients. J Acquir Immune Defic Syndr 57: 205–210.
21. Dao CN, Patel P, Overton ET, Rhame F, Pals SL, et al. (2011) Low vitamin D among HIV-infected adults: prevalence of and risk factors for low vitamin D Levels in a cohort of HIV-infected adults and comparison to prevalence among adults in the US general population. Clin Infect Dis 52: 396–405.
22. Arnsten JH, Freeman R, Howard AA, Floris-Moore M, Santoro N, et al. (2006) HIV infection and bone mineral density in middle-aged women. Clin Infect Dis 42: 1014–1020.
23. Bedimo R ZS, Drechsler H, Tebas P, Maalouf N (2011) Risk of Osteoporotic Fractures Associated with Cumulative Exposure to Tenofovir and Other Antiretroviral Agents. 6th IAS Conference on HIV Pathogenesis, Treatment and Prevention, July 17–20, 2011, Rome.
24. Triant VA, Brown TT, Lee H, Grinspoon SK (2008) Fracture prevalence among human immunodeficiency virus (HIV)-infected versus non-HIV-infected patients in a large U.S. healthcare system. J Clin Endocrinol Metab 93: 3499–3504.
25. Trombetti A, Herrmann F, Hoffmeyer P, Schurch MA, Bonjour JP, et al. (2002) Survival and potential years of life lost after hip fracture in men and age-matched women. Osteoporos Int 13: 731–737.
26. Aberg JA, Kaplan JE, Libman H, Emmanuel P, Anderson JR, et al. (2009) Primary care guidelines for the management of persons infected with human immunodeficiency virus: 2009 update by the HIV medicine Association of the Infectious Diseases Society of America. Clin Infect Dis 49: 651–681.
27. Watts NB, Lewiecki EM, Miller PD, Baim S (2008) National Osteoporosis Foundation 2008 Clinician's Guide to Prevention and Treatment of Osteoporosis and the World Health Organization Fracture Risk Assessment Tool (FRAX): what they mean to the bone densitometrist and bone technologist. J Clin Densitom 11: 473–477.
28. Kanis JA (1994) Assessment of fracture risk and its application to screening for postmenopausal osteoporosis: synopsis of a WHO report. WHO Study Group. Osteoporos Int 4: 368–381.
29. Marubini EV, MG editor (2004) Analysing Survival Data from Clinical Trials and Observational Studies.
30. Cooper C (1997) The crippling consequences of fractures and their impact on quality of life. Am J Med 103: 12S–17S; discussion 17S–19S.
31. McComsey GA, Tebas P, Shane E, Yin MT, Overton ET, et al. (2010) Bone disease in HIV infection: a practical review and recommendations for HIV care providers. Clin Infect Dis 51: 937–946.
32. Cazanave C (2010) Changes in Bone Mineral Density: 2-Years of follow up of the ANRS CO3 Aquitaine Cohort. CROI 2010.
33. Dolan SE, Kanter JR, Grinspoon S (2006) Longitudinal analysis of bone density in human immunodeficiency virus-infected women. J Clin Endocrinol Metab 91: 2938–2945.
34. Sharma (2010) Longitudinal Analysis of Bone Mineral Density in Aging Men with or at Risk for HIV Infection. CROI 2010.
35. Gourlay ML, Fine JP, Preisser JS, May RC, Li C, et al. (2012) Bone-density testing interval and transition to osteoporosis in older women. N Engl J Med 366: 225–233.
36. Kanis JA, Johnell O, Oden A, Dawson A, De Laet C, et al. (2001) Ten year probabilities of osteoporotic fractures according to BMD and diagnostic thresholds. Osteoporos Int 12: 989–995.
37. Gómez G, Calle M., Oller R., Langohr K. (2009) Tutorial on methods for interval-censored data and their implementation in R. Statistical Modelling 9: 259–297.

7

Metabolomic Profiles Delineate Signature Metabolic Shifts during Estrogen Deficiency-Induced Bone Loss in Rat by GC-TOF/MS

Bo Ma[1], Jiannan Liu[2], Qi Zhang[1]*, Hanjie Ying[3]*, Jiye A[4], Jianguo Sun[4], Di Wu[5,6], Yonglu Wang[1], Jing Li[1], Yinhui Liu[1]

1 School of Pharmaceutical Sciences, Nanjing University of Technology, Nanjing, People's Republic of China, **2** Department of Respiration, Jiangsu Geriatric Hospital, Nanjing, People's Republic of China, **3** School of Life Science and Pharmaceutical Engineering, Nanjing University of Technology, Nanjing, People's Republic of China, **4** Key Laboratory of Drug Metabolism and Pharmacokinetics, China Pharmaceutical University, Nanjing, People's Republic of China, **5** Laboratory for Systems Biology, Division of Clinical Pharmacology and Therapeutics, The Children's Hospital of Philadelphia, Philadelphia, Pennsylvania, United States of America, **6** Kinetic Modeling and Simulation (KMAS) Core, Institute of Translational Medicine and Therapeutics, University of Pennsylvania, Philadelphia, Pennsylvania, United States of America

Abstract

Postmenopausal osteoporosis is a complicated and multi-factorial disease. To study the metabolic profiles and pathways activated in osteoporosis, Eight rats were oophorectomized (OVX group) to represent postmenopausal osteoporosis and the other eight rats were sham operated (Sham group) to be the control. The biochemical changes were assessed with metabolomics using a gas chromatography/time-of-flight mass spectrometry. Metabolomic profile using serial blood samples obtained prior to and at different time intervals after OVX were analyzed by principal component analysis (PCA) and Partial least squares-discriminant analysis (PLS-DA). The conventional indicators (bone mineral density, serum Bone alkaline phosphatase (B-ALP) and N-telopeptide of type I collagen (NTx) of osteoporosis in rats were also determined simultaneously. In OVX group, the metabolomics method could describe the endogenous changes of the disease more sensitively and systematically than the conventional criteria during the progression of osteoporosis. Significant metabolomic difference was also observed between the OVX and Sham groups. The metabolomic analyses of rat plasma showed that levels of arachidonic acid, octadecadienoic acid, branched-chain amino acids (valine, leucine and isoleucine), homocysteine, hydroxyproline and ketone bodies (3-Hydroxybutyric Acid) significantly elevated, while levels of docosahexaenoic acid, dodecanoic acid and lysine significantly decreased in OVX group compared with those in the homeochronous Sham group. Considering such metabolites are closely related to the pathology of the postmenopausal osteoporosis, the results suggest that potential biomarkers for the early diagnosis or the pathogenesis of osteoporosis might be identified via metabolomic study.

Editor: Julie A. Chowen, Hosptial Infantil Universitario Niño Jesús, CIBEROBN, Spain

Funding: The study was supported by a grant from the "333 High Level Talent Cultivation Project" of Jiangsu Province (2012). The funders had no role in study design, data collection and analysis, decision to publish, or preparation of the manuscript.

Competing Interests: The authors have declared that no competing interests exist.

* E-mail: nancyzhang03@hotmail.com (QZ); yinghanjie134@163.com (HY)

These authors contributed equally to this work.

Introduction

Postmenopausal osteoporosis is a skeletal condition associated with reduced bone mineral and bone strength, involved in millions of people worldwide, especially those with pathological fracture. Osteoporosis is also called the "silent disease" in clinics because majority of people don't know they have got osteoporosis until it has progressed and diagnosed at the point of fracture, most frequently occurred in the hip, wrist or spine, and the fracture often causes dangerous conditions and leads to deformity, and even death.

Bone mineral density (BMD) as a "gold standard" has been used in osteoporosis for a long time [1,2]. BMD test can indicate bone density at the normal, relatively low or osteoporotic levels, and predict the risk of fracture at the certain points. However, alterations in bone mineral density are slow in the dynamic disease progress of osteoporosis. Recently, Gourlay et al [3] attempted to standardize the bone-density testing interval (The BMD testing interval was defined as the estimated time for 10% of women to make the transition to osteoporosis before having a hip or clinical vertebral fracture, with adjustment for estrogen use and clinical risk factors.) and transition process to osteoporosis in elder women. Their data indicated that the bone-density testing interval for women with normal bone density or mild osteopenia as well as advanced osteopenia are 15, 5 and 1 year, respectively. As a clinical biomarker, bone mineral density has the disadvantages of slow change and low sensitivity, even frequent BMD testing is unlikely to improve the prediction of fracture and osteoporosis. For this reason, simple, sensitive and specific biomarkers are needed to be discovered, validated and applied for early diagnose of postmenopausal osteoporosis in clinic.

An association between an imbalance of bone formation and bone resorption was identified in pathological study on bone loss. Specific biochemical indicators for bone turnover, including bone formation markers (B-ALP; Osteocalcin et al), and bone resorption markers (NTx; Tartrate-resistant acid phosphatase-5b, TRCAP-5b; and Carboxy-terminal collagen crosslinks, CTX etc), might be used as index for disease progression of osteoporosis[4–6]. These sensitive and validated biochemical markers can offer an alternative to well-accepted BMD test to monitor disease progression of osteoporosis and therapeutic treatment [7,8]. The disadvantage of the biochemical markers is that they only reflect the alteration of bone formation or bone resorption, while the incidence of osteoporosis is attributed to the dual outcomes of bone formation and resorption.

Metabolomics as an important component of systems biology, including genomics, transcriptomics and proteomics, provide a wide spectrum of information on the biochemical finger print in cell, tissue or organism levels to elucidate novel mechanisms by detecting and comparing small-molecule metabolite profiles under difference conditions [9]. Metabolomics is the endpoints of genotype functions and biochemical phenotype in body. Metabolic profiles detected by metabolomics in different conditions are linked closely to functions alteration in body [10]. Biomarkers obtained by metabolomics are more sensitive to disease etiology and progression compared with those obtained by proteinomics and genomics [11,12]. Metabolomics has been used in the early detection and diagnosis of disease progression and provided prognostic biomarkers as novel therapeutic targets [13–16]. Postmenopausal osteoporosis is known as a complex disease, and many pathophysiologic factors involve in its occurrence and progression, including estrogen receptor [17], OPG/RANK/RANKL system [18], inflammatory factor [19] and oxidative stress [20]. Considering there is no sensitive and specific biomarker indicating the pathogenesis of osteoporosis from a holistic point of view so far, metabolomics study might provide suitable approaches to investigate osteoporosis on disease etiology and progression, and identify a cluster of biomarkers of postmenopausal osteoporosis.

In our laboratory, metabolomic approach by using GC-MS or GC-TOF/MS has been successfully applied to the study of hypertension [21], hyperlipemia [22], chronic myeloid leukemia [23], colon carcinoma, and professional athletes [24] in serum or urine from rat or human. Metabolomic study on estrogen deficiency-induced obesity was performed recently and a series of biomarkers was identified to relate to estrogen deficiency [25]. Based on our previous work, the metabolic alterations occurred in osteoporosis induced by estrogen deficiency are examined by using GC-TOF/MS. The goals of study are listed as following. 1) Using GC-TOF/MS to delineate the metabolic profile and monitor the endogenous metabolomics in rat plasma during the process of estrogen deficiency-induced bone loss. 2) Identifying and characterizing specific metabolic pathways served as targets for treatment intervention or as substrates for molecular imaging in postmenopausal osteoporosis. 3) Exploring mechanisms of bone loss induced by estrogen deficiency from the perspective of metabolomics.

Materials and Methods

1. Chemicals and Reagents

Myristic-1,2-^{13}C2 acid, 99 atom %^{13}C, the stableisotopelabeled compound used as an internal standard (IS),Alkane series (C8–C40), MSTFA (N-methyl-N-trimethylsilyltrifluoroacetamid), and 1% TMCS (trimethylchlorosilane) were obtained from Sigma-Aldrich(St. Louis, MO, USA). HPLC-grade methanol and n-heptane were obtained from Merck (Damstadt, Germany). The reference substance octadecadienoic acid, arachidonic acid, docosahexaenoic acid, isoleucine, valine, leucine, homocysteine, hydroxyproline, tryptophan, cystine, succinic acid, citric acid, malic acid and lysine were purchased from Sigma-Aldrich (St. Louis, MO, USA). Purified water was produced by a Milli-Q system (Millipore, MA, USA).

2. Experimental Design

Sixteen virgin Sprague–Dawley female rats with specific pathogen free (SPF) (6 months old, body weight 260±20.0 g) were obtained from the Animal Center of Nanjing Medical University in this study. Rats were housed under controlled conditions, including room temperature kept at 22±1°C, and standard solid food with water ad libitum provided during the experiment. This study was reviewed and approved by the Animal Ethical Committee of Nanjing University of Technology.

After acclimatization for 7 days, all animals were anesthetized with 30 mg/kg pentobarbital sodium (Fluka, Germany), intraperitoneal injection. Eight rats were oophorectomized (OVX group) and the remaining eight rats were sham operated (Sham group). Prior to the experiment and at 9:00 am on the 3rd, 6th, 9th, 12th, 24th week after operation, 1 mL blood was collected and split equally into 2 tubes to separate serum and plasma. One aliquot whole blood was collected in the tube containing EDTA and placed for 15 min. Then plasma was immediately separated by centrifugation at 2000×g for 10 min at 4 °C. (no food but water ad libitum for 12 h). The serum was used for determinating bone alkaline phosphatase (B-ALP, an indicator of bone formation) and N-telopeptide of type I collagen (NTx) levels by ELISA method (Quantikine, R&D Systems, Minneapolis, MN, USA) following the manufacturer's instruction with 6.7% intra- and 8.4% inter-assay variabilities for B-ALP as well as 7.2% intra- and 5.7% inter-assay variabilities for NTx, respectively. The plasma sample was used for metabonomic study. All samples were stored at −80°C until analysis. BMD of the lumbar vertebrae (L1–L5) and left femur from anesthetized rats was measured (isoflurane) by dual-energy X-ray absorptiometry (GE, Lunar ProdigyTM) at the 12th 24th week post-operation. BMD was calculated by dividing the measured area by the bone mineral content (BMC), as previously reported [30]. Baseline of BMD was determined 1 week before surgery. All rats were weighed prior to surgical operation and monitored weekly post surgical operation. Uterine tissues were removed and weighed immediately to calculate uterus indexes by dividing the uterus weight by the body weight after rats were sacrificed. Meanwhile, the serum level of estradiol was analyzed immediately by ELISA method following the ELISA kit manufacturer's instruction.

3. Metabolomic Research

3.1 Sample preparation. A 50 μL aliquot of plasma in an eppendorf tube was spiked with 200 uL methanol containing internal standard myristic-1, 2-$^{13}C_2$ acid (12.5 μg/ml) to deproteinize. After the mixture was vortexed for 3 min, the mixture was centrifuged for 10 min at 12000×g at 4°C. One hundred microliter of the supernatant was transferred into a GC vial, followed by being evaporated to dryness under vacuum in speedvac concentrator (Thermo Fisher Scientific, Asheville, USA). Subsequently, The residue was reconstituted in 30 μl methoxyamine in pyridine (15 mg/ml) and vortexed for 2 min. Methoximation reaction was performed at room temperature for 16 h, before trimethylsilylation for 1 h by adding 30 μl MSTFA with 1% TMCS as catalyst. Finally, the solution was vortexed for 30 s after methyl myristate in heptane (30 μg/ml), the external standard, was added to the GC vial. One microliter of solution was used for GC-TOF/MS analysis.

3.2 GC-TOF/MS analysis. One microliter of the derivatized sample was injected into an Agilent 6980 GC equipped with an Agilent 7683 Series autosampler (Agilent, Atlanta, GA, USA).-Chromatographic separation was conducted on a fused-silica capillary column (10 m×0.18 mm ID) chemically bonded with a 0.18 μm DB5-MS stationary phase (J&W Scientific, Folsom, CA, USA). Helium was served as carrier gas through the column. Mass spectra were detected and obtained by using Pegasus III TOF/MS (Leco).The gas flow rate through the column was 1 mL/min. The column initial temperature was kept at 70°C for 2 min. Temperature was increased from 70°C to 310°C at a rate of 20°C/min and held for 2 min. The transfer line temperature and ion source temperature were controlled at 250°C and 200°C, respectively. Ion source voltage and current: 70 eV at a current of 3.0 mA. The MS data were acquired in scan mode over the range between m/z 50 and 800 at a rate of 20 spectra/s, the acceleration voltage was turned on after a solvent delay of 170 s and the acceleration voltage was turned on at1,650 v [26,27].

3.3 Data collection and processing. All GC/MS data was processed using ChromaTOF (version 3.25) software (Leco). Peak width in automatic peak detection and mass spectrum deconvolution were set to 2 s. Peaks with signal-to-noise (S/N) ratios lower than 30 were rejected. To obtain accurate peak areas for IS and specific peaks/compounds, one quant mass were specified for each peak and the data were reprocessed according to previous report, and each peak area was normalized using IS before multivariate data analysis. All compounds were identified and assigned by comparison of mass spectra and retention index of all detected compounds with the authentic reference standards and those in the NIST library 2.0 (2005), Wiley library, and in-house mass spectra library database established by the Key Laboratory of Drug Metabolism and Pharmacokinetics in China Pharmaceutical University [24,28].

Before multivariate data analysis, the peak area ratio of each compound to a corresponding internal standard was calculated as the response. Then, the data were imported to SIMCA-P v11.5 software (Umetrics AB, Sweden) for multivariate data analysis. Partial least squares-discriminant analysis (PLS-DA) and Principal component analysis (PCA) were used for modeling metabonomic data from Sham group and OVX group.

Data obtained from BMD, body weight, commercial assay kits were presented as the mean ± SD. The data were analyzed using one-way analysis of variance followed by a least significant difference (LSD) test at $P<0.01$ and $P<0.05$.

Results

1. Body Weight, Uterine Index and E2

The representative change tendency of body weight during the whole experiment period is listed in Table 1. The body weights of rats in OVX group were significantly higher than those in Sham group starting at 4th week post operation. Estrogen deficiency caused atrophy of uterine tissue, and serum E2 levels of rats in OVX group significantly deceased at the end of experiment compared with those in Sham group (shown in Table 1). Both data indicated the successful surgical procedure.

2. Bone Mineral Density Measurement

As shown in Table 1, at the12th week and 24th week after OVX, using DEXA analysis, significant decrease in BMD values for both the femur ($P<0.05$ for 12 weeks and $P<0.05$ for 24 weeks) and the lumbar vertebrae ($P<0.05$ for 12 weeks and $P<0.01$ for 24 weeks) were observed in rats in OVX group compared with those in Sham group.

3. Biochemical Studies

Estrogen deficiency resulted in gradual increase in serum B-ALP and NTx in OVX rats after surgery. B-ALP and NTx of rats in OVX group significantly increased since the 12th week ($P<0.05$) and 9th week ($P<0.05$) post operation, respectively, compared with those in Sham group(shown in Figure 1A and 1B). The results indicated that OVX rat had the characteristic of bone high turnover rate according to the previous reports [29,30].

4. Metabolic Changes in Plasma Samples by GC-TOF/MS

Distinct differences of the major metabolites levels between the OVX and Sham groups were observed in GC-TOF/MS chromatogram, shown in Figure 2A and Figure 2B. PCA (data not shown) and PLS-DA were performed to further discern the presence of inherent similarities in chromatographic profiles. The PLS-DA score plots (Figure 3A) and 3D plots (Figure 3B) of the metabolites showed the metabolomic movement during the periods of osteoporotic progression including pre-operation, the 3rd, 6th, 9th and 12th week post operation (these five time points were marked as M0, M3, M6, M9, and M12 in the figures respectively). The distinguished separations among M0, M3, M6, M9, and M12 were observed clearly. Postoperative plasma metabolomic profiles were observed to be distinguished from preoperative samples starting at the 3rd week. However, classical pathological indexes including BMD, plasma B-ALP and NTx did not appear significant changes still the 9th weeks.

In PLS-DA, the R2X, R2Y and Q2(cum) parameters were used for the model evaluation, representing the explanation, fitness and prediction power respectively. (R2X is the percentage of all GC/TOF-MS response variables explained by the model. R2Y is the percentage of all observation or sample variables explained by the model. Q2 is the percentage of all observation or sample variables predicted by the model). In the PLS-DA score plots (Figure 3A), two principal components (PC1 and PC2) were calculated with the R2X, R2Y and Q2 parameters of 0.449, 0.848 and 0.56, respectively.

Kinetics of metabolic changes in rat plasma before and after bilateral oophorectomy was shown in Figure 4. Plasma levels of alanine, citric acid, succinic acid, and docosahexaenoic acid decreased significantly while homocysteine, branched-chain amino acids (leucine, isoleucine and valine), fatty acids (arachidonic acid and octadecadienoic acid) and cholesterol increased significantly after OVX operation compared with those before operation. It's noted that the level of hydroxyproline was low at the 3rd week post operation, but unexpectedly and significantly increased at the 6th week. Figure 5C described the progression of the osteoporosis analyzed by PLS-DA, that plasma samples at the 12th week were well discriminated from those at the 24th week in OVX group.

The metabolic profiles of OVX and Sham groups at the same period were also analyzed and compared by PLS-DA. It's shown in Figure 5A and Figure 5B that metabolic profiles of OVX and Sham groups separated distinctly at the 12th week and 24th week post operation. Two principal components were calculated with the set of R2X, R2Y and Q2 parameters as 0.335, 0.946 and 0.714, and 0.325, 0.996 and 0.582 respectively. Metabolic changes were listed in Figure 6 and Table 2. In detail, the plasma level of arachidonic acid in OVX group elevated at 12th week (2.5-fold, $P=0.0050$) and 24th week (3.29-fold, $P=0.0023$), compared with that in the homeochronous Sham group. Omega-6 fatty acids-octadecadienoic acid also elevated at 12th week (1.19-fold, $P=0.5302$) and 24th week (1.85-fold, $P=0.0046$). Homocysteine

Table 1. Body weight, BMD, Uterine index, and Serum estradiol from the OVX and the Sham rats.

Parameters		The Sham group	The OVX group
Initial body weight (g)		252.62±11.47	250.72±16.35
Final body weight (g)		326.43±27.66	403.51±32.76**
Initial BMD(g/cm2)	*Femur*	0.210±0.012	0.211±0.010
The 12th week BMD(g/cm2)		0.224±0.019	0.201±0.010*
The 24th week BMD(g/cm2)		0.236±0.017	0.207±0.015*
Initial BMD(g/cm2)	*lumbar vertebrae*	0.202±0.011	0.201±0.015
The 12th week BMD(g/cm2)		0.213±0.016	0.188±0.017*
The 24th week BMD(g/cm2)		0.221±0.022	0.185±0.012**
Uterine index (mg/g)		2.312±0.252	0.532±0.124**
Serum estradiol (pk/mL)		35.53±6.45	13.53±5.47**

Values with a superscript are significantly different from the Sham group (*P<0.05, **P<0.01).

(1.53-fold at the 12th week, $P=0.042$; 1.98-fold at the 24th week $P=0.0442$) and Hydroxyproline (2.2-folds the 12th week, $P=0.0060$; 2.43-folds at the 24th week $P=0.0053$) concomitantly enhanced in plasma. However, the levels of omega-3 fatty acids (docosahexaenoic acid) in OVX group decreased (−1.22-fold P = 0.3508, −1.54-fold P = 0.0012) compared with those in the homeochronous Sham group. Elevated levels of branched-chain amino acids (leucine, isoleucine and valine), cholesterol, tryptophan, cystine and glycerol-3-phosphate were also found at the 12th week and 24thweek. Interestingly, a portion of metabolite changes were different in the12th week and 24th week. The levels of intermediate metabolites of TCA (succinic acid, citric acid and malic acid) significantly decreased at the 12th week, then gradually returned to the normal level at the 24th week.

Discussion

A rat model of estrogen deficiency-induced bone loss was chosen to simulate postmenopausal osteoporosis. Comprehensive analysis of changes in the plasma metabolic profile was performed to determine step-wise disease progression from normal conditions to estrogen deficiency and eventually to bone loss.

As shown in Fig. 3A and Fig. 3B, distinct changes were observed from GC-TOF/MS chromatograms in OVX and Sham groups. Further investigations in biomarkers identification were performed and significant differences were shown in Table 2. The alteration of these molecules including amino acids, carbohydrates, fatty acids and cholesterol suggested that they might play certain roles in the etiology of postmenopausal osteoporosis. The early detection of metabolic changes linked to the onset of disease suggested that metabolic alterations might precede BMD and other related diagnostic indexes, and metabolomics might be a sensitive technology to diagnose osteoporosis superior to the classical pathology indexes.

Metabolite fingerprinting obtained from metabolomics could be applied not only to early diagnosis of diseases, but also to identify the causes of disease via biomarker index. Metabolic biomarkers identified by GC-TOF/MS would be beneficial to systemically understand the mechanisms of postmenopausal osteoporosis and to design the target points of anti-osteoporosis drugs. A great many endogenous molecules including fatty acids, cholesterol, amino acids, and carbohydrates exhibited significant difference in OVX group compared with those in Sham group. In the process of bone loss, the metabolism of fatty acids (octadecadienoic acid,

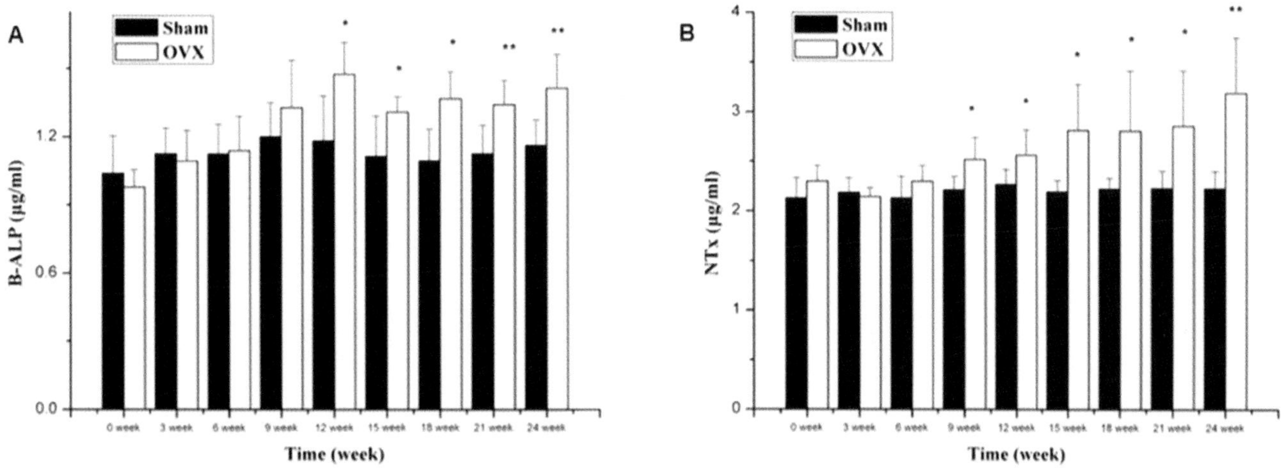

Figure 1. Biochemical parameters in serum. Biochemical parameters in serum from the Sham group and the OVX group over the whole experiment period. The values represent as the Means±SD. N = 8. (*P<0.05, **P<0.01 vs Sham).

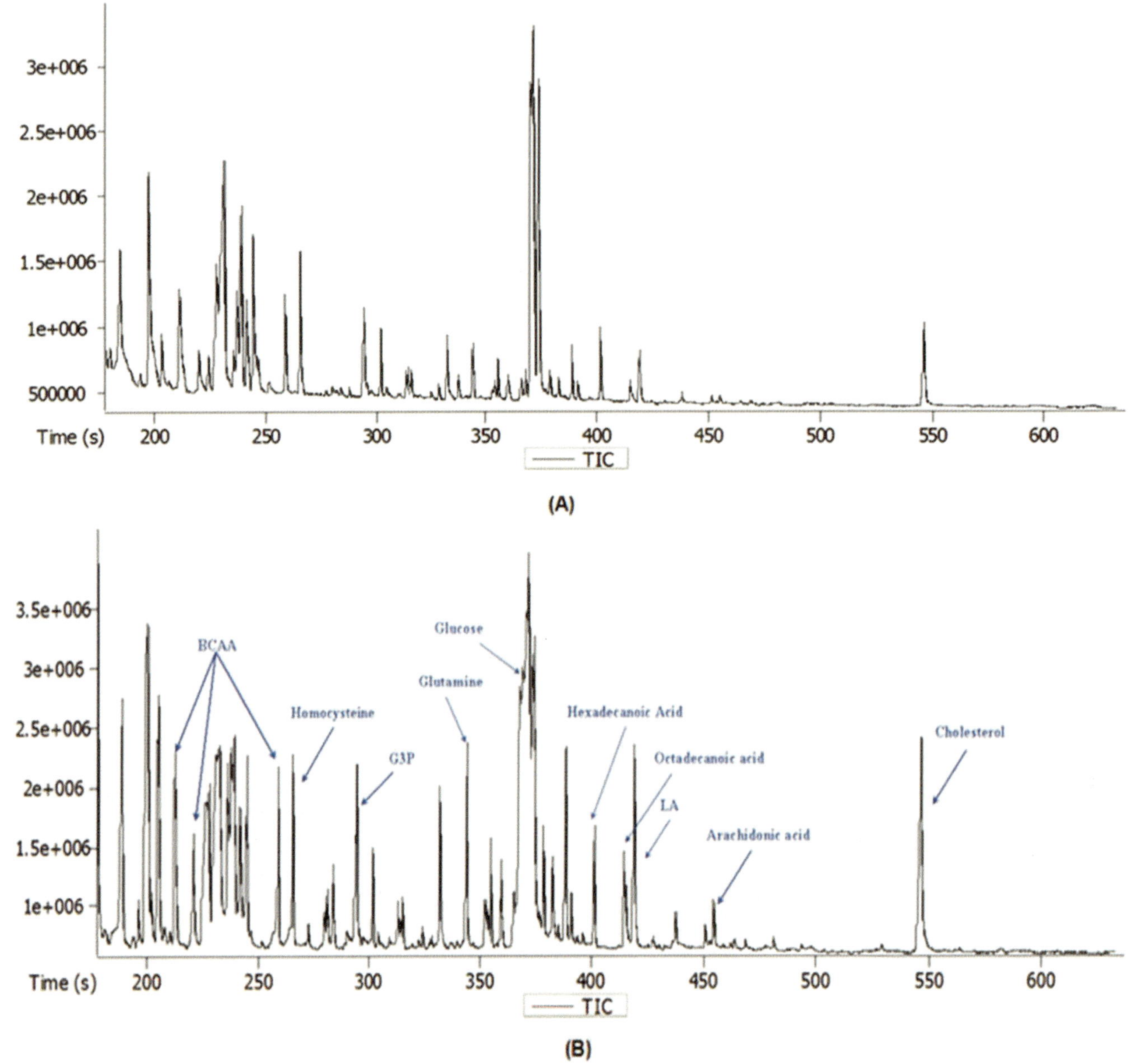

Figure 2. Typical GC-TOF/MS total ion chromatograms of rat plasma. Typical GC-TOF/MS total ion chromatograms of rat plasma obtained from the Sham group (A) and the OVX group (B).

arachidonic acid, oleic acid, docosahexaenoic acid, dodecanoic acid, aminomalonic acid, hexadecanoic acid), homocysteine, branched-chain amino acids (BCAA) and cholesterol were also significantly changed in our research.

Significant increase of the fatty acid levels in the process of bone loss are particularly noted in our metabolomic study. Arachidonic acid (AA, 20:4n-6), the n-6 long chain polyunsaturated fatty acid (LCPUFA), is a precursor of prostaglandins, thromboxanes, and leukotrienes. AA play an important role in the regulation of the metabolism on lipid protein, the body's inflammatory response, muscle growth, blood rheology, elasticity of blood vessels, white blood cell function and platelet activation[31–33]. Meanwhile, AA also affects the bone remodeling process. AA was found to promote osteoclastogenesis by stimulating RANK-L expression and inhibiting OPG secretion by osteoblasts. Its metabolites (prostaglandin and leukotrienes) also affect the bone formation and bone reabsorption. Coetzee et al, indicated that AA inhibited the secretion of OPG by osteoblasts, reduce the OPG/RANKL ratio and may increase osteoclastogenesis and prostaglandin E2 (PGE2), a pro-inflammatory lipid mediator derived from arachidonic acid by the activity of cyclooxygenase (COX), has similar effects on MG-63 and MC3T3-E1 osteoblast-like cells [34]. Moreover, leukotrienes, the fatty signaling molecules derived from arachidonic acid, and particularly IL-1 and IL-6 (potent bone-resorbing cytokines), have been implicated in bone remodeling and disease–specifically in osteoporosis and rheumatoid arthritis[35–37]. Abnormal metabolism pathway of AA due to estrogen deficiency might act as an important factor in the pathogenesis of osteoporosis based on our study data.

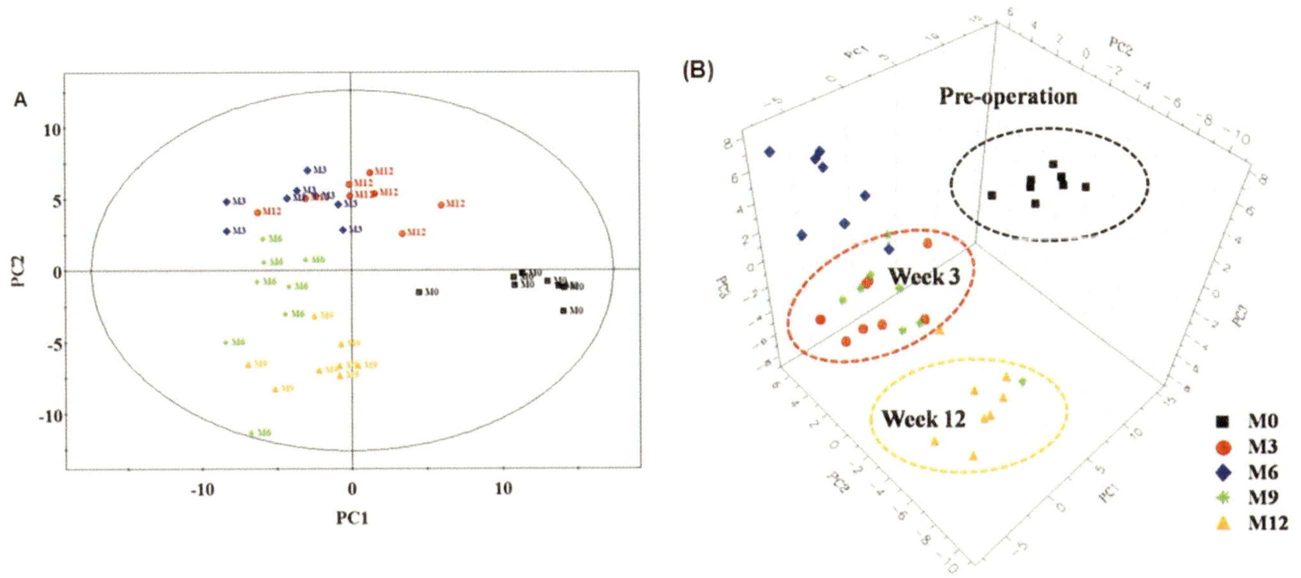

Figure 3. PLS-DA score plots and 3D plots. Partial least squares projection to latent structures and discriminant analysis (PLS-DA) score plots (A: PC1/PC2) and 3D plots (B: PC1/PC2/PC3) of the OVX group over the process of bone loss. X-axis, Y-axis and Z- axis were labeled with PC1 (the first principal component), PC2 (the second principal component), PC3 (the third principal component) respectively. Letters M denotes the OVX group. Numbers 0–12 represents different time points during the experiment: 0, before experiment; 3, week 3; 6, week 6 et al. M3 means the point from the sample in the OVX group at the 3rd week after the experiment. One data point stands for one subject: for instance, M3 and M6 mean the point from the sample in the OVX control rats at the 3rd and 6th week after surgery.

In contrast to AA, the levels of oleic acid and docosahexaenoic acid (DHA, 22:6n-3) decreased in plasma during bone loss induced by estrogen deficiency. An augmentation of the n-6/n-3 polyunsaturated fatty acid ratio was shown to lead to increased bone loss in both animal [38] and human [39]. The elevated levels of the n-6 polyunsaturated fatty acids (AA, Octadecadienoic acid)

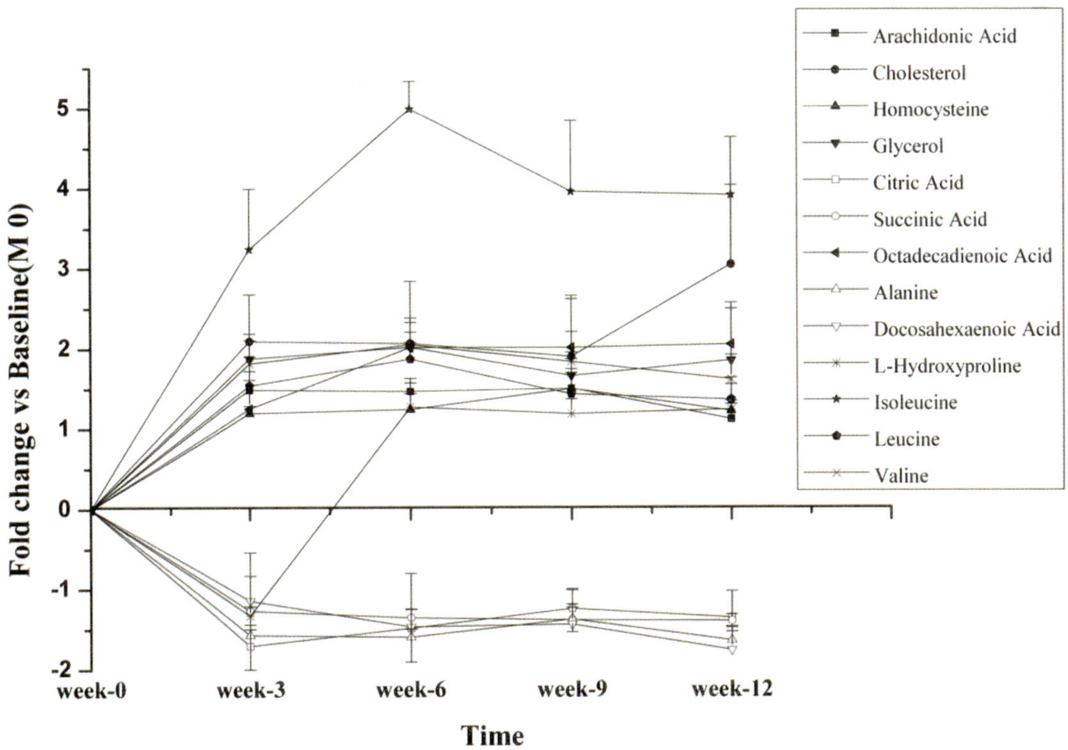

Figure 4. Kinetics of metabolic changes in the OVX plasma. Kinetics of metabolic changes in the OVX plasma over the 12 week post operation.

Table 2. Fold changes and P value of endogenous metabolites detected by GC/TOF-MS.

Metabolites	Retention index	Biological role	12 weeks after surgery		24 weeks after surgery	
			Fold change	*P*	Fold change	*P*
Cholesterol	3178.2	a sterol and a lipid found in the cell membranes	2.02	0.047	1.53	0.006
Octadecadienoic acid	2216.4	an unsaturated n-6 fatty acid and essential fatty acid	1.19	0.533	1.85	0.005
Arachidonic acid	2375.2	a polyunsaturated, essential fatty acid and precursor of prostaglandins, thromboxanes, and leukotrienes	2.25	0.005	3.29	0.002
Oleic acid	2215.3	An unsaturated fatty acid	1.09	0.793	1.72	0.013
9-(Z)-Hexadecenoic Acid	2029.7	an unsaturated fatty acid, a common constituent of the glycerides of adipose tissue	1.29	0.031	1.36	0.009
Hexadecanoic Acid	2049.2	a saturated fatty acid	−1.16	0.401	1.54	0.010
Octadecanoic Acid	2245.6	a saturated fatty acid	−1.10	0.340	1.18	0.047
Docosahexaenoic Acid	2566.9	an omega-3 fatty acid and associated with the heart disease	−1.22	0.350	−1.54	0.001
Glycerol	1282.4	an important component of triglycerides and of phospholipids, energy metabolism	1.18	0.362	1.43	0.013
Isoleucine	1305.8	Essential branched-chain aliphatic amino acid associated with energy metabolism and blood sugar regulation	1.24	0.012	1.78	0.018
Valine	1230.8		1.37	0.042	2.14	0.010
Leucine	1285.2		1.43	0.035	1.62	0.004
homocysteine	1437.9	sulfur-containing amino acid, associated with cardiovascular disease, Alzheimer's disease and fracture	1.53	0.042	1.98	0.044
L-Hydroxyproline	1522.4	a common non-proteinogenic amino acid and Paget's disease	2.20	0.006	2.43	0.005
Tryptophan	2244.0	an essential amino acid which is the precursor of serotonin	1.03	0.780	−1.44	0.001
Glutamine	1608.8	energy metabolism, nitrogen balances	1.01	0.969	−1.24	0.022
Cystine	1433.9	immune function and the synthesis of glutathione	1.61	0.030	1.44	0.226
Glycine	1438.4	a simple, nonessential amino acid	1.27	0.039	1.15	0.837
Alanine	1107.5	An important participant and regulator in glucose metabolism	−2.79	0.005	−2.77	0.017
Succinic Acid	1323.2	citric acid cycle, Glucose metabolism	−2.47	0.022	−1.14	0.814
Citric Acid	1844.1		−1.30	0.043	−1.21	0.071
Malic Acid	1502.8		−2.50	0.042	−1.26	0.797
Glucose	1935.6	a monosaccharide containing six carbon atoms	1.15	0.010	1.06	0.318
L-Lysine	1720.8	an essential amino acid	−1.89	0.011	−1.76	0.002
Ethanedioic Acid	1144.9	glyoxylic acid or ascorbic acid metabolism	1.79	0.004	1.25	0.302
2-Hydroxy-Butanoic Acid	1137.3	an organic acid that is involved in propanoate metabolism	−6.88	0.012	−2.26	0.007
Dodecanoic Acid	1656.1	a component of triglycerides	−1.54	0.023	1.24	0.026
2-Aminobutyric Acid	1185.5	a key intermediate in the biosynthesis of ophthalmic acid or ophthalmate.	−3.16	0.012	−3.67	0.003
3-Hydroxybutyric- Acid	1172.8	ketone body	−1.24	0.425	1.43	0.010
Glycerol-3-Phosphate	1787.1	a chemical intermediate in the glycolysis metabolic pathway	1.10	0.320	1.38	0.044

and decreased levels of n-3 polyunsaturated fatty acids (Docosahexaenoic acid) also supported these results.

In our previous study, significant elevated levels of plasma cholesterol were found in estrogen deficiency-induced obesity in ovariectomized rats [25]. Enhanced levels of cholesterol and increased body weight were also observed in bone loss rats induced by estrogen deficiency in the current study. Enhanced cholesterol uptake and biosynthesis or inhibition of cholesterol oxidation might explain the reason why estrogen deficiency increased total cholesterol accumulation in plasma. And, the negative relationship between estrogen and cholesterol might be an important index in the process of the menopause for the high incidence of cardiovascular disease, dementia, Alzheimer's disease, type 2 diabetes and osteoporosis in menopausal women [40]. Cholesterol and its metabolites would suppress the functional activity of osteoblasts and thereby induce reduced bone mineralization to decrease bone formation [41]. By the same token, high cholesterol diet increases the risk of osteoporosis, possible via inhibiting the differentiation and proliferation of osteoblasts in rats, as You et al observed [42]. At present, the drug treatment against osteoporosis can prevent bone loss, as well as lowering cholesterol levels. Arzoxifene, a new selective estrogen receptor modulator (SERM),

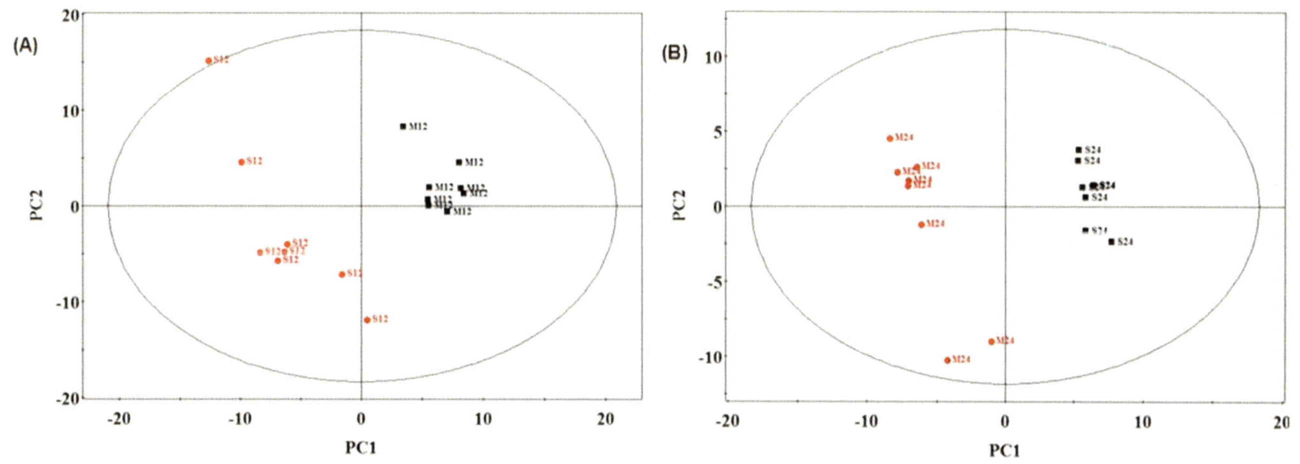

Figure 5. PLS-DA score plots of plasma samples. (A) PLS-DA score plots of OVX rats and sham rats at the 12th weeks post-surgery; (B) PLS-DA score plots of OVX rats and sham rats at the 24th weeks post-surgery; (C) PLS-DA score plots of OVX rats between the 12th weeks and 24th week post surgery. Letters M and S denotes the OVX group and the Sham group, respectively. Numbers 12 and 24 represents different time points during the experiment: 12, week 12; 24, week 24.

maintained bone formation, prevented bone loss by decreasing osteoclast number following by reducing serum cholesterol in OVX rats in Ma and co-workers' study [43]. Statins, the enzyme HMG-CoA reductase inhibitors, initially used for treating hyperlipidemia, were recently observed not only to prevent fractures, but also trigger significant bone re-growth. From the mechanistic point of views, statins were found to inhibit mevalonate synthesis, prevent the synthesis of cholesterol and indirectly further alter osteoblasts and osteoclast activity, its direct biologic action also affect on osteoblast activity by stimulating gene expression of bone morphogenetic protein-2 [44,45].

For the amino acids metabolism, above all, homocysteine levels significantly increased in OVX group compared to the Sham group. Homocysteine is a non-protein amino acid biosynthesized from methionine by the removal of its terminal Cε methyl group and recycled into methionine or converted into cysteine with the aid of B-vitamins. Homocysteine is still considered as part of a screen for people at the high risk of heart attack or stroke in clinics. A negative relationship between exogenous estrogen change and homocysteine levels was observed in post-menopause women, and estrogen blocking homocysteine-induced endothelial dysfunction in porcine coronary arteries was reported by Todd [46]. In our study, a gradually increasing homocysteine level followed by decreasing estrogen concentrations was found in plasma after ovaries removed. A positive correlation of homocysteine and osteoporosis was also observed in metabolomic profiles. The research led by McLean and Jacques indicated homocysteine could be a predictive factor for osteoporotic fracture in older persons [47]. For the correlation of homocysteine levels and osteoporosis, recent *in vitro* studies performed in mouse bone marrow cells have suggested that homocysteine directly stimulates osteoclast formation and activity (upregulated TRACP+ multinu-

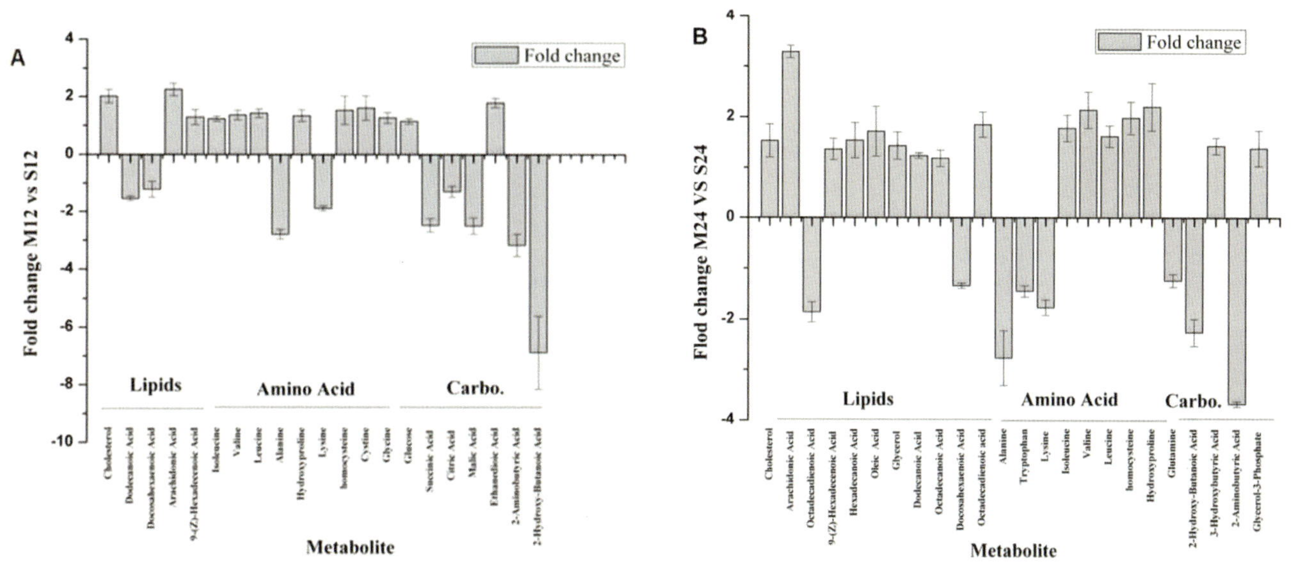

Figure 6. Relative changes of plasma metabolite levels. Relative changes of plasma metabolite levels in the sham group versus the OVX group at the 12th weeks and 24th weeks post surgery.

cleated cells and TRACP activity) by inducing p38 MAPK activity and intracellular reactive oxygen species (ROS) generation, which is a risk factor for osteoporosis and fracture [48]. An increased homocysteine level in plasma was mainly attributed to the lack of estrogen caused in postmenopausal osteoporosis. In terms of specific biochemistry pathways, estrogen influenced metabolism transformation between methionine and homocysteine, especially interfering with the transsulfuration pathway. Estrogen could enhance cystathionine-β-synthase activity and directed homocysteine metabolism to form cysteine and glutathione to eliminate homocysteine and prevent its accumulation, that may act as a key aspect in elucidating this phenomenon [49].

It suggested that homocysteine could be a potential biomarker in diagnosis, and treatment against postmenopausal osteoporosis. Some anti-osteoporosis drugs such as strontium ranelate [50], raloxifene [51] etc, could inhibit increased homocysteine levels in plasma induced by estrogen deficiency and reduce the risk of osteoporosis. Therefore, homocysteine enhancing excretion of amino acids might be a strong indicator in both post-menopause and osteoporosis, and could be a potential target point or a key factor of upper stream controller for anti-osteoporosis treatment.

Hydroxyproline is a major component of the protein collagen and plays key role for collagen stability. Some research suggested that increased serum and urine levels of hydroxyproline had been demonstrated in Paget's disease bone [52,53]. Meanwhile, mean plasma levels of branched-chain amino acids (BCAA, leucine, isoleucine, and valine) raised rapidly in the first three week after OVX and remained significantly elevated ($p<0.05$ versus sham-operated controls) for the entire 24 week. Overall, these observations indicated that increased homocysteine and hydroxyproline levels in OVX rats, besides increased accumulation of BCAA, may be potential biomarkers of postmenopausal osteoporosis.

Estrogen deficiency is the main reason of post-menopause osteoporosis. So, we used OVX rats, which are golden standard models of the post-menopause osteoporosis, to study the estrogen deficiency-induced bone loss and got the metabolomic profiles to delineate signature metabolic shifts during the progress of the estrogen deficiency. On the other hand, estrogen is involved in the regulation of many physiological functions of the body. Estrogen deficiency also induces other physical changes such as obesity. Therefore, on the basis of the current results, the further studies, that could link the metabolites found in this study to the osteoblasts or osteoclasts which are essential to the bone loss, should be carried out to confirm the specific biomarkers on estrogen deficiency-induced bone loss.

Conclusion

The global metabolomics approach applied in our research demonstrated that estrogen deficiency-induced bone loss resulted in a marked change in the plasma metabolic profile that appeared earlier than the known biomarkers of postmenopausal osteoporosis, such as BMD and serum B-ALP and NTx. In the preclinical osteoporosis model, significant changes of endogenous metabolites and specific metabolites were identified which not only regulated bone remodel effects, but also pointed to the mechanisms of disease etiology and progression. Further efforts should focuse on the validation of our findings and identification of genuine biomarkers from spurious biomarkers through preclinical and clinic study.

Author Contributions

Conceived and designed the experiments: QZ HJY. Performed the experiments: BM JNL JGS YLW JL YHL. Analyzed the data: JYA. Contributed reagents/materials/analysis tools: QZ HJY. Wrote the paper: BM JYA DW.

References

1. Villareal DT, Binder EF, Williams DB, Schechtman KB, Yarasheski KE, et al. (2001) Bone mineral density response to estrogen replacement in frail elderly women: a randomized controlled trial. JAMA 286: 815–820.
2. Hillier TA, Stone KL, Bauer DC, Rizzo JH, Pedula KL, et al. (2007) Evaluating the value of repeat bone mineral density measurement and prediction of fractures in older women: the study of osteoporotic fractures. Arch Intern Med 167: 155–160.
3. Gourlay ML, Fine JP, Preisser JS, May RC, Li C, et al. (2012) Bone-density testing interval and transition to osteoporosis in older women. N Engl J Med 366: 225–233.
4. Kahl KG, Rudolf S, Stoeckelhuber BM, Dibbelt L, Gehl HB, et al. (2005) Bone mineral density, markers of bone turnover, and cytokines in young women with borderline personality disorder with and without comorbid major depressive disorder. Am J Psychiatry 162: 168–174.
5. Bhattacharyya S, Siegel ER, Achenbach SJ, Khosla S, Suva LJ (2008) Serum biomarker profile associated with high bone turnover and BMD in postmenopausal women. J Bone Miner Res 23: 1106–1117.
6. Reginster JY, Collette J, Neuprez A, Zegels B, Deroisy R, et al. (2008) Role of biochemical markers of bone turnover as prognostic indicator of successful osteoporosis therapy. Bone 42: 832–836.
7. Vasikaran SD (2008) Utility of biochemical markers of bone turnover and bone mineral density in management of osteoporosis. Crit Rev Clin Lab Sci 45: 221–258.
8. Abe Y, Ishikawa H, Fukao A (2008) Higher efficacy of urinary bone resorption marker measurements in assessing response to treatment for osteoporosis in postmenopausal women. Tohoku J Exp Med 214: 51–59.
9. Nicholson JK, Lindon JC. (2008) Systems biology: Metabonomics. Nature 455: 1054–1056.
10. Leslie RD, Beyan H (2011) Metabolomics makes a mark: early changes associated with autoimmune diabetes. Diabetes 60: 2688–2690.
11. Patel VR, Eckel-Mahan K, Sassone-Corsi P, Baldi P (2012) CircadiOmics: integrating circadian genomics, transcriptomics, proteomics and metabolomics. Nat Methods 9: 772–773.
12. Patti GJ, Yanes O, Siuzdak G (2012) Innovation: Metabolomics: the apogee of the omics trilogy. Nat Rev Mol Cell Biol 13: 263–269.
13. Sreekumar A, Poisson LM, Rajendiran TM, Khan AP, Cao Q, et al. (2009) Metabolomic profiles delineate potential role for sarcosine in prostate cancer progression. Nature 457: 910–914.
14. Patti GJ, Yanes O, Shriver LP, Courade JP, Tautenhahn R, et al. (2012) Metabolomics implicates altered sphingolipids in chronic pain of neuropathicorigin. Nat Chem Biol 8: 232–234.
15. Shi X, Yao D, Chen C (2012) Identification of N-Acetyltaurine as a Novel Metabolite of Ethanol throughMetabolomics-guided Biochemical Analysis. J Biol Chem 287: 6336–6349.
16. Chen C, Shah YM, Morimura K, Krausz KW, Miyazaki M, et al. (2008) Metabolomics reveals that hepatic stearoyl-CoA desaturase 1 downregulation exacerbates inflammation and acute colitis. Cell Metab 7: 135–147.
17. Bonnelye E, Aubin JE (2005) Estrogen receptor-related receptor alpha: a mediator of estrogen response in bone. J Clin Endocrinol Metab 90: 3115–3121.
18. Hofbauer LC, Schoppet M (2004) Clinical implications of the osteoprotegerin/RANKL/RANK system for bone and vascular diseases. JAMA 292: 490–495.
19. Pacifici R, Vannice JL, Rifas L, Kimble RB (1993) Monocytic secretion of interleukin-1 receptor antagonist in normal and osteoporotic women: effects of menopause and estrogen/progesterone therapy. J Clin Endocrinol Metab;77: 1135–1141.
20. Wauquier F, Leotoing L, Coxam V, Guicheux J, Wittrant Y (2009) Oxidative stress in bone remodelling and disease. Trends Mol Med 15: 468–477.
21. Lu Y, A J, Wang G, Hao H, Huang Q, et al. (2008) Gas chromatography/time-of-flight mass spectrometry based metabonomic approach to differentiating hypertension- and age-related metabolic variation in spontaneously hypertensive rats. Rapid Commun Mass Spectrom 22: 2882–2888.
22. Zhang Q, Wang G, A J, Ma B, Dua Y, et al. (2010) Metabonomic profiling of diet-induced hyperlipidaemia in a rat model. Biomarkers 15: 205–216.
23. A J, Qian S, Wang G, Yan B, Zhang S, et al. (2010) Chronic myeloid leukemia patients sensitive and resistant to imatinib treatment show different metabolic responses. PLOS ONE 5: e13186.
24. Yan B, A J, Wang G, Lu H, Huang X, et al. (2009) Metabolomic investigation into variation of endogenous metabolites in professional athletes subject to strength-endurance training. J Appl Physiol 106: 531–538.

25. Ma B, Zhang Q, Wang GJ, A JY, Wu D, et al. (2011) GC-TOF/MS-based metabolomic profiling of estrogen deficiency-induced obesity in ovariectomized rats. Acta Pharmacol Sin 32: 270–278.
26. Liu L, Aa J, Wang G, Yan B, Zhang Y, et al. (2010) Differences in metabolite profile between blood plasma and serum. Anal Biochem 406: 105–112.
27. A J, Trygg J, Gullberg J, Johansson AI, Jonsson P, et al. (2005) Extraction and GC/MS analysis of the human blood plasma metabolome. Anal Chem 77: 8086–8094.
28. Jonsson P, Johansson AI, Gullberg J, Trygg J, A J, et al. (2005) High-throughput data analysis for detecting and identifying differences between samples in GC/MS-based metabolomic analyses. Anal Chem 77: 5635–5642.
29. Garnero P, Sornay-Rendu E, Chapuy MC, Delmas PD. (1996) Increased bone turnover in late postmenopausal women is a major determinant of osteoporosis. J Bone Miner Res 11: 337–349.
30. Ma B, Zhang Q, Wu D, Wang YL, Hu YY, et al. (2012) Strontium fructose 1,6-diphosphate prevents bone loss in a rat model of postmenopausal osteoporosis via the OPG/RANKL/RANK pathway. Acta Pharmacol Sin 33: 479–489.
31. Patel MI, Kurek C, Dong Q (2008) The arachidonic acid pathway and its role in prostate cancer development and progression. J Urol 179: 1668–1675.
32. Zordoky BN, El-Kadi AO (2010) Effect of cytochrome P450 polymorphism on arachidonic acid metabolism and their impact on cardiovascular diseases. Pharmacol Ther 125: 446–463.
33. Harizi H, Corcuff JB, Gualde N (2008) Arachidonic-acid-derived eicosanoids: roles in biology and immunopathology. Trends Mol Med 14: 461–469.
34. Coetzee M, Haag M, Kruger MC (2007) Effects of arachidonic acid, docosahexaenoic acid, prostaglandin E(2) and parathyroid hormone on osteoprotegerin and RANKL secretion by MC3T3-E1 osteoblast-like cells. J Nutr Biochem 2007 18: 54–63.
35. Tilg H, Moschen AR, Kaser A, Pines A, Dotan I (2008) Gut, inflammation and osteoporosis: basic and clinical concepts. Gut 57: 684–694.
36. Pacifici R, Rifas L, Teitelbaum S, Slatopolsky E, McCracken R, et al. (1987) Spontaneous release of interleukin 1 from human blood monocytes reflects bone formation in idiopathic osteoporosis. Proc Natl Acad Sci U S A 84: 4616–4620.
37. Abrahamsen B, Bonnevie-Nielsen V, Ebbesen EN, Gram J, Beck-Nielsen H (2000) Cytokines and bone loss in a 5-year longitudinal study–hormone replacement therapy suppresses serum soluble interleukin-6 receptor and increases interleukin-1-receptor antagonist: the Danish Osteoporosis Prevention Study. J Bone Miner Res 15: 1545–1554.
38. Watkins BA, Li Y, Allen KG, Hoffmann WE, Seifert MF (2000) Dietary ratio of (n-6)/(n-3) polyunsaturated fatty acids alters the fatty acid composition of bone compartments and biomarkers of bone formation in rats. J Nutr 130: 2274–2284.
39. Weiss LA, Barrett-Connor E, von Mühlen D (2005) Ratio of n-6 to n-3 fatty acids and bone mineral density in older adults: the Rancho Bernardo Study. Am J Clin Nutr 81: 934–938.
40. Omoigui S (2005) Cholesterol synthesis is the trigger and isoprenoid dependent interleukin-6 mediated inflammation is the common causative factor and therapeutic target for atherosclerotic vascular disease and age-related disorders including osteoporosis and type 2 diabetes. Med Hypotheses 65: 559–569.
41. Parhami F, Mody N, Gharavi N, Ballard AJ, Tintut Y (2002) Role of the cholesterol biosynthetic pathway in osteoblastic differentiation of marrow stromal cells. J Bone Miner Res 17: 1997–2003.
42. You L, Sheng ZY, Tang CL, Chen L, Pan L, et al. (2011) High cholesterol diet increases osteoporosis risk via inhibiting bone formation in rats. Acta Pharmacol Sin 32: 1498–1504.
43. Ma YL, Bryant HU, Zeng Q, Palkowitz A, Jee WS, et al. (2002) Long-term dosing of arzoxifene lowers cholesterol, reduces bone turnover, and preserves bone quality in ovariectomized rats. J Bone Miner Res 17: 2256–2264.
44. Whitney C, Warburton DE, Frohlich J, Chan SY, McKay H, et al. (2004) Are cardiovascular disease and osteoporosis directly linked. Sports Med 34: 779–807.
45. Jinno Y, Ayukawa Y, Ogino Y, Atsuta I, Tsukiyama Y, et al. (2009) Vertical bone augmentation with fluvastatin in an injectable delivery system: a rat study. Clin Oral Implants Res 20: 756–760.
46. Spencer TA, Chai H, Fu W, Ramaswami G, Cox MW, et al. (2004) Estrogen blocks homocysteine-induced endothelial dysfunction in porcine coronary arteries. J Surg Res 118: 83–90.
47. McLean RR, Jacques PF, Selhub J, Tucker KL, Samelson EJ, et al. (2004) Homocysteine as a predictive factor for hip fracture in older persons. N Engl J Med 350: 2042–2049.
48. Koh JM, Lee YS, Kim YS, Kim DJ, Kim HH, et al. (2006) Homocysteine enhances bone resorption by stimulation of osteoclast formation and activity through increased intracellular ROS generation. J Bone Miner Res 21: 1003–1011.
49. Dimitrova KR, DeGroot K, Myers AK, Kim YD (2002) Estrogen and homocysteine. Cardiovasc Res 53: 577–588.
50. Bayhan I, Uygur D, Ugurlu N, Ozaksit G (2009)Strontium ranelate decreases plasma homocysteine levels in postmenopausal osteoporotic women. Rheumatol Int 29: 263–266.
51. De Leo V, la Marca A, Morgante G, Lanzetta D, Setacci C, et al. (2001) Randomized control study of the effects of raloxifene on serum lipids and homocysteine in older women. Am J Obstet Gynecol 184: 350–353.
52. Ferrandez L, Martin M, Fernandez M (1990) Calcitonin, estradiol, and hydroxyproline as parameters in the early diagnosis of involutional osteoporosis. The importance of the "second calcitonin phenomenon". Arch Orthop Trauma Surg 109: 181–185.
53. Schmolke B (2001) Laboratory diagnosis of osteoporosis. Orthopade 30: 425–436.

Relationship between Bone Mineral Density and Serum Osteoprotegerin in Patients with Chronic Heart Failure

Ying-Hsien Chen[1,2], Yen-Wen Wu[1,2,3,6]❡, Wei-Shiung Yang[1,2], Shoei-Shen Wang[1,4], Chi-Ming Lee[1,2,5], Nai-Kuan Chou[1,4], Ron-Bin Hsu[1,4], Yen-Hung Lin[1,2], Mao-Shin Lin[1,2], Yi-Lwun Ho[1,2]*❡, Ming-Fong Chen[1,2]

1 National Taiwan University College of Medicine, Taipei, Taiwan, **2** Department of Internal Medicine, National Taiwan University Hospital, Taipei, Taiwan, **3** Department of Nuclear Medicine, National Taiwan University Hospital, Taipei, Taiwan, **4** Department of Surgery, National Taiwan University Hospital, Taipei, Taiwan, **5** Cardiovascular Center, National Taiwan University Hospital Yun-Lin Branch, Dou-Liu City, Taiwan, **6** Department of Nuclear Medicine, Far Eastern Memorial Hospital, New Taipei City, Taiwan

Abstract

Purpose: Heart failure (HF) had been reported with increased risk of hip fractures. However, the relationship between circulating biomarkers and bone mineral density (BMD) in chronic HF remained unclear.

Methods: This is a cross-sectional study which recruited stable chronic HF from registry of the Heart Failure Center of National Taiwan University Hospital. Patients underwent dual-energy x-ray absorptiometry (DEXA) measurements at hip and lumbar spines and biochemical assessments including B-type natriuretic peptide (BNP-32), myostatin, follistatin and osteoprotegerin (OPG).

Results: A total of 115 stable chronic HF individuals with left ventricular ejection fraction (EF) <45% (74% of male, mean age at 59) were recruited with 24 patients in NYHA class I, 73 patients in NYHA class II and 18 patients in NYHA class III. Results of BMD showed that Z scores of hip in NYHA III group (-0.12 ± 1.15) was significantly lower than who were NYHA II (0.58 ± 1.04). Serum OPG was significantly higher in subjects of NYHA III (9.3 ± 4.6 pmol/l) than NYHA II (7.4 ± 2.8 pmol/l) or NYHA I (6.8 ± 3.6 pmol/l) groups. There's a significant negative association between log transformed serum OPG and trochanteric BMD ($R=-0.299$, $P=0.001$), which remained significant after multivariate analysis.

Conclusions: Our study demonstrated an inverse association between serum OPG and trochanteric BMD in patients with HF. OPG may be a predictor of BMD and an alternative to DEXA for identifying at risk HF patients for osteoporosis.

Editor: Rajesh Mohanraj, UAE University, Faculty of Medicine & Health Sciences, United Arab Emirates

Funding: The work was supported by National Science Council of Taiwan [NSC 98-2314-B-002-145-MY2] to YW Wu and [NSC 99-2911-I-008-100] to YL Ho and Department of Health, Executive Yuan, R.O.C. [DOH 99-TD-B-111-001] to YL Ho. The funders had no role in study design, data collection and analysis, decision to publish, or preparation of the manuscript.

Competing Interests: The authors have declared that no competing interests exist.

* E-mail: ylho@ntu.edu.tw

❡ These authors contributed equally to this work.

Introduction

Heart failure (HF) and osteoporosis, both as disabling conditions, are two common chronic conditions in elderly which are gaining importance for healthcare recently due to the associated significant morbidity and mortality [1]. These two disabling conditions adversely affect quality of life especially in frail elderly individuals. From recent large epidemiological study, HF is associated with a substantial increase in osteoporotic fractures, particularly in the hip region [2]. In addition to decreased physical performance in HF and sharing a number of common risk factors [3] such as older age, smoking, renal insufficiency and type 2 diabetes, accelerated bone loss may also come from altered vitamin D levels, hyperparathyroidism [4] elevated aldosterone levels [5], elevated fibrotic markers [6] and loop diuretics use in subjects with HF [7]. Cardiac cachexia-related biomarkers including adiponection, follistatin and myostatin had been investigated in muscle, fat, and bone metabolism in heart failure metabolism [8], however, the relationship between circulating biomarkers and bone mineral density (BMD) in chronic HF remained unclear. To the best of our knowledge, HF is a clinical syndrome characterized by prolonged activation of the neuroendocrine system ranging from sympathoadrenal system, natriuretic peptides, renin-angiotensin-aldosterone system (RAAS) and to updated markers of osteoprotegerin (OPG) [9]. The higher OPG level predicts poor prognosis in subjects with HF with higher all-cause mortality and hospitalization for worsening of HF [10]. OPG has also been reported to be associated with neuroendocrine activation in elderly males with systolic HF [11] which makes believe that there were interaction among HF and osteoporosis through systemic hormonal activation. However, a direct causal association between these circulating biomarkers and osteoporosis or risk of fractures has not been established in elderly patients with chronic HF, nor does these associations hold true in all HF patients. Therefore, the present study was aimed to evaluate the associations between osteoporosis and HF in elderly patients, and to assess the circulating biomarkers on this association.

Methods

Patients

The registry of the specialized clinic of the Heart Failure Center of National Taiwan University Hospital since Aug. 2008 formed the basis for this study. All patients attending the clinic for the evaluation of heart failure were asked to participate in the registry and provide written informed consent for data storage and evaluation. The diagnosis of heart failure was based on the criteria of symptoms compatible with the diagnosis in the presence of objective evidence of systolic dysfunction which defined by left ventricular ejection fraction (LVEF) below 45% from echocardiography, radionuclide angiography and/or cine angiography. A total of 115 subjects with stable chronic systolic dysfunction were eligible and agreed to participate between January and October 2009. The main exclusion criteria were age <18 or >90 years old, residence outside the Great Taipei region, history of any non-traumatic fracture, metallic prosthesis/fixation at hip or lumbar spines, renal insufficiency with creatinine >3.0 mg/dL, advanced non-cardiac diseases or malignancy with an expected life expectancy less than 1 year, connective tissue or musculoskeletal diseases, significant liver, thyroid, adrenal gland or pituitary diseases, inability to ambulate, or taking hormone replacement therapy or steroids, unwillingness to participate or provide blood samples.

Ethics Statement

The study protocol was approved by the Institutional Review Board at National Taiwan university Hospital before the initiation of the study. Written form informed consent was obtained from all participating patients.

Study Design

A physical examination was performed to assess HF severity and New York Heart Association (NYHA) class and patients were classified accordingly. All participants were interrogated for cause of HF, medication history, smoking, alcohol abuse, additional comorbidities and previous falls and or fractures. Biochemical data within 3 months and echocardiography within six months were recorded. A priori medication classes of interest included angiotensin-converting enzyme inhibitors, angiotensin receptor blockers, beta-blockers, calcium channel blockers, lipid lower agents (statins, fibrates), antiplatelet agents, long-acting nitrate preparations, diuretics, spironolactone and thiazide diuretics.

Bone Mineral Density (BMD) Measurements

BMD measurements using Dual-Energy X-ray Absorptiometry (DEXA, Norland XR-26, USA) were performed according standard protocols by a single experienced operator. Hip with femoral neck, trochanter, Wards Triangle and lumbar spines over L2–L4 regions were measured and expressed as g/cm^2. The coefficient of variation of BMD measurement at the hip and lumbar spine was <1%. The difference between an individual's BMD and the mean BMD for a reference population are expressed in standard deviation (SD) units. Z- and T-scores were calculated where the Z-score is the S.D. of the individual's BMD compared to the mean BMD score of a similar sex-, age-, weight- and height matched population and the T-score is the S.D. of the individual's BMD compared with the mean BMD score in a young healthy population. The coefficient of variation for DEXA was less than 3% in our lab. [12]

Circulating Biomarkers Assessments

Peripheral venous blood was obtained at 8:00 AM after overnight fasting and refraining from smoking. Serum samples were immediately deep frozen and kept at −70°C until assay. Testing was performed using commercially available kits for brain natriuretic peptide 32 (BNP-32) (Phoenix Pharmaceuticals, Burlingame, CA, USA), high sensitivity C-Reactive Protein (hsCRP) (Chemicon International, Temecula, CA, USA), myostatin (Immundiagnostik AG, Bensheim, Germany), follistatin and Osteoprotegerin (R and D Systems, Minneapolis, MN, USA) following the manufacturer's instructions. The results were interpolated from the standard reference curve provided with each kit. The inter-assay and intra-assay coefficients of variation of all assays were ≤10%, and all laboratory work was undertaken by researchers who were blinded to the patient's clinical details. [13]

Statistical Analysis

Continuous variables are expressed as mean ± SD. One-way ANOVA was used to compare continuous data of three different NYHA functional classes. Categorical variables are compared by Chi-square analysis or Fisher's exact tests and summarized by proportion in each category. Pearson's correlation test was used to analyze the association between bone mineral density and other clinical determinants. Data of blood urea nitrogen, creatinine, fasting glucose, total cholesterol, triglyceride, follistatin, myostatin, high sensitivity C reactive protein, BNP-32, and osteoprotegerin were log-transformed due to non-normality which was tested by the Shapiro-Francia W' test. Significant determinants in the Pearson's correlation test ($P<0.05$) were then tested by a multivariate linear regression test with stepwise subset selection to identify independent factors predicting bone mineral density. All statistical analyses are completed using the STATA 11.0 and SPSS 17.0 software package. A two-sided $P<0.05$ was considered statistically significant.

Results

A total of 115 HF patients (74% of male, mean age at 59) who lived in Great Taipei Region were recruited in the outpatient clinics and grouped according to NYHA functional class. The majority of participants were of NYHA class I and II at the time of clinical evaluation (24 in the state of NYHA function class I, 73 in class II, 18 in class III and none in class IV). The clinical characteristics of patients according to NYHA class are presented in Table 1. There was a tendency of lower LVEF in advanced NYHA class ($P = 0.06$). The demographic characteristics, comorbidities, biochemical lab data and cardiac medications were not significantly different between groups except significantly lower rate of beta blocker use in advanced NYHA class (83% in NYHA class I, 60% in class II, vs. 44% in class III, $P = 0.03$), (Table 1).

Of various circulating biomarkers (Table 1 and Figure 1), only OPG was associated with higher NYHA class ($P = 0.04$). There were no significant group differences in levels of follistatin, hsCRP or BNP-32. The lower myostatin levels were associated with higher NYHA class, but not reaching statistical significance ($P = 0.10$).

BMD measurements of the hip and lumbar spines are shown in Table 1 and Figure 2. Comparisons of BMD of the femoral neck, trochanteric, Wards Triangle region of the hip and lumbar region revealed that a significant lower BMD over trochanteric region was observed in NYHA class III patients, with trochanteric BMD 0.60 ± 0.16 g/cm^2 comparing to NYHA class II 0.70 ± 0.13 g/cm^2 and NYHA class I 0.69 ± 0.12 g/cm^2 ($P = 0.02$). The hip Z-score in NYHA class III was -0.12 ± 1.15, comparing to NYHA class II

Table 1. Clinical parameters, laboratory data and cardiac medication in different NYHA functional classes.

	Total population N=115	NYHA I N=24	NYHA II N=73	NYHA III N=18	P value
Clinical parameters					
Gender, Male (n, %)	85, 74	21, 88	53,73	11, 61	0.14
Age, year	59.2a±14.7	56.8±12.9	59.5±14.9	61.0±16.4	0.62
Age >=60, (n, %)	58, 50.4	10, 41.7	39, 53.4	9, 50.0	0.61
Height, cm	165.2±8.4	167.4±6.1	165.0±9.3	163.0±6.7	0.22
Body weight, Kg	69.4±13.7	70.7±10.5	69.9±13.3	65.6±18.1	0.43
BMI, Kg/m^2	25.4±4.4	25.3±3.7	25.5±3.9	24.6±6.7	0.71
CAD (n, %)	55, 47	13, 54	32, 44	10, 56	0.53
DM (n, %)	34, 30	6, 25	22, 30	6, 33	0.83
Hypertension (n, %)	57, 50	14, 58	33, 45	10, 56	0.47
Af (n, %)	35, 30	8, 33	31, 43	4, 22	0.71
Smoking (n, %)	33, 29	7, 29	24, 33	2, 11	0.19
LVEF (n, %)	35.8±11.2	40.6±13.1	34.7±10.0	33.7±11.2	0.06
Lab data					
Blood urea nitrogen, mg/dL#	21.6±7.8	20.5±7.6	21.1±8.0	20.9±7.7	0.62
Creatinine, mg/dl#	1.2±0.4	1.3±0.4	1.2±0.3	1.3±0.6	0.47
Uric acid, mg/dL	6.8±1.9	6.1±1.4	7.0±1.8	6.7±2.5	0.13
Potassium, mmol/L	4.2±0.5	4.3±0.4	4.2±0.5	4.2±0.5	0.71
Fasting glucose, mg/dL#	111.2±42.2	109.4±33.7	110.6±42.7	116.8±52.6	0.91
Total cholesterol, mg/dL#	185.5±51.4	170.3±41.7	185.6±37.3	207.7±96.5	0.07
Triglyceride, mg/dL#	143.8±92.6	138.2±60.1	146.8±104.4	139.2±79.3	0.91
Cardiac Medications, (n,%)					
Diuretics	93, 80	19, 79	58, 79	16, 89	0.65
Spironolactone	47, 41	10, 42	27, 37	10, 56	0.36
Calcium channel blocker	9, 8	1, 4	5, 7	3, 17	0.29
Antiplatelet	62, 54	15, 63	35, 48	12, 67	0.24
Digoxin	56, 49	8, 33	37, 51	11, 61	0.18
ACEI	32, 28	6, 33	20, 27	4, 22	0.73
ARB	65, 57	15, 63	43, 59	3, 39	0.25
β-blockers	72, 63	20, 83	44, 60	8, 44	0.03
Statin	42, 37	11, 46	27, 37	4, 22	0.29
Fibrate	8, 7	1, 4	5, 7	2, 11	0.69
Anti-arrhythmics	28, 24	5, 21	20, 27	3, 17	0.58
Thiazolidinedione	4, 4	0, 0	4, 5	0, 0	0.31
Heart failure related biomarker					
Follistatin, pg/mL#	2109.4±973.2	1968.1±993.3	2135.6±973.3	2191.2±982.4	0.39
Myostatin, ng/mL#	7.2±4.0	8.3±4.4	7.2±3.9	5.6±3.1	0.10
hsCRP, ng/mL#	3.5±6.3	3.6±8.4	3.3±6.1	3.8±3.8	0.36
BNP-32, ng/mL#	1.95±0.89	1.99±0.74	1.94±0.98	1.87±0.71	0.74
Osteoprotegerin, pmol/L#	7.6±3.4	6.8±3.6	7.4±2.8	9.3±4.6*†	0.04
Bone mineral density					
Femoral neck BMD, g/cm2	0.82±0.18	0.80±0.13	0.84±0.19	0.76±0.17	0.15
Trochanteric BMD, g/cm2	0.68±0.14	0.68±0.12	0.70±0.13	0.60±0.16†	0.02
Ward triangle BMD, g/cm2	0.59±0.16	0.58±0.14	0.60±0.16	0.54±0.17	0.27
Hip Z score	0.37±1.05	0.12±0.86	0.58±1.04	−0.12±1.15†	0.017
Hip T score	−0.90±1.25	−1.13±1.05	−0.73±1.21	−1.29±1.53	0.14
L2 BMD, g/,m2	0.98±0.21	0.94±0.20	1.01±0.21	0.93±0.23	0.17
L3 BMD, g/cm2	1.03±0.24	1.02±0.23	1.06±0.22	0.94±0.28	0.16

Table 1. Cont.

	Total population	NYHA I	NYHA II	NYHA III	P value
	N = 115	N = 24	N = 73	N = 18	
L4 BMD, g/cm2	1.05±0.23	1.02±0.22	1.07±0.74	10.01±0.21	0.39
L2–4 BMD, g/cm2	1.03±0.22	0.99±0.21	1.04±0.22	0.98±0.21	0.33
L2–4 Z-Score	0.48±1.30	0.23±1.39	0.66±1.25	0.08±1.32	0.14
L2–4 T-Score	−0.02±1.65	−0.13±1.49	0.11±1.73	−0.43±1.50	0.43

Values given as n, percentage or mean±SD. BMI: body mass index, CAD: coronary artery disease, DM: diabetes mellitus, Af: atrial fibrillation, LVEF: left ventricle ejection fraction, ACEI: angiotensin-converting enzyme inhibitors, ARB: Angiotensin II receptor blockers, CRP: C-reactive protein, BNP-32: Brain natriuretic peptide 32, BMD: bone mineral density.

[#]Variables were not normally distributed, and were log transformed for statistical analysis.

*p<0.05 vs NYHA I,

[†]p<0.05 vs NYHA II.

Z-score: 0.58±1.04 and NYHA class I Z score: 0.12±0.86 (P = 0.017). While in lumbar region, there is no significant difference in BMD among different NYHA functional classes.

Among all the HF related biomarkers, there was a significant inverse correlation between log transformed serum OPG and trochanteric BMD in patients with HF (R = −0.299, P = 0.001) (Table 2), femoral neck BMD (R = −0.29, P = 0.002) and Ward triangle region of hip (R = −0.34, P<0.001) while there is no significant correlation between OPG and lumbar region BMD. The correlation between clinical variables and trochanteric BMD was shown on Table 2. In additional to log transformed serum OPG, hypertension, age equal or more than 60, male gender, body weight, body height and body mass index was correlated with trochanteric BMD. The correlation between HF related biomarker and BMD was not observed in hsCRP, myostatin, follistatin or BNP-32.

Log transformed serum OPG was positively correlated with age (R = 0.409, P<0.001), age equal or more than 60 (R = 0.325, P<0.001) and with an insignificant inverse correlation with BMI (R = −0.158, P = 0.09) and body weight (R = −0.181, P = 0.052). There is no significant correlation between log transformed follistatin, myostatin, OPG, BNP-32 and hsCRP.

Among all the BMD analysis, trochanteric BMD was inversely correlated with age (R = −0.351, P<0.001) as well as femoral neck BMD versus age (R = −0.458, P<0.001) and Ward Triangle region of the hip BMD versus age (R = −0.480, P<0.001). But

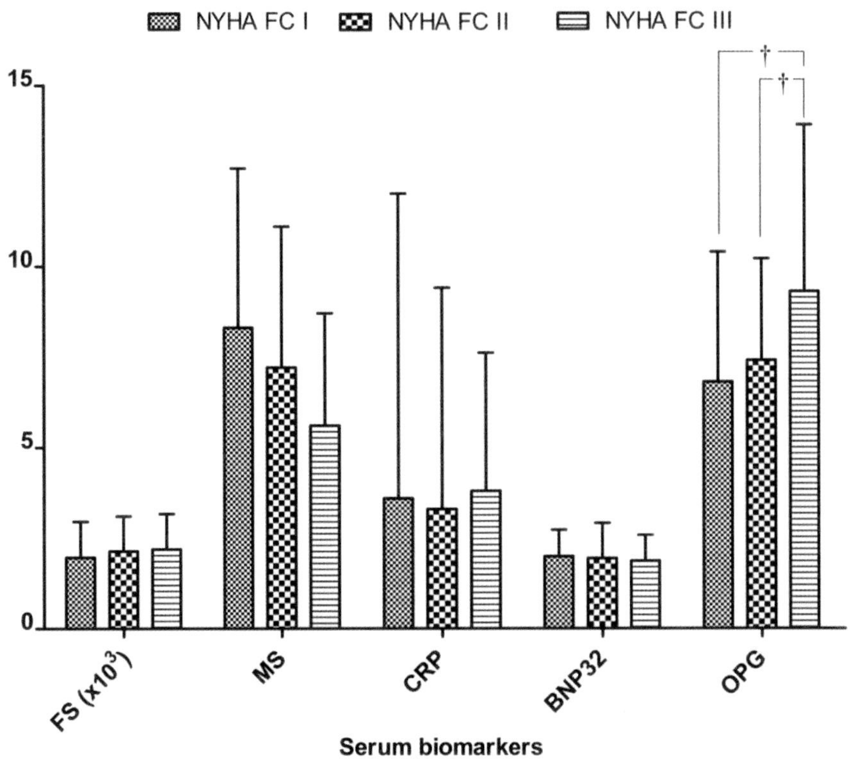

Figure 1. Heart failure related biomarker in different NYHA functional classes. FS: follistatin, MS: myostatin, BNP-32: Brain natriuretic peptide 32, CRP: high sensitivity C reactive protein, OPG: osteoprotegerin, †: p<0.05.

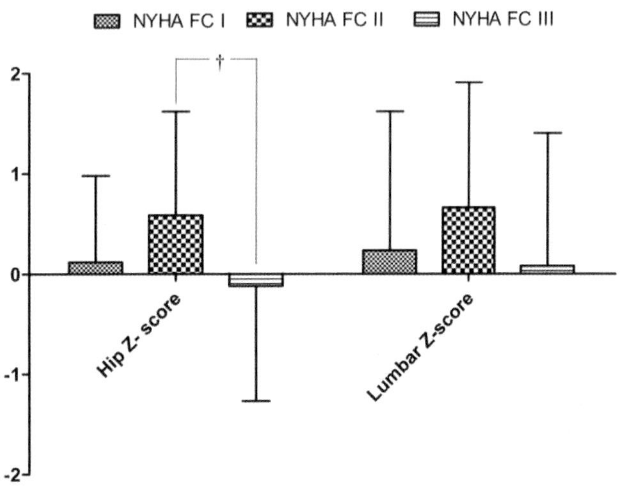

Figure 2. Hip and lumbar Z-score in different NYHA functional classes. A significant difference of hip Z-score was observed between NYHA functional class II and III, †: p<0.05.

there is no significant correlation between lumbar region BMD and age ($R=-0.109$, $P=0.24$). Trochanteric BMD in patients with HF was also significantly correlated with BMI ($R=0.456$, $P<0.001$), and also in femoral neck BMD versus BMI ($R=0.499$, $P<0.001$), Ward triangle region of the hip BMD versus BMI ($R=0.332$, $P<0.001$) and Lumbar BMD versus BMI ($R=0.251$, $P=0.007$). Multivariate analyses of impact of the OPG and clinical factors for trochanteric bone mineral density was conducted, and the inverse correlation of OPG to trochanteric BMD remained after adjusting male gender, age equal or more than 60, smoking, blood urea nitrogen, creatinine, medication of diuretics and body mass index (table 3).

Table 2. Factors associated with trochanteric bone mineral density.

	Pearson correlation coefficient	P value
Osteoprotegern#	−0.299	0.001
Male gender	0.420	<0.001
Age equal or more than 60	−0.2571	0.006
Hypertension	0.206	0.03
Smoking	0.181	0.05
Left ventricle systolic function	0.026	0.78
Diuretics	0.102	0.28
β-blockers	0.07	0.461
Blood urea nitrogen#	−0.173	0.06
Creatinine#	0.01	0.90
Hypertension	0.365	<0.001
Body height	0.362	<0.001
Body weight	0.563	<0.001
Body mass index	0.456	<0.001

#Value was log transformed for statistical analysis.

Table 3. Multivariate analyses for impact of the osteoprotegerin and clinical factors for trochanteric bone mineral density.

	Model 1	Model 2
	β coefficients	β coefficients
OPG#	−0.233‡	−0.202‡
Male gender	0.323‡	0.291†
Age equal or more than 60	−0.142	−0.080
Hypertension	0.181	0.042
Smoking	0.65	0.035
Creatinine#		0.134
Blood urea nitrogen#		−0.113
Diuretics		0.050
Body mass index		0.365*

OPG: osteoprotegerin.
*p<0.001,
†p<0. 01,
‡p<0.05.
#data was log transformed for statistic analysis.
Model 1, multivariate analysis after adjusting for male gender, age >=60, hypertension and smoking.
Model 2, multivariate analysis included in model 2 as well as adjusting for medication use of diuretics and body mass index.

Discussion

In our study with chronic systolic HF, we found that the worse the HF function classes, the lower the trochanteric BMD and the higher the circulating OPG. In addition, OPG was inversely correlated to the trochanteric BMD in HF patients.

OPG is secreted by osteoblast, mesenchymal stem cells, fibroblasts, endothelial cells and human fat tissue [14]. It is one of the members of the tumor necrosis factor (TNF) receptor super-family and has pleiotropic effects over bone metabolism as well as endocrine function. By binding the receptor activator of nuclear factor- kappa B ligand (RANKL) and acting as a decoy receptor to competitively inhibit RANKL interaction with its receptor activator of nuclear factor- kappa B (RANK), OPG subsequently inhibits the production and differentiation of osteoclasts, as a result, bone resorption is inhibited [15].

HF had been demonstrated with accelerated bone loss and therefore osteoporosis and increased risk of hip fracture [1,2], possibly attributed to either physical inactivity, increased loop diuretics use [7], similar comorbidities including renal disease, diabetes and altered neuroendocrine such as 25 hydroxyvitamin D [4], IL-1, IL-6 and TNF-alpha [3,16]. In our study, we had demonstrated an elevated OPG in chronic HF patients which was similar to the other clinical research [9]. In addition, we also found that OPG was inversely correlated to the trochanteric BMD in HF patients.

The reason for having higher circulating OPG level in HF osteoporotic patients may be attributed to several possible mechanisms. First, there may be regulatory pathways that involve bone metabolism other than the RANK-RANKL pathway. There are shared multiple pathophysiological mechanisms for heart failure and osteoporosis, through HF neuroendocrine activation matrix protein abnormalities, parathyroid hormone, adiponectin and leptin, etc [8,9]. These factors may entangle with OPG in the state of HF. Second, the cause of high OPG in HF may be deduced through similar observation in natriuretic peptides in HF.

While natriuretic peptides paralleled HF activity and was utilized in diagnosis, prognosis and monitoring treatment response, natriuretic peptides counteract the detrimental effects of the sympathetic nervous system through diuresis, vasodilatation, inhibition of renin and aldosterone production [17]. The cumulative effects of natriuretic peptides oppose the physiologic abnormalities of HF, instead of begetting HF.

However the relationship of OPG and BMD in distinct disease state is quite controversial from clinical observation. In patients with chronic obstructive lung disease (COPD), a positive correlation was observed between serum OPG and BMD in both lumbar spine L2–L4 and femoral neck region [18]. Adipose tissue OPG expressions are also positively correlated with femoral T score in patient with COPD [19]. On the other hand, in postmenopausal osteoporotic woman, the plasma RANKL, OPG, OPG/RANKL ratio were significant higher than sex-matched control group and circulating levels of OPG and RANKL are inversely related to BMD [20].

In consideration of increased fracture rate in patient with HF, one might expect to observe an osteoporotic range BMD result from HF patient. However, neither our clinical investigation nor other clinical report had yet demonstrated the inference [9]. This may be attributed to the fact that we had precludes initially immobilized, bed ridden, history of joint prosthesis, unable ambulation and renal insufficiency candidates which are the factors that had been associated with osteoporosis. In addition, we had enrolled less severe HF group. For end-stage HF awaiting cardiac transplantation patient, osteopenia and osteoporosis were observed approximately 42% and 19% respectively over femoral neck region [4]. In one study with serial bone mineral density scans over 2 years, accelerated bone loss which defined by a decline over 1% of bone mineral content annually was observed in 35% of HF male patients [21]. The disturbances in bone metabolism and the degree of bone loss may be only subtle in mild to moderate HF patients [22]. Diverse HF medical prescription, including angiotensin-converting enzyme inhibitors, thiazide diuretics, spironolactone and β-blockers with pros and cons effect over osteoporosis may also influence the BMD results in HF patients.

Lumbar spine BMD in our study was relative normal reflecting from Z score in the contrast to hip BMD. This is one interesting but not unique finding, in one study where cardiac transplant recipients and patients with HF awaiting transplantation, hip BMD were decreased while the spine BMD remained normal [23]. HF is associated with several factors that contribute to both reduced bone mineral density and increased risk of osteoporosis-related fractures. Therefore, in theory the systemic impact should bring equal risks to both axial bones and long bones. However, the risk of axial bone osteoporosis and vertebral compression fracture in heart failure was less addressed from the literature. It is postulated that the compressed osteopenic vertebrae bone led to falsely high vertebrae BMD. The discrepancy between femoral neck and lumbar spine BMD may be also caused by aortic calcifications, which may elevate lumbar spine BMD during measurement. In fact, vertebral compression fracture may be often overlooked in contrast to the hip fracture [24].

B-type natriuretic peptide (BNP) and myostatin are both are significantly increased in HF patients. However, there was no significant difference in myostatin among NYHA functional classes, as well as other heart failure associated biomarker such as BNP-32, follistatin in our study. Although Gruson et al. had demonstrated that myostatin may be significantly increased in HF patients and that myostatin may correlate with biomarkers related to HF severity [25]. Zamora et al. proposed that there was no relationship between the myostatin or myostatin propeptide level and any parameter of disease severity or prognosis in patients with chronic heart failure [26]. The insignificant change of myostatin in our heart failure patient may be attributed to the confounding effect of follistatin of which may antagonize myostatin during muscle mass regulation [27]. Angiotensin-converting enzyme inhibitors exert beneficial effects in lowering the risk of weight loss in HF patients and thus the body mass regulation had been altered. In a substudy from the SOLVD database, treatment with enalapril in contrast to placebo, was associated with significant lower risk of weight loss greater or equal than 6% [28]. In addition to the anabolic effect of beta-blockers on bone metabolism, beta-blocker had been also shown to reverse excess protein catabolism [29]. As a result, the absence of expected correlation between myostatin and heart failure severity in our study may be contributed by large portion of angiotensin-converting enzyme inhibitors and beta-blocker use.

There were several limitations to our study. First, this is a cross-sectional, observational association study, lack of clinical outcome. The study population was rather small, heterogeneous, with diversities of medication, which might confound the results. There were group differences in different NYHA classes, which imply that, HF as a disease spectrum, not a single disease. We did not enroll non-HF subjects as controls. This did not deter our observation because we adopted Z-scores from the same region with age-, sex-matched population as the historical controls. However, no serological biomarkers could be assessed. Although the inverse correlation between levels of OPG and BMD which may imply a potential link between HF and osteoporosis were found in the study, it is cautious to jump into conclusion for the causal relationship between them. Heart failure and osteoporosis are complex and multifactorial disorders, and we did not evaluate all potential biomarkers involved. Furthermore, the circulating levels may not reflect tissue levels.

OPG is gaining notice for being a prognostic role in cardiovascular disease. Serum OPG is an independent predictor of cardiovascular mortality in patients with stable coronary artery disease [30] and a markers of plaque instability in coronary artery disease [31]. In GISSI-HF trial, OPG may also pose a prognostic function in chronic HF [32]. Although it had been demonstrate the step up elevation of OPG in HF patients according to NYHA functional class [33], which is concordant with our study result. Few had addressed the change of OPG over the bone metabolism in HF patients. Our study further plots out the interaction between OPG and BMD in HF patients, which is mainly an inverse correlation. OPG may be use as an indicator for osteopenia or osteoporosis clinically. Instead of measuring bone mass directly, the assessment of bone turnover which reflect ongoing bone remodeling mat be alternative for identifying at risk HF patients for osteoporosis and taking preventive and therapeutic measures in time. Although it remains as an unanswered question whether heart failure leads to osteoporosis and frailty fractures, or just being an epiphenomenon as a passive participant in a population at risk for both diseases. However, the application or the mechanism underlies OPG and BMD in HF warrant further randomized prospective, outcome study in larger population and bench works.

Acknowledgments

We acknowledged the help from the Heart Failure Center of National Taiwan University Hospital and Mr. Yi-Hwen Huang, Ms. Pei-Chi Yu and Ms. Yu-Chiao Chi for the technical assistance.

Author Contributions

Conceived and designed the experiments: YHC YWW MFC WSY YLH. Performed the experiments: YHC YWW MFC WSY SSW CML NKC RBH YHL MSL YLH. Analyzed the data: YHC YWW YLH. Contributed reagents/materials/analysis tools: YHC YWW YLH. Wrote the paper: YHC YWW YLH.

References

1. Abou-Raya S, Abou-Raya A (2009) Osteoporosis and congestive heart failure (CHF) in the elderly patient: double disease burden. Arch Gerontol Geriatr 49: 250–254.
2. van Diepen S, Majumdar SR, Bakal JA, McAlister FA, Ezekowitz JA (2008) Heart failure is a risk factor for orthopedic fracture: a population-based analysis of 16,294 patients. Circulation 118: 1946–1952.
3. Carbone L, Buzkova P, Fink HA, Lee JS, Chen Z, et al. (2010) Hip fractures and heart failure: findings from the Cardiovascular Health Study. Eur Heart J 31: 77–84.
4. Shane E, Mancini D, Aaronson K, Silverberg SJ, Seibel MJ, et al. (1997) Bone mass, vitamin D deficiency, and hyperparathyroidism in congestive heart failure. Am J Med 103: 197–207.
5. Chhokar VS, Sun Y, Bhattacharya SK, Ahokas RA, Myers LK, et al. (2004) Loss of bone minerals and strength in rats with aldosteronism. Am J Physiol Heart Circ Physiol 287: H2023–2026.
6. Barasch E, Gottdiener JS, Aurigemma G, Kitzman DW, Han J, et al. (2009) Association between elevated fibrosis markers and heart failure in the elderly: the cardiovascular health study. Circ Heart Fail 2: 303–310.
7. Lim LS, Fink HA, Kuskowski MA, Taylor BC, Schousboe JT, et al. (2008) Loop diuretic use and increased rates of hip bone loss in older men: the Osteoporotic Fractures in Men Study. Arch Intern Med 168: 735–740.
8. Loncar G, Fulster S, von Haehling S, Popovic V (2011) Metabolism and the heart: An overview of muscle, fat, and bone metabolism in heart failure. Int J Cardiol.
9. Bozic B, Loncar G, Prodanovic N, Radojicic Z, Cvorovic V, et al. (2010) Relationship between high circulating adiponectin with bone mineral density and bone metabolism in elderly males with chronic heart failure. J Card Fail 16: 301–307.
10. Ueland T, Dahl CP, Kjekshus J, Hulthe J, Bohm M, et al. (2011) Osteoprotegerin predicts progression of chronic heart failure: results from CORONA. Circ Heart Fail 4: 145–152.
11. Loncar G, Bozic B, Cvorovic V, Radojicic Z, Dimkovic S, et al. (2010) Relationship between RANKL and neuroendocrine activation in elderly males with heart failure. Endocrine 37: 148–156.
12. Huang KC, Cheng WC, Yen RF, Tsai KS, Tai TY, et al. (2004) Lack of independent relationship between plasma adiponectin, leptin levels and bone density in nondiabetic female adolescents. Clin Endocrinol (Oxf) 61: 204–208.
13. Hwang JJ, Yang WS, Chiang FT, Chen MF, Lin HJ, et al. (2009) Association of circulating matrix metalloproteinase-1, but not adiponectin, with advanced coronary artery disease. Atherosclerosis 204: 293–297.
14. Witasp A, Carrero JJ, Hammarqvist F, Qureshi AR, Heimburger O, et al. (2011) Expression of osteoprotegerin in human fat tissue; implications for chronic kidney disease. Eur J Clin Invest 41: 498–506.
15. Boyle WJ, Simonet WS, Lacey DL (2003) Osteoclast differentiation and activation. Nature 423: 337–342.
16. Baldini V, Mastropasqua M, Francucci CM, D'Erasmo E (2005) Cardiovascular disease and osteoporosis. J Endocrinol Invest 28: 69–72.
17. Daniels LB, Maisel AS (2007) Natriuretic peptides. J Am Coll Cardiol 50: 2357–2368.
18. Kochetkova EA, Nevzorova VA, Maistrovskaia Iu V, Massard G (2010) [Osteoprotegerin and bone mineral density in patients with chronic obstructive pulmonary disease]. Ter Arkh 82: 10–14.
19. Pobeha P, Ukropec J, Skyba P, Ukropcova B, Joppa P, et al. (2011) Relationship between osteoporosis and adipose tissue leptin and osteoprotegerin in patients with chronic obstructive pulmonary disease. Bone 48: 1008–1014.
20. Jabbar S, Drury J, Fordham JN, Datta HK, Francis RM, et al. (2011) Osteoprotegerin, RANKL and bone turnover in postmenopausal osteoporosis. J Clin Pathol.
21. Jankowska EA, Jakubaszko J, Cwynar A, Majda J, Ponikowska B, et al. (2009) Bone mineral status and bone loss over time in men with chronic systolic heart failure and their clinical and hormonal determinants. Eur J Heart Fail 11: 28–38.
22. Zittermann A, Schleithoff SS, Koerfer R (2006) Markers of bone metabolism in congestive heart failure. Clin Chim Acta 366: 27–36.
23. Lee AH, Mull RL, Keenan GF, Callegari PE, Dalinka MK, et al. (1994) Osteoporosis and bone morbidity in cardiac transplant recipients. Am J Med 96: 35–41.
24. Lyons K, Majumdar SR, Ezekowitz JA (2011) The Unrecognized Burden of Osteoporosis-Related Vertebral Fractures in Patients with Heart Failure. Circ Heart Fail.
25. Gruson D, Ahn SA, Ketelslegers JM, Rousseau MF (2011) Increased plasma myostatin in heart failure. Eur J Heart Fail 13: 734–736.
26. Zamora E, Simo R, Lupon J, Galan A, Urrutia A, et al. (2010) Serum myostatin levels in chronic heart failure. Rev Esp Cardiol 63: 992–996.
27. Lee SJ (2004) Regulation of muscle mass by myostatin. Annu Rev Cell Dev Biol 20: 61–86.
28. Anker SD, Negassa A, Coats AJ, Afzal R, Poole-Wilson PA, et al. (2003) Prognostic importance of weight loss in chronic heart failure and the effect of treatment with angiotensin-converting-enzyme inhibitors: an observational study. Lancet 361: 1077–1083.
29. Herndon DN, Hart DW, Wolf SE, Chinkes DL, Wolfe RR (2001) Reversal of catabolism by beta-blockade after severe burns. N Engl J Med 345: 1223–1229.
30. Jono S, Otsuki S, Higashikuni Y, Shioi A, Mori K, et al. (2010) Serum osteoprotegerin levels and long-term prognosis in subjects with stable coronary artery disease. J Thromb Haemost 8: 1170–1175.
31. Shaker OG, El-Shehaby A, Nabih M (2010) Possible role of osteoprotegerin and tumor necrosis factor-related apoptosis-inducing ligand as markers of plaque instability in coronary artery disease. Angiology 61: 756–762.
32. Roysland R, Masson S, Omland T, Milani V, Bjerre M, et al. (2010) Prognostic value of osteoprotegerin in chronic heart failure: The GISSI-HF trial. Am Heart J 160: 286–293.
33. Ueland T, Yndestad A, Oie E, Florholmen G, Halvorsen B, et al. (2005) Dysregulated osteoprotegerin/RANK ligand/RANK axis in clinical and experimental heart failure. Circulation 111: 2461–2468.

9

Recognition of Morphometric Vertebral Fractures by Artificial Neural Networks: Analysis from GISMO Lombardia Database

Cristina Eller-Vainicher[1]*, Iacopo Chiodini[1], Ivana Santi[2], Marco Massarotti[3], Luca Pietrogrande[4], Elisa Cairoli[1], Paolo Beck-Peccoz[1], Matteo Longhi[5], Valter Galmarini[6], Giorgio Gandolini[7], Maurizio Bevilacqua[8], Enzo Grossi[9,10]

1 Endocrinology and Diabetology Unit, Medical Sciences Department, Fondazione Istituto di Ricovero e Cura a Carattere Scientifico Cà Granda Ospedale Maggiore Policlinico, Milan, Italy, **2** Istituto Geriatrico Azienda di Servizi alla Persona Istituti Milanesi Martinitt e Stelline e Pio Albergo Trivulzio, Milan, Italy, **3** Istituto di Ricovero e Cura a Carattere Scientifico Humanitas, Rozzano, Milan, Italy, **4** Orthopedic Clinic, Dipartimento di Medicina, Chirurgia e Odontoiatria San Paolo, University of Milan, Milan, Italy, **5** Unit of Reumathology, Istituto di Ricovero e Cura a Carattere Scientifico Istituto Ortopedico Galeazzi, Milan, Italy, **6** Azienda Ospedaliera Fatebenefratelli e Oftalmico, Milan, Italy, **7** Istituto di Ricovero e Cura a Carattere Scientifico Don Gnocchi, Milan, Italy, **8** Endocrinology and Diabetes Unit, Luigi Sacco Hospital (Vialba), University of Milan, Milan, Italy, **9** Bracco Medical Department, San Donato Milanese, Milan, Italy, **10** Semeion Research Centre, Rome, Italy

Abstract

Background: It is known that bone mineral density (BMD) predicts the fracture's risk only partially and the severity and number of vertebral fractures are predictive of subsequent osteoporotic fractures (OF). Spinal deformity index (SDI) integrates the severity and number of morphometric vertebral fractures. Nowadays, there is interest in developing algorithms that use traditional statistics for predicting OF. Some studies suggest their poor sensitivity. Artificial Neural Networks (ANNs) could represent an alternative. So far, no study investigated ANNs ability in predicting OF and SDI. The aim of the present study is to compare ANNs and Logistic Regression (LR) in recognising, on the basis of osteoporotic risk-factors and other clinical information, patients with SDI≥1 and SDI≥5 from those with SDI = 0.

Methodology: We compared ANNs prognostic performance with that of LR in identifying SDI≥1/SDI≥5 in 372 women with postmenopausal-osteoporosis (SDI≥1, n = 176; SDI = 0, n = 196; SDI≥5, n = 51), using 45 variables (44 clinical parameters plus BMD). ANNs were allowed to choose relevant input data automatically (TWIST-system-Semeion). Among 45 variables, 17 and 25 were selected by TWIST-system-Semeion, in SDI≥1 *vs* SDI = 0 (first) and SDI≥5 *vs* SDI = 0 (second) analysis. In the first analysis sensitivity of LR and ANNs was 35.8% and 72.5%, specificity 76.5% and 78.5% and accuracy 56.2% and 75.5%, respectively. In the second analysis, sensitivity of LR and ANNs was 37.3% and 74.8%, specificity 90.3% and 87.8%, and accuracy 63.8% and 81.3%, respectively.

Conclusions: ANNs showed a better performance in identifying both SDI≥1 and SDI≥5, with a higher sensitivity, suggesting its promising role in the development of algorithm for predicting OF.

Editor: Ulrich Thiem, Marienhospital Herne - University of Bochum, Germany

Funding: The authors have no support or funding to report.

Competing Interests: The authors have declared that no competing interests exist.

* E-mail: eller.vainicher@gmail.com

Introduction

Osteoporosis is a multi-factorial systemic skeletal disease, characterised by low bone mass and microarchitectural deterioration of bone tissue, with a consequent increase in bone fragility and susceptibility to fracture [1]. The diagnosis of osteoporosis relies on the measurement of bone mineral density (BMD), measured by dual energy X-ray absorptiometry (DXA), or on the presence of a fragility fracture. Nevertheless, the assessment of fracture risk with BMD shows several limitations. The bone microarchitecture, commonly named "bone quality", is difficult to assess by clinical parameters [2,3]. Also for this reason, the BMD detection rate for fragility fractures (sensitivity) is low, and the 96% of fragility fractures seems to arise in women without a densitometric diagnosis of osteoporosis [4]. The use of additional risk factors that, independently of BMD, add information on fracture risk, improves the BMD sensitivity in predicting fragility fracture [4,5]. Thus, recent efforts by the World Health Organization Metabolic Bone Disease Group have focused on developing a risk assessment tool (FRAX^{TM}) using clinical risk factors with and without femoral neck BMD to enhance fracture prediction [6].

Asymptomatic morphometric vertebral fractures (MVF) are considered the "prima facies" of osteoporosis, and are much more prevalent than clinical fractures [7]. Morphometric vertebral fractures are often overlooked by radiologist [8], although they represent one of the strongest clinical predictors of subsequent fractures [9]. Indeed, the risk of subsequent fractures increases with both the number and the severity of prior vertebral fractures [10–13]. Thus, it may be more relevant for an appropriate assessment of future fracture risk to assess all the fractures rather than to consider the spine as a whole, as a binary parameter (fracture Yes/No), as in FRAX^{TM}. The spinal deformity index (SDI) described by Minne [14] and Genant [15] is an assessment tool that integrates both the number and severity of fractures by summing the vertebral fracture grades along the spine from T4 to L4. Two studies suggested that SDI may be an accurate tool for vertebral fracture prediction and that baseline SDI was predictive of the 3-year incidence of subsequent vertebral fracture [16,17]. Recently, the SDI has been found to be negatively associated with functional outcome in women with hip fracture admitted consecutively to a rehabilitation hospital [18]. This is in line with histological data showing that microarchitectural deterioration is proportionally worse in women with increasing severity of vertebral fractures [19].

Recent studies suggest that FRAX^{TM} tool may have a poor sensitivity for fracture prediction and does not significantly improve the discriminatory value of hip BMD alone [20,21]. An explanation is that osteoporosis is a multi-factorial systemic skeletal disease, in which different factors and environments interact in stochastic, nonlinear biological mechanisms. Therefore, the link between bone mineral density, clinical risk factors and fragility fractures probably needs a special kind of mathematics, such as Artificial Neural Networks (ANNs), to be understood.

Artificial Neural Networks are artificial adaptive systems, inspired by the functioning processes of the human brain [22]. These mathematical informatics' systems are able to modify their internal structure in relation to a function objective. So, they are particularly suited for solving nonlinear problems, being able to reconstruct the fuzzy logic rules [23] that govern the optimal solution for these problems. The ability to learn through an adaptive way (i.e. extracting from the available data the information needed to gather a specific task and to generalise the acquired knowledge) is a characteristic that make the ANN models a very powerful tool for data analysis. The internal structure and functional organisation of such systems can be updated and modified with respect to the environmental changes enabling the ANN to create its own representation of the information. Moreover, these models are interesting also for their noise tolerance that allows accurate performances in presence of unreliability, wrong data or measurement errors.

Although ANNs offer promise for improving the predictive value of traditional statistical data analysis and have been successfully used in many areas of medicine [24], no reports have so far investigated the ability of ANNs in predicting osteoporosis fracture.

Methods

Objectives

The aim of the present study was to evaluate the capacity of ANNs, compared with Logistic Regression (LR), to recognise: 1) patients with or without morphometric vertebral fractures (SDI≥1 and SDI = 0 respectively) and 2) patients with SDI≥5 or without morphometric vertebral fractures (SDI≥5 and SDI = 0 respectively), on the basis of classical bone osteoporotic risk factors and other clinical information, routinely derived from the out-patient visits.

Participants

The study population included 430 patients consequently referred to 9 out-patient clinics for osteoporosis management belonging to *GISMO-Lombardia Group* (North-West of Italy), from 1st January to 31st March 2010. The majority of the patients had been referred from primary care. The inclusion criteria were: 1) female post-menopausal patients with osteopenia or osteoporosis defined by the presence of a T-score for spine BMD or hip BMD ≤−1.0>−2.5 and ≤−2.5 respectively. Exclusion criteria were: 1) patients who have been treated with bisphosphonates or other drugs for osteoporosis, or who have been taking these drugs for at least 1 year; 2) secondary forms of osteoporosis; 3) malignancies; 4) renal failure; 4) previous or present treatment with oral corticosteroids or any other drug known to affect bone metabolism. Eventually, data from 372 subjects were analyzed.

Information on menopausal age, number of pregnancies, breast feeding, smoking habits, and alcohol consumption were collected. In order to estimate this latter variable, all subjects were asked about quantity and type of drinks consumed and data were converted as Units per day (8 gr of pure alcohol) [25]. Patients with alcohol consumption >100 gr per day were excluded, as possibly affected by a secondary form of osteoporosis (see the above-mentioned exclusion criteria). Moreover, family history of osteoporosis and of all type of hip fractures was obtained from all subjects at consultation. The patients were also asked about previous clinical fragility fractures at spine, ribs, wrist and hip. Fractures of skull, jaw, coccyx, phalanx, ankle, cervical and thoracic vertebrae (C1 to T4), and of posterior arches of the vertebra were not considered as osteoporosis-related fractures and were excluded from the analysis. In all patients, the presence of previous fragility fractures was ascertained by self report and no additional validation of this information was conducted.

In all patients height and weight were measured and body mass index (BMI) was calculated. Calcium intake, expressed as mg/day, was assessed using a simplified questionnaire described in a previous paper [26]. In particular, usual calcium intake coming from some selected calcium-rich foods (milk and dairy products) was estimated by a 7-day food frequency questionnaire. The foods checked include milk, aged cheese, soft cheese, cottage cheese, and yoghurt. Portion sizes were quantified by means of household measures (slices, cups, glasses). To standardize the slice weight, three cardboard samples of different size were used (about 100, 50 and 25 g). The number of standardized servings was assessed, each containing approximately 300 mg of calcium (a glass of milk, a cup of yoghurt, a portion of about 100 g of cottage cheese, a 50 g slice of soft cheese and a 25 g slice of aged cheese [26]. Patients were asked about co-morbidities (i.e. arterial hypertension, dyslipidemia, gastric/esophagus disease, anxiety, depression, chronic obstructive pulmonary disease (COPD), osteoarthritis, kidney stones, type 2 diabetes mellitus) (Table 1).

Since ANNs cannot analyze missing values, patients who missed one or more information were excluded. Eventually, 372 post-menopausal patients were considered for the analysis.

Description of investigations undertaken

Dual energy X-ray absorptiometry (DXA) scans were carried out to measure BMD at the spine and hip with the instrument available locally: Hologic Discovery (Watham MA, USA) in 73% and Lunar GE (Lunar Pty Ltd., Madison, Wisconsin, USA) in 27% of the centres. All patients had at least one measurement among hip or spine and were classified as having or not a low BMD (T-score > or ≤−2.5 at least at one site, respectively). No cross-calibration was undertaken between the Hologic and Lunar machines.

Conventional spinal radiographs in lateral (T5–L4) and anterior-posterior (AP) projection (L1–L4) were obtained in all subjects with standardised technique. The vertebrae were

Table 1. Variables used in the analysis and variables selected by TWIST system in the subsequent analysis: SDI = 0 vs SDI≥1 (SDI≥1) and SDI = 0 vs SDI≥5 (SDI≥5).

	SDI≥1	SDI≥5
Age	x	
Age<68 years	x	x
Age≥68 years		x
Body Mass Index (BMI) Kg/m^2	x	
BMI≤21	x	x
BMI>21<30		
BMI≥30	x	x
Years since menopause (YSM)	x	x
YSM<18		x
YSM≥18		x
Number of pregnancies		x
Months of breast feeding		
Current smoking yes	x	x
Current smoking no	x	
Previous smoking yes	x	
Previous smoking no		
Alcohol yes		x
Alcohol no		x
Bone mineral density T-score ≤−2.5 yes		
Bone mineral density T-score ≤−2.5 no		
Previous fragility fracture yes	x	x
Previous fragility fracture no		x
Familiar history of femoral fracture yes		x
Familiar history of femoral fracture no		
Calcium intake mg/day	x	x
Calcium intake ≤300 mg/day yes		x
Calcium intake ≤300 mg/day no	x	x
Arterial hypertension yes	x	
Arterial hypertension no		x
Dyslipidemia yes		
Dyslipidemia no	x	x
Gastric/oesophagus disease yes		x
Gastric/oesophagus disease no		x
Anxiety/depression yes	x	x
Anxiety/depression no		x
Chronic pulmonary obstructive disease (COPD) yes		
Chronic pulmonary obstructive disease (COPD) no		x
Osteoarthritis yes		
Osteoarthritis no		
History of kidney stones yes	x	
History of kidney stones no		
Type 2 Diabetes Mellitus (T2D) yes	x	x
Type 2 Diabetes Mellitus (T2D) no		
SDI = 0		
SDI≥1		
SDI≥5		

SDI≥1: Variables selected by TWIST system in the analysis aimed to differentiate patients with SDI≥1 from those with SDI = 0 (the number 17, reported in Table 4a, refers to a maximisation of these variables); SDI≥5: Variables selected by TWIST system in the analysis aimed to differentiate patients with SDI≥5 from those with SDI = 0 (the number 25, reported in Table 4b, refers to a maximisation of these variables).
Twist system can easily select just one of the two binary forms of the variables since that choosing one option implies also the information of its complement.

identified and evaluated by the clinicians of the osteoporosis centres by using dedicated software for quantitative morphometry (MorphoXpress, Optasia Medical, Warner Chilcott, Rockaway, NJ, USA) [27]. In brief the MorphoXpress operates as follows: original lateral vertebral radiographs are digitised using a TWAIN scanner (UMAX Power Look 1000, Techville, Dallas, TX, USA). Analysis is then initialised by the manual targeting of the centres of the upper and lower vertebrae to be analysed. The software then automatically finds the positions of landmarks for a standard 6-point morphometry measurement. The software then allows these points to be moved by the operator, if deemed necessary, before the points are confirmed as being correct. The positions of the confirmed points are then used by the software to calculate anterior, middle and posterior vertebral heights, which may also be used for the determination of deformity shape [27]. Before beginning the study in each participating centre, adequate training was given to a single operator in order to standardise the use of quantitative morphometry. In each centre, the operator read at least 15 radiographs more than once to assess how reliable within himself he was. In order to assess the correct identification of thoracic vertebral fractures, copies of the X-rays from 50 patients randomly taken from centres were sent to an experienced radiologist. Inter-reader reliability between results obtained in various centres and central assessment by the experienced radiologist, summarised by the kappa statistics (k) test, was 0.85. The fractures were defined as intact (SQ grade 0) or as having approximately mild (20–25% compression), moderate (25–40% compression), or severe (>40% compression) deformity (SQ grades 1, 2 and 3, respectively). Subsequently, for each subject the spinal deformity index (SDI) was calculated by summing the SQ grade for each of the 13 vertebrae from T5 to L4 (SDI = SQT4+...+SQT12+SQL1+...+SQL4) (17).

Ethics

Ethics Committee approval was not required since data were collected as part of the standard care for the patients and the data sets available to researchers were fully de-identified.

Statistical methods

The 9 out-patient clinics for osteoporosis management belonging to GISMO-Lombardia Group have been working altogether since September 2005 using the same protocols for data collection. The homogeneity between the 9 centres has been checked by specific investigators meetings twice yearly, but a Inter-rater Cohen's k of agreement was not obtained.

We performed the analysis, both the traditional and ANNs, using two different end-points: 1) SDI≥1 (This identifies eligibility for full reimbursement for osteoporosis treatment according to the Italian rules: "Nota 79") [28]; 2) SDI≥5. This latter end-point was chosen considering that there is an almost linear relationship between SDI and fracture risk, not influenced by the particular fracture configurations, till a SDI of 5 [16].

Logistic Regression Analysis

Statistical analysis was performed by SPSS version 12.0 statistical package (SPSS Inc., Chicago, IL, USA). The normality of distribution was checked by Kolmogorov-Smirnov test. The results are expressed as mean±SD if not differently specified. Comparison of continuous variables between groups was performed using Student's t-test or Mann-Whitney test on the basis of the normality of distribution. Categorical variables between the two groups were compared by χ^2test. The bivariate associations between SDI and all the variables were tested by Pearson product moment association or Spearman correlation as appropriate. In all patients, logistic regression analysis assessed the association between the presence of SDI≥1 or SDI≥5 as dependent variables (expressed as categorical variables) and the presence of previous fragility fracture, arterial hypertension, chronic obstructive pulmonary disease, low BMD (T-score ≤−2.5) and dyslipidemia (independent variables, expressed as categorical variables) and years since menopause and daily calcium intake (independent variables, expressed as continuous variables). We decided to include in the logistic regression model those variables, which were found to be different between fractured and not fractured subjects.

Bone mineral density data were categorized on the basis of a T-score > or ≤2.5, which is the commonly used threshold to define osteoporosis [1,2], to avoid the possible influence of having used two different instruments for determining BMD.

The alcohol consumption was collected as a categorical variable (presence of alcohol consumption < or ≥3 alcohol units/day), as persons consuming more than 3 alcohol units per day have been demonstrated to have an higher risk of fractures compared to abstainers, while a precise range of beneficial alcohol consumption has not been determined so far, although available evidence suggest a favourable effect of 0.9–1.8 alcohol units per day [29].

We employed a classical multivariable logistic regression including all variables and then building the final model using forward stepwise logistic regression. A significance level of 0.3 was required to allow a variable into the model, and a significance level of 0.35 was required for a variable to stay in the model. In addition, the data set has been re-analyzed also building a multiple model including in the logistic regression analysis only the variables with p<0.25 in bivariate analysis. P values of ≤0.05 were considered significant.

Artificial neural networks analysis

Advanced intelligent systems based on novel coupling of artificial neural networks and evolutionary algorithms have been applied. In this study we applied TWIST system and supervised ANNs in order to develop a model able to predict with a high degree of accuracy the diagnostic class starting from available data. Supervised ANNs are networks which learn by examples, calculating an error function during the training phase and adjusting the connection strengths in order to minimize the error function. [30]. The learning constraint of the supervised ANNs makes their own output coincide with the predefined target. The general form of these ANNs is: $y = f(x,w^*)$, where w^* constitutes the set of parameters which best approximate the function.

The trained ANN generates a single output which is a continuous variable that can range between 0 and 1. However, as our 'real' dependent variables are binary (0 or 1), the ANN output needs to be reduced to 0 or 1 using a specific threshold. If the ANN gives as output values from 0 to 0.5 then the output is considered as 0 (e.g SD 5 absent therefore SD 1); while is the output is comprised from 0.51 to 1 then the output is considered as 1(e.g SD 5 present therefore SD 5). The ROC curve, which measures sensitivity and 1-specificity (the false positive rate) across different cutoffs, is then generated varying the threshold for binary classification.

Data analysis was performed using a re-sampling system named TWIST developed by Semeion Research Centre. The TWIST system consists in an ensemble of two previously described systems: Training & Testing (T&T) and Input Selection (I.S) [31]. The T&T system is a robust data re-sampling technique that is able to arrange the source sample into sub-samples that all possess a similar probability density function. In this way, the data is split into two or more sub-samples in order to train, test and validate the ANN models more effectively. The IS system is an evolutionary wrapper system able to reduce the amount of data while conserving the largest amount of information available in the dataset. The combined action of these two systems allow us to solve two frequent problems in managing Artificial Neural Networks, i.e. the optimal splitting of the data set in training and testing subsets containing a balanced distribution of outliers and the optimal selection of variables with maximal amount of information relevant to the problem under investigation. Both systems are based on a Genetic Algorithm, the Genetic Doping Algorithm (GenD) developed at Semeion Research Centre [32,33]. After this processing, the features that were most significant for the classification were selected and at the same time the training set and the testing set were created with a function of probability distribution similar to the one that provided the best results in the classification. Twin supervised Multi Layer Perceptron, with four hidden units, were then used for the classification task employing a crossover training-testing procedure (named a–b; b–a, where the a-subset first function as training data and b-subset as testing data, then they are reversed) The twin ANNs which were trained and tested on the new data set generated by TWIST systems are "virgin" and operate independently and blindly from each other and from TWIST system.

The validation protocol is a procedure to verify the models' ability to generalize the results reached in the testing phase. Among the different protocols reported in literature, the selected model is the protocol with the greatest generalization ability on data unknown to the model itself. The procedural steps in developing the validation protocol are: 1) subdividing the dataset randomly into two sub-samples: the first called Training Set, and the second, called Testing Set; 2) choosing a fixed ANNs (and/or Organism) which is trained on the Training Set. In this phase, the ANNs learns to associate the input variables with those that are indicated as targets; 3) saving the weight matrix produced by the ANNs at the end of the training phase, and freezing it with all of the parameters used for the training; 4) showing the Testing Set to the ANNs, so that in each case, the ANNs can express an evaluation based on the training just performed. This procedure takes place for each input vector but every result (output vector) is not communicated to the ANNs; in this way, the ANNs is evaluated only in reference to the generalization ability that it has acquired during the Training phase; 5) constructing a new ANNs with identical architecture to the previous one and repeating the procedure from point 1. This protocol is applied once starting from the first subsample and once starting from the second subsample taken as training set obtaining in this way 2 independent classification experiments. This procedure was repeated 10 times according to 5×2 cross-validation protocol [34]. In this procedure the study sample is five-time randomly divided into two sub-samples, always different but containing similar distribution of cases and controls. Training and testing sets are then reversed and consequently 10 independent models carried out [34].

We estimated for each strategy sensitivity, specificity, and overall accuracy. We also calculated the areas under the receiver operating curve (ROC) in an empirical (non-parametric) approach, which were used for comparison among the different strategies [35]. The statistical comparison among ROC curves was performed as described elsewhere [36]. The ROC represents the relationship between sensitivity and specificity for the prediction of each of the considered outcomes.

Differences were considered significant at a 5% probability level.

Results

Clinical characteristics of patients (all, SDI 0, SDI≥1 and SDI≥5) are reported in Table 2. The patients with SDI≥1 were older and farer from menopause than patients with SDI = 0. Moreover, they showed a higher prevalence of arterial hypertension and a lower prevalence of anxiety/depression in respect with SDI = 0 patients. Similarly, as compared with SDI = 0 patients, SDI>5 subjects were older, farer from menopause, and had a higher prevalence of calcium intake ≤300 mg/day, arterial hypertension, previous fragility fractures and COPD and a lower prevalence of dyslipidemia.

The linear correlation index between the input variables and the Spinal Deformity Index was generally very low (range R: 0.000–0.384). The SDI was significantly and positively associated with age ($R = 0.374$, $p = 0.0001$), and with years since menopause (YSM) ($R = 0.384$, $p = 0.0001$). Logistic regression analysis showed that YSM and the absence of dyslipidemia were independently associated with SDI≥1, regardless for the presence of low BMD (Table 3A). Moreover, this analysis showed that YSM, COPD and the absence of dyslipidemia were independently associated (and the presence of a previous fragility fracture borderline associated) with the presence of SDI≥5, regardless of low BMD (Table 3B).

The variables selected by TWIST system, at the end of its evolution, for the analysis aimed to identify patients with a SDI≥1 and a SDI≥5, are reported in Table 1.

The sensitivity, specificity and accuracy of ANNs and LR (by Forward Stepwise method) in discriminating patients with SDI = 0 from those with SDI≥1 and from those with SDI>5 are reported in table 4A and 4B, respectively. The sensitivity, specificity and accuracy of ANNs represent the mean of the ten experiments for each target prediction according to five per two cross-validation protocol (tables 5A and 5B) [34]. In both the analysis the overall accuracy of ANNs as evaluated with ROC AUC was significantly superior to that of LR (table 4A and 4B and figures 1a and 1b).

The analysis performed by a multiple model including in LR only the variables with p<0.25 in bivariate analysis, showed less satisfactory results than those obtained with the Forward Stepwise method (data not shown).

Discussion

The present study showed that Artificial Neural Networks have a better capacity of discriminating between patients without morphometric vertebral fractures (SDI = 0) and patients with at least 1 morphometric vertebral fractures (SDI≥1) and patients with a SDI≥5, than logistic regression analysis. Moreover, in our sample, the LR showed a low sensitivity in identifying SDI≥1 and SDI≥5. This result is in keeping with some previous studies suggesting that the algorithm using classical statistical approach, like FRAX™, have a low sensitivity [20,21], probably due to the limitations of a linear analytical approach in explaining a complex multifactorial disease, like osteoporosis.

To our knowledge, this is the first study which aimed to evaluate the capacity of ANNs, compared with Logistic Regression (LR), to recognise patients with fragility vertebral fractures. The present

Table 2. Clinical characteristics of all patients, patients without morphometric vertebral fractures, SDI≥1 and SDI≥5.

	All (n = 372)	SDI = 0 (n = 196)	SDI≥1 (n = 176)	SDI≥5 (n = 51)	*P	#P
Age (years)	68.0±8.5	65.3±8.1	71.1±7.8	75.2±6.1	0.0001	0.0001
YSM (years)	18 (1–50)	16 (1–44)	22.5 (3–50)	27 (8–50)	0.0001	0.0001
BMI (Kg/m^2)	23.0 (16–41)	23 (16–41)	23 (16–36)	24 (16–36)	0.374	0.160
Calcium intake (mg/day)	636±404	640±382	632±429	596±458	0.861	0.486
n. of pts with calcium intake≤300 mg/day (%)	73 (19.6)	32 (16.3)	41 (23.3)	16 (31.4)	0.116	0.027
n. of pregnancies	2 (0–5)	2 (0–5)	2 (0–4)	2 (0–4)	0.795	0.383
BF months	3 (0–72)	3 (0–60)	3 (0–72)	3 (0–72)	0.255	0.352
n. of smokers (%)	57 (15.3)	28 (14.3)	29 (16.5)	5 (9.8)	0.568	0.494
n. of ex-smokers (%)	38 (10.2)	22 (11.2)	16 (9.1)	4 (7.8)	0.608	0.613
n. of patients consuming alcohol ≥3 units/day (%)	124 (33.3)	63 (32.1)	61 (34.7)	19 (37.3)	0.660	0.507
n. of patients with previous clinical fracture (%)	33 (8.9)	14 (7.1)	19 (10.8)	10 (19.6)	0.273	0.014
n. of patients with familiar history of hip fracture (%)	64 (17.2)	35 (17.9)	29 (16.5)	9 (17.6)	0.784	1.000
n. of patients with kidney stones (%)	17 (4.6)	10 (5.1)	7 (4.0)	1 (2.0)	0.630	0.468
n. of patients with arterial hypertension (%)	110 (29.6)	47 (24.0)	63 (35.8)	20 (39.2)	0.017	0.035
n. of patients with dyslipidemia (%)	55 (14.8)	35 (17.9)	20 (11.4)	2 (3.9)	0.081	0.014
n. of patients with gastric/esophagus disease (%)	84 (22.6)	47 (24.0)	37 (21.0)	8 (15.7)	0.536	0.258
n. of patients with anxiety/depression (%)	50 (13.4)	33 (16.8)	17 (9.7)	9 (17.6)	0.048	0.837
n. of patients with COPD (%)	14 (3.8)	4 (2.0)	10 (5.7)	5 (9.8)	0.099	0.020
n. of patients with Osteoarthritis (%)	80 (21.5)	46 (23.5)	34 (19.3)	11 (21.6)	0.377	0.854
n. of patients with T2D (%)	14 (3.8)	8 (4.3)	6 (3.4)	1 (2.0)	0.791	0.690
n. of patients with Low BMD (T-score ≤−2.5) (%)	242 (65.1)	127 (64.8)	115 (65.3)	35 (68.6)	1.000	0.741
SDI	0 (0–24)	0 (0–0)	2 (1–24)	8 (5–24)		

Data are expressed as mean±SD, and median (range) for not normally distributed variables, if not differently specified.
*SDI = 0 vs SDI≥1; #SDI = 0 vs SDI≥5; SDI: Spinal Deformity Index; YSM: Years since menopause; BMI: Body Mass Index: weight (Kg)/height ^{2} (m^2); BF: breast feeding expressed in months; COPD: chronic obstructive pulmonary disease; T2D: Type 2 diabetes mellitus; SDI: Spinal Deformity Index calculated according to the method described by Crans (see Methods);

Table 3. OR for detecting morphometric vertebral fracture (SDI$\geq$: A and SDI$\geq$5: B) for Potential Risk Factors using the multivariable Logistic Regression Model.

	OR	95% CI	p
A			
Years since menopause	1.07	1.04–1.09	0.0001
Previous fragility fracture	1.28	0.60–2.75	0.522
Arterial Hypertension	1.54	0.93–2.55	0.093
COPD	2.63	0.74–9.31	0.134
Daily calcium intake (mg/day)	1.00	1.00–1.00	0.664
Low BMD (T-score $\leq$−2.5)	1.06	0.67–1.67	0.811
Dyslipidemia (absence)	2.21	1.15–4.24	0.017
B			
Years since menopause	1.13	1.08–1.19	0.0001
Previous fragility fracture	2.93	0.98–8.75	0.054
Arterial Hypertension	1.81	0.80–4.11	0.154
COPD	7.11	1.12–45.19	0.038
Daily calcium intake (mg/day)	1.00	1.00–1.00	0.134
Low BMD (T-score $\leq$−2.5)	1.22	0.55–2.73	0.629
Dyslipidemia (absence)	12.5	2.21–71.43	0.004

results are similar to those obtained in previous studies in other medicine fields [37–42], suggesting that this kind of statistical approach may be better than the traditional one, to understand complex topics like human diseases.

The comparison of results obtained with two different analytical approaches (logistic regression and TWIST system), points out the need to employ systems that are really able to handle the disease complexity instead of treating the data with reductionist approaches that are unable to detect multiple contribution of smaller effect in predisposing to the disease. Moreover, ANNs are able to identify variables combinations that are likely to produce accurate predictions of outcomes for a single individual, a very important property for the clinician facing every day with decision to be taken in a specific patient. The superiority of ANNs vs LR may be also due to the fact that ANNs build up models with higher number of variables, since they can manage also variables with a very poor linear correlation index. Another novelty of this study is the possibility of identifying the presence of a morphometric vertebral fracture (SDI$\geq$1) as a binary parameter (fracture Yes/No), but also the presence of a high SDI (SDI$\geq$5), that is known to be associated with a higher risk of new vertebral fractures [16], regardless for BMD. This is an important point since it has been demonstrated that also the risks of hip and any non vertebral fractures increase with SDI [43]. Thus, the use of SDI combined with other risk factors, particularly if with an ANNs algorithm, may consent to better identify patients at high risk of fractures. It must be considered that an histomorphometric study showed that the SDI is inversely associated with bone volume, therefore suggesting SDI as a surrogate marker of bone quality [19].

The presence of a fragility fracture was found to be associated with hypertension by the ANNs analyses (tending to the statistical significance also by LR analysis) and with the absence of dyslipidemia by both the LR and ANNs analyses (Table 3A). This result, although not a declared end-point deserves particular interest. Indeed, the link between arterial hypertension, BMD and fractures is debated and may be possibly explained by the use of antihypertensive drugs. Several studies showed an association between the use of antihypertensive drugs, such as diuretic loops, and BMD loss, probably due to an increase in urinary calcium excretion, but the effect on fracture risk is still controversial [44,45]. On the other hand, another study suggested that there was no association between BMD and hypertension after correction for several confounding factors [46]. Recently, the sensitivity to glucocorticoids has been suggested as a possible link between hypertension and osteoporosis. Indeed, the combination of hypertension and vertebral fractures has been shown to be associated with the sensitizing polymorphisms of the glucocorticoid receptor in patients with a subtle cortisol excess [47].

Similarly, the association between the dyslipidemia and fractures risk probably has a reference to the use of statins. Statins inhibits cholesterol synthesis by blocking the initial part of the mevalonate metabolic pathway, which is the same metabolic pathway inhibited, more downstream, by bisphosphonates. Moreover, lipophilic statins seem to influence bone formation influencing the expression of bone morphogenetic protein 2 (BMP-2) [48]. Finally, in several clinical trials the use of statins had been associated with a reduction in the risk of fracture [49,50].

The relatively small sample size is a limitation of the present study. However, as the prevalence of morphometric vertebral fractures is higher than that of clinical fractures, the use of the formers as end point, allows reducing the sample size saving the statistic power of the study. It is well known that ANNs, at

Table 4. Sensitivity, Specificity and overall accuracy in identifying patients with a SDI$\geq$1 (A) and SDI$\geq$5 (B) by artificial neural networks analysis and traditional statistics.

	n° of variables	SN (%)	SP (%)	Accuracy (%)	ROC AUC
		(95% CI)	(95% CI)	(95% CI)	(95%CI)
A					
ANNs	17	72.5 (65.91–79.09)	78.5 (72.75–84.00)	75.5 (71.13–79.87)	0.714** (0.673–0.755)
LR	45	35.8 (30.22–44.38)	76.5 (70.40–83.61)	56.2 (51.78–60.62)	0.616 (0.576–0.656)
B					
ANNs	25	74.8 (62.89–80.72)	87.8 (83.22–92.38)	81.3 (76.44–86.16)	0.823** (0.780–0.866)
LR	45	37.3 (25.14–49.46)	90.3 (86.16–94.44)	63.8 (57.88–69.72)	0.699 (0.657–0.741)

ANNs: artificial neural networks; LR: logistic regression analysis; SN: sensitivity; SP: specificity; ROC: receiver operating characteristic; AUC: area under the curve.
**: $p<0.01$.

Table 5. Goodness of fit test for ANNs in identifying patients with a SDI≥1 (A) and SDI≥5 (B).

	Testing on subset	Sensitivity (%)	Specificity (%)	Overall accuracy (%)
A	1a	73.4	78.9	76.2
	1b	71.7	79.2	75.5
	2a	72.0	77.5	74.8
	2b	73.2	77.9	75.6
	3a	74.0	78.0	76.0
	3b	71.2	79.2	75.2
	4a	72.3	77.9	75.1
	4b	72.9	78.7	75.8
	5a	72.2	78.8	75.5
	5b	72.1	78.9	75.5
	Average	72.5	78.5	75.5
B	1a	77.3	87.9	82.6
	1b	72.4	87.6	80.0
	2a	73.2	88.4	80.8
	2b	74.5	88.2	81.4
	3a	74.5	87.6	81.1
	3b	74.2	87.5	80.9
	4a	76.6	87.8	82.2
	4b	78.0	88.2	83.1
	5a	75.4	87.3	81.4
	5b	72.3	87.3	79.8
	Average	74.8	87.8	81.3

5×2 cross validation protocol.
A: Chi square = 0.10; N.S.; B: Chi square = 0.23; N.S.

variance with the classical statistical tests, can manage complexity even with relatively small samples and the subsequent unbalanced ratio between variables and records. Indeed, it is important to note that adaptive learning algorithms of inference, based on the principle of a functional estimation like artificial neural networks, can partially overcome the problem of dimensionality. Moreover, the cross-sectional design of the study does not consent to look at the incidence of fractures and to compare, head to head, this approach with FRAX. Another limit of the study may be related to the lack of a cross-calibration of different devices for measuring BMD. However, this possible error should have been corrected, at least in part, by the use of the T-score for expressing bone mineral density data and by having dichotomized the variable on the basis of a T-score > or ≤2.5. Similarly, it must be note that a inter-rater Cohen's k of agreement was not obtained between results obtained in various centers. However, the 9 out-patient clinics for osteoporosis management belonging to GISMO-Lombardia Group have been working altogether since September 2005 using the same protocols for data collection, and the homogeneity between the 9 centers has been checked by specific investigators meetings twice yearly. Finally, we do not have information about pharmacological history other than anti-osteoporotic drugs. It must be also considered that the study was conducted in female osteoporosis clinic patients, and, therefore, the extrapolation of the results to other groups should be done with caution. In the future, wider longitudinal studies could help to confirm our data and to better understand causal relationship between variables.

Notwithstanding these limitations, the present study shows, for the first time, that ANNs have a better capacity, in respect with LR, in identifying the presence of morphometric vertebral fractures and the presence of a high risk SDI. The use of ANNs in developing algorithms for predicting the fracture risk in the individual subject may be an important advance in assessing the most cost-effective therapeutic threshold in the field of osteoporosis.

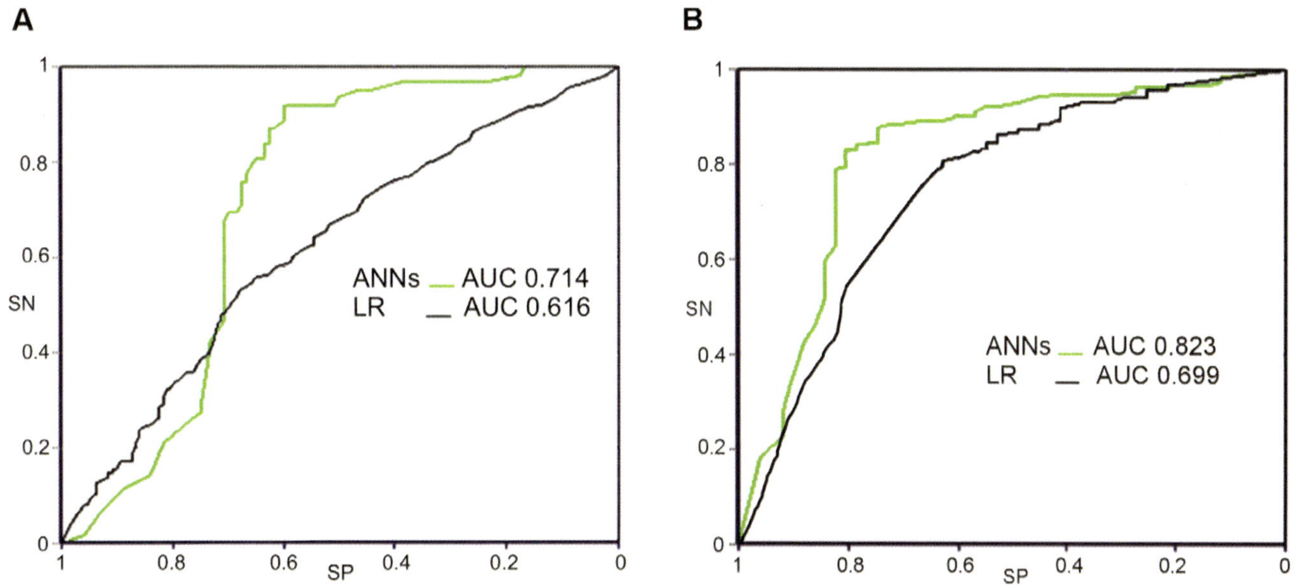

Figure 1. ROC curve for artificial neural networks and logistic regression analysis in identifying SDI≥1 and SDI≥5. The ANN AUC is significantly superior to LR AUC both in identifying SDI≥1 ($p<0.01$) (A) and SDI≥5 ($p<0.001$) (B). ROC: Receiver operating characteristic, SN: sensitivity, SP: specificity. ANNs: artificial neural networks; AUC: area under the curve; LR: logistic regression analysis.

Acknowledgments

Fazio Rosa (Milano), Arioli Giovanni (Pieve di Coriano MN), Aversa Annamaria (Milano), Broggini Marco (Varese), Capponi Aldo (Ponte S.Pietro BG), Cavaiani Paola (Abbiategrasso MI), Davoli Camillo (Cremona), Dughi Silvia (Rovato BS), Fezzi Paolo (Merate LC), Galimberti Gianluca (Rozzano MI), Gipponi Claudio (Orzinuovi BS), Giustina Andrea (Brescia), Locati Maurizio (Saronno VA), Melchioretti Renata (Lonato BS), Pagano Patrizia (Trescore Balneario BG), Pezzali Francesco (Leno BS), Pirola Luigi (Melzo MI), Poccobelli Umberto (Corsico MI), Resmini Giuseppina (Treviglio BG), Rondena Maurizio (Legnano MI), Sileo Fulvio (Bergamo), Varenna Massimo (Milano).

Author Contributions

Conceived and designed the experiments: CEV IC GG MB EG. Performed the experiments: CEV IC EG. Analyzed the data: CEV IC EG. Contributed reagents/materials/analysis tools: CEV IC IS MM LP PBP ML VG GG MB EG EC. Wrote the paper: CEV IC PBP EG EC.

References

1. NIH Consensus Statement (2000) Osteoporosis prevention, diagnosis, and therapy. Mar 27–29 17(1): 1–45.
2. World Health Organization (2007) Assessment of osteoporosis at the primary health care level. Summary Report of a WHO Scientific Group. WHO, Geneva. Available: http://www.who.int/chp/topics/rheumatic/en/index.html. Accessed 2011 Sep 1.
3. Marshall D, Johnell O, Wedel JJ (1996) Meta-analysis of how well measures of bone mineral density predict occurrence of osteoporotic fractures. Br Med J 312: 1254–1259.
4. Kanis JA, Johnell O, Oden A, De Laet C, Jonsson B, et al. (2002) Ten-year risk of osteoporotic fracture and the effect of risk factors on screening strategies. Bone 30: 251–258.
5. De Laet C, Oden A, Johansson H, Johnell O, Jonsson B, et al. (2005) The impact of the use of multiple risk indicators for fracture on case-finding strategies: a mathematical approach. Osteoporos Int 16: 313–318.
6. Kanis JA, Johnell O, Oden A, Johansson H, McCloskey E (2008) FRAX and the assessment of fracture probability in men and women from the UK. Osteoporos Int 19(4): 385–397.
7. Cummings SR, Melton LJ, 3rd (2002) Epidemiology and outcomes of osteoporotic fractures. Lancet 359: 1761–67.
8. Gehlbach SH, Bigelow C, Heimisdottir M, May S, Walker M, et al. (2000) Recognition of vertebral fracture in a clinical setting. Osteoporos Int 11: 577–82.
9. Klotzbuecher CM, Ross PD, Landsman PB, Abbott TA, III, Berger M (2000) Patients with prior fractures have an increased risk of future fractures: a summary of the literature and statistical synthesis. J Bone Miner Res 15: 721–39.
10. Ross PD, Davis JW, Epstein RS, Wasnich RD (1991) Pre-existing fractures and bone mass predict vertebral fracture incidence in women. Ann Intern Med 1: 919–23.
11. Black DM, Arden NK, Palermo L, Pearson J, Cummings SR (1999) Prevalent vertebral deformities predict hip fractures and new vertebral deformities but not wrist fractures. Study of Osteoporotic Fractures Research Group. J Bone Miner Res 14: 821–8.
12. Lindsay R, Silverman SL, Cooper C, Hanley DA, Barton I, et al. (2001) Risk of new vertebral fracture in the year following a fracture. JAMA 285: 320–323.
13. Melton LJ, 3rd, Wenger DE, Atkinson EJ, Achenbach SJ, Berquist TH, et al. (2006) Influence of baseline deformity definition on subsequent vertebral fracture risk in post menopausal women. Osteoporos Int 17: 978–985.
14. Minne HW, Leidig G, Wüster C, Siromachkostov L, Baldauf G, et al. (1988) A newly developed spine deformity index (SDI) to quantitate vertebral crush fractures in patients with osteoporosis. Bone Miner 3: 335–49.
15. Genant HK, Wu CY, Van Kujik C, Nevitt MC (1993) Vertebral fracture assessment using a semiquantitative technique. J Bone Miner Res 8: 1137–48.
16. Crans GG, Genant HK, Krege JH (2005) Prognostic utility of a semiquantitative spinal deformity index. Bone 37: 175–9.
17. Kerkeni S, Kolta S, Fechtenbaum J, Roux C (2009) Spinal deformity index (SDI) is a good predictor of incident vertebral fractures. Osteoporos Int 20: 1547–1552.
18. Di Monaco M, Vallero F, Di Monaco R, Franza G, Tappero R (2011) The burden of prevalent vertebral fractures is negatively associated with functional outcome in women with hip fracture. Am J Phys Med Rehabil 90: 1–7.
19. Genant HK, Delmas PD, Chen P, Jiang Y, Eriksen EF, et al. (2007) Severity of vertebral fracture reflects deterioration of bone microarchitecture. Osteoporos Int 18: 69–76.
20. Trémollieres FA, Pouillès JM, Drewniak N, Laparra J, Ribot JA, et al. (2010) Fracture risk prediction using BMD and clinical risk factors in early postmenopausal women. Sensitivity of the who FRAX™ tool. J Bone Miner Res 25(5): 1002–9.
21. Sornay-Rendu E, Munoz F, Delmas P, Chapurlat R (2010) The FRAX(R) tool in French women: how well does it describe the real incidence of fracture in the OFELY cohort. J Bone Miner Res 25(10): 2101–7.
22. McCulloch WS, Pitts WH (1943) A logical calculus of the ideas immanent in nervous activity. Bull Math Biophys 5: 115–133.
23. Zadeh LA (1997) Torwards a theory of fuzzy information granulation and its centrality in human reasoning and fuzzy logic. Fuzzy Sets Syst 90: 11–27.
24. Lisboa JP (2002) A review of evidence of health benefit from artificial neural networks in medical intervention. Neural Netw 15: 11–39.
25. National Institute on Alcohol Abuse and Alcoholism, U.S. Dept of Health and Human Services (2005) Description for standard drinks chart. Available: http://pubs.niaaa.nih.gov/publications/Practitioner/PocketGuide/pocket_guide2.htm. Accessed 2007 June 28.
26. Varenna M, Binelli L, Zucchi F, Ghiringhelli D, Sinigaglia L (2001) Unbalanced diet to lower serum cholesterol level is a risk factor for postmenopausal osteoporosis and distal forearm fracture. Osteoporos Int 12(4): 296–301.
27. Guglielmi G, Stoppino LP, Placentino MG, D'Errico F, Palmieri F (2007) Reproducibility of a semi-automatic method for 6-point vertebral morphometry in a multi-centre trial. Eur J Radiol 69(1): 173–8.
28. Agenzia Italiana per il Farmaco: Nota AIFA 79. Available: http://www.agenziafarmaco.gov.it/it/content/nota-79 Accessed 2011 Sep 1.
29. Berg KM, Kunins HV, Jackson JL, Nahvi S, Chaudhry A, et al. (2008) Association between alcohol consumption and both osteoporotic fracture and bone density. Am J Med 121: 406–418.
30. Rumelhart DE (1986) A general framework for parallel distributed processing. In: Rumelhart DE, Mc Clelland JL. Parallel: Distributed Processing: Explorations in the Microstructure of Cognition. vol. 1: Cambridge, MA: Foundations, MIT Press. pp 45–76.
31. Buscema M, Grossi E, Intraligi M, Garbagna N, Andriulli A, et al. (2005) An optimized experimental protocol based on neuro-evolutionary algorithms application to the classification of dyspeptic patients and to the prediction of the effectiveness of their treatment. Artif Intell Med 34: 279–305.
32. Buscema M (2004) Genetic Doping Algorihm (GenD): theory and applications. Expert Systems 21: 63–79.
33. Buscema M, Capriotti M, Bergami F, Babiloni C, Rossini P, et al. (2007) The implicit function as squashing time model: a novel parallel nonlinear EEG analysis technique distinguishing mild cognitive impairment and Alzheimer's disease subjects with high degree of accuracy. Comput Intell Neurosci 35021: 1–15.
34. Dietterich TG (1998) Approximate statistical tests for comparing supervised classification learning algorithms. Neural Computation 10: 1885–1924.
35. Hanley JA, Mcneil BJ (1982) The meaning and use of the area under a receiver operating characteristic (ROC) curve. Radiology 143: 29–36.
36. Hanley JA, McNeil BJ (1983) A method of comparing the areas under receiver operating characteristic curves derived from the same cases. Radiology 148: 839–843.
37. Andriulli A, Grossi E, Buscema M, Festa V, Intraligi NM, et al. (2003) NUD LOOK Study Group. Contribution of artificial neural networks to the classification and treatment of patients with uninvestigated dyspepsia. Dig Liver Dis 35(4): 222–31.
38. Caocci G, Baccoli R, Vacca A, Mastronuzzi A, Bertaina A, et al. (2010) Comparison between an artificial neural network and logistic regression in predicting acute graft-vs-host disease after unrelated donor hematopoietic stem cell transplantation in thalassemia patients. Exp Hematol 38(5): 426–33.
39. Ottenbacher KJ, Linn RT, Smith PM, Illig SB, Mancuso M, et al. (2004) Comparison of logistic regression and neural network analysis applied to predicting living setting after hip fracture. Ann Epidemiol 14(8): 551–9.
40. Nilsson J, Ohlsson M, Thulin L, Höglund P, Nashef SA, et al. (2006) Risk factor identification and mortality prediction in cardiac surgery using artificial neural networks. J Thorac Cardiovasc Surg 132(1): 12–9.
41. Eftekhar B, Mohammad K, Ardebili HE, Ghodsi M, Ketabchi E (2005) Comparison of artificial neural network and logistic regression models for prediction of mortality in head trauma based on initial clinical data. BMC Med Inform Decis Mak 15(5): 3.
42. Snow PB, Kerr DJ, Brandt JM, Rodvold DM (2001) Neural network and regression predictions of 5-year survival after colon carcinoma treatment. Cancer 91(8 Suppl): 1673–8.
43. Delmas PD, Genant HK, Crans GG, Stock JL, Wong M, et al. (2003) Severity of prevalent vertebral fractures and the risk of subsequent vertebral and nonvertebral fractures: results from the MORE trial. Bone 22: 522–532.
44. Lim LS, Fink HA, Blackwell T, Taylor BC, Ensrud KE (2009) Loop diuretic use and rates of hip bone loss and risk of falls and fractures in older women. J Am Geriatr Soc 57(5): 855–62.
45. Rejnmark L, Vestergaard P, Heickendorff L, Andreasen F, Mosekilde L (2006) Loop diuretics increase bone turnover and decrease BMD in osteopenic postmenopausal women: results from a randomized controlled study with bumetanide. J Bone Miner Res 21(1): 163–70.
46. Mussolino ME, Gillum RF (2006) Bone mineral density and hypertension prevalence in postmenopausal women: results from the Third National Health and Nutrition Examination Survey. Ann Epidemiol 16(5): 395–9.

47. Morelli V, Donadio F, Eller-Vainicher C, Cirello V, Olgiati L, et al. (2010) Role of glucocorticoid receptor polymorphism in adrenal incidentalomas. Eur J Clin Invest 40(9): 803–11.
48. Garrett I, Escobedo A, Esparza J, Mundy G (1999) Cerivastatin increase BMP-2 expression in vivo and bone formation in concentration of two orders of magnitude lower than other statins. J Bone Miner Res 14(Suppl 1): S180.
49. Reid IR, Hague W, Emberson J, Baker J, Tonkin A, et al. (2001) Effect of pravastatin on frequency of fracture in the LIPID study: secondary analysis of a randomised controlled trial. Long term intervention with pravastatin in ischemic disease. Lancet 357: 509–12.
50. Bauer DC, Mundy GR, Jamal SA, Black DM, Cauley JA, et al. (2004) Use of statins and fracture: results of 4 prospective studies and cumulative meta-analysis of observational studies and controlled trials. Arch Intern Med 164: 146–52.

10

Bivariate Genome-Wide Association Analyses Identified Genes with Pleiotropic Effects for Femoral Neck Bone Geometry and Age at Menarche

Shu Ran[2], Yu-Fang Pei[2], Yong-Jun Liu[1], Lei Zhang[2], Ying-Ying Han[2], Rong Hai[3], Qing Tian[1], Yong Lin[2], Tie-Lin Yang[4], Yan-Fang Guo[5], Hui Shen[1], Inderpal S. Thethi[1], Xue-Zhen Zhu[2], Hong-Wen Deng[1,2]*]

1 School of Public Health and Tropical Medicine, Tulane University, New Orleans, Louisiana, United States of America, **2** Center of System Biomedical Sciences, School of Medical Instrument and Food Engineering, University of Shanghai for Science and Technology, Shanghai, P. R. China, **3** Inner Mongolia People's Hospital, Hohhot, P. R. China, **4** School of Life Science and Technology, Xi'an Jiaotong University, Xi'an, Shanxi, P. R. China, **5** School of Basic Medical Science, Institute of Bioinformatics, Southern Medical University, Guangzhou, Guangdong, P. R. China

Abstract

Femoral neck geometric parameters (FNGPs), which include cortical thickness (CT), periosteal diameter (W), buckling ratio (BR), cross-sectional area (CSA), and section modulus (Z), contribute to bone strength and may predict hip fracture risk. Age at menarche (AAM) is an important risk factor for osteoporosis and bone fractures in women. Some FNGPs are genetically correlated with AAM. In this study, we performed a bivariate genome-wide association study (GWAS) to identify new candidate genes responsible for both FNGPs and AAM. In the discovery stage, we tested 760,794 SNPs in 1,728 unrelated Caucasian subject, followed by replication analyses in independent samples of US Caucasians (with 501 subjects) and Chinese (with 826 subjects). We found six SNPs that were associated with FNGPs and AAM. These SNPs are located in three genes (i.e. NRCAM, IDS and LOC148145), suggesting these three genes may co-regulate FNGPs and AAM. Our findings may help improve the understanding of genetic architecture and pathophysiological mechanisms underlying both osteoporosis and AAM.

Editor: Yi-Hsiang Hsu, Harvard Medical School, United States of America

Funding: The study was partially supported by startup funds from Shanghai University of Science and Technology and Shanghai Leading Academic Discipline Project (S30501). The investigators of this work were partially supported by grants from NIH (R01AG026564, RC2DE020756, R01AR057049, R01AR050496 and R03TW008221), a SCOR (Specialized Center of Research) grant (P50AR055081) supported by National Institute of Arthritis and Musculoskeletal and Skin Diseases (NIAMS) and the Office of Research on Women's Health (ORWH), and the Edward G. Schlieder Endowment and the Franklin D. Dickson/Missouri Endowment. Lei Zhang was also supported by the National Natural Science Foundation of China project (31100902). The funders had no role in study design, data collection and analysis, decision to publish, or preparation of the manuscript.

Competing Interests: The authors have declared that no competing interests exist.

* E-mail: hdeng2@tulane.edu

Introduction

Bone strength at the hip is directly related to the risk of hip fracture, the most serious and disabling type of osteoporotic fractures [1]. Femoral neck geometry is a major determinant of the mechanical resistance of the hip and plays an important role, independent of bone mineral density (BMD), in determining bone strength and osteoporotic fractures [2]. Femoral neck geometric parameters (FNGPs) measure bone structural properties (such as shape, size, and microarchitecture) and are believed to be as good as BMD in predicting hip fracture risk [3]. FNGPs, including cortical thickness (CT), periosteal diameter (W), buckling ratio (BR), cross-sectional area (CSA), and section modulus (Z), can be conveniently and accurately inferred from dual energy X-ray absorptiometry (DXA) measurements.

FNGPs have strong genetic determination with heritability ranging from 40–50% [4–7]. Earlier studies, including ours in Caucasians and Chinese, have identified some promising candidate genes associated with FNGPs [8–12].

Menarche is the first menstrual cycle in female human beings, which occurs when thickened endometrial tissue undergoes a sudden death because of fluctuations of estrogen levels. Age at menarche (AAM) is an important factor that affects women's health. Late AAM is related with higher risk of osteoporosis in women, which may partially due to the less exposure to estrogen [13,14]. It has been shown that AAM is under strong genetic control and heritability of AAM is as high as 50–70% [15,16].

Since FNGPs and AAM are heritable traits highly related to risk of osteoporosis and women's health, it would be interesting to investigate whether there are pleiotropic genes that influence variation in both FNGPs and AAM. Previous studies were largely conducted on FNGPs or AAM separately using univariate analysis method which does not consider potential correlations between them [7,17]. This problem could be addressed by performing multivariate analysis which analyzes correlated traits simultaneously. Compared to univariate analysis, multivariate analysis has an advantage in detecting pleiotropic genes by considering the correlations between traits in the model. In addition, the multiple testing problems caused by testing different traits separately in univariate analysis can be alleviated in multivariate analysis.

Here we report the first bivariate genome-wide association study (GWAS) for FNGPs and AAM in a sample of 1,728 unrelated US

Table 1. Basic characteristics of the study subjects.

Traits	Discovery Caucasians (n = 1728)	Replication Caucasians (n = 501)	Replication Chinese (n = 826)
Age (years)	51.58 (12.92)	50.15 (17.69)	37.46 (13.77)
Height (cm)	163.28 (6.27)	163.85 (6.51)	158.38 (5.22)
Weight (kg)	71.45 (16.04)	71.32 (15.92)	54.63 (8.09)
AAM (years)	12.92 (1.58)	12.90 (1.49)	13.91 (1.61)
CT (cm)	0.15 (0.02)	0.15 (0.03)	0.14 (0.02)
W (cm)	3.30 (0.34)	3.36 (0.25)	3.11 (0.35)
BR	11.46 (2.42)	11.61 (2.74)	11.07 (2.76)
CSA (cm^2)	2.45 (0.48)	2.48 (0.45)	2.24 (0.38)
Z (cm^3)	1.45 (0.36)	1.49 (0.31)	1.26 (0.29)

Note:
All the values are presented as mean (standard deviation).

Caucasian female subjects followed by replication analyses in independent Caucasians and Chinese samples. We identified three genes (i.e. NRCAM, IDS and LOC148145) that were associated with both FNGPs and AAM, suggesting their roles in co-regulating FNGPs and AAM. Our findings may help improve the understanding of genetic architecture and pathophysiological mechanisms underlying both osteoporosis and AAM.

Table 2. Results of bivariate GWAS for AAM and three FNGPs ($p<10^{-5}$ in the discovery sample).

Traits pair	SNP	Chr	Position	Gene	*P* value in discovery sample	*P* value in replication Caucasian	*P* value in replication Chinese	Combined *p* value[1]	Combined *p* value[2]
AAM-CT									
	rs8113142	19	33704761	LOC148145	3.87×10^{-7}	–	0.73	–	4.54×10^{-6}
	rs4141232	**19**	**33727396**	**LOC148145**	$\mathbf{4.12\times10^{-7}}$	**0.03**	0.89	2.37×10^{-7}	5.80×10^{-6}
	rs4805257	19	33822305	LOC148145	1.62×10^{-6}	–	0.58	–	1.40×10^{-5}
	rs6578985	11	2094715	IGF2	1.06×10^{-6}	0.36	0.18	6.02×10^{-6}	3.14×10^{-6}
	rs6578987	11	2098162	IGF2	1.28×10^{-6}	–	0.14	–	2.96×10^{-6}
	rs6578986	11	2094728	IGF2	1.28×10^{-6}	–	0.34	–	6.81×10^{-6}
	rs4929957	11	2084885	IGF2	4.97×10^{-6}	–	0.08	–	6.26×10^{-6}
AAM-W									
	rs7929583	11	86904123	RAB38	4.35×10^{-6}	0.85	0.85	5.00×10^{-5}	5.00×10^{-5}
	rs12146626	11	86907172	RAB38	4.25×10^{-6}	0.92	0.84	5.26×10^{-5}	4.83×10^{-5}
	rs10898723	11	86904392	RAB38	8.58×10^{-6}	0.84	0.87	9.25×10^{-5}	9.56×10^{-5}
	rs6975557	**7**	**107760533**	**NRCAM**	$\mathbf{2.82\times10^{-5}}$	$\mathbf{8.33\times10^{-5}}$	0.45	$\mathbf{4.84\times10^{-8}}$	1.56×10^{-4}
	rs13230316	**7**	**107778803**	**NRCAM**	$\mathbf{5.58\times10^{-5}}$	$\mathbf{1.10\times10^{-4}}$	0.58	1.22×10^{-7}	3.67×10^{-4}
	rs5980450	**X**	**148285691**	**IDS**	$\mathbf{6.76\times10^{-5}}$	–	**0.05**	–	4.60×10^{-5}
	rs4844014	**X**	**148212344**	**IDS**	$\mathbf{7.31\times10^{-5}}$	0.39	**0.05**	3.27×10^{-4}	4.94×10^{-5}
	rs7064959	**X**	**148294515**	**IDS**	$\mathbf{8.64\times10^{-5}}$	–	**0.05**	–	5.77×10^{-5}
AAM-BR									
	rs4141232	19	33727396	LOC148145	6.99×10^{-7}	0.96	0.87	1.02×10^{-5}	9.31×10^{-6}
	rs7929583	11	86904123	RAB38	3.54×10^{-6}	0.84	0.58	4.08×10^{-5}	2.89×10^{-5}
	rs12146626	11	86907172	RAB38	4.36×10^{-6}	0.44	0.58	2.72×10^{-5}	3.51×10^{-5}
	rs10898723	11	86904392	RAB38	7.43×10^{-6}	0.35	0.62	3.69×10^{-5}	6.12×10^{-5}

Note:
Combined *p* value[1]: Combined *p* values by joint analyses of the Caucasian discovery and the Caucasian replication samples.
Combined *p* value[2]: Combined *p* values by joint analyses of the Caucasian discovery and the Chinese replication samples.
–: *p* value not available.
Bold: SNPs that were replicated in the replication samples.

Table 3. Characteristics of SNPs bivariately associated with FNGPs and AAM.

SNP	Chr	Position	Gene	Role	Allele[a]	MAF[b]	MAF[c]	MAF[d]	MAF[e]	MAF[f]	AAM-CT	AAM-W	AAM-BR
rs4141232	19	33727396	LOC148145	upstream	C/T	0.16	0.15	0.18	0.20	0.23	4.12×10^{-7}	1.09×10^{-3}	6.99×10^{-7}
rs6975557	7	107760533	NRCAM	intron	G/A	0.28	0.26	0.26	0.45	0.41	6.29×10^{-3}	2.82×10^{-5}	5.31×10^{-4}
rs13230316	7	107778803	NRCAM	intron	G/C	0.27	0.26	0.25	0.45	0.38	7.14×10^{-3}	5.58×10^{-5}	6.63×10^{-4}
rs5980450	X	148285691	IDS	downstream	A/G	0.06	–	0.03	0.15	0.15	0.44	6.76×10^{-5}	6.07×10^{-3}
rs4844014	X	148212344	IDS	downstream	C/A	0.06	0.06	0.03	0.14	0.15	0.55	7.31×10^{-5}	6.91×10^{-3}
rs7064959	X	148294515	IDS	downstream	G/A	0.06	–	0.04	0.13	0.15	0.75	8.64×10^{-5}	0.01

Note:
[a]The first allele represents the minor allele of each locus.
[b]Minor allele frequency calculated in our discovery Caucasian sample (n = 1728).
[c]Minor allele frequency calculated in our replication Caucasian sample (n = 501).
[d]Minor allele frequency reported for Caucasians in the public database of HapMap CEU.
[e]Minor allele frequency calculated in our replication Chinese subjects.
[f]Minor allele frequency reported for Chinese in the public database of HapMap.
–: MAF not available.

Methods

Subjects

The discovery sample contained 1,728 unrelated Caucasian female subjects recruited in Midwestern US (Kansas City, MO, and Omaha, NE) for studies of osteoporosis and related health problems. All the identified subjects were US Caucasians of European origin. The replication samples included Caucasians and Chinese. The Caucasian replication sample included 501 unrelated female subjects living in Omaha, NE, USA, and its surrounding areas. There was no overlap between the discovery and replication Caucasian samples. The Chinese replication sample included 826 unrelated female subjects living in Changsha or Xi'an, China.

The study was approved by Institutional Review Boards of Creighton University, University of Missouri-Kansas City, Hunan Normal University of China and Xi'an Jiaotong University of China. All the subjects signed informed-consent documents and completed structured questionnaires. The exclusion criteria were detailed in our previous publications [18]. Briefly, subjects with chronic diseases and conditions that might affect bone metabolism and AAM were excluded from this study.

Areal BMD (g/cm^2) and region area (cm^2) of FN were measured using dual-energy X-ray absorptiometry scanners Hologic QDR 4500 W (Hologic Inc., Bedford, MA, USA). The machines were calibrated daily. The coefficient of variation (CV) values obtained from the DXA measurements for FN bone size and FN BMD were 1.94% and 1.87%. Bone geometric parameters were calculated using the DXA-derived FN BMD and bone size. The methods for calculating these variables were detailed elsewhere [7,19,20]. The five estimated FNGPs are CT, W, BR, CSA, and Z. CT is an estimate of mean cortical thickness, W is the outer diameter of the bone, BR is an index of cortical instability indicating the risk of fracture by buckling, CSA is an indicator of bone axial compression strength, and Z is an index of bone bending strength indicating the bending resistance of a tube.

Genotyping

For each study subject, we extracted genomic DNA from peripheral blood leukocytes using standard protocols, and genotyping experiments were performed strictly following the standard protocol recommended by related manufacturer. The subjects of the discovery sample and the Chinese replication sample were genotyped using Affymetrix Genome-wide Human SNP 6.0 genotyping arrays (Affymetrix, Santa Clara, CA, USA) which include 909,622 SNPs [21]. The Caucasian replication sample was genotyped using Affymetrix Human Mapping 500 K arrays which included 500,567 SNPs.

Quality Control

In order to obtain high quality genotyping data, we followed strict quality control procedures. Samples with a minimum call rate of 95% were included in the analyses. For the Caucasian sample, the final mean call rate reached a level of 98.93%. We discarded SNPs that deviated from Hardy-Weinberg equilibrium ($p<0.0001$) and those with a minor allele frequency (MAF) <0.01. After quality control, the numbers of SNPs available for association analysis were 760,794 in the discovery sample, 702,413 in the Chinese replication sample, and 407,192 in the Caucasian replication sample.

Statistical Analyses

The five FNGPs were adjusted by age, height and weight [22], while AAM was adjusted by height and weight [23,24] using Minitab (Minitab Inc., State College, PA, USA). The covariates-adjusted phenotypic values were used in subsequent association analyses. We tested the phenotypic correlation between FNGPs and AAM using bivariate correlation analysis in Minitab.

The association analyses between genotype and the covariates-adjusted traits were performed using a bivariate linear regression

Table 4. Proportions of phenotype correlation explain correlations coefficients of three trait pairs.

	AAM-CT	AAM-W	AAM-BR
corr1	−0.05	0.04	0.08
corr2	−0.04	0.03	0.07
corrp	18.52%	25.26%	12.99%

Note:
Corr1: The original phenotype correlation coefficients.
Corr2: The phenotype correlation coefficients after adjusted by the SNPs.
Corrp: The proportion of correlations between each trait pairs explained by the reported SNPs, which is calculated by $corrp = (corr1 - corr2)/corr1$.

Table 5. Results of univariate association analyses for the six SNPs in the discovery sample and the replication samples.

SNP	Univariate p value discovery sample (n = 1728)				Univariate p value Replication Chinese sample (n = 826)				Univariate p value Replication Caucasian sample (n = 501)			
	AAM	CT	W	BR	AAM	CT	W	BR	AAM	CT	W	BR
rs4141232	3.48×10^{-3}	7.70×10^{-6}	6.67×10^{-3}	5.88×10^{-6}	0.82	0.95	0.63	0.81	0.46	0.01	0.96	0.66
rs6975557	0.02	0.03	8.62×10^{-5}	7.57×10^{-4}	0.28	7.57×10^{-4}	0.53	7.57×10^{-4}	0.63	0.66	2.09×10^{-5}	0.57
rs13230316	0.03	0.02	1.25×10^{-4}	6.30×10^{-4}	0.36	6.30×10^{-4}	0.65	6.30×10^{-4}	0.75	0.59	2.49×10^{-5}	0.68
rs5980450	0.47	0.40	2.36×10^{-5}	3.70×10^{-3}	0.02	3.70×10^{-3}	0.39	3.70×10^{-3}	–	–	–	–
rs4844014	0.77	0.39	1.91×10^{-5}	3.13×10^{-3}	0.02	3.13×10^{-3}	0.43	3.13×10^{-3}	0.17	0.40	0.93	0.91
rs7064959	0.86	0.51	1.79×10^{-5}	5.00×10^{-3}	0.03	0.42	0.33	0.32	–	–	–	–

Note:
–: p value not available.

model. The model is represented by $\mathbf{y}_{1i} = \boldsymbol{\mu} + \boldsymbol{\beta} x_i + \boldsymbol{\varepsilon}_i$, where $\boldsymbol{y}_i$ is the vector of the two traits for individual i; $\boldsymbol{\mu}$ is the vector of grand means; $\boldsymbol{\beta}$ is the vector of its effects, and x_i is the genotype score for individual i. ε_i is the vector of residues following a multivariate normal distribution with mean zero. The genotype x_i was encoded with an additive mode of inheritance. The association was examined by testing the significance of $\boldsymbol{\beta}$, and the test was performed with R package *lm*. Individual p values achieved in the three studied samples were then combined by fisher's method [25]. Genomic control approach was used to evaluate population effect and control potential population stratification that may lead to spurious association results. The p value of 5×10^{-8} was used as the threshold to claim significant associations at the genome-wide level, after accounting for multiple-testing by applying Bonferroni correction. Since Bonferroni correction is quite conservative, we reported SNPs that achieved a p value of 10^{-5} or less in the discovery stage. For replication, due to the prior evidence of association, we used a threshold of the nominal p level of 0.05.

We evaluated the proportion of phenotype correlations between each trait pairs explained by the reported SNPs. We define corr1 as the original phenotype correlation coefficients and corr2 as the phenotype correlation coefficients after adjusted by the SNPs. The proportion of correlations between each trait pairs explained by the reported SNPs (corrp) was calculated by the formula: $corrp = {(corr1 - corr2)}/{corr1}$.

For the SNPs showing potential pleiotropic effects, we further investigated the effect direction and causal relationship. The effect direction of the SNPs was evaluated using a linear regression model implemented in PLINK [26]. The causal relationship of the SNPs was examined by comparing adjusted/conditional models in bivariate linear regression analyses, in which the genotype of each of the reported SNPs was adjusted as a covariate in turn.

For comparison purpose, we also performed univariate association analyses for each trait using a univariate linear regression model with the R package *lm*. To compare statistical power between univariate and bivariate association analyses, we performed power analyses using the *GEE* (Generalized Estimation Equation) implemented in R. The power analyses were based on the sample sizes of 1,728, 826, and 501 unrelated subjects as used in the present study for discovery and replication analyses. Simulation analysis was performed to calculate the power.

The coefficient of linkage disequilibrium (LD) between specific SNPs was obtained from the Haploview system [27]. We used the FASTSNP program (http://fastsnp.ibms.sinica.edu.tw) to explore potential functions of the reported SNPs [28].

Results

The basic characteristics of the discovery and replication samples are summarized in Table 1. Correlation analysis of the study traits showed that AAM was significantly correlated with FNGPs. In the discovery sample, significant correlations were observed between AAM and three FNGPs (CT, W, and BR), and the correlation coefficients were -0.054 ($p = 0.028$) for AAM and CT, 0.043 ($p = 0.082$) for AAM and W, 0.077 ($p = 0.002$) for AAM and BR, respectively. The significant correlations observed here are consistent with previous findings of others [29,30]. We subsequently focused biviarate analyses on AAM and these three FNGPs.

We identified six SNPs that were associated with both FNGPs and AAM in the discovery sample ($p<10^{-5}$). These SNPs were replicated in independent Caucasian and/or Chinese replication samples (Table 2). Among them, rs4141232 is located in the upstream of the LOC148145 gene ($p = 4.12\times10^{-7}$ for AAM-CT), rs6975557 and rs13230316 are located in the intron of the NRCAM (neuronal cell adhesion molecule isoform A) gene ($p = 2.82\times10^{-5}$ and 5.58×10^{-5} for AAM-W, respectively), and the other three SNPs, rs5980450, rs4844014, and rs7064959, are located in the downstream of the IDS (Iduronate-2-sulfatase) gene ($p = 6.76\times10^{-5}$, 7.31×10^{-5} and 8.64×10^{-5} for AAM-W, respectively). Three SNPs (rs4141232, rs6975557 and rs13230316) were replicated in the Caucasian sample ($p = 0.03$, 8.33×10^{-5} and 1.10×10^{-4}, respectively). The other three SNPs (rs5980450, rs4844014, and rs7064959) near the IDS gene were replicated in the Chinese sample ($p = 0.05$) (Table 2). Combined p values of meta-analyses are also shown in Table 2.

The characteristics of the six SNPs bivariately associated with FNGPs and AAM are shown in Table 3. The proportions of phenotype correlation explained by the six SNPs were 18.52% for AAM-CT, 25.26% for AAM-W, and 12.99% for AAM-BR, respectively (Table 4).

Based on SNPs genotyped in GWAS, we estimated inflation factor (λ) which is a measure of population stratification. Generally, for a homogenous population with no stratification the value of λ should be equal or close to 1. In our GWAS cohorts, the estimated λ values for AAM, CT, W, and BR were 0.938, 0.982, 0.934, and 0.936, respectively, suggesting no or very modest population stratification, if any.

We performed univariate association analyses for the six identified SNPs in the three studied samples. As presented in Table 5, p values of univariate association analyses were less

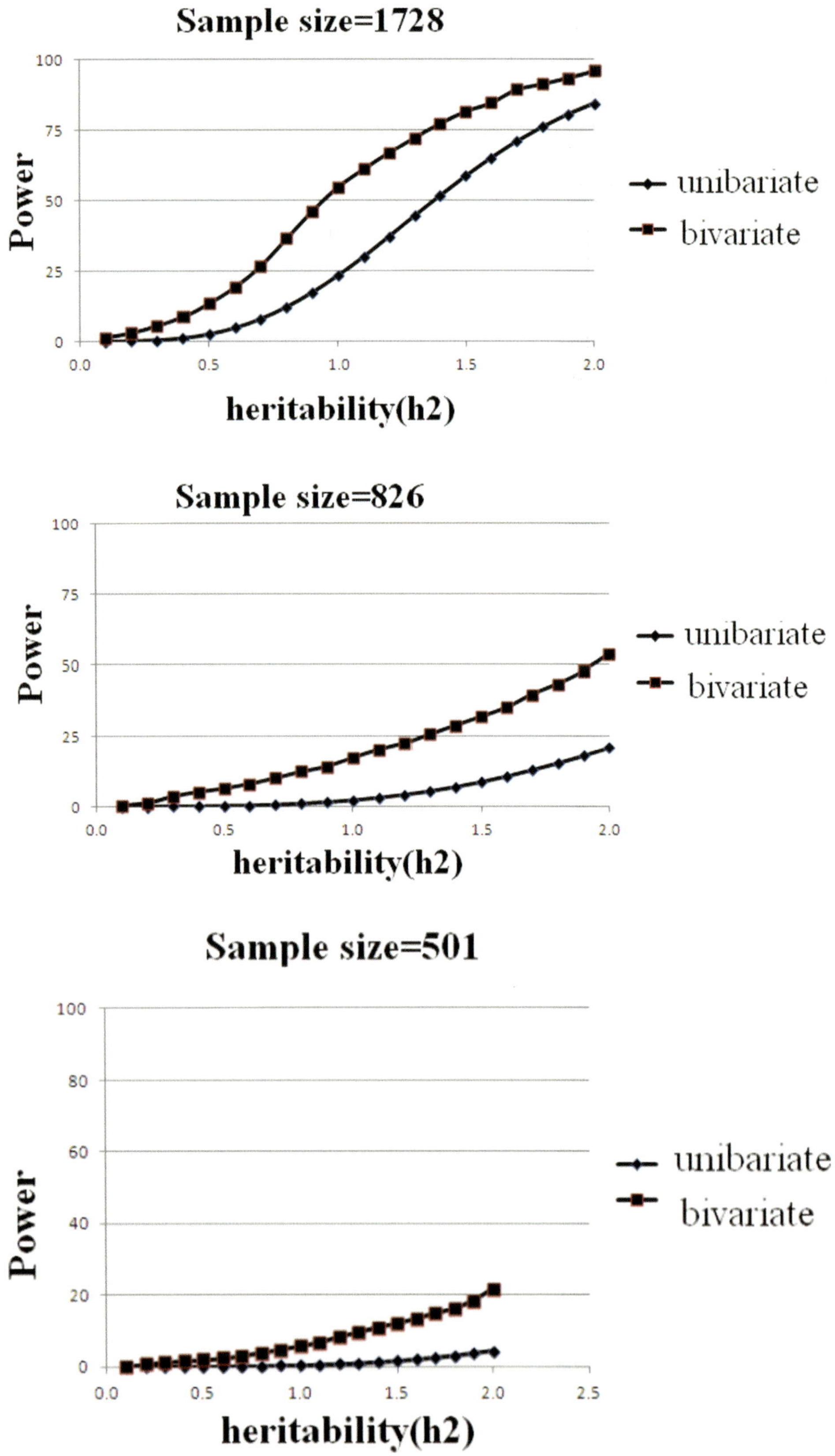

Figure 1. Comparison of statistical power of bivariate vs. univariate association analyses in three samples of this study. The Y axis shows the expected power, and the X axis shows the heritability. Type 1 error was set at 0.05 and minor allele frequency (MAF) was set at 0.1. The sample sizes were 1728 (discovery Caucasians), 826 (replication Chinese) and 501 (replication Caucasians), respectively.

Table 6. The effect direction of the SNPs in discovery and replication samples.

	Gene	Discovery Caucasian sample (n = 1728)					Replication Chinese sample (n = 826)			
		β/AAM	β/CT	β/W	β/BR	Minor allele	β/AAM	β/CT	β/W	β/BR
rs4141232	LOC148145	−0.13	0.20	−0.13	−0.21	C	0.02	−0.004	0.02	0.01
rs6975557	NRCAM	0.10	−0.09	0.16	0.13	G	−0.05	−0.04	0.03	0.07
rs13230316	NRCAM	0.09	−0.09	0.16	0.13	G	−0.03	−0.04	0.02	0.06
rs5980450	IDS	−0.07	−0.06	0.30	0.21	A	0.21	0.04	−0.06	−0.07
rs4844014	IDS	−0.06	−0.06	0.30	0.22	C	0.19	0.03	−0.05	−0.06
rs7064959	IDS	−0.03	−0.05	0.32	0.21	G	0.21	0.06	−0.06	−0.07

Note:
The effect direction was assessed using a linear regression model. A positive/negative regression coefficients (β) value means that the minor allele is associated with a higher/lower trait value. The three FNGP phenotypes were adjusted by age, height and weight while AAM was adjusted by height and weight.

significant than those of bivariate analyses. Power calculation showed that bivariate analysis exhibited consistently higher statistical power than univariate analysis did for any of the three samples (Fig. 1).

The effect directions of these SNPs are presented in Table 6. A positive beta value means that the minor allele is associated with a higher trait value. Since these SNPs were not included in the SNP arrays scanned in the Caucasian replication sample, their effect directions are not available for this sample. The effect direction for AAM was contrary between discovery and Chinese replication samples. For CT, W and BR, two SNPs of the NRCAM gene had the same effect direction in both samples, while three SNPs near the IDS gene had contrary effect directions between the two samples.

We examined the causal relationships of the six SNPs (Table 7). It can be seen that for the SNPs located in the same gene, using the genotype of one SNP as a covariate, the association signals disappeared, suggesting these SNPs are in linkage disequilibrium.

Table 7. The causal relationship of the six SNPs for three trait pairs in the discovery sample.

	Covariate	Gene	rs4141232	rs6975557	rs13230316	rs5980450	rs4844014	rs7064959
AAM-CT								
	rs4141232	LOC148145	–	4.67×10^{-3}	4.63×10^{-3}	0.54	0.67	0.85
	rs6975557	NRCAM	4.26×10^{-7}	–	0.96	0.55	0.64	0.77
	rs13230316	NRCAM	2.90×10^{-7}	0.91	–	0.56	0.41	0.64
	rs5980450	IDS	8.10×10^{-7}	9.09×10^{-3}	8.89×10^{-3}	–	0.84	0.83
	rs4844014	IDS	1.02×10^{-6}	7.95×10^{-3}	9.05×10^{-3}	0.88	–	0.98
	rs7064959	IDS	1.38×10^{-6}	8.69×10^{-3}	9.90×10^{-3}	0.91	0.99	–
AAM-W								
	rs4141232	LOC148145	–	2.43×10^{-5}	4.39×10^{-5}	9.03×10^{-5}	9.33×10^{-5}	1.30×10^{-4}
	rs6975557	NRCAM	4.04×10^{-4}	–	1.00	7.64×10^{-5}	5.60×10^{-5}	5.87×10^{-5}
	rs13230316	NRCAM	2.76×10^{-4}	0.94	–	6.98×10^{-5}	8.78×10^{-5}	9.29×10^{-5}
	rs5980450	IDS	7.82×10^{-4}	4.83×10^{-5}	1.02×10^{-4}	–	0.82	0.81
	rs4844014	IDS	7.76×10^{-4}	5.00×10^{-5}	1.15×10^{-4}	0.86	–	0.91
	rs7064959	IDS	1.20×10^{-3}	4.57×10^{-5}	1.07×10^{-4}	0.88	0.90	–
AAM-BR								
	rs4141232	LOC148145	–	2.58×10^{-4}	2.81×10^{-4}	8.40×10^{-3}	8.94×10^{-3}	0.02
	rs6975557	NRCAM	3.66×10^{-7}	–	0.97	7.67×10^{-3}	6.17×10^{-3}	0.01
	rs13230316	NRCAM	2.74×10^{-7}	0.92	–	6.42×10^{-3}	2.43×10^{-3}	6.94×10^{-3}
	rs5980450	IDS	1.21×10^{-6}	8.43×10^{-4}	9.51×10^{-4}	–	0.77	0.83
	rs4844014	IDS	1.34×10^{-6}	7.92×10^{-4}	1.07×10^{-3}	0.83	–	0.97
	rs7064959	IDS	2.37×10^{-6}	7.78×10^{-4}	1.06×10^{-3}	0.88	0.93	–

Note:
The causal relationship of the SNPs was examined by comparing adjusted/conditional models in bivariate linear regression analyses, in which the genotype of each of the six SNPs was adjusted as a covariate in turn. *P* values of the analyses are shown in the table.

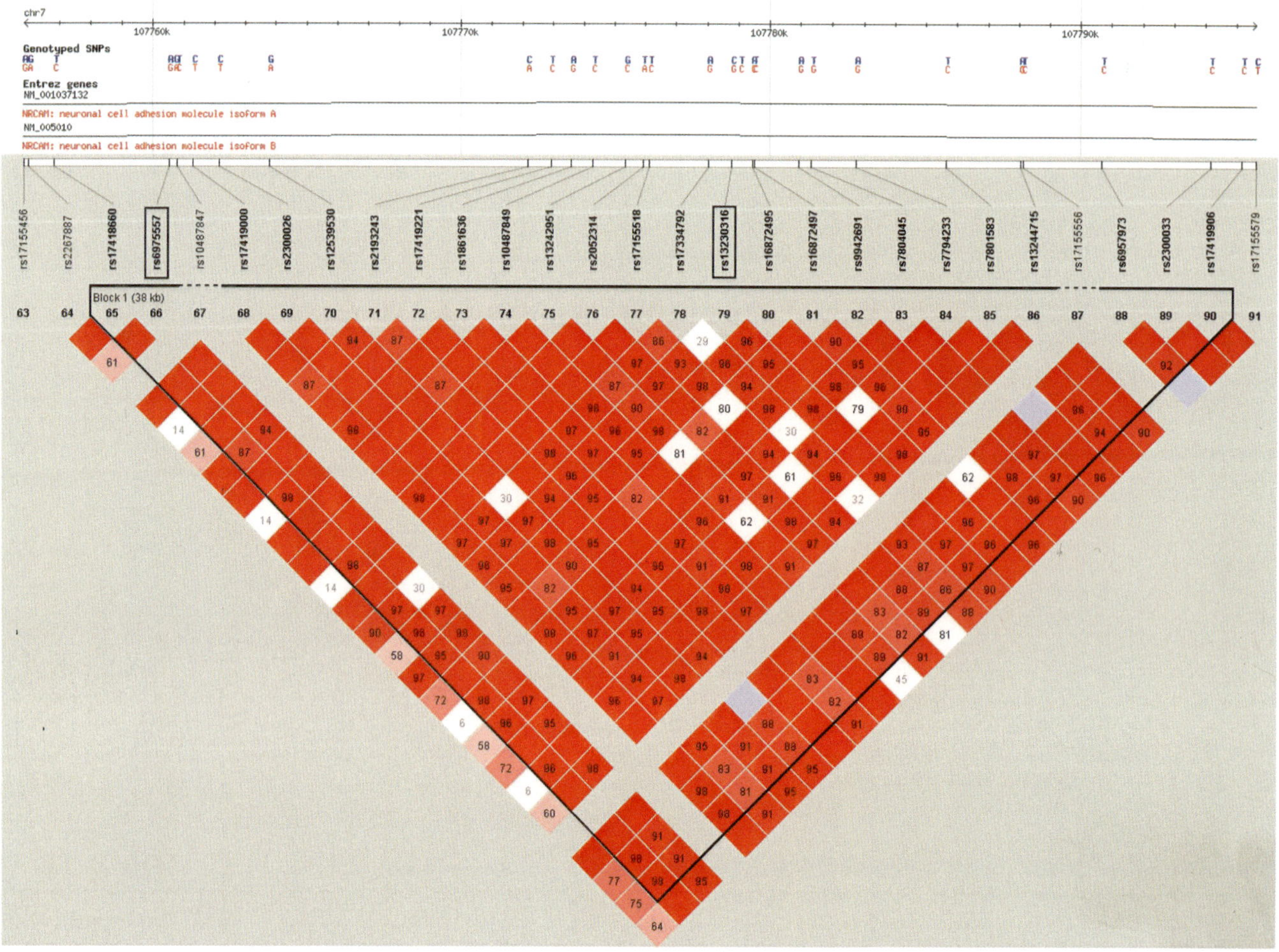

Figure 2. LD structure of the NRCAM gene in the discovery Caucasian sample. The region demarcated in red indicates that r^2>0.9. The region includes only one LD block as indicated by triangle with black lines. SNP rs6975557 and rs13230316 are located within one block.

When the genotypes of the SNPs located in different genes were used as a covariate, the association signals remained, suggesting they are independent. From biology point of view, the concept of causality is more complex than comparison of adjusted/conditional models as used here. The causal effects of the variants need to be further explored and validated via deep re-sequencing of the gene locus and subsequent molecular functional studies.

Analysis using the software Haploview in the Caucasian sample showed that SNPs rs6975557 and rs13230316 located in the NRCAM gene are in the same LD block ($r^2 \geq 0.97$) (Fig. 2). The SNPs rs8113142, rs4141232, and rs4805257 near the LOC148145 gene are in two LD blocks ($r^2 = 0.93$, and 0.88, respectively) (Fig. 3). The SNPs rs5980450, rs4844014, and rs7064959 near the IDS gene are not available in the Haploview.

Using the FASTSNP program, we investigated the potential functions of these six SNPs. The SNPs rs6975557 and rs13230316 are located at potential transcription factor-binding sites and thus may have a role in transcription regulation. A G→A change at rs6975557 may result in the elimination of the binding sites for transcription factor GATA-1, while a G→C change at rs13230316 may produce a change in the binding sites of S8 and OCT-1. The other four SNPs (i.e., rs4141232, rs5980450, rs4844014, and rs7064959) did not show known functions according to the FASTSNP program.

Discussion

To the best of our knowledge, this is the first bivariate GWAS for FNGPs and AAM, which identified three novel genes (i.e., NRCAM, IDS and LOC148145) which may contribute to co-variation of FNGPs and AAM. GWAS were largely performed by analyzing individual traits separately in a univariate framework. Although univariate analysis is effective for discovering novel genes responsible for a specific disease or trait, the approach generally ignores the potential genetic co-predisposition to human diseases. Bivariate analysis considers the correlation between traits and has an advantage in identifying genes with pleiotropic effects. The approach may help reveal the interconnected pathophysiological networks for a spectrum of common human diseases [31,32].

The gene NRCAM encodes a neuronal cell adhesion molecule [33]. Early studies showed that NRCAM gene expression increased during osteogenic and chondrogenic differentiation [34], suggesting it may function in osteoblasts and chondrocytes and probably be master control gene. The NRCAM gene is located on the chromosome 7q31, a region showed significant association with BMD in a published GWAS [35]. NRCAM is also a gene involved in regulation of estrogen. As one of the oocyte-specific genes, the NRCAM possess embryogenesis cellular growth and differentiation identified from the human primordial follicles cDNA library [36].

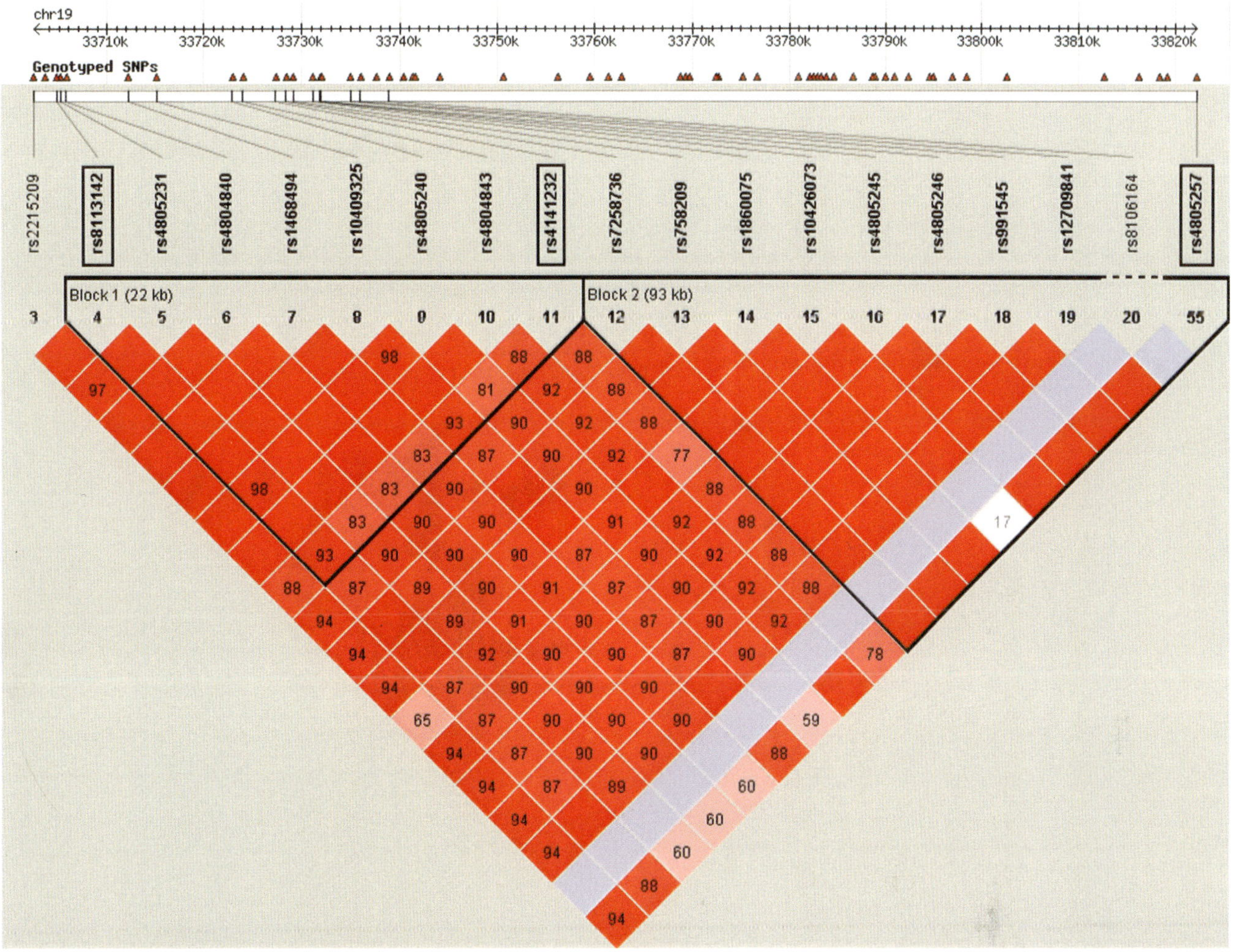

Figure 3. LD structure of the upstream of LOC148145 gene in the discovery Caucasian sample. The region demarcated in red indicates that $r^2>0.9$. The region includes two LD blocks (Block1 and Block2) marked by triangles with black lines. SNPs rs8113142 and rs4141232 are located in Block1, and the SNP rs4805257 is located in Block 2.

The IDS gene encodes Iduronate-2-sulfatase which is required for the lysosomal degradation of heparan sulfate and dermatan sulfate [37]. Mutations in the gene that result in enzymatic deficiency may lead to the sex-linked Mucopolysaccharidosis Type II [38]. Since glycosaminoglycans are fundamental in connective tissue structure and function, mucopolysaccharidosis disorders are characterized by severe skeletal abnormality including abnormal bone structure, growth failure and severe articular cartilage and joint problems [39]. The IDS gene also has relationship to AAM. IDS plays an important role in metabolism of steroid hormones such as estrone and estradiol [40]. Significant declines in activity of IDS was observed in the mammary cell lines MCF7 and T47D with estrogen exposure, with higher doses of estradiol associated with more significant declines [41]. The collective evidence suggests that IDS is important for both bone metabolism and AAM.

The LOC148145 gene locates on the chromosome 19q12. It is the non-coding RNA gene. The biological function of this gene is currently unclear and thus the exact mechanisms by which LOC148145 is involved in co-regulation of bone and AAM await discovery.

For the six SNPs associated with FNGPs and AAM, the effect directions were not completely consistent in the discovery and replication studies. The inconsistency could be explained by several reasons. First, it may be caused by genetic heterogeneity. For instance, allele frequencies of genetic variants could be different among diverse populations due to different evolution histories, which results in different genotype phenotype associations [42]. Recent studies showed that replicable findings in specific populations might be more generalizable in other populations, and such variants are more likely to be causal in nature [43]. Second, GWAS is an indirect association method based on linkage disequilibrium between SNP markers. Significant associations may be found at genetic markers that are in linkage disequilibrium with causal variants, rather than the causal variants *per se*. Therefore, inconsistency of the effect directions could be a result of different patterns of linkage disequilibrium in different populations.

Interestingly, there was an overlap between the results of this study and those of some published studies. Elks et al. reported the largest meta-analysis of GWAS for AAM in 87,802 women of European ancestry [44]. In that study, the SNP rs6589964 was strongly associated with AAM ($p=1.9\times10^{-12}$). In our study, this

SNP achieved *p* values of 6.64×10^{-4} to 8.79×10^{-4} for three trait pairs in the Caucasian discovery sample and p values of 2.86×10^{-3} to 6.27×10^{-3} in the Chinese replication sample.

In the current study, FNGPs were calculated based on DXA-derived FN BMD and bone size. This is a convenient method to obtain bone geometric indices using the areal BMD with the assumption that the mineral in the cross section is confined to an annular cortical region. However, the DXA measured BMD is restricted to two dimensions, and the resolution and accuracy of the structural parameters are affected. Despite this, studies showed that the geometry of femoral neck cross sections was reasonably well characterized by DXA compares to a more rigorous 3D finite element technique [45]. In particular, due to the wide availability of DXA scanners and the low radiation exposure of scanning, DXA is still the most popular method in clinical settings and bone research.

In summary, by performing a bivariate GWAS, we identified three novel genes (NRCAM, IDS and LOC148145) that may co-regulate FNGPs and AAM. Our findings need to be validated in different populations and molecular functional studies. Once confirmed, our findings may help improve our understanding of genetic architecture and pathophysiological mechanisms underlying osteoporosis and fracture risk. Our findings also furnish a foundation for further molecular and functional analyses of the genes in regulating timing of menarche and women's health in general.

Author Contributions

Conceived and designed the experiments: HWD YJL HS. Performed the experiments: SR YYH RH TLY HS XZZ. Analyzed the data: YFP LZ QT YL YFG. Wrote the paper: SR YJL IST HWD.

References

1. Kannus P, Parkkari J, Sievanen H, Heinonen A, Vuori I, et?al. (1996) Epidemiology of hip fractures. Bone 18: 57S–63S.
2. Turner CH, Hsieh YF, Muller R, Bouxsein ML, Baylink DJ, et al. (2000) Genetic regulation of cortical and trabecular bone strength and microstructure in inbred strains of mice. J Bone Miner Res 15 (6): 1126–1131.
3. Melton LJ, Beck TJ, Amin S, Khosla S, Achenbach SJ, et?al. (2005) Contributions of bone density and structure to fracture risk assessment in men and women. Osteoporos Int 16 (5): 460–467.
4. Demissie S, Dupuis J, Cupples LA, Beck TJ, Kiel DP, et?al. (2007) Proximal hip geometry is linked to several chromosomal regions: genome-wide linkage results from the Framingham Osteoporosis Study. Bone 40 (3): 743–750.
5. Shen H, Long JR, Xiong DH, Liu YJ, Liu YZ, et al. (2005) Mapping quantitative trait loci for cross-sectional geometry at the femoral neck. J Bone Miner Res 20 (11): 1973–1982.
6. Xiong DH, Shen H, Xiao P, Guo YF, Long JR, et al. (2006) Genome-wide scan identified QTLs underlying femoral neck cross-sectional geometry that are novel studied risk factors of osteoporosis. J Bone Miner Res 21 (3): 424–437.
7. Zhao LJ, Liu XG, Liu YZ, Liu YJ, Papasian CJ, et al. (2010) Genome-wide association study for femoral neck bone geometry. J Bone Miner Res 25 (2): 320–329.
8. Qureshi AM, McGuigan FE, Seymour DG, Hutchison JD, Reid DM, et al. (2001) Association between COLIA1 Sp1 alleles and femoral neck geometry. Calcif Tissue Int 69 (2): 67–72.
9. Rivadeneira F, Houwing-Duistermaat JJ, Beck TJ, Janssen JA, Hofman A, et al. (2004) The influence of an insulin-like growth factor I gene promoter polymorphism on hip bone geometry and the risk of nonvertebral fracture in the elderly: the Rotterdam Study. J Bone Miner Res 19 (8): 1280–1290.
10. Moffett SP, Zmuda JM, Oakley JI, Beck TJ, Cauley JA, et al. (2005) Tumor necrosis factor-alpha polymorphism, bone strength phenotypes, and the risk of fracture in older women. J Clin Endocrinol Metab 90 (6): 3491–3497.
11. Xiong DH, Liu YZ, Peng YL, Zhao LJ, Deng HW (2005) Association analysis of estrogen receptor alpha gene polymorphisms with cross-sectional geometry of the femoral neck in Caucasian nuclear families. Osteoporos Int 16 (12): 2113–2122.
12. Jiang H, Lei SF, Xiao SM, Chen Y, Sun X, et al. (2007) Association and linkage analysis of COL1A1 and AHSG gene polymorphisms with femoral neck bone geometric parameters in both Caucasian and Chinese nuclear families. Acta Pharmacol Sin 28 (3): 375–381.
13. Roy DK, O'Neill TW, Finn JD, Lunt M, Silman AJ, et al. (2003) Determinants of incident vertebral fracture in men and women: results from the European Prospective Osteoporosis Study (EPOS). Osteoporos Int 14 (1): 19–26.
14. Silman A J (2003) Risk factors for Colles' fracture in men and women: results from the European Prospective Osteoporosis Study. Osteoporos Int 14 (3): 213–218.
15. Anderson CA, Duffy DL, Martin NG, Visscher PM (2007) Estimation of variance components for age at menarche in twin families. Behav Genet. 37 (5): 668–677.
16. van den Berg SM, Boomsma DI (2007) The familial clustering of age at menarche in extended twin families. Behav Genet 37 (5): 661–667.
17. Liu YZ, Guo YF, Wang L, Tan LJ, Liu XG, et al. (2009) Genome-wide association analyses identify SPOCK as a key novel gene underlying age at menarche. PLoS Genet 5: e1000420.
18. Deng HW, Deng HY, Liu YJ, Liu YZ, Xu FH, et al. (2002) A genomewide linkage scan for quantitative-trait loci for obesity phenotypes. Am J Hum Genet 70 (5): 1138–1151.
19. Beck T. (2003) Measuring the structural strength of bones with dual-energy X-ray absorptiometry: principles, technical limitations, and future possibilities. Osteoporos Int 14 Suppl 5: S81–S88.
20. Chen Y, Xiong DH, Guo YF, Pan F, Zhou Q, et al. (2010) Pathway-based genome-wide association analysis identified the importance of EphrinA-EphR pathway for femoral neck bone geometry. Bone 46 (1): 129–136.
21. McCarroll SA, Kuruvilla FG, Korn JM, Cawley S, Nemesh J, et al. (2008) Integrated detection and population-genetic analysis of SNPs and copy number variation. Nat Genet 40: 1166–1174.
22. Zhang F, Tan LJ, Lei SF, et al. (2009) The differences of femoral neck geometric parameters: effects of age, gender and race. Osteoporos Int 21: 1205–1214.
23. Onland-Moret NC, Peeters PH, van Gils CH, Clavel-Chapelon F, Key T, et al. (2005) Age at menarche in relation to adult height: The EPIC study. Am J Epidemiol 162: 623–632.
24. Wellens R, Malina RM, Roche AF, Chumlea WC, Guo S, et al. (1992) Body size and fatness in young adults in relation to age at menarche. Am J Hum Biol 4: 783–787.
25. RA F (1948) Combining independent tests of significance. The American Statistician 2: 30.
26. Purcell S, Neale B, Todd-Brown K, Thomas L, Ferreira MA, et al. (2007) PLINK: a tool set for whole-genome association and population-based linkage analyses. Am J Hum Genet 81: 559–575.
27. Barrett JC, Fry B, Maller J, Daly MJ (2005) Haploview: analysis and visualization of LD and haplotype maps. Bioinformatics 21: 263–265.
28. Yuan HY, Chiou JJ, Tseng WH, Liu CH, Liu CK, et al. (2006) FASTSNP: an always up-to-date and extendable service for SNP function analysis and prioritization. Nucleic Acids Res 34: W635–W641.
29. Rauch F, Klein K, Allolio B, Schonau E (1999) Age at menarche and cortical bone geometry in premenopausal women. Bone 25 (1): 69–73.
30. Petit MA, Beck TJ, Lin HM, Bentley C, Legro RS, et al. (2004) Femoral bone structural geometry adapts to mechanical loading and is influenced by sex steroids: the Penn State Young Women's Health Study. Bone 35 (3): 750–759.
31. Liu YZ, Pei YF, Liu JF, Yang F, Guo Y, et al. (2009) Powerful bivariate genome-wide association analyses suggest the SOX6 gene influencing both obesity and osteoporosis phenotypes in males. PLoS One 4 (8): e6827.
32. Liu J, Pei Y, Papasian CJ, Deng HW (2009) Bivariate association analyses for the mixture of continuous and binary traits with the use of extended generalized estimating equations. Genet Epidemiol 33: 217–227.
33. Marui T, Funatogawa I, Koishi S, Yamamoto K, Matsumoto H, et al. (2009) Association of the neuronal cell adhesion molecule (NRCAM) gene variantswith autism. Int J Neuropsychopharmacol 12: 1–10.
34. Baksh D, Song L, Tuan RS (2004) Adult mesenchymal stem cells: characterization, differentiation, and application in cell and gene therapy. J Cell Mol Med 8 (3): 301–316.
35. Hsu YS, Nandakumar K, and Karasik D (2011) Musculoskeletal Genetics and -Omics: Meeting Report from the 32nd Annual Meeting of the American Society for Bone and Mineral Research. IBMS BoneKEy 8 (2): 112–122.
36. Serafica MD, Goto T, Trounson AO (2005) Transcripts from a human primordial follicle cDNA library. Hum Reprod 20 (8): 2074–2091.
37. Tuschl K, Gal A, Paschke E, Kircher S, Bodamer OA (2005) Mucopolysaccharidosis type II in females: case report and review of literature. Pediatr Neurol 32: 270–272.
38. Morini SR, Steiner CE, Gerson LB (2010) Mucopolysaccharidosis type II: skeletal-muscle system involvement. J Pediatr Orthop B 19 (4): 313–317.
39. Marucha J, Jurecka A, Syczewska M, Rozdzynska-Swiatkowska A, Tylki-Szymanska A. (2011) Restricted joint range of motion in patients with MPS II: correlation with height, age and functional status. Acta Paediatr 101 (4): e183–e188.
40. Bhattacharyya S, Tobacman JK (2007) Steroid sulfatase, arylsulfatases A and B, galactose-6-sulfatase, and iduronate sulfatase in mammary cells and effects of sulfated and non-sulfated estrogens on sulfatase activity. J Steroid Biochem Mol Biol 103 (1): 20–34.

41. Tobacman JK, Bhattacharyya S (2005) Sulfatase enzyme activity in MCF-7 and MCF-10a cells following exposure to estrogenic hormones. AACR Meeting Abstracts.
42. Economou M, Trikalinos TA, Loizou KT, Tsianos EV, Ioannidis JP (2004) Differential effects of NOD2 variants on Crohn's disease risk and phenotype in diverse populations: a metaanalysis. Am J Gastroenterol 99: 2393–2404.
43. Zuo L, Gelernter J, Zhang CK, Zhao H, Lu L, et al. (2012) Genome-Wide Association Study of Alcohol Dependence Implicates KIAA0040 on Chromosome 1q. Neuropsychopharmacology 37: 557–566.
44. Elks CE, Perry JR, Sulem P, Chasman DI, Franceschini N, et al. (2010) Thirty new loci for age at menarche identified by a meta-analysis of genome-wide association studies. Nat Genet 42: 1077–1085.
45. Danielson ME, Beck TJ, Karlamangla AS, Greendale GA, Atkinson EJ, et al. (2012) A comparison of DXA and CT based methods for estimating the strength of the femoral neck in post-menopausal women. Osteoporos Int. Jul 19.

11

The Transcriptional Profile of Mesenchymal Stem Cell Populations in Primary Osteoporosis Is Distinct and Shows Overexpression of Osteogenic Inhibitors

Peggy Benisch[1], Tatjana Schilling[1], Ludger Klein-Hitpass[2], Sönke P. Frey[3], Lothar Seefried[1], Nadja Raaijmakers[1], Melanie Krug[1], Martina Regensburger[1], Sabine Zeck[1], Thorsten Schinke[4], Michael Amling[4], Regina Ebert[1], Franz Jakob[1]*

1 Orthopedic Center for Musculoskeletal Research, University of Wuerzburg, Wuerzburg, Germany, **2** Institute of Cell Biology (Tumor Research), University Hospital Essen, Essen, Germany, **3** Department of Trauma, Hand-, Plastic- and Reconstructive Surgery, University Hospital of Wuerzburg, Wuerzburg, Germany, **4** Department of Osteology and Biomechanics, University Medical Center Hamburg Eppendorf, Hamburg, Germany

Abstract

Primary osteoporosis is an age-related disease characterized by an imbalance in bone homeostasis. While the resorptive aspect of the disease has been studied intensely, less is known about the anabolic part of the syndrome or presumptive deficiencies in bone regeneration. Multipotent mesenchymal stem cells (MSC) are the primary source of osteogenic regeneration. In the present study we aimed to unravel whether MSC biology is directly involved in the pathophysiology of the disease and therefore performed microarray analyses of hMSC of elderly patients (79–94 years old) suffering from osteoporosis (hMSC-OP). In comparison to age-matched controls we detected profound changes in the transcriptome in hMSC-OP, e.g. enhanced mRNA expression of known osteoporosis-associated genes (*LRP5, RUNX2, COL1A1*) and of genes involved in osteoclastogenesis (*CSF1, PTH1R*), but most notably of genes coding for inhibitors of WNT and BMP signaling, such as Sclerostin and MAB21L2. These candidate genes indicate intrinsic deficiencies in self-renewal and differentiation potential in osteoporotic stem cells. We also compared both hMSC-OP and non-osteoporotic hMSC-old of elderly donors to hMSC of ~30 years younger donors and found that the transcriptional changes acquired between the sixth and the ninth decade of life differed widely between osteoporotic and non-osteoporotic stem cells. In addition, we compared the osteoporotic transcriptome to long term-cultivated, senescent hMSC and detected some signs for pre-senescence in hMSC-OP. Our results suggest that in primary osteoporosis the transcriptomes of hMSC populations show distinct signatures and little overlap with non-osteoporotic aging, although we detected some hints for senescence-associated changes. While there are remarkable inter-individual variations as expected for polygenetic diseases, we could identify many susceptibility genes for osteoporosis known from genetic studies. We also found new candidates, e.g. *MAB21L2*, a novel repressor of BMP-induced transcription. Such transcriptional changes may reflect epigenetic changes, which are part of a specific osteoporosis-associated aging process.

Editor: Xing-Ming Shi, Georgia Health Sciences University, United States of America

Funding: This work was supported by the German Research Foundation [FOR793 JA506/9-1](http://www.dfg.de/index.jsp). The funder had no role in study design, data collection and analysis, decision to publish, or preparation of the manuscript.

Competing Interests: The authors have read the journal's policy and have the following conflicts: F. Jakob has received honoraria and travel grants for lectures, advice and expert testimony from Lilly, Amgen, Novartis, Merck Sharp and Dohme (MSD), Nycomed, Servier, Medtronic and Roche. He has received unrestricted research grants from Novartis and is involved in clinical studies related to osteoporosis drugs initiated by Lilly, Amgen, Servier and Novartis. L. Seefried has received honoraria and travel grants for lectures from Lilly, Amgen and Novartis. He is involved in clinical studies related to osteoporosis drugs initiated by Amgen, Servier and Novartis. R. Ebert received honoraria and travel grants for lectures from Lilly and Novartis.

* E-mail: f-jakob.klh@uni-wuerzburg.de

Introduction

Primary osteoporosis is a polygenetic disease characterized by low bone mineral density and microarchitectural deteriorations, leading to an increased risk of fragility fractures of vertebrae, femoral neck and other typical localizations of lower incidence [1]. Advanced age, gender and immobilization are major risk factors for developing osteoporosis besides a series of other contributors, e.g. diminished sex steroid production in elderly individuals and after menopause [2,3]. During the first decades of osteoporosis research the main focus has been the imbalance of bone resorption over bone formation as a consequence of pathologically enhanced osteoclast development and function [4]. Hence, antiresorptive treatment, targeting mature osteoclasts and the osteoclastogenesis promoting RANK (Receptor Activator of NF-κB)/RANKL (RANK ligand) pathway has evolved as a standard therapy over the last decades [1,5]. In contrast, research on presumptive deficiencies in bone anabolism has been relatively neglected. Little is known about the impact of bone forming osteoblasts on the pathophysiology of osteoporosis in humans, although evidence was found for reduced activity [6] and enhanced apoptosis [7,8]. Osteoblasts derive from mesenchymal stem cells (MSC), which can also give rise to other mesodermal cell types, such as adipocytes, chondrocytes and fibroblasts [9]. Despite of MSC as the source for bone regeneration it is currently unknown if intrinsic deficiencies in these cells contribute to osteoporotic bone loss.

Three major signaling pathways have been identified to govern bone regeneration with an intense intracellular crosstalk: a) Bone morphogenetic protein (BMP) signaling, b) WNT signaling and c) signaling through parathyroid hormone receptor (PTH1R) activation. Recent research has highlighted the relevance of inhibitors of the respective pathways for the regulation of bone mass and thereby suggested new targets for the treatment of bone loss [1].

BMP proteins belong to the TGFβ superfamily and activation of BMP receptors leads to induction of transcription through either MAP kinase signaling or phosphorylation of SMAD1/5/8 proteins [10,11]. Signaling through BMP proteins is regulated by either extracellular antagonists such as Noggin and Gremlin [12,13] or by intracellular inhibitors, e.g. inhibitory SMAD proteins [14] or nuclear MAB21L2 (Mab-21-like 2), a recently discovered BMP4 inhibitor [15].

Depending on coreceptors WNT signaling can be divided into canonical and non-canonical pathways. Canonical signaling is induced by binding of WNT ligands to the receptors of the Frizzled (FZD) family and LRP5/6 coreceptors, which results in activation of WNT-specific gene transcription by stabilization and nuclear translocation of β-Catenin. Non-canonical WNT signaling is transduced through FZD and ROR2/RYK coreceptors, which leads to the activation of G-protein or Ca^{2+}-dependent cascades [16]. In MSC canonical signaling through WNT2, WNT3 or WNT3a induces proliferation and keeps the cells in an undifferentiated state, whereas non-canonical signaling, e.g. by WNT5a, WNT5b or WNT11, supports osteogenesis [17,18,19].

The osteocyte-specific factor Sclerostin (*SOST*) was described as an inhibitor of canonical WNT signaling, whereas there is ongoing discussion about its putative inhibitory effect on BMP signaling [20,21]. Sclerostin leads to reduced bone formation [22] and loss of function mutations are responsible for the high bone mass syndromes Van Buchem disease and sclerosteosis [23]. A neutralizing antibody against Sclerostin is a new, upcoming therapeutic treatment for osteoporosis [1,24].

Intermittent treatment with parathyroid hormone (PTH) is another therapeutical approach for osteoporosis and activates the third major signaling pathway in bone regeneration. However, continuous activation of PTH receptor has negative effects on bone homeostasis because subsequently enhanced RANKL expression on maturing osteoblasts stimulates osteoclast formation and bone resorption [25,26].

Interestingly, the genetic loci of proteins involved in the signaling pathways mentioned above, e.g. LRP5, LRP4, Sclerostin, PTH, BMPs or BMP receptor BMPR1B, have already been linked to the polygenetic nature of primary osteoporosis by whole-genome association studies and meta-analyses [27,28,29,30].

Besides genetic predisposition, advanced age is another strong risk factor for developing osteoporosis with adult stem cells being the restrictive parameter for unlimited tissue regeneration. *In vitro*, cells exhibit limited dividing capacity and enter replicative senescence, a state of irreversible G1 phase arrest, after about 50 population doublings [31,32]. It is caused by multiple factors like telomere shortening, oxidative stress, deficiencies in DNA repair and epigenetic changes. Currently it is still controversial, whether clock-driven, organismic aging is caused by the loss of self-regeneration due to replicative senescence of stem cells or by extrinsic environmental factors [33].

The impact of presumptive deficiencies of hMSC in elderly, osteoporotic patients has not been studied intensely yet and to our knowledge changes at the gene expression level have not been examined before. Therefore, we performed microarray analyses of hMSC of elderly donors with and without osteoporosis to detect disease-associated changes in gene expression. With osteoporosis being an age-related disease, we also investigated the impact of aging on hMSC in general by analyzing the transcriptome of *in vivo*-aged and *in vitro*-aged, senescent cells. We discovered that hMSC of patients suffering from severe osteoporosis display a disease-specific gene expression pattern that is distinct from the effects of organismic aging *per se*. Besides the induced expression of inhibitors of bone formation we detected promising new candidate genes for osteoporosis and even found evidence for reduced stem cell function.

Results

Osteoporosis-induced changes in gene expression

In this study, we compared the transcriptome of hMSC from 5 patients (79–94 years old) suffering from primary osteoporosis (hMSC-OP) with hMSC of the age-matched control group (hMSC-old; donor age 79–89 years) (Table 1). Genome-wide gene expression patterns were examined by employing microarray hybridizations; the obtained data was compared by SAM method (GEO accession number GSE35958). Fold changes (FC) in gene expression were regarded as significant at a threshold of at least 2fold and a false discovery rate (FDR) of less than 10%. We detected 2477 gene products with higher and 1222 gene products with reduced expression in osteoporotic hMSC-OP in comparison to non-osteoporotic hMSC-old (Figure 1A, Table S1).

Osteoporosis as a polygenetic disease has been studied intensively on gene level, resulting in the detection of gene loci and polymorphisms associated with low bone mineral density (BMD), osteoporosis and fracture risk. In contrast to these approaches, our data represents the effects of both genetic and epigenetic changes in hMSC during the development of osteoporosis.

To see if our results coincide at least partly with the genes associated to BMD by specific single nucleotide polymorphisms (SNP) and copy number variations, we searched the NCBI data base for genome-wide association studies, meta-analyses and candidate gene association studies. The genes listed in these studies were compared to all gene products differentially expressed in the approach hMSC-OP versus hMSC-old.

We identified enhanced expression of 39 genes in hMSC-OP and reduced expression of 16 genes that are already described as reliable or promising candidates for osteoporosis, including susceptibility genes like *LRP5*, *SPP1* (Osteopontin), *COL1A1* and *SOST* (Table 2).

Effects of osteoporosis are independent of clock-driven aging

One of the main risk factors for developing primary osteoporosis is advanced age. Therefore, in the next step, we focused on gene expression patterns that were identical in hMSC-OP of elderly patients suffering from osteoporosis and hMSC-old of non-osteoporotic, elderly donors. As a new control group for microarray comparisons, we used hMSC of middle-aged donors (hMSC-C; donor age 42–67 years).

In the comparison of hMSC-OP versus hMSC-C (GEO accession number GSE35956) we detected 630 gene products with higher and 368 gene products with reduced expression due to osteoporosis and advanced donor age. By comparing hMSC-old with hMSC-C (GEO accession number GSE35955) we obtained gene expression changes due to advanced age *per se* and found

Table 1. Human MSC populations used for microarray hybridization.

hMSC group	hMSC-C	hMSC-OP	hMSC-old	hMSC-senescent
Donors (n)	5	5	4	5
Average donor age (years)	57.6±9.56	86.2±5.89	81.75±4.86	56.4±8.96
Donors showed signs of osteoporosis	no	yes	no	no
Gender	4x f, 1x m	5x f	3x f, 1x m	3x f, 2x m
RNA of hMSC used in passage	4x P1, 1x P2	4x P1, 1x P2	P1	Px

hMSC-C = control hMSC; hMSC-OP = osteoporotic hMSC; hMSC-old = hMSC of non-osteoporotic, elderly donors; hMSC-senescent = long term-cultivated hMSC in the state of replicative senescence; standard deviations are indicated by ±; n = number; f = female; m = male; P = passage; Px = senescent passage.

enhanced expression of 540 gene products and decreased expression of 1741 gene products in hMSC-old.

Due to the fact that we used hMSC-C as a control in both SAM approaches we could compare the differentially gene expression

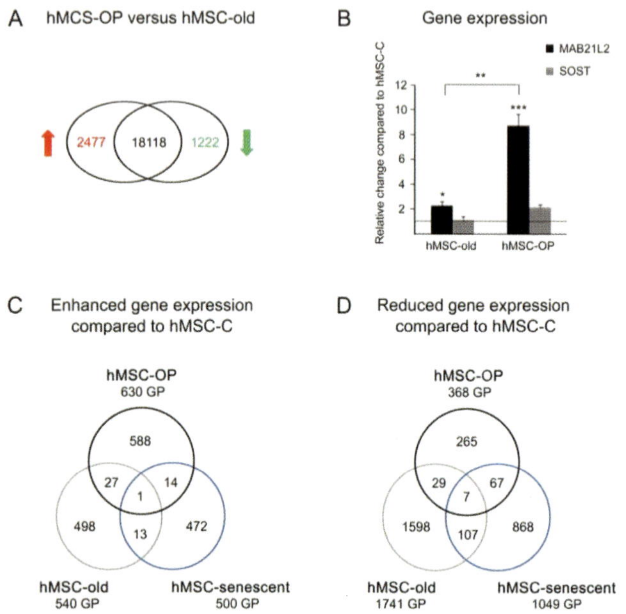

Figure 1. Differential gene expression of osteoporotic and aged hMSC. (A) Microarray comparison of hMSC-OP of elderly patients suffering from primary osteoporosis to age-matched control group hMSC-old. The numbers indicate the number of gene products with enhanced expression (red) and reduced expression (green) in hMSC-OP (for gene names see Table S1). Black numbers mark expressed gene products without significant change in expression. (B) Quantitative PCR of relative change in gene expression of *SOST* (Sclerostin) and *MAB21L2* (Mab-21-like 2) in hMSC-old and osteoporotic hMSC-OP in comparison to hMSC-C. Complementary DNA of hMSC-OP of patients suffering from primary osteoporosis (n = 12, including 4 samples also used for microarray hybridization; age 84.2±6.3), hMSC-old from non-osteoporotic donors of advanced age (n = 13, including 4 samples also used for microarray hybridization; age 82.3±3.6) and hMSC-C of middle-aged, healthy donors (n = 11, including one sample also used for microarray hybridization; age 41.6±2.6) was used. Asterisks indicate significant differences as analyzed by Mann-Whitney U test (*$p<0.05$, **$p<0.01$, ***$p<0.001$). (C–D) Comparison of differential gene expression patterns of hMSC-OP, hMSC-old and hMSC-senescent when compared to hMSC-C of middle-aged, healthy donors by microarray analyses. The numbers indicate the number of gene products (GP) with significantly enhanced (C) or reduced (D) expression, respectively (for gene names see Table S2).

patterns of hMSC-OP and hMSC-old (Figure 1C and D). Surprisingly we detected a minority of 28 gene products with enhanced and 36 gene products with reduced expression in both approaches (for gene names see Table S2).

One of the genes that was enhanced expressed due to osteoporosis but also due to advanced age was *MAB21L2* with FC[hMSC-old versus hMSC-C] = 2.7 and FC[hMSC-OP versus hMSC-C] = 14.4. By performing qPCR analysis with up to 13 samples per hMSC group we confirmed that the expression of *MAB21L2* is significantly higher in osteoporotic hMSC-OP than in hMSC-old when compared to hMSC-C of the middle-aged control group (Figure 1B).

In contrast, *SOST*, the gene coding for Sclerostin, is not associated with advanced age (no significant FC), but both microarray analysis (FC[hMSC-OP versus hMSC-C] = 7.3) and qPCR revealed the enhanced expression of the gene in osteoporotic hMSC-OP (Figure 1B).

Osteoporotic stem cells show few signs of replicative senescence

Because donors of osteoporotic cells were of highly advanced age (79+ years old) and due to the hypothesis that aging is caused by stem cells losing their self-renewal capacity due to replication limits, we investigated whether hMSC-OP showed any signs of replicative senescence. Therefore, we performed long-term cultivation of hMSC from healthy donors of medium age (42–64 years old) until they entered senescence (hMSC-senescent), proved by proliferation stop and positive senescence-associated β-galactosidase staining (data not shown).

Microarray analyses of hMSC in senescent passage Px revealed 500 gene products with enhanced and 1049 gene products with reduced expression when compared to the previously used control group hMSC-C of early passages (GEO accession number GSE35957).

By using hMSC-C as control cells for all three SAM datasets we could compare the differential gene expression pattern of hMSC-OP, hMSC-old and hMSC-senescent to find parallels in gene expression. We detected small overlap for gene products with enhanced expression when comparing hMSC-OP with hMSC-senescent (15) and hMSC-old with hMSC-senescent (14) (Figure 1C). More senescence-associated gene products were found reduced expressed in hMSC-old (114) and hMSC-OP (74) (Figure 1 D, Table S2). Few genes were differentially expressed in all three datasets: *TMEFF1* showed induced expression, whereas *MED13L*, *ANLN*, *ZWILCH*, *CMPK2*, *DDX17*, *MCM2* and *MCM8* showed diminished expression in hMSC-OP, hMSC-old and hMSC-senescent when compared to hMSC-C.

By generating a heat map for gene products at least 2fold differentially expressed in hMSC-OP compared to hMSC-C we

Table 2. Differentially expressed genes in hMSC-OP in comparison to hMSC-old with known association to BMD or fracture risk.

Symbol	Gene name	Probeset ID	FC	FDR (%)	Reference
Enhanced expression in hMSC-OP					
AAS	achalasia, adrenocortical insufficiency, alacrimia	218075_at	3.57	0.08	[58]
ANKH	ankylosis, progressive homolog	223094_s_at	3.60	0.26	[27]
		1560369_at	3.40	0.35	
ARHGAP1	Rho GTPase activating protein 1	216689_x_at	7.06	0.00	[58]
ASPH	aspartate beta-hydroxylase	205808_at	7.80	0.00	[28]
ASXL2	additional sex combs like 2	1555266_a_at	9.07	0.00	[59]
		218659_at	2.39	0.33	[59]
CAMK1G	calcium/calmodulin-dependent protein kinase IG	217128_s_at	2.45	0.44	[60]
CKAP5	cytoskeleton associated protein 5	1555278_a_at	2.78	0.26	[58]
COL1A1	collagen, type I, alpha 1	217430_x_at	22.19	0.00	[27]
CRTAP	cartilage associated protein	1554464_a_at	2.44	0.86	[61]
CUL7	cullin 7	203558_at	4.09	0.00	[28]
		241747_s_at	3.41	0.35	
		36084_at	3.07	0.08	
DBP	D site of albumin promoter (albumin D-box) binding protein	209782_s_at	2.87	2.45	[27]
DIO2	deiodinase, iodothyronine, type II	231240_at	4.48	0.00	[62]
DMWD	dystrophia myotonica, WD repeat containing	213231_at	4.11	0.26	[59]
		33768_at	3.11	0.23	
		1554429_a_at	2.71	0.19	
E2F7	E2F transcription factor 7	241725_at	2.21	0.86	[63]
ERCC2	excision repair cross-complementing rodent repair deficiency, complementation group 2	213468_at	2.97	0.08	[59]
ERLIN1	ER lipid raft associated 1	202444_s_at	4.33	0.08	[58]
FOXC2	forkhead box C2 (MFH-1, mesenchyme forkhead 1)	214520_at	6.24	0.00	[27]
FZD1	frizzled homolog 1	204452_s_at	2.85	0.35	[27]
GSR	glutathione reductase	205770_at	2.10	2.06	[64]
GSTM1	glutathione S-transferase mu 1	204550_x_at	3.57	0.19	[64]
		215333_x_at	3.19	0.35	
HMGA2	high mobility group AT-hook 2	1558682_at	3.33	0.63	[27]
HSD11B1	hydroxysteroid (11-beta) dehydrogenase 1	205404_at	2.15	9.00	[65]
IBSP	integrin-binding sialoprotein	207370_at	9.41	0.00	[29,66]
		236028_at	4.88	0.26	
KPNA4	karyopherin alpha 4 (importin alpha 3)	209653_at	4.04	0.19	[58]
LRP5	low density lipoprotein receptor-related protein 5	209468_at	3.54	0.33	[27]
MRPL2	mitochondrial ribosomal protein L2	218887_at	2.07	0.73	[28]
ND2	mitochondrially encoded NADH dehydrogenase 2 (MTND2)	1553551_s_at	2.66	0.14	[67]
PDE7B	phosphodiesterase 7B	220343_at	3.39	0.55	[28]
PRR16	proline rich 16	1554867_a_at	2.12	2.72	[68]
PTPRD	protein tyrosine phosphatase, receptor type, D	213362_at	3.07	3.21	[69]
		205712_at	2.91	1.67	
RARG	retinoic acid receptor, gamma	204189_at	3.85	0.26	[58]
RERE	arginine-glutamic acid dipeptide (RE) repeats	221643_s_at	5.26	0.00	[27]
RUNX2	runt-related transcription factor 2	216994_s_at	11.86	0.00	[27]
SIX5	SIX homeobox 5	229009_at	2.69	0.26	[59]
SOST	sclerostin	223869_at	4.60	1.00	[27]
SOX4	SRY (sex determining region Y)-box 4	201418_s_at	2.23	2.72	[29]
SP1	Sp1 transcription factor	1553685_s_at	4.19	0.08	[58]
		214732_at	3.49	0.35	
SPP1	secreted phosphoprotein 1	209875_s_at	2.53	4.15	[70]

Table 2. Cont.

Symbol	Gene name	Probeset ID	FC	FDR (%)	Reference
TBC1D1	TBC1 (tre-2/USP6, BUB2, cdc16) domain family, member 1	1568713_a_at	4.11	0.35	[58]
Reduced expression in hMSC-OP					
CTNNB1	catenin (cadherin-associated protein), beta 1, 88 kdf	201533_at	0.44	1.67	[66]
		1554411_at	0.23	0.23	
FAM3C	family with sequence similarity 3, member C	236316_at	0.44	9.00	[27]
FBXL17	F-box and leucine-rich repeat protein 17	227203_at	0.32	0.55	[68]
FGF14	fibroblast growth factor 14	230231_at	0.50	5.82	[68]
FGFR2	fibroblast growth factor receptor 2	208229_at	0.20	0.73	[70]
IFNAR2	interferon (alpha, beta and omega) receptor 2	204786_s_at	0.43	2.72	[71]
ITIH5	inter-alpha (globulin) inhibitor H5	1553243_at	0.30	2.72	[69]
JAG1	Jagged 1 (Alagille syndrome)	231183_s_at	0.33	2.06	[72]
NHS	Nance-Horan syndrome	242800_at	0.38	2.72	[28]
PLCL1	phospholipase C-like 1	205934_at	0.25	5.82	[27]
PTN	pleiotrophin	211737_x_at	0.49	6.81	[70]
		209465_x_at	0.46	5.82	
PTPRM	protein tyrosine phosphatase, receptor type, M	1555578_at	0.47	6.81	[28]
RAPGEF4	Rap guanine nucleotide exchange factor (GEF) 4	205651_x_at	0.46	3.67	[69]
SERPINE2	Serpin peptidase inhibitor, clade E, member 2	227487_s_at	0.44	4.93	[28]
SFRP4	secreted frizzled-related protein 4	204052_s_at	0.26	3.67	[73]
SMAD1	SMAD family member 1	227798_at	0.47	3.21	[71]

FC = fold change; FDR = false discovery rate.

could highlight the difference between hMSC-OP, hMSC-old and hMSC-senescence (Figure 2). Osteoporotic cells exhibit a distinct gene expression profile independent of both clock-driven aging and cellular aging.

Relevance of transcriptional changes for stem cell function

To unravel if changes in gene expression profile could cause deficiencies in cellular processes we carried out gene function and pathway identifications by Gene Ontology classification and by searching within the NCBI database for literature. By comparing functions of genes differentially expressed in hMSC-OP, hMSC-old and hMSC-senescent when compared to hMSC-C we detected differences in the effect of osteoporosis, age and senescence on stem cell characteristics. Hereby we focused on genes with known relevance in the following 4 processes: (1) osteoblastogenesis, (2) osteoclastogenesis, (3) proliferation and (4) DNA repair (Table 3). These categories play important roles in sustaining bone homeostasis by influencing bone formation, bone resorption and self-renewal of stem cells.

In hMSC-OP we found enhanced expression of gene products with relevance in osteoblastogenesis by autocrine and paracrine stimulation, respectively (*PTH1R*, *IBSP*, *IGF2*, *VEGFA* and *VEGFB*). In senescent hMSC and hMSC-old we detected reduced expression of genes coding for enhancers of osteoblast differentiation and matrix mineralization (*SPP1*, *ALPL*, *EFNB2*, *COL1A1*, *RUNX2* and *ANKH*).

Genes coding for inhibitors of WNT signaling (*SOST*, *KREMEN1*) showed enhanced expression in hMSC-OP in comparison to hMSC-C, whereas activators of canonical WNT signaling that indirectly inhibit osteogenic differentiation by augmenting proliferation, were more highly expressed in *in vitro*- aged and senescent hMSC (*WNT2*, *WNT3*, *CTNNB1*). Next to *MAB21L2*, which codes for a repressor of BMP-induced transcription, another negative regulator of osteoblastogenesis was enhanced expressed in hMSC-OP and hMSC-old: Follistatin (*FST*), which is associated with inhibition of Activin.

Genes linked to bone resorption were differentially expressed in all three hMSC groups with senescent cells exhibiting strongly diminished potential for inducing osteoclastogenesis by decreased expression of secreted ligands (*TGFB*, *VEGF*, *IL7*, *IL1A*) and other stimulators like *TNFSF11* (RANKL). The gene coding for the osteoclast inhibitor Osteoprotegerin (*TNFRSF11B*) was expressed to a higher extent in hMSC-senescent. *In vivo*-aged hMSC-old showed a similar gene expression pattern whereas osteoporotic hMSC-OP revealed enhanced expression of genes indirectly (*PTH1R*, *PTGS2* and *IGF2*) as well as directly (*CSF1*, *VEGFA* and *VEGFB*) involved in promoting osteoclast formation.

By examining the expression of genes related to proliferation we found a substantial number of repressed genes that code for proteins important for cell division, like several Cyclins, CDC2 and CDC25 proteins in hMSC-senescent. Markers for cellular senescence and genes described as mediators of cell cycle were also differentially expressed in these cells, e.g. *CDKN2A* (P16), several *PSG*, *PTN*, *ARHGAP29* (*PARG1*), *HMMR* and *HELLS*. Clock-driven aging and osteoporosis showed less negative effects on proliferative capacity of stem cells, but in hMSC-OP the expression of a second well known marker of replicative senescence – besides P16 – was increased: *CDKN1A*, which codes for P21.

DNA repair is one of the reasons for cell cycle arrest at the G1, S or G2 checkpoints of mitosis to prevent the accumulation of DNA damage or mutations that could result in tumor development. Again hMSC-senescent exhibited the most severe deficien-

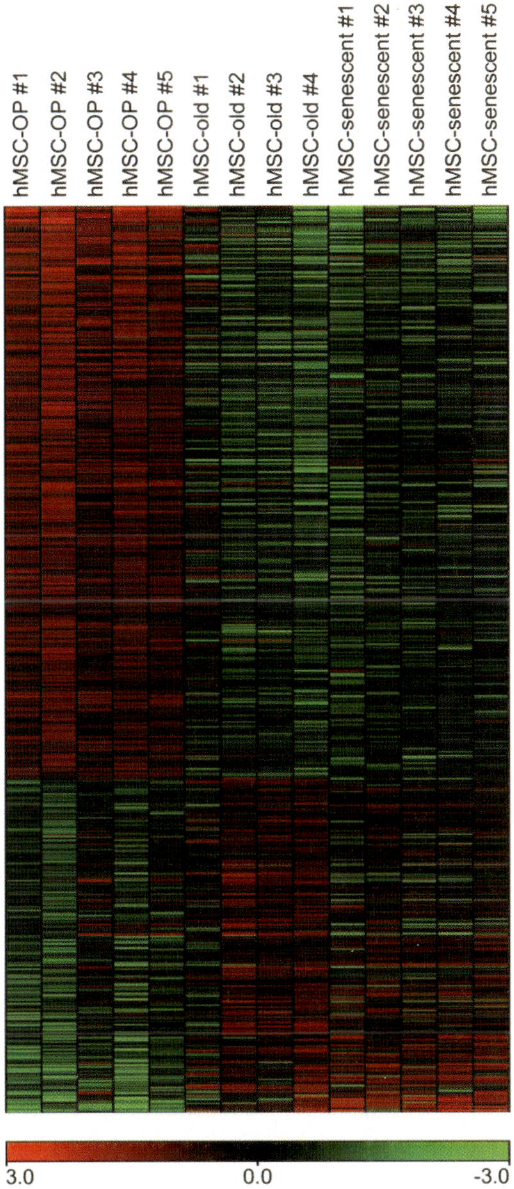

Figure 2. Heat map of microarray results of osteoporotic and aged hMSC. Color-coded microarray hybridization signals (green to red = low to high signals) of hMSC-OP, hMSC-old and hMSC-senescent. The 998 gene products depicted showed at least 2fold differential gene expression (630 enhanced, 368 reduced; FDR < 10%) in SAM comparison of hMSC-OP versus hMSC-C (for gene names see Table S2).

cies with a diminished expression of genes involved in DNA repair like *TOP2A*, *EXO1* and several DNA polymerases. Osteoporotic and aged hMSC showed minor changes.

Discussion

During aging, a continuous decrease in bone mass and bone density occurs and peaks in the development of primary osteoporosis in one of three women and one of eight men over the age of 50 [2,27]. Induced by a variety of risk factors like advanced age, loss of sex steroid production and unhealthy life style [2,3,34], recent research has largely unraveled the polygenetic nature and the multifaceted pathophysiology of this syndrome [27,29,35]. Hitherto, approaches for studying the disease mostly consisted of whole genome association studies of BMD-associated gene loci as well as of manipulating expression of candidate genes in animal models or cells *in vitro*, followed by characterization of phenotypes [36,37,38]. However, bone loss associated with increasing age is a continuous process not only caused by gene polymorphisms but very likely also by epigenetic modulations of gene expression changes that accompany aging [39]. So far, analyses of these changes in primary cells of osteoporotic patients or in whole bone samples have been almost neglected.

We analyzed the effect of primary osteoporosis on the source of bone regeneration and performed microarray hybridizations of hMSC of elderly patients suffering from severe osteoporosis (hMSC-OP) and of donors of advanced age without any indication for the syndrome (hMSC-old). We detected several genes connected to BMD with either reduced (16) or increased (39) expression in hMSC-OP including well-investigated susceptibility genes like *LRP5*, *SPP1* (Osteopontin), *COL1A1* and *SOST* (Table 2) [27]. The latter codes for the osteocyte-specific protein Sclerostin, which acts as a WNT antagonist and is also controversially discussed as a BMP inhibitor [20,22,23]. Upon release, the protein inhibits proliferation of MSC and osteoblasts, blocks osteogenic differentiation and even induces apoptosis in osteoblasts [23,40]. Direct connections between the protein and osteoporosis have already been described: serum levels of Sclerostin were found enhanced in postmenopausal women [41] and one of the upcoming treatments for osteoporosis is the application of anti-Sclerostin-antibodies [24,42]. It is conceivable that the premature expression of *SOST* in osteoporotic stem cells auto-inhibits proliferation and self-renewal of hMSC-OP and thereby leads to the reduced ratios of formation to resorption observed in primary osteoporosis [43].

Furthermore we also found higher expression of *MAB21L2* (Mab-21-like 2) in hMSC-OP in comparison to hMSC-old. QPCR revealed that, even though the expression was induced by advanced donor age itself, the transcription of *MAB21L2* was even more triggered in osteoporotic stem cells (Figure 1B). In *Xenopus laevis* gastrulae it was shown that MAB21L2 antagonizes the effects of BMP4 by repressing the BMP-induced gene expression. The nuclear protein binds SMAD1, the transducer of BMP2/4/7 signaling, but so far it is still unknown if MAB21L2 exerts its effects in a DNA-binding or a non-binding fashion [15]. Our data of age- and osteoporosis-induced expression of *MAB21L2* in hMSC made us hypothesize that BMP-signaling in stem cells is less effective in advanced age and even less so in primary osteoporosis due to transcriptional repression of BMP-target genes.

Despite high inter-individual variability in the gene expression level, as demonstrated in our heat map (Figure 2), we could validate the microarray results for both *SOST* and *MAB21L2* in qPCR analysis with up to 13 different hMSC-OP and hMSC-old populations. We hereby demonstrate the reliability of our microarray approach, which was performed with a comparably low number of samples. Being inhibitors of WNT and BMP signaling, our two leading candidates are major hubs in blocking differentiation programs right at the beginning. Hereby, our data support the results of Rodriguez *et al.* and Dalle Carbonare *et al.*, who demonstrated *in vitro* that osteoporotic hMSC exhibit diminished osteogenic differentiation potential [44,45]. Future research will have to unravel how many of the genes differentially expressed in osteoporotic hMSC-OP (Table S1) are downstream *SOST* or *MAB21L2* over-expression.

Table 3. Functional clustering of differentially expressed genes of hMSC-OP, hMSC-old and hMSC-senescent when compared to hMSC-C.

Symbol	Gene name	hMSC-OP	hMSC-old	hMSC-senescent	Reference
(1) Osteoblastogenesis					
positive					
PTH1R	parathyroid hormone 1 receptor	↑			[74]
IBSP	integrin-binding sialoprotein	↑			[75]
INHA	inhibin, alpha	↑			[76]
IGFBP2	insulin-like growth factor binding protein 2	↑			[77]
IGF2	insulin-like growth factor 2	↑		↓	[77]
VEGFB	vascular endothelial growth factor B	↑	↓		[78]
VEGFA	vascular endothelial growth factor A	↑	↓	↓	[78]
FOXC2	forkhead box C2 (MFH-1, mesenchyme forkhead 1)	↑	↓		[79]
COL1A1	collagen, type I, alpha 1		↓		[75]
RUNX2	runt-related transcription factor 2		↓		[75]
ANKH*	ankylosis, progressive homolog	↓	↓		[80]
SMAD3[B]	SMAD family member 3		↓		[81]
SPP1	secreted phosphoprotein 1			↓	[75]
EFNB2	ephrin-B2			↓	[82]
ALPL	alkaline phosphatase, liver/bone/kidney			↓	[80]
CYP2R1	cytochrome P450, family 2, subfamily R, polypeptide 1			↓	[80,83]
FOXC1	forkhead box C1		↑	↓	[84]
IL6ST	interleukin 6 signal transducer (Oncostatin M receptor)		↓	↑	[85]
PDGFA	platelet-derived growth factor alpha polypeptide		↑		[11]
VDR	vitamin D receptor		↑		[80]
FGFR2*	fibroblast growth factor receptor 2		↑	↓	[86]
BMP6[B]	bone morphogenetic protein 6			↑	[11]
ROR1[W]	receptor tyrosine kinase-like orphan receptor 1	↓		↑	[87]
ANKRD6[W]	ankyrin repeat domain 6			↑	[16,18]
negative					
TGFB1	transforming growth factor, beta 1	↑	↓		[88]
MAB21L2[B]	mab-21-like 2	↑	↑		[15]
FST	follistatin	↑	↑		[89,90]
FSTL3	follistatin-like 3	↑			[91]
KREMEN1[W]	kringle containing transmembrane protein 1	↑			[38]
SOST[W B]	sclerostin	↑			[23]
FGFR1	fibroblast growth factor receptor 1	↑			[92]
IGFBP5	insulin-like growth factor binding protein 5	↑		↑	[11]
IGFBP4	insulin-like growth factor binding protein 4		↓		[11]
EGFR	epidermal growth factor receptor		↓		[93]
GREM2[B]	gremlin 2, cysteine knot superfamily, homolog	↓	↓		[94]
NOG[B]	noggin		↑		[11]
CTNNB1[W]	catenin, beta 1		↑		[17,18]
SFRP4[W]	secreted frizzled-related protein 4			↑	[95]
WNT2[W]	wingless-type MMTV integration site family, member 2			↑	[17,18]
WNT3[W]	wingless-type MMTV integration site family, member 3			↑	[17,18]
(2) Osteoclastogenesis					
positive					
PTH1R	parathyroid hormone 1 receptor	↑			[25]
CSF1	colony stimulating factor 1	↑			[4]
PTGS2	prostaglandin-endoperoxide synthase 2	↑		↓	[96]

Table 3. Cont.

Symbol	Gene name	hMSC-OP	hMSC-old	hMSC-senescent	Reference
IGF2	insulin-like growth factor 2	↑		↓	[97]
TNFSF11	tumor necrosis factor superfamily, member 11			↓	[98]
SPP1	secreted phosphoprotein 1			↓	[99]
IL7	interleukin 7			↓	[100]
THBS1	thrombospondin 1			↑	[101]
IL1A*	interleukin 1, alpha		↓	↑	[67]
TNFSF10	tumor necrosis factor superfamily, member 10		↓	↓	[102]
TGFB2	transforming growth factor, beta 2		↓	↓	[103]
VEGFA	vascular endothelial growth factor A	↑	↓	↓	[46]
VEGFB	vascular endothelial growth factor B	↑	↓		[46]
TGFB1	transforming growth factor, beta 1	↑	↓		[47]
RUNX2	runt-related transcription factor 2		↓		[104]
negative					
TNFRSF11B	tumor necrosis factor receptor superfamily, member 11b			↑	[98]
FSTL3	follistatin-like 3	↑			[105]
(3) Proliferation					
positive					
HMMR	hyaluronan-mediated motility receptor	↓		↓	[49]
HELLS	helicase, lymphoid-specific			↓	[106]
PTN	pleiotrophin			↓	[107]
SOD2	superoxide dismutase 2, mitochondrial		↓	↑	[108]
CCNB2	cyclin B2			↓	[109]
CDC2	cell division cycle 2, G1 to S and G2 to M	↓		↓	[109]
CCNA2	cyclin A2	↓	↓	↓	[109]
CCNE2	cyclin E2	↓	↓	↓	[109]
CCNF	cyclin F			↓	[110]
CCND1	cyclin D1			↑	[109]
CCND2	cyclin D2			↑	[109]
CDC25A	cell division cycle 25 homolog A			↓	[111]
CDC25B	cell division cycle 25 homolog B			↓	[112]
CDC25C	cell division cycle 25 homolog C			↓	[113]
CDK2	cyclin-dependent kinase 2		↓		[109]
negative					
PSG1	pregnancy specific beta-1-glycoprotein 1			↑	[114]
PSG2	pregnancy specific beta-1-glycoprotein 2			↑	[114]
PSG3	pregnancy specific beta-1-glycoprotein 3		↓	↑	[114]
PSG4	pregnancy specific beta-1-glycoprotein 4			↑	[114]
PSG6	pregnancy specific beta-1-glycoprotein 6			↑	[114]
PSG7	pregnancy specific beta-1-glycoprotein 7			↑	[114]
ARHGAP29	Rho GTPase activating protein 29	↓		↑	[107]
CDKN2A	cyclin-dependent kinase inhibitor 2A			↑	[107]
CDKN1A	cyclin-dependent kinase inhibitor 1A	↑			[50]
(4) DNA-repair					
positive					
POLD1	polymerase (DNA directed), delta 1, catalytic subunit 125kDa			↓	[115]
POLE2	polymerase (DNA directed), epsilon 2 (p59 subunit)	↓		↓	[115]
POLQ	polymerase (DNA directed), theta			↓	[115]
POLH	polymerase (DNA directed), eta		↓		[115]
POLK	polymerase (DNA directed) kappa		↓		[115]

Table 3. Cont.

Symbol	Gene name	hMSC-OP	hMSC-old	hMSC-senescent	Reference
MRE11A	MRE11 meiotic recombination 11 homolog A		↓		[116]
PARP3	poly (ADP-ribose) polymerase family, member 3		↓		[117]
RAD50	RAD50 homolog	↓			[116]
RAD51	RAD51 homolog			↓	[116]
RAD51AP1	RAD51 associated protein 1	↓		↓	[118]
TOP2A	topoisomerase (DNA) II alpha 170 kDa	↓		↓	[119]
EXO1	exonuclease 1			↓	[116]
CHEK1	CHK1 checkpoint homolog			↓	[120]
HMGB2	high-mobility group box 2			↓	[121]

arrows pointing downward = at least 2fold reduced expression in comparison to hMSC-C; arrows pointing upward = at least 2fold enhanced expression in comparison to hMSC-C;
[W] = gene associated with WNT signaling;
[B] = gene associated with BMP signaling;
* = probesets that refer to the gene are not identical in the indicated comparisons.

Furthermore, we detected indications for osteoporotic stem cells actively enhancing osteoclastogenesis and therefore bone resorption. Besides the enhanced expression of genes coding for osteoclast stimulating ligands, e.g. VEGF, TGFB and CSF1 [4,46,47], we also detected the osteoporosis-induced expression of Parathyroid hormone receptor *PTH1R*. Activation of PTH1R triggers osteoblast maturation and induces RANKL expression which leads to osteoclast precursor differentiation and activation [26]. The enhanced expression of osteoclastogenesis promoting factors has already been described in fragility fractured bone [48] and is in general consistent with the enhanced bone resorption described for osteoporosis [2].

Because high age is one of the main risk factors for developing osteoporosis, we tried to dissect effects of aging from effects of primary osteoporosis by using hMSC from middle-aged donors as control cells (hMSC-C) for comparisons with hMSC-OP and hMSC-old, respectively, of elderly individuals (Figure 1C and 1D, Table S2). Surprisingly, the patterns of the differential gene expression in aged and osteoporotic hMSC differed widely. Only a few gene products with identical expression profiles in hMSC-old and hMSC-OP were observed and we therefore conclude that osteoporosis-associated changes are very distinct and independent of effects of clock-driven aging. We hypothesize that donors of advanced age who suffered from osteoarthritis but not from osteoporosis, aged in a healthier way than osteoporotic patients, or *vice versa* that osteoporosis is a distinct syndrome of premature aging.

One hypothetical reason for aging is the loss of tissue regeneration due to replicative senescence of stem cells, which accumulates over time and ends in organ failure and death of the organism [33]. Due to the fact that donors of hMSC-OP were of advanced age we analyzed whether these cells exhibited signs of replicative senescence by comparing them to the gene expression pattern of long term-cultivated, senescent hMSC. Thereby we detected a small overlap of genes differentially expressed in hMSC-OP and hMSC-senescent when compared to the identical control group hMSC-C (Figure 1C and D). Despite the distinct gene expression pattern, we found some markers for replicative senescence in osteoporotic hMSC-OP, like the reduced expression of Hyaluronan receptor *HMMR*, which was described as inversely regulated to tumor suppressor P53 [49], and the induction of *CDKN1A*, which codes for P21, another inhibitor of cyclin-dependent kinases (Table 3) [50]. In contrast, analyses of non-osteoporotic hMSC-old of the age-matched donor group revealed no expression of markers for senescence and highlighted even more the differences between aging with and without primary osteoporosis. Our findings suggest that osteoporotic stem cells exhibit deficiencies in proliferation and might already be prone to a pre-senescent state. So far, reduction in proliferative activity in osteoporotic cells has only been described for osteoblasts [51,52]. For confirmation, more detailed investigations of hMSC-OP on protein level and by proliferation or senescence studies are needed.

In summary, this study indicates that intrinsic alterations in stem cell biology are involved in the pathophysiology of osteoporosis. By microarray analyses, we detected significant differences between hMSC of elderly donors with and without osteoporosis, suggesting that primary osteoporosis causes distinct transcriptional changes, which differ from age-related changes in non-osteoporotic donors. Next to indications for a pre-senescent state we detected enhanced transcription of inhibitors of WNT and BMP signaling in osteoporotic hMSC-OP, which can lead to functional deficiencies, such as autoinhibition of osteogenic differentiation and loss of self-renewal. Our data facilitate the importance of well-known susceptibility genes of osteoporosis such as *SOST*, *COL1A1* and *LRP5*, and additionally, we detected new candidate genes for further investigations, e.g. *MAB21L2*. Our study confirms that disturbed bone homeostasis by inhibition of osteogenic regeneration is at least an equally important feature of primary osteoporosis besides enhanced bone resorption. Therefore, "inhibition of inhibitors" of bone regeneration by using, e.g. SOST antibodies, is a mechanistically plausible treatment of the syndrome and will get even more attention in the future.

Materials and Methods

Ethics Statement

Bone material was used under agreement of the local Ethics Committee of the Medical Faculty of the University of Wuerzburg with written informed consent of each patient.

Cell culture

Human MSC of non-osteoporotic donors were obtained from bone marrow of femoral heads according to the described protocol [53] after total hip arthroplasty due to osteoarthritis and/or hip dysplasia. MSC of patients suffering from osteoporosis were isolated from femoral heads after low-energy fracture of the femoral neck. Additional criteria for confirming primary osteoporosis in these donors were vertebrae fractures and advanced age.

Cell culture medium, fetal calf serum (FCS), trypsin-EDTA and antibiotics were obtained from PAA Laboratories GmbH, Linz, Austria. Human MSC were selected by surface adherence and expanded in DMEM/Ham's F-12 (1:1) medium supplemented with 10% heat-inactivated FCS, 1 U/ml penicillin, 100 µg/ml streptomycin and 50 µg/ml L-ascorbic acid 2-phosphate (Sigma Aldrich GmbH, Schnelldorf, Germany).

For long term cultivation, cells were expanded at 70–90% confluence by trypsinization with 1× trypsin-EDTA and reseeding in a ratio of 1:3. This procedure was repeated for up to x passages when the hMSC did not become confluent within 3 weeks due to replicative senescence.

RNA isolation

At 80–90% confluence human MSC monolayers were lysed directly in the cell culture flask in passage (P) 1 or 2 and the last, senescent passage Px, respectively. Total RNA was isolated using the NucleoSpin RNA II Purification Kit (Macherey-Nagel, Düren, Germany) according to the manufacturer's instructions including DNase digestion.

Microarray analysis

For microarray analyses total RNA of hMSC-C, hMSC-senescent and hMSC-OP (Table 1) was amplified and labeled according to the GeneChip One-Cycle cDNA Synthesis Kit (Affymetrix, High Wycombe, United Kingdom). Total RNA of hMSC-old was amplified and labeled according to the Affymetrix GeneChip 3′IVT Express Kit. Following fragmentation, 10 µg of cRNA were hybridized for 16 hr at 45°C on Affymetrix GeneChips Human Genome U133_Plus_2.0. GeneChips were washed and stained in the Affymetrix Fluidics Station 450 using the Affymetrix Hybridization, Wash and Stain Kit. Hybridization signals were detected with Affymetrix Gene Chip Scanner 3000 and global scaling was performed by Affymetrix GeneChipOperatingSoftware 1.4 using the MAS5 algorithm. Microarray data of all 4 hMSC groups have been published in Gene Expression Omnibus (GEO, http://www.ncbi.nlm.nih.gov/geo/) and are accessible through GEO superSeries accession number GSE35959. Gene expression patterns of two groups of hMSC populations were compared with the significance analysis of microarrays (SAM) approach by using the SAM software of Stanford University, Palo Alto, USA (http://www-stat.stanford.edu/~tibs/SAM/) [54]. For data interpretation we only took those gene products into account that provided present hybridization signals in at least 3 of x hMSC populations in at least one of the two groups compared. Furthermore, only gene products (probesets) with fold changes (FC) ≤0.5 or ≥2.0, and a false discovery rate (FDR) <10% were considered as significantly, differentially expressed.

Heat maps were generated by CARMAweb using globally normalized data [55].

Differentially expressed gene products were assigned to protein function by Gene Ontology classification (http://www.geneontology.org/) and NCBI PubMed literature search (http://www.ncbi.nlm.nih.gov/sites/entrez). Genes with at least one differentially expressed probeset were taken into account.

Additionally, SAM data was compared to publically available data from genome-wide association studies, meta-analyses or candidate gene association studies obtained by a NCBI PubMed search for reviews and original publications from 2010 and later with the following search terms: genome-wide association/polymorphism/meta-analysis+osteoporosis or+bone mineral density.

Quantitative PCR analysis

One microgram of total RNA was reverse-transcribed with Oligo(dT)15 primers (peqlab Biotechnologie GmbH, Erlangen, Germany) and MMLV reverse transcriptase (Promega GmbH, Mannheim, Germany) according to the manufacturer's instructions. Quantitative real-time PCR (qPCR) was performed in triplets in 20 µl with 16 ng cDNA, 5 µl KAPA SYBR FAST Universal 2× qPCR Master Mix (peqlab Biotechnologie GmbH) and 0.25 pmol of sequence specific primers obtained from biomers.net GmbH, Ulm, Germany. The following primer sequences were used (5′-3′ forward and reverse, respectively): RPLP0 (ribosomal protein, large, P0) as housekeeping gene (NM_001002.3) [56], TGCATCAGTACCCCATTCTATCAT and AGGCAGATGGATCAGCCAAGA; SOST (NM_025237.2), CAGGCGTTCAAGAATGATGC and TACTCGGACACGTCTTTGGTC; and MAB21L2 (NM_006439.4), TGGGTGCTACAGTTCG and CAGGCAGGAGATGAGC. QPCR was performed with Opticon DNA Engine (MJ Research, Waltham, USA) and the following conditions: 95°C for 3 min; 40 cycles: 95°C for 15 s; 60°C for 15 s; 72°C for 10 s; followed by melting curve analysis. Results were calculated with the $\Delta\Delta C_T$ method.

Senescence-associated β-galactosidase staining

To confirm replicative senescence in the last, non-confluent passage of hMSC after long time cultivation, senescence-associated β-galactosidase staining was performed as described [57]. After each passage 2×10^5 cells were seeded on coverslips in 9.6 cm^2 petri dishes and cultured to 70–90% confluence. After fixation in 2% formaldehyde/0.2% glutaraldehyde for 5 min the coverslips were stored at 4°C. Staining was performed for hMSC in P1and Px simultaneously by incubating the cells for 16 h at 37°C (normal air CO_2) with 1 ml staining solution (1 mg/ml 5-bromo-4-chloro-3-indolyl β-D-galactosidase (Sigma Aldrich GmbH), 40 mM citric acid/sodium phosphate (pH 6.0), 5 mM potassium ferrocyanide, 5 mM potassium ferricyanide, 150 mM NaCl and 2 mM $MgCl_2$). Counterstaining with nuclear fast red was performed after washing twice with ddH_2O.

Supporting Information

Table S1 Gene products with significant expression changes in hMSC-OP compared to hMSC-old. FC = fold change (at least 2fold); FDR = false discovery rate (<10%).

Table S2 Gene products differentially expressed in hMSC-OP, hMSC-old and hMSC-senescent when compared to hMSC-C. arrows pointing downward = significant, reduced expression in comparison to hMSC-C; arrows pointing upward = significant, enhanced expression in comparison to hMSC-C; FC = fold change (at least 2fold); FDR = false discovery rate (<10%); — = no expression in both hMSC groups compared.

Acknowledgments

We are grateful to the Orthopedic Surgeons U. Nöth and A. Steinert (Wuerzburg, Germany) who supplied us with explanted human femoral heads.

Author Contributions

Conceived and designed the experiments: PB FJ. Performed the experiments: MK MR SZ LKH. Analyzed the data: LKH PB RE. Contributed reagents/materials/analysis tools: T. Schilling SPF LS NR. Wrote the paper: PB. Critical revision/substantial impulses: MA T. Schinke T. Schilling.

References

1. Rachner TD, Khosla S, Hofbauer LC (2011) Osteoporosis: now and the future. Lancet 377: 1276–1287.
2. Seeman E (2008) Bone quality: the material and structural basis of bone strength. J Bone Miner Metab 26: 1–8.
3. Pietschmann P, Rauner M, Sipos W, Kerschan-Schindl K (2009) Osteoporosis: an age-related and gender-specific disease–a mini-review. Gerontology 55: 3–12.
4. Manolagas SC (2000) Birth and death of bone cells: basic regulatory mechanisms and implications for the pathogenesis and treatment of osteoporosis. Endocr Rev 21: 115–137.
5. Khosla S (2001) Minireview: the OPG/RANKL/RANK system. Endocrinology 142: 5050–5055.
6. Misof B, Gamsjaeger S, Cohen A, Hofstetter B, Roschger P, et al. (2012) Bone material properties in premenopausal women with idiopathic osteoporosis. J Bone Miner Res.
7. Jilka RL (2003) Biology of the basic multicellular unit and the pathophysiology of osteoporosis. Med Pediatr Oncol 41: 182–185.
8. Duque G (2008) Bone and fat connection in aging bone. Curr Opin Rheumatol 20: 429–434.
9. Valtieri M, Sorrentino A (2008) The mesenchymal stromal cell contribution to homeostasis. J Cell Physiol 217: 296–300.
10. Rawadi G, Vayssiere B, Dunn F, Baron R, Roman-Roman S (2003) BMP-2 controls alkaline phosphatase expression and osteoblast mineralization by a Wnt autocrine loop. J Bone Miner Res 18: 1842–1853.
11. Canalis E (2009) Growth factor control of bone mass. J Cell Biochem 108: 769–777.
12. Gazzerro E, Pereira RC, Jorgetti V, Olson S, Economides AN, et al. (2005) Skeletal overexpression of gremlin impairs bone formation and causes osteopenia. Endocrinology 146: 655–665.
13. Devlin RD, Du Z, Pereira RC, Kimble RB, Economides AN, et al. (2003) Skeletal overexpression of noggin results in osteopenia and reduced bone formation. Endocrinology 144: 1972–1978.
14. Estrada KD, Retting KN, Chin AM, Lyons KM (2011) Smad6 is essential to limit BMP signaling during cartilage development. J Bone Miner Res 26: 2498–2510.
15. Baldessari D, Badaloni A, Longhi R, Zappavigna V, Consalez GG (2004) MAB21L2, a vertebrate member of the Male-abnormal 21 family, modulates BMP signaling and interacts with SMAD1. BMC Cell Biol 5: 48.
16. Katoh M (2007) WNT signaling pathway and stem cell signaling network. Clin Cancer Res 13: 4042–4045.
17. Boland GM, Perkins G, Hall DJ, Tuan RS (2004) Wnt 3a promotes proliferation and suppresses osteogenic differentiation of adult human mesenchymal stem cells. J Cell Biochem 93: 1210–1230.
18. Ling L, Nurcombe V, Cool SM (2009) Wnt signaling controls the fate of mesenchymal stem cells. Gene 433: 1–7.
19. Cho HH, Kim YJ, Kim SJ, Kim JH, Bae YC, et al. (2006) Endogenous Wnt signaling promotes proliferation and suppresses osteogenic differentiation in human adipose derived stromal cells. Tissue Eng 12: 111–121.
20. Krause C, Korchynskyi O, de Rooij K, Weidauer SE, de Gorter DJ, et al. (2010) Distinct modes of inhibition by sclerostin on bone morphogenetic protein and Wnt signaling pathways. J Biol Chem 285: 41614–41626.
21. van Bezooijen RL, Svensson JP, Eefting D, Visser A, van der Horst G, et al. (2007) Wnt but not BMP signaling is involved in the inhibitory action of sclerostin on BMP-stimulated bone formation. J Bone Miner Res 22: 19–28.
22. Winkler DG, Sutherland MK, Geoghegan JC, Yu C, Hayes T, et al. (2003) Osteocyte control of bone formation via sclerostin, a novel BMP antagonist. EMBO J 22: 6267–6276.
23. ten Dijke P, Krause C, de Gorter DJ, Lowik CW, van Bezooijen RL (2008) Osteocyte-derived sclerostin inhibits bone formation: its role in bone morphogenetic protein and Wnt signaling. J Bone Joint Surg Am 90 Suppl 1: 31–35.
24. Ominsky MS, Vlasseros F, Jolette J, Smith SY, Stouch B, et al. (2010) Two doses of sclerostin antibody in cynomolgus monkeys increases bone formation, bone mineral density, and bone strength. J Bone Miner Res 25: 948–959.
25. Potts JT (2005) Parathyroid hormone: past and present. J Endocrinol 187: 311–325.
26. Datta NS, Abou-Samra AB (2009) PTH and PTHrP signaling in osteoblasts. Cell Signal 21: 1245–1254.
27. Li WF, Hou SX, Yu B, Li MM, Ferec C, et al. (2010) Genetics of osteoporosis: accelerating pace in gene identification and validation. Hum Genet 127: 249–285.
28. Koller DL, Ichikawa S, Lai D, Padgett LR, Doheny KF, et al. (2010) Genome-wide association study of bone mineral density in premenopausal European-American women and replication in African-American women. J Clin Endocrinol Metab 95: 1802–1809.
29. Duncan EL, Danoy P, Kemp JP, Leo PJ, McCloskey E, et al. (2011) Genome-wide association study using extreme truncate selection identifies novel genes affecting bone mineral density and fracture risk. PLoS Genet 7: e1001372.
30. Rivadeneira F, Styrkarsdottir U, Estrada K, Halldorsson BV, Hsu YH, et al. (2009) Twenty bone-mineral-density loci identified by large-scale meta-analysis of genome-wide association studies. Nat Genet 41: 1199–1206.
31. Hayflick L (1965) The Limited in Vitro Lifetime of Human Diploid Cell Strains. Exp Cell Res 37: 614–636.
32. Wagner W, Horn P, Castoldi M, Diehlmann A, Bork S, et al. (2008) Replicative senescence of mesenchymal stem cells: a continuous and organized process. PLoS One 3: e2213.
33. Sethe S, Scutt A, Stolzing A (2006) Aging of mesenchymal stem cells. Ageing Res Rev 5: 91–116.
34. Kawaguchi H (2006) Molecular backgrounds of age-related osteoporosis from mouse genetics approaches. Rev Endocr Metab Disord 7: 17–22.
35. Richards JB, Kavvoura FK, Rivadeneira F, Styrkarsdottir U, Estrada K, et al. (2009) Collaborative meta-analysis: associations of 150 candidate genes with osteoporosis and osteoporotic fracture. Ann Intern Med 151: 528–537.
36. Albers J, Schulze J, Beil FT, Gebauer M, Baranowsky A, et al. (2011) Control of bone formation by the serpentine receptor Frizzled-9. J Cell Biol 192: 1057–1072.
37. Schulze J, Seitz S, Saito H, Schneebauer M, Marshall RP, et al. (2010) Negative regulation of bone formation by the transmembrane Wnt antagonist Kremen-2. PLoS One 5: e10309.
38. Ellwanger K, Saito H, Clement-Lacroix P, Maltry N, Niedermeyer J, et al. (2008) Targeted disruption of the Wnt regulator Kremen induces limb defects and high bone density. Mol Cell Biol 28: 4875–4882.
39. Fraga MF, Ballestar E, Paz MF, Ropero S, Setien F, et al. (2005) Epigenetic differences arise during the lifetime of monozygotic twins. Proc Natl Acad Sci U S A 102: 10604–10609.
40. Sutherland MK, Geoghegan JC, Yu C, Turcott E, Skonier JE, et al. (2004) Sclerostin promotes the apoptosis of human osteoblastic cells: a novel regulation of bone formation. Bone 35: 828–835.
41. Mirza FS, Padhi ID, Raisz LG, Lorenzo JA (2010) Serum sclerostin levels negatively correlate with parathyroid hormone levels and free estrogen index in postmenopausal women. J Clin Endocrinol Metab 95: 1991–1997.
42. Li X, Ominsky MS, Warmington KS, Niu QT, Asuncion FJ, et al. (2011) Increased bone formation and bone mass induced by sclerostin antibody is not affected by pretreatment or cotreatment with alendronate in osteopenic, ovariectomized rats. Endocrinology 152: 3312–3322.
43. Teitelbaum SL (2007) Osteoclasts: what do they do and how do they do it? Am J Pathol 170: 427–435.
44. Rodriguez JP, Garat S, Gajardo H, Pino AM, Seitz G (1999) Abnormal osteogenesis in osteoporotic patients is reflected by altered mesenchymal stem cells dynamics. J Cell Biochem 75: 414–423.
45. Dalle Carbonare L, Valenti MT, Zanatta M, Donatelli L, Lo Cascio V (2009) Circulating mesenchymal stem cells with abnormal osteogenic differentiation in patients with osteoporosis. Arthritis Rheum 60: 3356–3365.
46. Yang Q, McHugh KP, Patntirapong S, Gu X, Wunderlich L, et al. (2008) VEGF enhancement of osteoclast survival and bone resorption involves VEGF receptor-2 signaling and beta3-integrin. Matrix Biol 27: 589–599.
47. Fox SW, Lovibond AC (2005) Current insights into the role of transforming growth factor-beta in bone resorption. Mol Cell Endocrinol 243: 19–26.
48. Hopwood B, Tsykin A, Findlay DM, Fazzalari NL (2009) Gene expression profile of the bone microenvironment in human fragility fracture bone. Bone 44: 87–101.
49. Sohr S, Engeland K (2008) RHAMM is differentially expressed in the cell cycle and downregulated by the tumor suppressor p53. Cell Cycle 7: 3448–3460.
50. Bringold F, Serrano M (2000) Tumor suppressors and oncogenes in cellular senescence. Exp Gerontol 35: 317–329.
51. Trost Z, Trebse R, Prezelj J, Komadina R, Logar DB, et al. (2010) A microarray based identification of osteoporosis-related genes in primary culture of human osteoblasts. Bone 46: 72–80.
52. Giner M, Rios MA, Montoya MA, Vazquez MA, Naji L, et al. (2009) RANKL/OPG in primary cultures of osteoblasts from post-menopausal women. Differences between osteoporotic hip fractures and osteoarthritis. J Steroid Biochem Mol Biol 113: 46–51.
53. Limbert C, Ebert R, Schilling T, Path G, Benisch P, et al. (2010) Functional signature of human islet-derived precursor cells compared to bone marrow-derived mesenchymal stem cells. Stem Cells Dev 19: 679–691.
54. Tusher VG, Tibshirani R, Chu G (2001) Significance analysis of microarrays applied to the ionizing radiation response. Proc Natl Acad Sci U S A 98: 5116–5121.
55. Rainer J, Sanchez-Cabo F, Stocker G, Sturn A, Trajanoski Z (2006) CARMAweb: comprehensive R- and bioconductor-based web service for microarray data analysis. Nucleic Acids Res 34: W498–503.

56. Boukhechba F, Balaguer T, Michiels JF, Ackermann K, Quincey D, et al. (2009) Human primary osteocyte differentiation in a 3D culture system. J Bone Miner Res 24: 1927–1935.
57. Dimri GP, Lee X, Basile G, Acosta M, Scott G, et al. (1995) A biomarker that identifies senescent human cells in culture and in aging skin in vivo. Proc Natl Acad Sci U S A 92: 9363–9367.
58. Cheung CL, Sham PC, Xiao SM, Bow CH, Kung AW (2011) Meta-analysis of gene-based genome-wide association studies of bone mineral density in Chinese and European subjects. Osteoporos Int.
59. Farber CR, Bennett BJ, Orozco L, Zou W, Lira A, et al. (2011) Mouse genome-wide association and systems genetics identify Asxl2 as a regulator of bone mineral density and osteoclastogenesis. PLoS Genet 7: e1002038.
60. Saint-Pierre A, Kaufman JM, Ostertag A, Cohen-Solal M, Boland A, et al. (2011) Bivariate association analysis in selected samples: application to a GWAS of two bone mineral density phenotypes in males with high or low BMD. Eur J Hum Genet 19: 710–716.
61. Li GH, Kung AW, Huang QY (2010) Common variants in FLNB/CRTAP, not ARHGEF3 at 3p, are associated with osteoporosis in southern Chinese women. Osteoporos Int 21: 1009–1020.
62. Heemstra KA, Hoftijzer H, van der Deure WM, Peeters RP, Hamdy NA, et al. (2010) The type 2 deiodinase Thr92Ala polymorphism is associated with increased bone turnover and decreased femoral neck bone mineral density. J Bone Miner Res 25: 1385–1391.
63. Paternoster L, Lorentzon M, Vandenput L, Karlsson MK, Ljunggren O, et al. (2010) Genome-wide association meta-analysis of cortical bone mineral density unravels allelic heterogeneity at the RANKL locus and potential pleiotropic effects on bone. PLoS Genet 6: e1001217.
64. Mlakar SJ, Osredkar J, Prezelj J, Marc J (2011) Opposite effects of GSTM1 - and GSTT1 - gene deletion variants on bone mineral density. Dis Markers 31: 279–287.
65. Hwang JY, Lee SH, Kim GS, Koh JM, Go MJ, et al. (2009) HSD11B1 polymorphisms predicted bone mineral density and fracture risk in postmenopausal women without a clinically apparent hypercortisolemia. Bone 45: 1098–1103.
66. Ralston SH, Uitterlinden AG (2010) Genetics of osteoporosis. Endocr Rev 31: 629–662.
67. Guo Y, Yang TL, Liu YZ, Shen H, Lei SF, et al. (2011) Mitochondria-wide association study of common variants in osteoporosis. Ann Hum Genet 75: 569–574.
68. Zhang YP, Deng FY, Chen Y, Pei YF, Fang Y, et al. (2010) Replication study of candidate genes/loci associated with osteoporosis based on genome-wide screening. Osteoporos Int 21: 785–795.
69. Karasik D, Hsu YH, Zhou Y, Cupples LA, Kiel DP, et al. (2010) Genome-wide pleiotropy of osteoporosis-related phenotypes: the Framingham Study. J Bone Miner Res 25: 1555–1563.
70. Cheung CL, Xiao SM, Kung AW (2010) Genetic epidemiology of age-related osteoporosis and its clinical applications. Nat Rev Rheumatol 6: 507–517.
71. Yerges LM, Klei L, Cauley JA, Roeder K, Kammerer CM, et al. (2010) Candidate gene analysis of femoral neck trabecular and cortical volumetric bone mineral density in older men. J Bone Miner Res 25: 330–338.
72. Mitchell BD, Yerges-Armstrong LM (2011) The genetics of bone loss: challenges and prospects. J Clin Endocrinol Metab 96: 1258–1268.
73. Lee DY, Kim H, Ku SY, Kim SH, Choi YM, et al. (2010) Association between polymorphisms in Wnt signaling pathway genes and bone mineral density in postmenopausal Korean women. Menopause 17: 1064–1070.
74. Pountos I, Georgouli T, Henshaw K, Bird H, Jones E, et al. (2010) The effect of bone morphogenetic protein-2, bone morphogenetic protein-7, parathyroid hormone, and platelet-derived growth factor on the proliferation and osteogenic differentiation of mesenchymal stem cells derived from osteoporotic bone. J Orthop Trauma 24: 552–556.
75. Komori T (2010) Regulation of bone development and extracellular matrix protein genes by RUNX2. Cell Tissue Res 339: 189–195.
76. Perrien DS, Nicks KM, Liu L, Akel NS, Bacon AW, et al. (2011) Inhibin A enhances bone formation during distraction osteogenesis. J Orthop Res.
77. Palermo C, Manduca P, Gazzerro E, Foppiani L, Segat D, et al. (2004) Potentiating role of IGFBP-2 on IGF-II-stimulated alkaline phosphatase activity in differentiating osteoblasts. Am J Physiol Endocrinol Metab 286: E648–657.
78. Street J, Lenehan B (2009) Vascular endothelial growth factor regulates osteoblast survival - evidence for an autocrine feedback mechanism. J Orthop Surg Res 4: 19.
79. Park SJ, Gadi J, Cho KW, Kim KJ, Kim SH, et al. (2011) The forkhead transcription factor Foxc2 promotes osteoblastogenesis via up-regulation of integrin beta1 expression. Bone 49: 428–438.
80. Orimo H (2010) The mechanism of mineralization and the role of alkaline phosphatase in health and disease. J Nippon Med Sch 77: 4–12.
81. Dingwall M, Marchildon F, Gunanayagam A, Louis CS, Wiper-Bergeron N (2011) Retinoic acid-induced Smad3 expression is required for the induction of osteoblastogenesis of mesenchymal stem cells. Differentiation 82: 57–65.
82. Zhao C, Irie N, Takada Y, Shimoda K, Miyamoto T, et al. (2006) Bidirectional ephrinB2-EphB4 signaling controls bone homeostasis. Cell Metab 4: 111–121.
83. Schuster I (2011) Cytochromes P450 are essential players in the vitamin D signaling system. Biochim Biophys Acta 1814: 186–199.
84. Rice R, Rice DP, Thesleff I (2005) Foxc1 integrates Fgf and Bmp signalling independently of twist or noggin during calvarial bone development. Dev Dyn 233: 847–852.
85. Shin HI, Divieti P, Sims NA, Kobayashi T, Miao D, et al. (2004) Gp130-mediated signaling is necessary for normal osteoblastic function in vivo and in vitro. Endocrinology 145: 1376–1385.
86. Miraoui H, Severe N, Vaudin P, Pages JC, Marie PJ (2010) Molecular silencing of Twist1 enhances osteogenic differentiation of murine mesenchymal stem cells: implication of FGFR2 signaling. J Cell Biochem 110: 1147–1154.
87. Fukuda T, Chen L, Endo T, Tang L, Lu D, et al. (2008) Antisera induced by infusions of autologous Ad-CD154-leukemia B cells identify ROR1 as an oncofetal antigen and receptor for Wnt5a. Proc Natl Acad Sci U S A 105: 3047–3052.
88. Zhou S (2011) TGF-beta regulates beta-catenin signaling and osteoblast differentiation in human mesenchymal stem cells. J Cell Biochem 112: 1651–1660.
89. Gaddy-Kurten D, Coker JK, Abe E, Jilka RL, Manolagas SC (2002) Inhibin suppresses and activin stimulates osteoblastogenesis and osteoclastogenesis in murine bone marrow cultures. Endocrinology 143: 74–83.
90. Abe Y, Abe T, Aida Y, Hara Y, Maeda K (2004) Follistatin restricts bone morphogenetic protein (BMP)-2 action on the differentiation of osteoblasts in fetal rat mandibular cells. J Bone Miner Res 19: 1302–1307.
91. Sidis Y, Mukherjee A, Keutmann H, Delbaere A, Sadatsuki M, et al. (2006) Biological activity of follistatin isoforms and follistatin-like-3 is dependent on differential cell surface binding and specificity for activin, myostatin, and bone morphogenetic proteins. Endocrinology 147: 3586–3597.
92. Jacob AL, Smith C, Partanen J, Ornitz DM (2006) Fibroblast growth factor receptor 1 signaling in the osteo-chondrogenic cell lineage regulates sequential steps of osteoblast maturation. Dev Biol 296: 315–328.
93. Zhu J, Shimizu E, Zhang X, Partridge NC, Qin L (2011) EGFR signaling suppresses osteoblast differentiation and inhibits expression of master osteoblastic transcription factors Runx2 and Osterix. J Cell Biochem 112: 1749–1760.
94. Ideno H, Takanabe R, Shimada A, Imaizumi K, Araki R, et al. (2009) Protein related to DAN and cerberus (PRDC) inhibits osteoblastic differentiation and its suppression promotes osteogenesis in vitro. Exp Cell Res 315: 474–484.
95. Nakanishi R, Akiyama H, Kimura H, Otsuki B, Shimizu M, et al. (2008) Osteoblast-targeted expression of Sfrp4 in mice results in low bone mass. J Bone Miner Res 23: 271–277.
96. Kaji H, Sugimoto T, Kanatani M, Fukase M, Kumegawa M, et al. (1996) Prostaglandin E2 stimulates osteoclast-like cell formation and bone resorbing activity via osteoblasts: role of cAMP-dependent protein kinase. J Bone Miner Res 11: 62–71.
97. Avnet S, Salerno M, Quacquaruccio G, Granchi D, Giunti A, et al. (2011) IGF2 derived from SH-SY5Y neuroblastoma cells induces the osteoclastogenesis of human monocytic precursors. Exp Cell Res 317: 2147–2158.
98. Perez-Sayans M, Somoza-Martin JM, Barros-Angueira F, Rey JM, Garcia-Garcia A (2010) RANK/RANKL/OPG role in distraction osteogenesis. Oral Surg Oral Med Oral Pathol Oral Radiol Endod 109: 679–686.
99. Shapses SA, Cifuentes M, Spevak L, Chowdhury H, Brittingham J, et al. (2003) Osteopontin facilitates bone resorption, decreasing bone mineral crystallinity and content during calcium deficiency. Calcif Tissue Int 73: 86–92.
100. Roato I, Brunetti G, Gorassini E, Grano M, Colucci S, et al. (2006) IL-7 up-regulates TNF-alpha-dependent osteoclastogenesis in patients affected by solid tumor. PLoS One 1: e124.
101. Carron JA, Wagstaff SC, Gallagher JA, Bowler WB (2000) A CD36-binding peptide from thrombospondin-1 can stimulate resorption by osteoclasts in vitro. Biochem Biophys Res Commun 270: 1124–1127.
102. Brunetti G, Oranger A, Mori G, Sardone F, Pignataro P, et al. (2011) TRAIL effect on osteoclast formation in physiological and pathological conditions. Front Biosci (Elite Ed) 3: 1154–1161.
103. Shaarawy M, Zaki S, Sheiba M, El-Minawi AM (2003) Circulating levels of osteoclast activating cytokines, interleukin-11 and transforming growth factor-beta2, as valuable biomarkers for the assessment of bone turnover in postmenopausal osteoporosis. Clin Lab 49: 625–636.
104. Geoffroy V, Kneissel M, Fournier B, Boyde A, Matthias P (2002) High bone resorption in adult aging transgenic mice overexpressing cbfa1/runx2 in cells of the osteoblastic lineage. Mol Cell Biol 22: 6222–6233.
105. Bartholin L, Destaing O, Forissier S, Martel S, Maguer-Satta V, et al. (2005) FLRG, a new ADAM12-associated protein, modulates osteoclast differentiation. Biol Cell 97: 577–588.
106. Sun LQ, Arceci RJ (2005) Altered epigenetic patterning leading to replicative senescence and reduced longevity. A role of a novel SNF2 factor, PASG. Cell Cycle 4: 3–5.
107. Wagner W, Bork S, Lepperdinger G, Joussen S, Ma N, et al. (2010) How to track cellular aging of mesenchymal stromal cells? Aging (Albany NY) 2: 224–230.
108. Longo VD (2004) Ras: the other pro-aging pathway. Sci Aging Knowledge Environ 2004: pe36.
109. Musgrove EA (2006) Cyclins: roles in mitogenic signaling and oncogenic transformation. Growth Factors 24: 13–19.
110. Kong M, Barnes EA, Ollendorff V, Donoghue DJ (2000) Cyclin F regulates the nuclear localization of cyclin B1 through a cyclin-cyclin interaction. EMBO J 19: 1378–1388.

111. Sandhu C, Donovan J, Bhattacharya N, Stampfer M, Worland P, et al. (2000) Reduction of Cdc25A contributes to cyclin E1-Cdk2 inhibition at senescence in human mammary epithelial cells. Oncogene 19: 5314–5323.
112. Dalvai M, Mondesert O, Bourdon JC, Ducommun B, Dozier C (2011) Cdc25B is negatively regulated by p53 through Sp1 and NF-Y transcription factors. Oncogene 30: 2282–2288.
113. Bonnet J, Coopman P, Morris MC (2008) Characterization of centrosomal localization and dynamics of Cdc25C phosphatase in mitosis. Cell Cycle 7: 1991–1998.
114. Endoh M, Kobayashi Y, Yamakami Y, Yonekura R, Fujii M, et al. (2009) Coordinate expression of the human pregnancy-specific glycoprotein gene family during induced and replicative senescence. Biogerontology 10: 213–221.
115. Hubscher U, Maga G, Spadari S (2002) Eukaryotic DNA polymerases. Annu Rev Biochem 71: 133–163.
116. Mimitou EP, Symington LS (2011) DNA end resection–unraveling the tail. DNA Repair (Amst) 10: 344–348.
117. Boehler C, Gauthier LR, Mortusewicz O, Biard DS, Saliou JM, et al. (2011) Poly(ADP-ribose) polymerase 3 (PARP3), a newcomer in cellular response to DNA damage and mitotic progression. Proc Natl Acad Sci U S A 108: 2783–2788.
118. Modesti M, Budzowska M, Baldeyron C, Demmers JA, Ghirlando R, et al. (2007) RAD51AP1 is a structure-specific DNA binding protein that stimulates joint molecule formation during RAD51-mediated homologous recombination. Mol Cell 28: 468–481.
119. Nitiss JL (2009) DNA topoisomerase II and its growing repertoire of biological functions. Nat Rev Cancer 9: 327–337.
120. Ranuncolo SM, Polo JM, Melnick A (2008) BCL6 represses CHEK1 and suppresses DNA damage pathways in normal and malignant B-cells. Blood Cells Mol Dis 41: 95–99.
121. Thomas JO (2001) HMG1 and 2: architectural DNA-binding proteins. Biochem Soc Trans 29: 395–401.

12

Soluble Rank Ligand Produced by Myeloma Cells Causes Generalised Bone Loss in Multiple Myeloma

Clive Henry Buckle[1¶], Evy De Leenheer[1¶], Michelle Anne Lawson[1], Kwee Yong[2], Neil Rabin[2], Mark Perry[3], Karen Vanderkerken[4], Peter Ian Croucher[1,5]*

1 Department of Human Metabolism, University of Sheffield Faculty of Medicine, Dentistry and Health, Sheffield, United Kingdom, **2** Department of Haematology, University College London, London, United Kingdom, **3** Department of Anatomy, University of Bristol, Bristol, United Kingdom, **4** Department of Haematology and Immunology, Vrije Universiteit Brussel, Brussels, Belgium, **5** Garvan Institute for Medical Research, Sydney, Australia

Abstract

Patients with multiple myeloma commonly develop focal osteolytic bone disease, as well as generalised osteoporosis. The mechanisms underlying the development of osteoporosis in patients with myeloma are poorly understood. Although disruption of the RANKL/OPG pathway has been shown to underlie formation of focal osteolytic lesions, its role in the development of osteoporosis in myeloma remains unclear. Increased soluble RANKL in serum from patients with myeloma raises the possibility that this molecule plays a key role. The aim of the present study was to establish whether sRANKL produced by myeloma cells contributes directly to osteoporosis. C57BL/KaLwRij mice were injected with either 5T2MM or 5T33MM murine myeloma cells. 5T2MM-bearing mice developed osteolytic bone lesions ($p<0.05$) with increased osteoclast surface ($p<0.01$) and reduced trabecular bone volume ($p<0.05$). Bone volume was also reduced at sites where 5T2MM cells were not present ($p<0.05$). In 5T2MM-bearing mice soluble mRANKL was increased ($p<0.05$), whereas OPG was not altered. In contrast, 5T33MM-bearing mice had no changes in osteoclast surface or trabecular bone volume and did not develop osteolytic lesions. Soluble mRANKL was undetectable in serum from 5T33MM-bearing mice. In separate experiments, RPMI-8226 human myeloma cells were transduced with an human RANKL/eGFP construct, or eGFP alone. RPMI-8226/hRANKL/eGFP cells, but not RPMI-8226/eGFP cells, stimulated osteoclastic bone resorption ($p<0.05$) *in vitro*. Sub-cutaneous injection of NOD/SCID mice with RPMI-8226/hRANKL/eGFP or RPMI-8226/eGFP cells resulted in tumour development in all mice. RPMI-8226/hRANKL/eGFP-bearing mice exhibited increased serum soluble hRANKL ($p<0.05$) and a three-fold increase in osteoclast number ($p<0.05$) compared to RPMI-8226/eGFP-bearing mice. This was associated with reduced trabecular bone volume (27%, $p<0.05$), decreased trabecular number (29%, $p<0.05$) and increased trabecular thickness (8%, $p<0.05$). Our findings demonstrate that soluble RANKL produced by myeloma cells causes generalised bone loss, suggesting that targeting RANKL may prevent osteoporosis in patients with myeloma.

Editor: Denise Pires de Carvalho, Universidade Federal do Rio de Janeiro, Brazil

Funding: These studies were supported by grants from the following organisations: Leukaemia and Lymphoma Research - (no 09021) (leukaemialymphomaresearch.org.uk) - provided support for staff and recurrent costs to support the project; the Fonds voor Wetenschappelijk Onderzoek (FWO) - Vlaanderen, Onderzoeksraad-VUB (www.fwo.be) - provided support for staff and recurrent costs to support the project; The Multiple Myeloma Research Foundation - contract 10/2003 (www.themmrf.org) - provided support for maintaining the mouse models of myeloma used in this project; and the Ernest Heine Family Foundation and Mrs Janice Gibson (no url or number) provide support for PIC. The authors confirm that the funders had no role in study design, data collection and analysis, decision to publish, or preparation of the manuscript.

Competing Interests: The authors have declared that no competing interests exist.

* E-mail: p.croucher@garvan.org.au

¶ These authors contributed equally to this work.

Introduction

An important clinical feature of multiple myeloma is the development of a bone disease characterised by the presence of osteolytic lesions, bone pain and pathological fractures. Patients with myeloma also develop generalised bone loss, or osteoporosis, independent of the focal osteolytic bone lesions [1]. There is a two-fold increase in risk of osteoporotic fractures in patients with myeloma [2] and individuals with monoclonal gammopathy of underdetermined significance have an increased risk of axial fractures prior to development of myeloma [3]. Although it is widely recognised that increased osteoclastic resorption accounts for the development of osteolytic bone disease, the cellular and molecular mechanism responsible for the generalised bone loss is poorly understood. Furthermore, studies aimed at clarifying the importance of osteoporosis in the bone disease associated with multiple myeloma, as well as the mechanism(s) involved, will help provide the rationale for targeting this component of the disease.

The identification of the ligand for receptor activator of NFκB (RANKL) [4,5,6], and the demonstration that RANKL plays a critical role in normal osteoclast formation [7], raises the possibility that abnormal expression of this molecule may stimulate osteoclast formation and bone resorption in myeloma. RANKL expression is increased in bone marrow stromal cells in patients with myeloma [8,9] and may also be expressed directly by both murine and human myeloma cells [10,11,12,13,14]. Furthermore, RANKL may be upregulated in T lymphocytes derived from the bone marrow of patients with myeloma [15]. The soluble decoy receptor for RANKL, osteoprotegerin (OPG), prevents RANKL-association with receptor activator of NFκB (RANK) and blocks osteoclast formation and bone resorption [10]. Studies have demonstrated that myeloma cells down-regulate OPG production in stromal cells and osteoblasts in a contact dependent manner [8,9,16] and that serum concentrations of OPG are decreased in patients with myeloma [17,18,19]. Furthermore, targeting RANKL can prevent the development of myeloma bone disease demonstrating that RANKL plays a pivotal role [9,10,20,21].

RANKL exists principally as a membrane-bound molecule, although a soluble form (sRANKL) is generated by either proteolytic processing, or alternative mRNA splicing [22,23,24]. The soluble form of RANKL can induce osteoclastogenesis *in vitro* [5,25] and may be produced by T cells isolated from patients with myeloma [15]. Furthermore, myeloma cells have been shown to express the mRNA encoding the sRANKL isoform [23] and increases in the concentration of sRANKL, and the ratio of sRANKL/OPG, have both been detected in the serum of patients with multiple myeloma. However, the importance of sRANKL and its role in the development of osteoporosis associated with myeloma bone disease remains unclear. Therefore, the aim of the present study was to determine whether sRANKL causes osteoporosis in murine models of multiple myeloma.

Materials and Methods

The 5T2MM and 5T33MM Models of Myeloma

The 5T2MM and 5T33MM murine models of myeloma originated spontaneously in C57BL/KaLwRij mice [26,27]. 5T2MM or 5T33MM cells were isolated from bone marrow of disease-bearing animals, purified and injected into recipient mice [28]. These models closely reflect many aspects of the disease seen in humans. For example, they include the growth of myeloma in bone, the dependency of the myeloma on the bone microenvironment for its growth and survival, the development of a paraprotein that reflects myeloma burden and, in the case of 5T2MM, the characteristic osteolytic bone disease. Animals were housed under conventional conditions and had free access to food and tap water. All procedures involving these mice were approved by the local ethics committee at the Free University of Brussels (Belgium). Male C57BL/KaLwRij mice were injected with either 5T2MM or 5T33MM cells, or left un-injected (naïve). Serum paraprotein was monitored using standard electrophoretic techniques throughout the development of the disease [29]. All animals, including the respective uninjected, non-tumour bearing, control groups, were sacrificed at 12 weeks for the 5T2MM

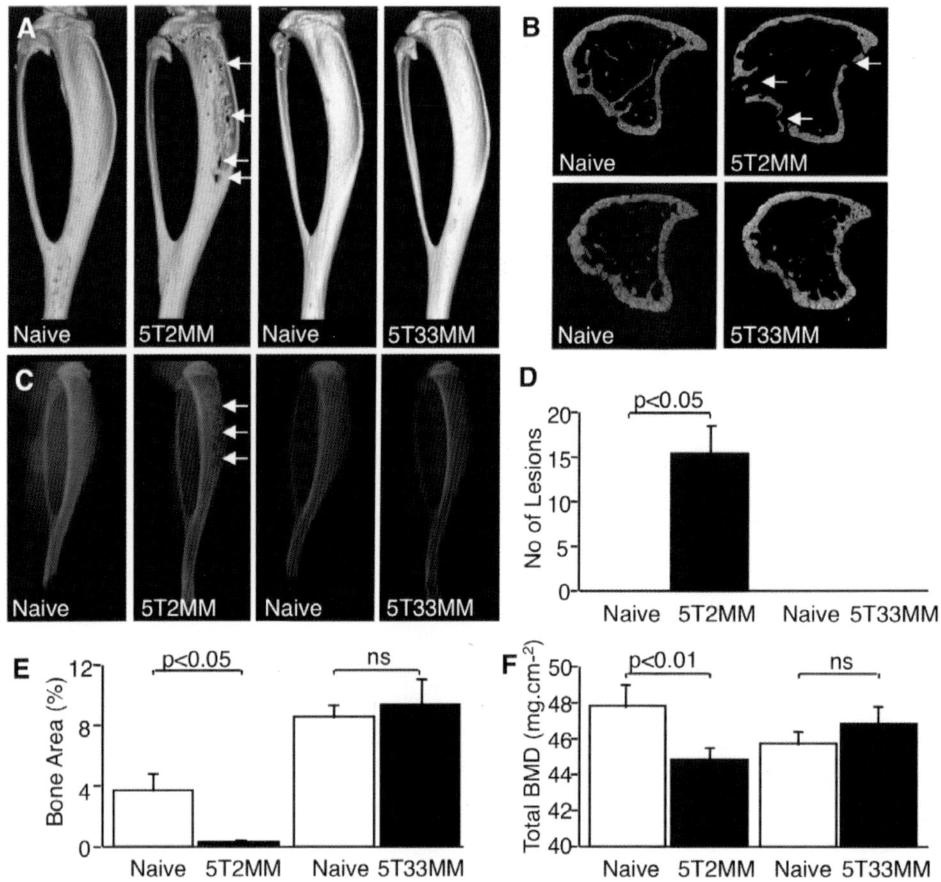

Figure 1. 5T2MM, but not 5T33MM cells cause osteolytic bone disease and tumour-induced bone loss. A. Reconstructed 3-dimensional micro-CT images of the tibia of naïve mice, mice bearing 5T2MM cells and mice bearing 5T33MM cells. Lesions in the tibia of 5T2MM bearing animals are arrowed. B. Transverse sections of micro-CT images of tibiae from naïve mice, mice bearing 5T2MM cells and mice bearing 5T33MM cells. Lesions are arrowed. C. Radiographs of the tibia of naïve mice, mice bearing 5T2MM cells and mice bearing 5T33MM cells. Lesions are arrowed. D. Number of lesions in the tibia of naïve mice and 5T2MM or 5T33MM bearing mice. E. Trabecular bone area as a proportion of total tissue area in the tibia of naïve mice, and mice bearing 5T2MM or 5T33MM cells. F. Total bone mineral density of naïve mice, and 5T2MM or 5T33MM bearing mice. Statistical analysis by Mann-Whitney U test. Data = mean ± S.E.M.

bearing mice (n = 12, naïve control n = 9) and 4 weeks for the 5T33MM bearing mice (n = 7, naïve control n = 9).

NOD/SCID Xenograft Model of Myeloma

Following whole body γ-irradiation of NOD/SCID mice (3.0 Gy per mouse, at a rate of 1Gy per 21.0 secs, using an IBL 437C ^{137}Cs gamma source, CIS BioInternational) at day −1, RPMI-8226 myeloma cells (American Type Culture Collection (ATCC), Manassas, VA, USA) were injected subcutaneously (10^7 per mouse) at day 0 (mice aged 8 weeks at day 0, and all male). The following tumour cells were injected into irradiated mice: RPMI-8226/hRANKL/eGFP (n = 8/group), RPMI- 8226/eGFP (n = 8/group), RPMI-8226-wild-type (n = 7/group). Subcutaneous tumour progression was monitored via both eGFP-imaging (LightTools®, Synopsis Inc., Pasadena, CA) and caliper measurement and mice were sacrificed once the tumour had reached 1 cm^3. All procedures involving these mice were undertaken at the University of Sheffield, with written UK Home Office licence approval (ref. PPL402901).

Radiogaphic, Densitometric and MicroCT Analysis of Myeloma Bone Disease To assess the number of osteolytic bone lesions induced by the presence of myelomacells the femora and tibiae were radiographed using a Faxitron x-ray system (Hewlett Packard, McMinnville, Oregon). The radiographs were scanned using a UMAX PowerLook 1100 scanner. Images were enlarged using Adobe Photoshop 5.0 LE software and the numbers of lytic bone lesions in the proximal tibiae and distal femora were counted manually on the digital image. Total bone mineral density (BMD) was measured by dual-energy x-ray absorptiometry (DXA) using a PIXImus scanner (Lunar, Madison, WI).

In some studies tibiae were scanned using a microCT scanner (Skyscan 1172) at 50 kV, 200 uA, using a detection pixel size of 4.3 um^2 and a 0.5 mm aluminium filter, capturing images (×2) every 0.7° through 180° rotation. Reconstruction was performed using Skyscan Recon software and images analysed using Skyscan CT analysis software. A 1 mm^3 volume of trabecular bone, 0.2 mm distal to the growth plate, was selected as a region of interest (ROI), and trabecular volume as a proportion of tissue volume (BV/TV, %), and trabecular number (Tb. N, mm^{-1}) was assessed in this area.

Histomorphometric Analysis of Myeloma Bone Disease

The femora, tibiae, calvariae and lumbar vertebrae were dissected free of soft tissues and processed for histological analysis. Bones were decalcified in EDTA and embedded in paraffin. Sections were cut and stained with haematoxylin and eosin. Trabecular bone area as a proportion of the total area (Cn.Ar/T.Ar,%) was determined in the distal femoral metaphysis and proximal tibial metaphysis and lumbar vertebrae, on a minimum of two separate sections, using a Leica QWin image analysis system (Leica Microscope Systems, Milton Keynes, UK). The medullary area in the calvariae was measured using the Leica Qwin system and expressed as a proportion of total tissue area or as an absolute area. To identify osteoclasts, sections were reacted for the presence of tartrate resistant acid phosphatase (TRAP) and counterstained with Mayer's Haematoxylin. The number of osteoclasts and/or the proportion of surface occupied by osteoclasts on the cortical-endosteal bone surface (N.Oc/CE; Oc.S/CE,%) were determined and, where appropriate, the trabecular bone surface (N.Oc/Ca; Oc.S/Ca,%).

Measurement of Soluble RANKL and OPG in Serum

At sacrifice, blood samples were obtained from naïve animals (n = 8 as control for 5T2MM; n = 9 as control for 5T33MM) and animals bearing 5T2MM (n = 12) or 5T33MM (n = 7) tumour

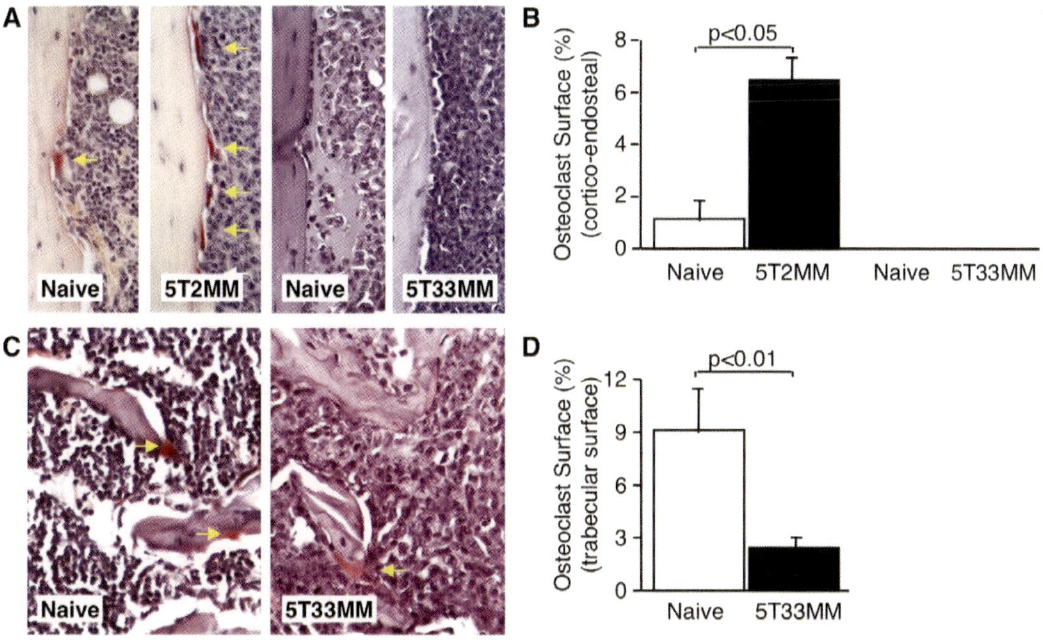

Figure 2. 5T2MM, but not 5T33MM murine myeloma cells promote osteoclast formation in C57BL/KaLwRij mice. A. Photomicrographs of sections of the tibia reacted for TRAP activity from naive, 5T2MM and 5T33MM bearing mice showing the cortico-endosteal bone surface. TRAP-positive osteoclasts are arrowed. Original magnification ×40. B. The proportion of the cortical-endosteal bone surface occupied by osteoclasts, expressed as the percentage of the total bone surface, from naive mice and mice bearing 5T2MM or 5T33MM myeloma cells. C. Photomicrographs of sections of the tibia stained for TRAP activity from naive and 5T33MM bearing mice showing areas of trabecular bone. TRAP-positive osteoclasts are arrowed. Original magnification ×40. D. The proportion of trabecular bone covered by osteoclasts in naïve and 5T33MM bearing mice. Statistical analysis by Mann-Whitney U test. Data = mean± S.E.M.

cells. Serum was separated by centrifugation and murine sRANKL, and murine OPG, were each measured by commercially available ELISA (R&D Systems, Abingdon, UK), according to the manufacturer's instructions.

Production of RPMPI-8226/hRANKL/eGFP myeloma cells

cDNA encoding full-length human RANKL (hRANKL) was originally isolated from the SAOS2 osteosarcoma cell line (ATCC, Manassas, VA, USA). Its sequence corresponds to AF053712 (NCBI). hRANKL was cloned into the pCL10.1 bicistronic expression vector upstream of the sequence encoding enhanced green fluorescent protein (eGFP - *Aequorea victoria*), in which co-expression is controlled by the murine stem cell virus promoter. Self-inactivating lentiviral particles were produced as described previously [30]. Briefly, 293T human embryonal kidney cells (ATCC, Manassas, VA, USA) were co-transfected using a four plasmid-system, which introduced lentiviral *gag-pol* genes, the vesicular stomatitis virus envelope glycoprotein gene, reverse transcriptase and the expression cassette from pCL10.1. Titre was determined by limiting dilution on HeLa cells (ATCC, Manassas, VA, USA). RPMI-8226 human myeloma cells were plated at 5×10^4 cells per well in six-well plates, then exposed to viral supernatant (MOI 10) for 12 hours, in the presence of polybrene (8 μg.ml^{-1}). Transduced RPMI-8226 expressing hRANKL/eGFP, or eGFP alone, were expanded in culture, and used for *in vitro* and *in vivo* experiments.

Detection of hRANKL expression

Transduction was assessed using flow cytometry (anti-hRANKL-PE, eBioscience Inc. Cat. No. 12-6619, mouse IgG2b-PE isotype control Cat. No. 12-4732), end-point polymerase chain reaction (PCR) (using primers directed at hRANKL: FOR 5′-TAGGAGAATTAAACAGGCCTTTC-3′, REV 5′-CAAAAAC-TGGGGCTCAATC-3′) and western blot (performed using anti-hRANKL, R&D Systems Cat. No. AF626, 0.1 ug.ml^{-1}, and detected with anti-goat-HRP, Dako Cat. No. P0449, 1/30000; abcam anti-RNA polymerase II antibody, Cat. No. ab5408, 1/2000, detected with anti-mouse-HRP, Amersham Biosciences Cat. No. NA931V, 1/15000, was used as a loading control). ELISA, directed at hRANKL (Biomedica Gruppe, Wien, Austria) (performed according to the manufacturer's instructions), was used to quantify hRANKL in culture supernatant produced using transduced cells, as well as control cells. Where appropriate, SaOS2 and MG63 human osteoblast like cells (ATCC, Manassas, VA, USA) were included as bone cell controls.

Determining whether over-expressed hRANKL is biologically active in vitro

Freshly isolated mouse peripheral blood mononuclear cells were plated in medium conditioned with RPMI-8226/hRANKL/eGFP cells, and supplemented with rmM-CSF at 25 ng.ml^{-1} (using 6-well plates). Media conditioned using either wild-type or eGFP-transduced cells were used as controls. Alpha-MEM, supplemented with rmM-CSF (see above) and rhRANKL at 0.5 ngml^{-1}, in order to match the concentration detected in the conditioned medium, was included as a positive control. The number of TRAP-positive multinuclear (3+) cells was determined at 7, 14 and 21-day time points, via light microscopy.

In order to determine whether the multinuclear TRAP-positive cells could resorb bone, freshly-isolated mouse PBMC were cultured on dentine slices in medium conditioned with RPMI-8226/hRANKL/eGFP, as above (using 96-well plates). eGFP-only and wild-type controls were also included. At 21-days, slices were stained, using toluidine blue, and resorption pits visualised and scored, using light microscopy.

Statistical Analysis

Data were expressed as the mean ± SEM. Comparison between groups was performed by Mann-Whitney U test, Chi-square analysis or Student's unpaired t test, as appropriate. Comparisons between distributions were performed using a Kolmogorov-Smirnov test.

Results

5T2MM but not 5T33MM Myeloma Cells Promote the Development of Myeloma Bone Disease in the Tibiae and Femora in vivo

Injection of 5T2MM and 5T33MM cells into the tail vein of syngeneic C57BL/KaLwRij mice resulted in growth of myeloma cells in the bone marrow. Both 5T2MM and 5T33MM bearing mice had detectable levels of paraprotein in the serum (1.25±0.25 g.L^{-1}, at 12 weeks, in the case of the 5T2MM-bearing mice). MicroCT, as well as radiographic analysis, of the long bones of mice bearing 5T2MM cells was used to demonstrate the presence of osteolytic bone lesions in the tibia and femur, which are areas in which increased osteoclast activity results in focal bone loss (Figure 1A–C). On a digitised radiographic image of a mouse tibia, the osteolytic bone lesions can be distinguished from surrounding intact bone as darker regions in which the bone has been removed. Assessment of the numbers of lesions in the

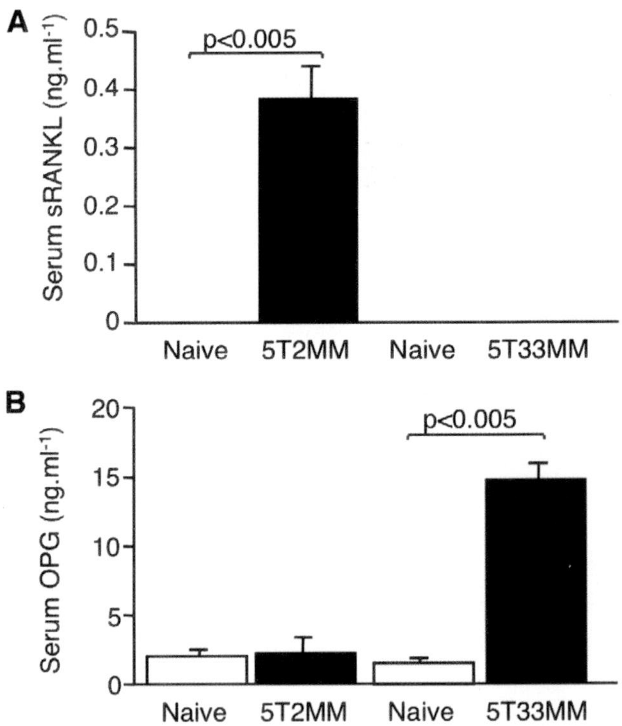

Figure 3. Serum concentrations of sRANKL and OPG are abnormally regulated in mice bearing 5T2MM and 5T33MM cells, respectively. Serum concentrations of sRANKL and OPG are abnormally regulated in mice bearing 5T2MM and 5T33MM cells, respectively. A. Serum concentrations of sRANKL in naive mice and mice bearing 5T2MM or 5T33MM cells. B. Serum concentrations of OPG in naive animals and animals bearing 5T2MM or 5T33MM cells. Statistical analysis by Mann-Whitney U test. Data = mean± S.E.M.

tibia showed a significant increase in 5T2MM bearing animals when compared to naïve animals ($p<0.05$)(Figure 1D), whereas no lesions were observed in mice bearing 5T33MM cells (Figures 1C and 1D). Histomorphometric analysis of the long bones of 5T2MM bearing mice demonstrated a significant decrease in the trabecular bone area in the tibia and femur when compared to un-injected naïve animals ($p<0.05$). In contrast, trabecular bone area in mice bearing 5T33MM cells was not significantly different from naïve, uninjected mice (Figure 1E). Total BMD in the tibiae was also lower in 5T2MM bearing mice when compared to naïve, un-injected animals ($p<0.01$). There was no difference in total BMD in the tibiae in naïve mice and mice bearing 5T33MM cells (Figure 1F).

Histomorphometric analysis demonstrated that the proportion of cortico-endosteal bone surface covered by osteoclasts was significantly increased in 5T2MM bearing animals when compared to control ($p<0.05$). In contrast, osteoclasts were not identified on the cortico-endosteal surface of naïve mice or mice bearing 5T33MM cells (Figure 2A and 2B). Analysis of the trabecular bone surfaces of 5T33MM bearing mice showed a

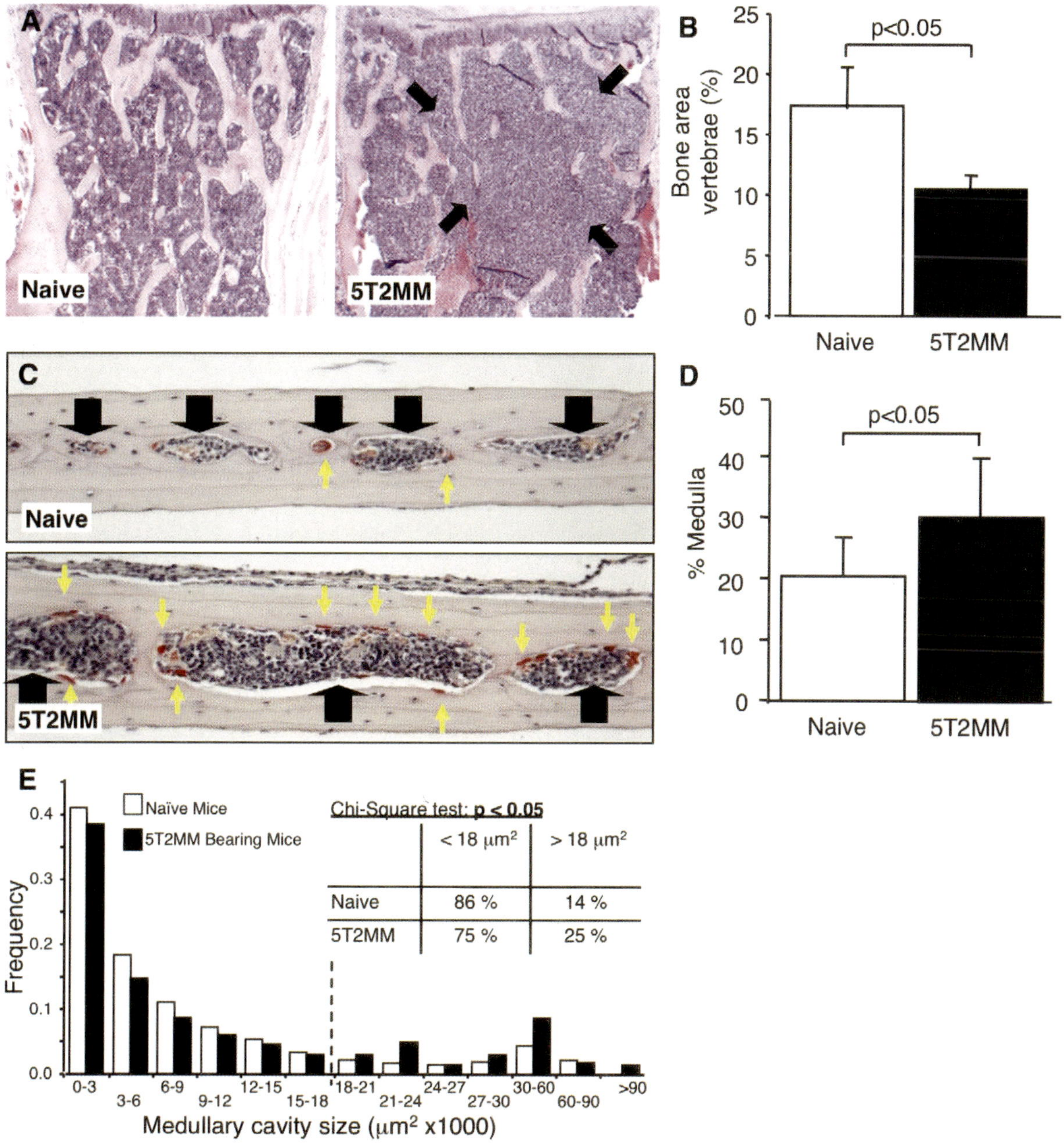

Figure 4. 5T2MM bearing mice have increased bone loss in the lumbar vertebrae and calvariae. A. Photomicrographs of the vertebrae from naïve and 5T2MM bearing mice. Tumour infiltration is identified with black arrows. B. The proportion of trabecular bone area in the vertebrae from naïve and 5T2MM-bearing mice. C. Photomicrographs of the calvariae of naïve and 5T2MM bearing mice. Medullary spaces are identified with black arrows, and OC with yellow arrows. Non tumour-containing spaces are shown. D. The proportion of medullary area as a percentage of total tissue area in naïve and 5T2MM-bearing mice. E. Distribution of medullary spaces in naïve and 5T2MM-bearing mice, showing significant differences in distribution (KS test, $p<0.02$). Chi-square analysis demonstrated that 5T2MM-bearing mice had significantly fewer, smaller spaces and more, larger spaces than naïve mice ($p<0.05$). Data = mean ± S.E.M. (B and D).

decrease in the proportion of trabecular bone surface covered by osteoclasts ($p<0.01$) (Figure 2C and 2D). It was not possible to analyse the trabecular bone surface occupied by osteoclasts in 5T2MM bearing mice as the trabecular bone had been almost completely resorbed.

Serum Concentrations of Soluble RANKL and OPG Are Abnormally Regulated in 5T2MM and 5T33MM Bearing Mice Compared to Non-Tumour Bearing, Naïve Mice

We next measured serum concentrations of sRANKL and OPG in mice bearing 5T2MM and 5T33MM cells and compared them to non-tumour bearing, naïve mice. sRANKL was not detectable in the serum of naïve mice or mice bearing 5T33MM cells. However, significant concentrations of sRANKL were measured in the serum of mice bearing 5T2MM cells (379.0±58.4 pg/ml, shown in Figure 3A). In contrast, serum concentrations of OPG in 5T2MM bearing animals and naïve animals were not significantly different (1.86±0.08 and 1.77±0.13 ng/ml respectively), whereas serum OPG was significantly increased in mice bearing 5T33MM cells when compared to naïve, un-injected animals (14.97±1.09 and 1.33±0.13 ng/ml respectively, $p<0.005$) (Figure 3B). There was no significant correlation between sRANKL and OPG in 5T2MM bearing mice.

5T2MM Bearing Mice Have Increased Bone Loss in the Vertebrae and Calvariae

High serum concentration of sRANKL would be consistent with the bone loss observed in the tibia and the development of osteolytic bone lesions. However, alterations in circulating sRANKL would also be expected to promote more generalised bone loss. We therefore examined bones isolated from other sites for evidence of generalised osteoporosis in 5T2MM bearing mice. Histomorphometric examination of lumbar vertebrae demonstrated a significant decrease in trabecular bone in 5T2MM bearing mice compared to non-tumour bearing, naïve mice (Figure 4A and 4B), although, bone loss was also associated with significant infiltration of 5T2MM tumour cells. However, analysis of the medullary area in the calvariae demonstrated a significant increase in area in 5T2MM bearing mice compared to naïve mice ($p<0.05$), consistent with increased bone loss (Figure 4C, 4D). In the 5T2MM-bearing mice tumour infiltration was seen in only a limited number of medullary spaces (13%). Comparison of the medullary spaces from naïve and 5T2MM-bearing mice, but excluding those showing evidence of tumour infiltration, demonstrated a significant difference in the distribution of medullary space size ($p<0.02$) (Figure 4E). Chi-square analysis demonstrated that 5T2MM-bearing mice had significantly more, larger spaces and fewer, smaller spaces than naïve mice ($p<0.05$). In contrast, 5T33MM bearing mice showed no difference in the distribution of their medullary spaces when compared to naïve mice ($p=0.42$; data not shown) and Chi-square analysis failed to show any difference in the proportion of larger medullary spaces when compared to naïve mice.

RPMI-8226/hRANKL/eGFP human myeloma cells express biologically active soluble hRANKL

To determine whether myeloma cell derived RANKL could induce systemic bone loss we generated myeloma cells over-expressing hRANKL (RPMI-8226/hRANKL/eGFP). Using end-

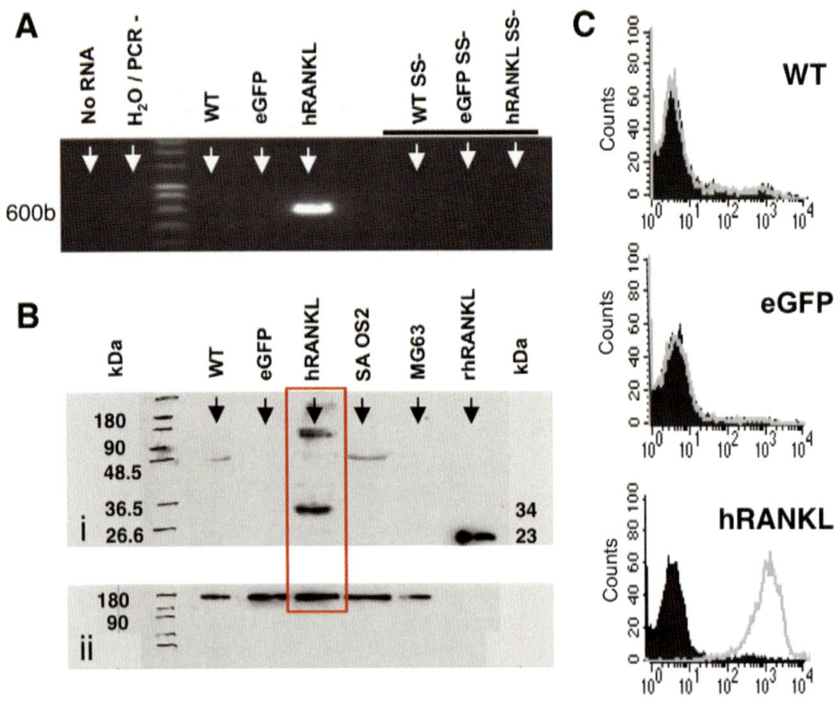

Figure 5. RPMI-8226/hRANKL/eGFP cells express hRANKL. A. End-point PCR demonstrating that human RANKL mRNA is present in RPMI-8226/hRANKL/eGFP cells (labeled hRANKL). hRANKL mRNA was not detected in the corresponding eGFP-only control cell line (labeled eGFP), or in wild-type cells (labeled WT). No product was amplified in the absence of RNA (labelled no RNA) or the superscript enzyme (labeled SS-). B. Western Blot analysis detected the hRANKL monomer (~34 kDa) in culture supernatant from RPMI-8226/hRANKL/eGFP cells - red outline. (i) Wild-type and eGFP-only expressing cell controls are included, and the rhRANKL antibody-control is also shown (~23 kDa). (ii) Ribosomal RNA loading controls were included. C. Flow cytometric analysis of the RPMI-8226/hRANKL/eGFP-expressing cells. Representative plots showing cells stained with anti-hRANKL-PE antibody (eBioScience, 1/50 dilution) (transparent profile) and isotype control (solid profile).

point PCR, hRANKL mRNA was detected in RPMI-8226/hRANKL/eGFP (Figure 5A). In contrast, no expression was detected in the vector-only control, or wild-type cells. Following western blot, normalised using ribosomal RNA loading controls, hRANKL protein was detected in culture medium conditioned by RPMI-8226/hRANKL/eGFP cells (Figure 5B), but not in medium conditioned by wild-type or vector only control cells, as well as medium conditioned using osteoblast cell lines SAOS2 and MG63. In addition, flow cytometric analysis, using an antibody directed at hRANKL along with its corresponding isotype control, demonstrates that the RPMI-8226/hRANKL/eGFP cells express hRANKL at the cell surface (Figure 5C), whereas the RPMI-8226/eGFP and wild-type cells do not. Soluble hRANKL was detected in medium conditioned using the RPMI-8226/hRANKL/eGFP cells (circa 0.4 ng.ml^{-1}), determined by ELISA. Soluble RANKL was not detected in wild-type or RPMI-8226/eGFP control cells (Figure 6A).

When freshly isolated mouse PBMC were cultured in medium conditioned with RPMI-8226/hRANKL/eGFP cells, multinucleate TRAP-positive cells were observed. No such cells formed in the cultures treated with medium conditioned using RPMI-8226/eGFP cells (Figure 6B). In separate *in vitro* experiments, where mouse PBMC were cultured on dentine slices, in the presence of medium conditioned by RPMI-8226/hRANKL/eGFP cells, resorption trails were observed (Figure 6C). No pits were observed on dentine slices cultured with medium conditioned using RPMI-8226/eGFP control cells (Figure 6C).

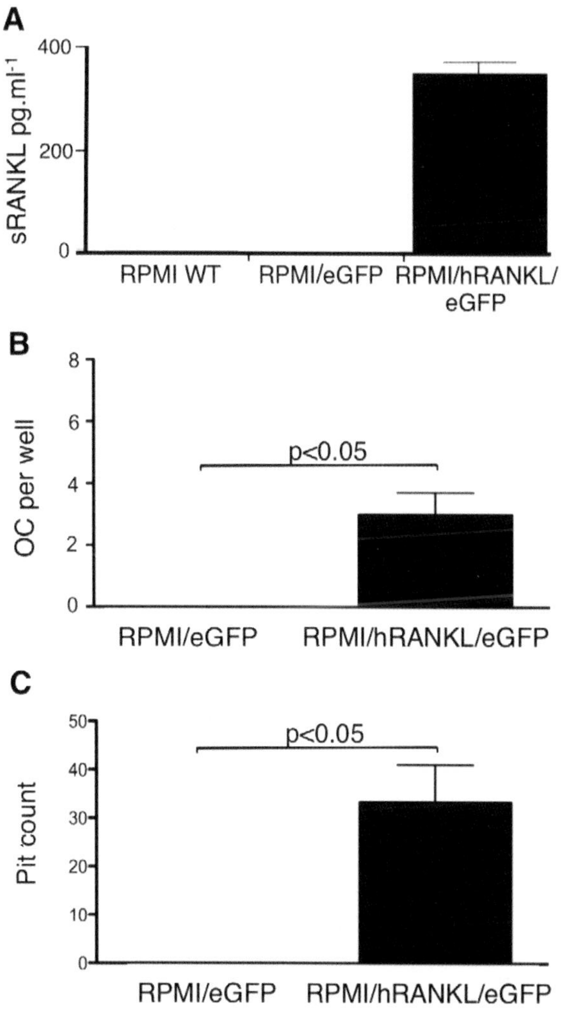

Figure 6. Transduced RPMI-8226 human myeloma cells express biologically active soluble hRANKL. A. shRANKL is detected by ELISA (Biomedica Gruppe, Wien, Austria), at a concentration of ~0.4 ng.ml^{-1}, in medium conditioned using RPMI-8226/hRANKL/eGFP cells, but not in controls. B. Multinucleated TRAP-positive cells (osteoclasts) formed in a culture of mouse PBMC cultured in medium conditioned with RPMI-8226/hRANKL/eGFP, supplemented with M-CSF (50 ng.ml^{-1}). No osteoclasts were observed in control wells containing conditioned media from wild-type cells (data not shown) or RPMI-8226/eGFP. C. Resorption trails formed on the surface of dentine slices cultured in the presence of freshly prepared mouse PBMC, using medium conditioned with RPMI-8226/hRANKL/eGFP. No trails formed on slices cultured in medium conditioned by RPMI-8226/eGFP (or wild-type - data not shown). Statistical analysis performed using unpaired t-test. Data = mean± S.E.M.

RPMI-8226/hRANKL/eGFP-bearing mice have increased osteoclast number, elevated serum soluble RANKL and reduced trabecular bone volume and number

Sub-cutaneous injection of NOD/SCID mice with RPMI-8226/hRANKL/eGFP, or RPMI-8226/eGFP cells, resulted in palpable tumour development in all mice. The mice bearing RPMI-8226/hRANKL/eGFP cells also exhibited increased serum soluble hRANKL ($p<0.05$) compared to RPMI-8226/eGFP cells (Figure 7A), although not all mice had detectable sRANKL. Following sacrifice, histological analysis of the tibiae from all mice showed that marrow space was not infiltrated with myeloma cells. However, histomorphometric analysis demonstrated that RPMI-8226/hRANKL/eGFP-bearing mice exhibited a three-fold increase in osteoclast number ($p<0.05$) along the cortico-endosteal surface compared to RPMI-8226/eGFP-bearing mice (Figure 7B and 7C). MicroCT analysis of tibiae of RPMI-8226/hRANKL/eGFP-bearing mice, with detectable sRANKL in the serum, was associated with reduced trabecular bone volume (27%, $p<0.05$) (Figure 7D and 7E), decreased trabecular number (29%, $p<0.05$) (Figure 7F), and increased trabecular thickness (8%, $p<0.05$ - data not shown).

Discussion

In the present study we examined the ability of two syngeneic models of multiple myeloma, the 5T2MM and the 5T33MM models, to cause both osteolytic bone disease and osteoporosis. In 5T2MM bearing mice this was characterised by the presence of osteolytic bone lesions on radiographs, loss of trabecular bone, a reduction in total bone mineral density and an increase in the proportion of bone surface covered by osteoclasts. This mimics the features of the bone disease seen in patients with multiple myeloma. In contrast, injection of 5T33MM cells had little effect on bone. 5T33MM cells did not promote the development of osteolytic bone lesions, had no effect on trabecular bone area or total bone mineral density and did not increase osteoclast formation. Indeed, histomorphometric analysis demonstrated that osteoclast surface on trabecular bone was significantly reduced in mice bearing 5T33MM cells. These data contrast with a previous study in which 5T33MM cells were reported to promote the development of a myeloma bone disease [31]. The reason for the difference between the two studies is unclear. However, the 5T33MM cells have been maintained independently, in different laboratories for many years and therefore, this may reflect the selection of different clones of 5T33MM cells over time.

In addition to focal osteolytic bone lesions, generalised osteoporosis was observed in the bones of 5T2MM bearing mice in which tumour cells were not present. In the calvariae of these

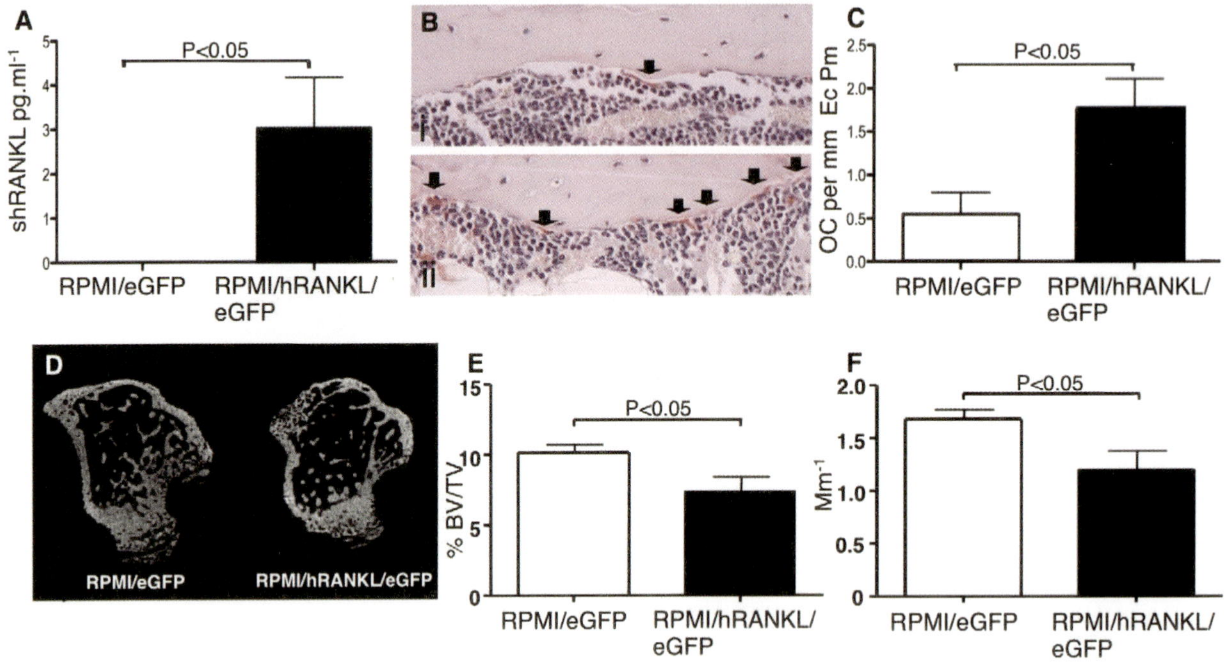

Figure 7. RPMI-8226/hRANKL/eGFP-bearing mice have elevated serum soluble RANKL, increased osteoclast number and reduced trabecular bone volume. A. ELISA demonstrating significantly increased serum sRANKL in mice bearing RPMI-8226/hRANKL/eGFP cells, compared to RPMI-8226/eGFP-bearing animals, as well as wild-type cells (data not shown). B. Photomicrographs of sections of mouse tibiae demonstrating that mice bearing RPMI-8226/hRANKL/eGFP (ii) have increased OC number at the CE-surface, compared to mice bearing RPMI-8226/eGFP control cells (i). OC are arrowed. Original magnification ×40. C. Increased OC number is observed at the CE surface in mice bearing RPMI-8226/hRANKL/eGFP cells. D. MicroCT images showing reduced bone volume in tibiae of mice bearing RPMI-8226/hRANKL/eGFP, as opposed to wild-type cells. E. RPMI-8226/hRANKL/eGFP-treated mice have decreased trabecular bone volume (27%) when compared to RPMI-8226/eGFP cell-bearing animals. F. RPMI-8226/hRANKL/eGFP-treated mice have reduced trabecular number (29%), when compared to RPMI-8226/eGFP-bearing animals. Statistical analysis performed using unpaired t-test. Data = mean± S.E.M.

mice, significant bone loss was observed, which is consistent with the hypothesis that bone loss also occurs independently of local induction by tumour cells, and results from systemic induction of osteoclastogenesis. In support of this, studies have shown that a significant proportion of patients with multiple myeloma develop osteopenia or osteoporosis independent of lytic bone lesions [2]. The molecular mechanism responsible for the development of osteoporosis in myeloma is unknown.

Measurement of sRANKL in serum showed that 5T2MM-bearing mice had high circulating levels of sRANKL in all tumour-bearing mice. In contrast, sRANKL was not detectable in the serum of naïve mice, or mice bearing 5T33MM cells. This is consistent with the demonstration of increased serum concentrations of sRANKL in patients with myeloma and that an increase in the ratio of RANKL/OPG is associated with lytic bone lesions [32]. The source of sRANKL remains unclear, but may reflect production by cells within the bone marrow microenvironment, such as stromal cells and T-cells, or production by 5T2MM cells, since we have shown previously that these cells express RANKL [10]. Furthermore, the mechanism responsible for generating sRANKL is unknown, but may include proteolytic cleavage of a membrane-bound RANKL isoform, as myeloma cells can shed membrane bound molecules [33,34] and express ADAM17, a proteinase capable of shedding RANKL [35]. Alternatively, circulating sRANKL may be generated by differential mRNA splicing, which has been reported in myeloma cells [13]. Treatment of the RPMI8226/eGFP/hRANKL cells with phorbol 12-myristate 13-acetate, which has been shown to activate membrane shedding activity, had no effect on membrane RANKL expression and did not increase sRANKL in the culture supernatent (data not shown). This may argue against proteolytic processing of the membrane bound form being the main mechanism of production. Irrespective of the source, these data support the notion that sRANKL, as a key regulator of osteoclastic bone resorption, drives the development of osteoporosis.

Serum concentrations of OPG were unchanged in 5T2MM-bearing mice, but were elevated in those mice bearing 5T33MM cells. This may account for the observed inhibition of osteoclast formation, the lack of detectable bone disease seen in the 5T33MM model and explain the difference between the present study and data reported by Garrett *et al.* [31]. The failure to affect BMD in 5T33MM bearing mice is likely to reflect the short timeframe of this model (4 weeks) and the relatively small contribution attributable to trabecular bone.

In order to investigate the hypothesis that osteoporosis is caused, at least in part, by elevated systemic sRANKL, experiments were performed using a mouse xenograft system in which the tumour cells were engineered to over-express hRANKL. Mice were injected subcutaneously with RPMI-8226/hRANKL/eGFP cells and growth shown to be restricted to the site of implant. Significant increases in serum sRANKL were observed in mice bearing RPMI-8226/hRANKL/eGFP cells, compared to control, myeloma cell bearing animals. Histological examination demonstrated that this increase was associated with elevated numbers of osteoclasts in bones from RPMI-8226/hRANKL/eGFP bearing animals, despite the absence of tumour cells in the bone marrow. These findings are associated with a significant reduction in bone volume and trabecular number in those animals. Taken together these data demonstrate that RANKL expressed by myeloma cells, and released as soluble RANKL, stimulates osteoclast formation and promotes bone loss at distant sites in the skeleton. In support of this, both OPG [10] and a soluble receptor activator of NF_kB-Fc construct (data not shown) were able to prevent osteoclast formation and the development of bone disease in the 5T2MM model.

In conclusion, using mouse models of myeloma we have been able to demonstrate that myeloma is associated with both focal osteolytic bone disease and osteoporosis, and this is associated with increased serum concentrations of sRANKL. Furthermore, myeloma cells that express RANKL also produce soluble RANKL *in vivo* and this is able to promote osteoclast formation and osteoporosis. This supports the hypothesis that elevated serum soluble RANKL contributes to the development of osteoporosis in myeloma. Therefore, inhibiting RANKL may have therapeutic potential not only for the treatment of osteolytic bone lesions but also the generalised osteoporosis. Furthermore, this raises the possibility of using novel treatments such as the monoclonal antibody Denosumab, a fully human monoclonal antibody that targets the RANK-RANKL interaction [36]. This agent has been in development for the treatment of osteolytic bone disease in patients with multiple myeloma, for the treatment of bone disease in bone metastases and for osteoporosis in post- menopausal women [37,38,39]. Its role in the treatment of osteoporosis in myeloma is unclear but the data presented would argue that consideration should be given to its use in this setting. Thus, treatments such as Denosumab, which have been used successfully for the treatment of post-menopausal osteoporosis, could be considered as potential treatment of both the focal osteolytic disease [39,40] and the generalised osteoporosis seen in patients with multiple myeloma.

Acknowledgments

Our thanks go to Mike Blundell, Angelo Willems, Sandy Cordiner-Lawrie, Orla Gallagher, Holly Evans, Julia Hough, Jenny Down and Matt Prideaux for expert technical assistance.

Author Contributions

Conceived and designed the experiments: CHB EDL KV PIC. Performed the experiments: CHB EDL MAL MP KV. Analyzed the data: CHB EDL MAL MP KV PIC. Contributed reagents/materials/analysis tools: KLY NR. Wrote the paper: CHB EDL PIC.

References

1. McCloskey EV (2004) Bone Disease. In Gharton G, Durie Brian GM, Samson D (Eds). Multiple Myeloma and Related Disorders. London: Arnold.
2. Melton LJ, 3rd, Kyle RA, Achenbach SJ, Oberg AL, Rajkumar SV (2005) Fracture risk with multiple myeloma: a population-based study. J Bone Miner Res 20: 487–493.
3. Melton LJ, 3rd, Rajkumar SV, Khosla S, Achenbach SJ, Oberg AL, et al (2004) Fracture risk in monoclonal gammopathy of undetermined significance. Journal of bone and mineral research : the official journal of the American Society for Bone and Mineral Research 19: 25–30.
4. Anderson DM, Maraskovsky E, Billingsley WL, Dougall WC, Tometsko ME, et al. (1997) A homologue of the TNF receptor and its ligand enhance T-cell growth and dendritic-cell function. Nature 390: 175–179.
5. Lacey DL, Timms E, Tan HL, Kelley MJ, Dunstan CR, et al. (1998) Osteoprotegerin ligand is a cytokine that regulates osteoclast differentiation and activation. Cell 93: 165–176.
6. Wong BR, Rho J, Arron J, Robinson E, Orlinick J, et al. (1997) TRANCE is a novel ligand of the tumor necrosis factor receptor family that activates c-Jun N-terminal kinase in T cells. J Biol Chem 272: 25190–25194.
7. Kong YY, Yoshida H, Sarosi I, Tan HL, Timms E, et al. (1999) OPGL is a key regulator of osteoclastogenesis, lymphocyte development and lymph-node organogenesis. Nature 397: 315–323.
8. Giuliani N, Bataille R, Mancini C, Lazzaretti M, Barille S (2001) Myeloma cells induce imbalance in the osteoprotegerin/osteoprotegerin ligand system in the human bone marrow environment. Blood 98: 3527–3533.
9. Pearse RN, Sordillo EM, Yaccoby S, Wong BR, Liau DF, et al. (2001) Multiple myeloma disrupts the TRANCE/osteoprotegerin cytokine axis to trigger bone destruction and promote tumor progression. Proc Natl Acad Sci U S A 98: 11581–11586.
10. Croucher PI, Shipman CM, Lippitt J, Perry M, Asosingh K, et al. (2001) Osteoprotegerin inhibits the development of osteolytic bone disease in multiple myeloma. Blood 98: 3534–3540.
11. Sezer O, Heider U, Jakob C, Zavrski I, Eucker J, et al. (2002) Immunocytochemistry reveals RANKL expression of myeloma cells. Blood 99: 4646–4647; author reply 4647.
12. Heider U, Langelotz C, Jakob C, Zavrski I, Fleissner C, et al. (2003) Expression of Receptor Activator of Nuclear Factor kappaB Ligand on Bone Marrow Plasma Cells Correlates with Osteolytic Bone Disease in Patients with Multiple Myeloma. Clin Cancer Res 9: 1436–1440.
13. Farrugia AN, Atkins GJ, To LB, Pan B, Horvath N, et al. (2003) Receptor activator of nuclear factor-kappaB ligand expression by human myeloma cells mediates osteoclast formation in vitro and correlates with bone destruction in vivo. Cancer Res 63: 5438–5445.
14. Shipman CM, Holen I, Lippitt JM, E V, Croucher PI (2000) Tumour cells isolated from patients with multiple myeloma express the critical osteoclastogenic factor, RANKL. Blood 96: 1552 (Abstr).
15. Giuliani N, Colla S, Sala R, Moroni M, Lazzaretti M, et al. (2002) Human myeloma cells stimulate the receptor activator of nuclear factor-kappa B ligand (RANKL) in T lymphocytes: a potential role in multiple myeloma bone disease. Blood 100: 4615–4621.
16. Shipman CM, Croucher PI (2003) Osteoprotegerin Is a Soluble Decoy Receptor for Tumor Necrosis Factor-related Apoptosis-inducing Ligand/Apo2 Ligand and Can Function as a Paracrine Survival Factor for Human Myeloma Cells. Cancer Res 63: 912–916.
17. Seidel C, Hjertner O, Abildgaard N, Heickendorff L, Hjorth M, et al. (2001) Serum osteoprotegerin levels are reduced in patients with multiple myeloma with lytic bone disease. Blood 98: 2269–2271.
18. Lipton A, Ali SM, Leitzel K, Chinchilli V, Witters L, et al. (2002) Serum osteoprotegerin levels in healthy controls and cancer patients. Clin Cancer Res 8: 2306–2310.
19. Terpos E, de la Fuente J, Szydlo R, Hatjiharissi E, Viniou N, et al. (2003) Tartrate-resistant acid phosphatase isoform 5b: a novel serum marker for monitoring bone disease in multiple myeloma. Int J Cancer 106: 455–457.
20. Yaccoby S, Pearse RN, Johnson CL, Barlogie B, Choi Y, et al. (2002) Myeloma interacts with the bone marrow microenvironment to induce osteoclastogenesis and is dependent on osteoclast activity. Br J Haematol 116: 278–290.
21. Heath DJ, Vanderkerken K, Cheng X, Gallagher O, Prideaux M, et al. (2007) An osteoprotegerin-like peptidomimetic inhibits osteoclastic bone resorption and osteolytic bone disease in myeloma. Cancer research 67: 202–208.
22. Schlondorff J, Lum L, Blobel CP (2001) Biochemical and pharmacological criteria define two shedding activities for TRANCE/OPGL that are distinct from the tumor necrosis factor alpha convertase. J Biol Chem 276: 14665–14674.
23. Nakashima T, Kobayashi Y, Yamasaki S, Kawakami A, Eguchi K, et al. (2000) Protein expression and functional difference of membrane-bound and soluble receptor activator of NF-kappaB ligand: modulation of the expression by osteotropic factors and cytokines. Biochem Biophys Res Commun 275: 768–775.
24. Ikeda T, Kasai M, Utsuyama M, Hirokawa K (2001) Determination of three isoforms of the receptor activator of nuclear factor-kappaB ligand and their differential expression in bone and thymus. Endocrinology 142: 1419–1426.
25. Matsuzaki K, Udagawa N, Takahashi N, Yamaguchi K, Yasuda H, et al. (1998) Osteoclast differentiation factor (ODF) induces osteoclast-like cell formation in human peripheral blood mononuclear cell cultures. Biochem Biophys Res Commun 246: 199–204.
26. Radl J, De Glopper ED, Schuit HR, Zurcher C (1979) Idiopathic paraproteinemia. II. Transplantation of the paraprotein- producing clone from old to young C57BL/KaLwRij mice. J Immunol 122: 609–613.
27. Radl J, Croese JW, Zurcher C, Van den Enden-Vieveen MH, de Leeuw AM (1988) Animal model of human disease. Multiple myeloma. Am J Pathol 132: 593–597.
28. Vanderkerken K, Asosingh K, Braet F, Van Riet I, Van Camp B (1999) Insulin-like growth factor-1 acts as a chemoattractant factor for 5T2 multiple myeloma cells. Blood 93: 235–241.
29. Vanderkerken K, Asosingh K, Willems A, De Raeve H, Couck P, et al. (2005) The 5T2MM murine model of multiple myeloma: maintenance and analysis. Methods Mol Med 113: 191–205.
30. Hanawa H, Kelly PF, Nathwani AC, Persons DA, Vandergriff JA, et al. (2002) Comparison of various envelope proteins for their ability to pseudotype lentiviral vectors and transduce primitive hematopoietic cells from human blood. Mol Ther 5: 242–251.
31. Garrett IR, Dallas S, Radl J, Mundy GR (1997) A murine model of human myeloma bone disease. Bone 20: 515–520.

32. Terpos E, Szydlo R, Apperley JF, Hatjiharissi E, Politou M, et al. (2003) Soluble receptor activator of nuclear factor kappaB ligand-osteoprotegerin ratio predicts survival in multiple myeloma: proposal for a novel prognostic index. Blood 102: 1064–1069.
33. Hargreaves PG, Wang F, Antcliff J, Murphy G, Lawry J, et al. (1998) Human myeloma cells shed the interleukin-6 receptor: inhibition by tissue inhibitor of metalloproteinase-3 and a hydroxamate-based metalloproteinase inhibitor. Br J Haematol 101: 694–702.
34. Holen I, Drury NL, Hargreaves PG, Croucher PI (2001) Evidence of a role for a non-matrix-type metalloproteinase activity in the shedding of syndecan-1 from human myeloma cells. Br J Haematol 114: 414–421.
35. Lum L, Wong BR, Josien R, Becherer JD, Erdjument-Bromage H, et al. (1999) Evidence for a role of a tumor necrosis factor-alpha (TNF-alpha)- converting enzyme-like protease in shedding of TRANCE, a TNF family member involved in osteoclastogenesis and dendritic cell survival. J Biol Chem 274: 13613–13618.
36. Dougall WC, Chaisson M (2006) The RANK/RANKL/OPG triad in cancer-induced bone diseases. Cancer metastasis reviews 25: 541–549.
37. McClung MR, Lewiecki EM, Cohen SB, Bolognese MA, Woodson GC, et al. (2006) Denosumab in postmenopausal women with low bone mineral density. The New England journal of medicine 354: 821–831.
38. Cummings SR, San Martin J, McClung MR, Siris ES, Eastell R, et al. (2009) Denosumab for prevention of fractures in postmenopausal women with osteoporosis. The New England journal of medicine 361: 756–765.
39. Body JJ, Facon T, Coleman RE, Lipton A, Geurs F, et al. (2006) A study of the biological receptor activator of nuclear factor-kappaB ligand inhibitor, denosumab, in patients with multiple myeloma or bone metastases from breast cancer. Clinical cancer research 12: 1221–1228.
40. Body JJ, Lipton A, Gralow J, Steger GG, Gao G, et al. (2010) Effects of denosumab in patients with bone metastases with and without previous bisphosphonate exposure. Journal of bone and mineral research 25: 440–446.

13

Bisphosphonates and Risk of Upper Gastrointestinal Cancer — A Case Control Study Using the General Practice Research Database (GPRD)

Ellen Wright*, **Peter T. Schofield, Paul Seed, Mariam Molokhia**

Department of Primary Care and Public Health Sciences, King's College London, London, United Kingdom

Abstract

Background: Concerns have been raised as to the safety of bisphosphonates; in particular a possible link between bisphosphonate use and upper gastrointestinal (GI) cancer. Two published studies using different study populations but drawn from earlier versions of the same national UK database, reached differing conclusions: one finding no evidence for an increase in the risk of gastric or oesophageal cancer in bisphosphonate users and one finding a small but significantly increased risk of oesophageal cancer linked to duration of bisphosphonate use.

Methodology/ Principal Findings: Design-A case control study comparing bisphosphonate prescribing in cases of upper GI cancer from 1995 to 2007 using UK primary care electronic health records (GPRD). Main Outcome Measure-Relative Risk (approximated to Odds Ratio for rare events) for oesophageal and gastric cancer development in bisphosphonate users compared to non–users. The odds of being a case of oesophageal cancer, adjusted for smoking status, were significantly increased in women who had had one or more bisphosphonate prescriptions, odds ratio 1·54 (95% CI 1·27–1·88) compared to non-users. There was no significant effect on gastric cancer in women, odds ratio adjusted for smoking status, 1.06 (95% CI 0.83–1.37) and also no apparent risk in men for either oesophageal or gastric cancer, odds ratio adjusted for smoking status 0.78 (95%CI 0.56–1.09) and 0.87 (95% CI 0.55–1.36) respectively.

Conclusions/ Significance: Our results support a small but significant increased risk of oesophageal cancer in women prescribed bisphosphonates and is based on the largest number of exposed cases to date in the UK.

Editor: Georgina L Hold, University of Aberdeen, United Kingdom

Funding: This research is supported by the National Institute for Health Research (NIHR) Biomedical Research Centre at Guy's and St Thomas' NHS Foundation Trust and King's College London. The GPRD dataset for this study was obtained under the collaborative research licence funded by the Medical Research Council and the study was approved by the Independent Scientific Advisory Committee of the GPRD (protocol number 09_093R). The funders had no role in study design, data collection and analysis, decision to publish, or preparation of the manuscript.

Competing Interests: MM has received grants from AstraZeneca and Pfizer and from the Serious Adverse Events Consortium (collaboration of academia & industry) for studies of adverse drug reactions.

* E-mail: ellen.wright@kcl.ac.uk

Introduction

There has been a 20-fold rise in the prescribing of bisphosphonates in general and alendronate in particular in recent years. In 1992 0·2% of women over 40 included in the UK General Practice Research Database (GPRD) were prescribed a bisphosphonate but by 2005 this had risen to 4·1%. At the same time there has been a parallel reduction in hormone replacement therapy (HRT) prescribing from 8·2% in 1991 to 7·0% in 2005, with a 50% fall since 2002, largely driven by concerns over excess risk of breast cancer (and to a lesser degree ovarian cancer) and cardiovascular events.[1]

Bisphosphonates and particularly alendronate are well known to cause both dyspepsia and inflammatory changes such as erosive oesophagitis, delayed healing, and mucosal abnormalities.[2] Multinucleated giant cells have been detected in oesophageal inflammatory exudates. Whether these can undergo malignant transformation is not known but concerns have been raised as to a possible link between bisphosphonate use and upper GI cancer.[3,4]

Wysowski[3], in her report to the US Federal Drug Administration (FDA), noted that since the initial marketing of alendronate in 1995 the FDA had received 23 reports of patients who developed oesophageal tumours after taking the drug. Typically 2 years elapsed between the time patients started taking the drug and the onset of oesophageal cancer. In Europe and Japan a further 31 cases had been reported linking oesophageal cancer and bisphosphonate use. The FDA reporting did not include any denominator data. Wysowski suggested distal oesophageal carcinoma might be associated with bisphosphonate use but recommended more rigorous study approaches with sufficient size, length of follow up, inclusion of a control group, and control for confounding variables. In the meantime the authors advised that the drugs should not be used in patients with Barrett's oesophagus (an abnormal change in the cells of the lower portion of the oesophagus, thought to be due mainly to chronic acid reflux from the stomach, its main significance is an increased risk of developing adenocarcinoma of the oesophagus). However, Merck (the makers of alendronate) have not reported any cases of oesophageal cancer linked to bisphosphonate use in their clinical database of 17,000 patients.

Following the FDA reports, rapid communications of studies using a large national database in Denmark and Medicare beneficiaries in the US concluded there was no evidence for an increased risk of oesophageal cancer in bisphosphonate users[5,6]. However, again the follow up period was short (2 years). Because of the relative rarity of these conditions and the limited number of patients, the confidence intervals were wide and it was impossible to conclude whether there could be a clinically important association. Two published studies using the UK General Practice Research Database (GPRD) reached differing conclusions. Cardwell et al.[7] in a retrospective cohort study found no evidence of an increase in the combined risk for gastric and oesophageal cancer in bisphosphonate users compared to non-users, Hazard Ratio 0·96, (95% CI 0·74–1·49) but again confidence intervals were wide (i.e. study is also consistent with a fairly substantial effect). Green et al.[8] carried out a nested case control study using a sample drawn from the same database and found an overall increased risk of oesophageal cancer in bisphosphonate users (Relative Risk 1·30, 95% CI 1·02–1·66). This increased with more than ten prescriptions or longer than three years use (RR 1·93). Although these studies appear to give different results, the relatively wide confidence intervals overlap substantially, so results could be consistent with a similar magnitude of risk. In Cardwell's study a relatively small proportion of exposed cases were included limiting power and precision.

Dixon and Solomon [9] have reviewed in detail the conflicting results of these two studies and concluded similarly that even when confining the comparison to patients with greater than three years exposure to bisphosphonates (allowing for induction and latency periods) the confidence intervals of the relative risks for both studies included the possibility of a 50% increase in risk. At less than three years exposure, although neither study found an increase in relative risk of oesophageal cancer with bisphosphonate use, Dixon and Solomon point out that the confidence intervals of both span one and, therefore, one should say that the results are 'inconclusive' rather than "there is no effect". The upper limits of the RR's of 3 years' exposure are 1.73 and 1.81 respectively according to the 95% confidence intervals of the two analyses. They note "it is, therefore, plausible in both studies that, despite the best guess being of 'no increased risk', there may be as much as a 70% increase in baseline risk."

Haber et al[10] concluded after reviewing both Green and Cardwell's studies and the observational study on the incidence of oesophageal cancer in patients with Barrett's oesophagus taking bisphosphonates by Nugyen[11], as well as the case reports in Wysowski's article, that "the evidence on the use of bisphosphonates and risk of esophageal cancer is weak and conflicting".

Our primary aim was to carry out a retrospective case control study with the greatest possible power using a large UK primary care database (the GPRD), to determine whether any association exists between prescribing of alendronate specifically (and bisphosphonates in general) and the development of upper GI malignancy. We were particularly concerned to have enough statistical power to detect a small increase in a rare, but serious disease and, therefore, chose to do a matched case control study using all known cases of oesophageal and gastric cancer. Although this is the third study using data drawn from the GRPD, it uses a later and significantly larger version of the database and it is substantially more powerful.

Methods

Source population

The study population included all adults (men & women) registered with up to standard GP (General Practitioner) practices in the UK General Practice Research Database (GPRD) from 1/1/1995 to 31/12/2007. The GPRD is a primary care database holding approximately 5 million longitudinal anonymised records of patients registered with a national health service (NHS) GP.[12] Only UK general practices with data of approved quality can contribute to the database. Strict protocols are followed by practices for data entry. The accuracy and completeness of GPRD data, particularly with respect to prescribing (almost 100%) and cancer diagnosis (95%) is high and has been confirmed in validation studies.[13,14]. The data extraction was performed from the May 2010 version of the GPRD.

Case and control definition

Cases had a clinical or referral record of incident upper GI (UGI) malignancy in the study period and their registration period.

UGI cancer events were identified by the following READ codes: (See appendix S1 for full list)

B11 + all daughter codes–malignant neoplasm of stomach

B10 + all daughter codes–malignant neoplasm of oesophagus

BB55–linitis plastica

BB5C–gastrinoma and carcinoma

B105–malignant neoplasm of lower third of oesophagus

B10z–oesophageal cancer

B11-1–gastric neoplasm

For every case, four control patients matched on age (+/−2 years) and gender and with no record of UGI cancer were selected from the database. Observation window matching was used: i.e. observation of all four controls started before that of the case, and ended after that of the case. The observation times of the controls matched exactly those of their matched cases. Control events outside the observation window of the case were ignored. The period of follow up was earliest of: death, last medical record, practice transfer, or end of study period.

Exposure assessment. (bisphosphonate use)

Bisphosphonate use was defined as any patient ever prescribed a bisphosphonate during the study period. We excluded patients with prescriptions for bisphosphonates licensed to treat Paget's disease or bone metastases (pamidronate, ibandronate) in the sensitivity analysis as these patients would already be suffering from cancer or Paget's disease. Duration of bisphosphonate use was the time between first and last prescription. We categorized bisphosphonate use by number of prescriptions issued in the study period into low (<10 prescriptions) and high (>10 prescriptions).

Covariates

As covariates and potential confounders we evaluated the presence of smoking as a major risk factor for UGI cancer. Smoking was defined as any record of use from 1980. We also adjusted for alcohol intake, dyspepsia, proton pump inhibitor (PPI) use, *Helicobacter pylori* (*H. pylori*) status and body mass index (BMI) although previous studies had not shown an effect.[8]

Sample size calculation

Typically for rare diseases case control studies are used to maximize efficiency and power to provide a valid estimate of risk or hazard ratio. Using multiple controls per case can increase power, although the gain in power beyond 4 controls is relatively small. With 8,000 cases & 32,000 controls, we calculated we would have 89% power to detect a difference of 2% (50% compared to 52%) in the rate of bisphosphonate use in the two arms. If the rate of bisphosphonate use was lower, the minimum detectable odds ratio would be increased; but its clinical importance would be similar. For example, for 4% use in controls (a more realistic figure based on recent figures) [8] and 4·8% use in cases, we would be able to detect an odds ratio of 1·21 with 88% power. We used a matched (age and gender) design to reduce confounding.

Statistical methods

Taking into account the matched study design we used conditional logistic regression to calculate unadjusted and adjusted odds ratios (ORs) and corresponding 95% confidence intervals (CIs) for the association between bisphosphonate use and UGI cancer. We adjusted for the main confounder smoking, as well as alcohol intake, dyspepsia, proton pump inhibitor (PPI) use, *H. pylori* status and body mass index (BMI). We tested for the interaction between gender and bisphosphonate use and risk of upper GI cancer. We restricted analyses to oesophageal cancer, gastric cancer and alendronate alone. We carried out sensitivity analyses as follows: excluding bisphosphonates used to treat bone metastases; excluding bisphosphonates commenced 6 months or less before the diagnosis of UGI cancer and excluding cases where the READ code for UGI cancer was uncertain. All analyses were conducted using Stata version 11 (Stata Corporation, USA).

Results

We received data on 8,636 cases of UGI cancer where the cancer diagnosis date was between January 1, 1995, and December 31, 2007, and 34,544 controls, 4 per case, matched on age (+/−2 years) and sex. We initially analyzed the complete data set and then looked at the subsets of oesophageal and gastric cancer cases and controls. Table 1 gives summary descriptive statistics separately for the cases and controls.

Statistical Analysis

Risk of all bisphosphonates on UGI cancer

We initially investigated the effect of all bisphosphonates on UGI cancer in both men and women and found an Odds Ratio (OR) of 1·13 (95% CI 0·99–1·28) for men and women combined (appendix S2). The OR for the effect of all bisphosphonates on UGI cancer in women adjusted for smoking status was 1·34 (95% CI 1·14–1·56) and 0·81 (95% CI 0·62–1·06) for men.

Risk of all bisphosphonates on oesophageal cancer and gastric cancer

When we analysed the effects of all bisphosphonates on oesophageal cancer only we found an OR of 1·43 (95% CI 1·18–1·72) in women and 0·87 (95% CI 0·65–1·18) in men. The corresponding results for gastric cancer were OR 1.06 (95% CI 0.83–1.35) in women and OR 0.77 (95% CI 0.50–1.20) in men. Adjusting the analyses for smoking status did not change the results significantly. The OR for the effect of all bisphosphonates on oesophageal cancer adjusted for smoking status was 1·54 (95% CI 1·27–1·88) for women and 0·78 (95% CI 0·56–1·09) for men (tables 2 and 3).

Risk of alendronate alone on oesophageal cancer

When we restricted to alendronate alone we found corresponding ORs of 1.37 (95% CI 1.07–1.75) for women and 0.78 (95% CI 0.50–1.22). The OR for alendronate alone on oesophageal cancer adjusted for smoking status was 1·42 (95% CI 1·10–1·83) for women and 0·73 (95% CI 0·46–1·17) for men (table 4).

Interaction of bisphosphonate use and oesophageal cancer risk with gender

We looked at the interaction of bisphosphonate use and oesophageal cancer risk with gender, which gave an OR of 1·27 (95% CI 1·10–1·47) for women (Table 2) and 0·84 (95% CI 0·66–1·07) for men (Table 3); in other words there appeared to be an effect in women but not in men. The interaction between bisphosphonate use and gender, using the likelihood-ratio test (LRT) was statistically significant, p = 0.0011.

Sensitivity analyses

We performed three sensitivity analyses none of which significantly altered the results (table 5). Firstly we excluded bisphosphonates licensed to treat bone metastases, as these patients by definition would already be suffering from cancer. The corresponding ORs for the effect of all bisphosphonates on UGI cancer adjusted for smoking status were 1·34 (95% CI 1·14–1·57) for women and 0·80 (95% CI 0·61–1·05) for men. Secondly we excluded prescriptions of bisphosphonates commenced six months or less before the UGI diagnosis date on the grounds that the time interval was too short for bisphosphonates to be causative. The subsequent ORs adjusted for smoking status were 1·30 (95% CI 1·10–1·53) for women and 0·77 (95% CI 0·58–1·04) for men. Finally we excluded cases where the READ code for UGI cancer diagnosis was uncertain. The ORs adjusted for smoking in these cases were 1·34 (95% CI 1·14–1·56) for women and 0·81 (95% CI 0·62–1·06) for men.

Discussion

Summary of main findings

The results show that female cases of oesophageal cancer were significantly more likely to have been prescribed a bisphosphonate than controls. This effect was more pronounced when we looked at alendronate rather than all bisphosphonates. The risk remained significant after adjusting for to the effect of smoking. There was no significant apparent effect in men although the confidence intervals did not exclude this. There was also no effect on gastric cancer. Adjusting for covariates – dyspepsia, PPI use, BMI, alcohol intake and *H. pylori* status did not alter the result.

Excluding bisphosphonates prescribed for bone metastases; bisphosphonates commenced 6 months or less before the diagnosis of upper GI cancer and cases where there was uncertainty regarding the READ coding of the case did not significantly alter the results.

From the data, 95 out of 4442 female cases of upper GI cancer annually in the UK could be linked to bisphosphonate use (based on an OR of 1·34 for bisphosphonates in women for UGI cancer, 4442 new cases of UGI cancer in women in 2007 and 8·43% of female cases of UGI cancer being prescribed a bisphosphonate).[15]

How our studies differed from other findings

Solomon et al[6] in their response to Wysowski's article used SEER (Surveillance, Epidemiology and End Results) registry data to compare rates of oesophageal cancer in persons receiving oral bisphosphonates with those receiving other medications for osteoporosis and the general incidence rate in the SEER registry. They did not find a difference but, as they admitted, due to the rarity of oesophageal cancer, the confidence intervals were very wide and compatible with an effect as well as no effect.

Nugyen et al[11] performed a nested case-control study examining bisphosphonate use in oesophageal cancer cases and controls in patients with Barrett's oesophagus. The data came from the National Department of Veterans Affairs database. They

Table 1. Summary descriptive statistics for cases and controls.

Characteristics	OES CA CASES'	OES CA CONTROLS	GASTRIC CANCER CASES	GASTRIC CANCER CONTROLS	All UGI CA CASES	All UGI CA CONTROLS
Male	3,412	13,648	2,084	8,336	5,496	21,984
Female	1,814	7,256	1,326	5,304	3,140	12,560
Total (male and female)	5,226	20,904	3,410	13,640	8,636	34,544
Mean Age (at time of diagnosis of case)	63·4	63·4	66.5	66.5	64·7	64·7
Mean age men	61·6	61·6	65.6	65.6	63·1	63·1
Mean age women	67·0	67·0	68.1	68.1	67·5	67·5
Mean years observed in data base	6·3	6·3	5.7	5.7	6·1	6·1
Smoking-any positive record of smoking (%)	2,229 (51.5)	8,437 (45.4)	1,303 (46.5)	5,274 (43.9)	3,532 (49.5)	13,711 (44.9)
Dyspepsia–any record up to 12 mths before cancer diagnosis in cases and equivalent date in controls (%)	1,169 (22.3)	4,184 (20.0)	827 (24.3)	2,910 (21.3)	1,996 (23.1)	7,094 (20.5)
PPI-any use within study window (%)	1,100 (21.1)	3,215 (15.4)	728 (21.4)	2,073 (15.2)	1,828 (21.2)	5,288 (15.3)
H. pylori positive–any record	121 (2.3)	491 (2.4)	128 (3.8)	321 (2.4)	249 (2.9)	812 (2.4)
BMI>30 (%)	88 (1.7)	1,621 (7.8)	58 (1.8)	948 (6.7)	146 (1.7)	2,569 (7.44)
Alcohol intake–any record greater than recommended limits (%)	620 (11.9)	2,293 (11.0)	286 (8.4)	1,345 (9.9)	906 (10.5)	3,638 (10.5)
Prescribed bisphosphonate-male and female (%)	225 (4·3)	749 (3·6)	117 (3.4)	478 (3.5)	342 (4·0)	1227 (3·6)
Men (%)	54 (1.6)	246 (1.8)	24 (1.2)	124 (1.5)	78 (1.4)	370 (1.7)
Women (%)	171 (7.8)	503 (6.9)	93 (7.0)	354 (6.7)	264 (8.4)	857 (6.8)
Prescribed alendronate (%)	119 (2·3)	410 (2·0)	72 (2.1)	252 (1.9)	191 (2·2)	662 (1·9)
Men (%)	24 (0.7)	122 (0.9)	14 (0.7)	68 (0.8)	38 (0.7)	190 (0.9)
Women (%)	95 (5.2)	288 (4.0)	58 (4.4)	184 (3.5)	153 (4.9)	472 (3.8)
Prescribed bisphosphonate–xcluding those used to treat metastases (%)	218 (4·2)	726 (3·5)	113 (3.3)	461 (3.4)	331 (3·8)	1,187 (3·5)
Prescribed bisphosphonates-less than 10 prescriptions-mean number per time observed in database	3·8	4·0	3.9	3.8	3·8	3·9
Prescribed bisphosphonates–more than 10 prescriptions–mean number per time observed in database	26·5	26·2	23.0	26.0	25·4	26·1

did not find a significant difference between the groups but the number of cases and controls were relatively small (116 and 696 respectively) and the number of bisphosphonate users in both groups was small which the authors admit limits the power to detect significant differences between the groups.

Abrahamsen and colleagues have reported two cohort studies using data from national registries in Denmark. The first in 2009[5], published as a response to Wysowski's case reports, looked at 13,678 patients with fractures who had used bisphosphonates and compared them with 27,356 controls of the same sex and similar age and fracture type. They found a reduced incidence of oesophageal cancer in the bisphosphonate group and no difference in gastric cancer between the two groups. However, the follow up period was relatively short (2.2 years) and the total number of cases identified small (37 and 48 for gastric and oesophageal cancer respectively). In November 2010 they reported

Table 2. Risk of bisphosphonates on oesophageal and gastric cancer in women.

	Oesophageal Cancer Odds Ratio (95% CI)	Gastric Cancer Odds Ratio (95% CI)	All UGI Cancer Odds Ratio (95% CI)
Women taking bisphosphonates	1.43 (1.18–1.72) (171 cases, 503 controls)	1.06 (0.83–1.35) (93 cases, 354 controls)	1·27(1.10–1.47) (264 cases, 857 controls)
Adjusted for smoking	1.54 (1.27–1.88)	1.06 (0.83–1.37)	1.34 (1.14–1.56)
Adjusted for smoking, alcohol intake, PPI, *H. pylori* status, dyspepsia andBMI	1.43 (1.16–1.75)	0.98 (0.76–1.27)	1.24 (1.06–1.45)

Table 3. Risk of bisphosphonates on oesophageal and gastric cancer in men.

	Oesophageal Cancer Odds Ratio (95% CI)	Gastric Cancer Odds Ratio (95% I)	All UGI Cancer Odds Ratio (95%CI)
Men taking bisphosphonates	0.87 (0.65–1.18) (54 cases, 246 controls)	0.77 (0.50–.20) (24 cases, 124 controls)	0·84 (0.66–1.07) (78 cases, 370 controls)
Adjusted for smoking	0.78 (0.56–1.09)	0.87 (0.55–1.36)	0.81 (0.62–1.06)
Adjusted for smoking, alcohol intake, PPI, *H. pylori*, dyspepsia andBMI	0.73 (0.53–1.03)	0.77 (0.49–1.21)	0.75 (0.57–0.98)

a further study, which compared 30,606 alendronate users with 122,424 matched controls[16]. This time they found a lower risk of gastric cancer in the alendronate group (OR 0.61; 95% CI 0.39–0.97) and no increased risk for oesophageal cancer (OR 0.71; 95% CI 0.43–1.19), however the confidence interval for oesophageal cancer is quite wide and is compatible with an effect as well as no effect. They also found that alendronate users were more likely to have had a recent upper endoscopy.

Vestargaard[17] carried out another cohort study of Danish patients but with significantly larger numbers. 103,562 patients using drugs for osteoporosis were compared with 310,683 age and gender matched controls. They found an excess risk with alendronate and etidronate for oesophageal cancer (RR 2.32 and 2.00 respectively) which was most pronounced for low doses and short duration but still present at higher doses and longer durations.

Chen et al[18] have used claims data from the National Health Insurance Database of Taiwan (NHIRD) to carry out a case control study comparing alendronate prescriptions in 282 cases of oesophageal cancer and 2,811 controls. They found 31.2% of the cases had been prescribed alendronate and 27.1% of the controls which equated to an adjusted OR of 0.61; 95% CI 0.21–1.75 with a p-value of 0.36. The confidence interval, as in other studies, is compatible with a modest effect (e.g. 50% increase or decrease) as well as no effect.

Ho et al[19] recently published another study from Taiwan using the same claims database (NHIRD). This was a large case control study comparing oral bisphosphonate prescribing in 16,204 cases of oesophageal cancer with 64,816 controls. Overall they found bisphosphonates had been prescribed to 7.8% of the cases versus 3.6% of the controls, however they then break the analysis down by frequency of use of bisphosphonates and find a decreasing trend of ORs from rare to regular users of 3.86 to 2.68 and also with time observed and conclude that there is no effect. Unfortunately no confidence intervals are reported and the numbers of frequent and regular bisphosphonate users are very small overall; the authors rely on the basic error of comparing p-values between unequal-sized groups rather than carrying out a valid test.[20] If one looks at the rare user group which has the largest numbers of cases and controls for the three observation periods then the OR's are 3.86, 2.58 and 2,27 for one year, three years and five years respectively with a p value of 0.001.

This last study illustrates the problem of studies on side effects of drugs where the outcome is a rare disease (oesophageal cancer, incidence 9.8:100,000 UK age standardized rate 2008)[15] and the exposure is also relatively small (average prescribing of bisphosphonates in the UK 4.1% in 2005)[1].

The two previous studies using this data set (GPRD) followed different approaches and had substantially smaller numbers of exposed oesophageal cancer cases (79 Cardwell, 90 Green) than ours. Their confidence intervals are correspondingly wider, and indeed overlap. (Cardwell: adjusted HR 1·07 (95% CI 0·77–1·49); Green: RR1·30 (95% CI 1·02–1·66). In the context of a rare disease, the tiny numerical difference between Hazard Ratio, Risk Ratio and Odds Ratio can be ignored. A formal test for a difference is not possible as the studies draw on the same data. However, there is a substantial overlap of Cardwell & Green's results from 1·02 to 1·49.

In the present study, with 225 exposed oesophageal cancer cases, over twice as many, the OR for oesophageal cancer, for men and women adjusted for smoking, is 1·30 (95% CI 1.21–1·39), which is within the overlap noticed above, but the confidence interval is much narrower.

Possible mechanisms for association of bisphosphonates with oesophageal cancer and why this may vary by gender

The mechanism may be via inflammatory changes to the oesophageal mucosa, well known already as a side effect of bisphosphonates.[21,22]The apparent lack of an effect in men may be a) due to the much smaller numbers of men (25% of total) prescribed bisphosphonates (and hence the difficulty of demonstrating an effect on a rare disease), however, the significant interaction test strongly suggests that the difference is real; b) the observation that the average age of the men prescribed bisphosphonates (67·8) was less than the women (69·7) and the incidence of UGI cancer increases significantly with age. When we reduced the whole sample size to 25% of the original and re-ran the analysis, the effect in women, although present (OR1.2) was no longer significant (p = 0.2). Women are usually prescribed

Table 4. Effect of alendronate on oesophageal cancer for men and women (mean number of observations 19,991.

	Odds Ratio	P value	95% confidence interval
Women on alendronate (95 cases, 288 controls)	1·37	0·014	1·07–1·75
Adjusted for smoking	1·42	0·007	1·10–1·83
Men on alendronate (24 cases and 122 controls)	0·78	0·28	0·50–1·22
Adjusted for smoking	·0·73	0·19	0·46–1·17

Table 5. Sensitivity Analyses: excluding bisphosphonates used to treat bone metastases; excluding prescriptions for bisphosphonates commenced 6 months or less before diagnosis of all UGI cancer; excluding cases where the READ code for UGI cancer diagnosis was uncertain.

UGI Cancer Odds Ratio (95% CI)		
	Women	Men
Excluding bisphosphonates used to treat bone metastases, adjusted for smoking status	1.34 (1.14–1.57)	0.80 (0.61–1.05)
Excluding prescriptions for bisphosphonates commenced 6 months or less before diagnosis of all UGI cancer, adjusted for smoking status	1·30 (1·10–1·53)	0·77 (0·58–1·04)
Excluding cases where the READ code for UGI cancer diagnosis was uncertain, adjusted for smoking	1·34 (1·14–1·56)	0.81 (0·62–1·06)

bisphosphonates for osteoporosis occurring idiopathically whereas men are more likely to be prescribed bisphosphonates for iatrogenically caused osteoporosis, typically from steroids prescribed for chronic obstructive pulmonary disease, or even prophylactically if on high dose steroids for more than three months. Some of the risk factors, apart from prolonged steroid use, for developing osteoporosis – smoking, heavy alcohol intake, anorexia/low BMI, and poor nutrition – also are risk factors for upper GI cancer. Although correcting for these factors in the analysis did not alter the results it may be that as a group women with osteoporosis are at higher risk than men of a similar age for upper GI cancer.

Strengths and limitations

The main strength of our study is that it is based on one of the most reliable population samples to date and uses electronic patient records rather administrative claims data (Zhang et al[23] have described the problems related to using the latter). It is also based on the largest number of cases giving a relatively precise confidence interval. We were confident from our sample size calculations about being able to detect even quite small differences and that a negative result would be strong evidence against an adverse effect that was important from a public health perspective.

Limitations of our study are that adherence to bisphosphonates was not formally measured (but this is a general difficulty with large anonymised database studies) and although the accuracy of the GPRD cancer codes is likely to be high they were not formally validated. Walker[24] has recently published a study on the accuracy of identification of oesophageal cancer in the GPRD and concluded that while essentially all cases bearing a code for the condition had oesophageal cancer the clinical onset might be significantly earlier than the first code recorded in the GPRD. This could affect cohort studies with short follow up times but not case control studies.

With any retrospective longitudinal study there are also always limitations due to incomplete data recording; prescriptions issued not dispensed/taken; missing data; unmeasured confounders etc.

Oesophageal cancer is rare but often fatal and associated with significant morbidity. Bisphosphonates in general and alendronate in particular are being recommended, by current osteoporosis prevention guidelines, to increasing numbers of men and women in predominantly older age groups. Our data supports a small increased risk of oesophageal cancer in women prescribed bisphosphonates. With a rare disease such as this (incidence of oesophageal cancer in 60–79 age group is 10/100,100) it would need very large prospective cohort studies, with sufficiently long follow up to confirm and clarify the size of the association and none have been published to date, however, Vinogradova et al[25] have recently published a protocol for a large nested case-control study using the Qrisk research database (significantly larger than GPRD) which will look at the association between bisphosphonate prescribing and the 10 most common primary cancers diagnosed in patients between 1996 and 2011.

In the presence of an association and with a plausible mechanism to account for possible causation (irritation of the gastric and oesophageal mucosa) it would be sensible to exercise caution in prescribing bisphosphonates to patients with pre-existing risk factors for upper GI cancer (although unfortunately many of these are also risk factors for developing osteoporosis) and to have a lower threshold for investigating such patients, if on bisphosphonates, should they develop symptoms suggestive of upper GI cancer.

Supporting Information

Appendix S1 List of Read/OXMIS codes as evidence of upper GI malignancy.

Appendix S2 Effect of bisphosphonates on UGI cancer for men and women.

Author Contributions

Conceived and designed the experiments: EW PS. Performed the experiments: EW PS PTS. Analyzed the data: PTS PS. Contributed reagents/materials/analysis tools: PTS. Wrote the paper: EW. Data interpretation: MM EW PTS. Revised article critically for important intellectual content: MM. Original hypothesis and study design: EW. Literature search: EW. Final manuscript editing: EW. Contributions to final manuscript: PS PTS.

References

1. Watson J, Wise L, Green J (2007) Prescribing of hormone therapy for menopause, tibolone, and bisphosphonates in women in the UK between 1991 and 2005. Eur J Clin Pharmacol 63: 843–849.
2. Parfitt JR, Driman DK (2007) Pathological effects of drugs on the gastrointestinal tract: a review. Hum Pathol 38: 527–536.
3. Wysowski DK (2009) Reports of esophageal cancer with oral bisphosphonate use. N Engl J Med 360: 89–90.
4. Wysowski DK (2010) Oral bisphosphonates and oesophageal cancer. BMJ 341.
5. Abrahamsen B, Eiken P, Eastell R (2009) More on reports of esophageal cancer with oral bisphosphonate use. N Engl J Med 360: 1789; author reply 1791–1782.

6. Solomon DH, Patrick A, Brookhart MA (2009) More on reports of esophageal cancer with oral bisphosphonate use. N Engl J Med 360: 1789–1790; author reply 1791–1782.
7. Cardwell CR, Abnet CC, Cantwell MM, Murray LJ (2010) Exposure to oral bisphosphonates and risk of esophageal cancer. JAMA 304: 657–663.
8. Green J, Czanner G, Reeves G, Watson J, Wise L, et al. (2010) Oral bisphosphonates and risk of cancer of oesophagus, stomach, and colorectum: case-control analysis within a UK primary care cohort. BMJ 341: c4444.
9. Dixon WG, Solomon DH (2011) Bisphosphonates and esophageal cancer-a pathway through the confusion. Nat Rev Rheumatol 7: 369–372.
10. Haber SL, McNatty D (2012) An Evaluation of the Use of Oral Bisphosphonates and Risk of Esophageal Cancer. The Annals of Pharmacotherapy 46: 419–423.
11. Nguyen D, Schwartz J, Richardson P, El-Serag H (2010) Oral Bisphosphonate Prescriptions and the Risk of Esophageal Adenocarcinoma in Patients with Barrett's Esophagus. Digestive Diseases and Sciences 55: 3404–3407.
12. GPRD (2010) The Database.
13. Herrett E, Thomas SL, Schoonen WM, Smeeth L, Hall AJ (2010) Validation and validity of diagnoses in the General Practice Research Database: a systematic review. Br J Clin Pharmacol 69: 4–14.
14. Khan NF, Harrison SE, Rose PW (2010) Validity of diagnostic coding within the General Practice Research Database: a systematic review. Br J Gen Pract 60: e128–136.
15. CancerResearchUK Cancer Statistics.
16. Abrahamsen B, Pazianas M, Eiken P, Russell RG, Eastell R (2011) Esophageal and gastric cancer incidence and mortality in alendronate users. J Bone Miner Res.
17. Vestergaard P (2011) Occurrence of gastrointestinal cancer in users of bisphosphonates and other antiresorptive drugs against osteoporosis. Calcif Tissue Int 89: 434–441.
18. Chen Y-M, Tsai Y-W, Liu C-L, Chen Y-T, Chang L-C, et al. (2011) Alendronate and Risk of Esophageal Cancer: A Nationwide Population-Based Study in Taiwan.
19. Ho YF, Lin JT, Wu CY (2012) Oral bisphosphonates and risk of esophageal cancer: a dose-intensity analysis in a nationwide population. Cancer Epidemiol Biomarkers Prev 21: 993–995.
20. Altman D (1991) Practical Statistics in Medical Research.[16.4.3 Errors in Analysis]. London: Chapman & Hall.
21. Colina RE, Smith M, Kikendall JW, Wong RK (1997) A new probable increasing cause of esophageal ulceration: alendronate. Am J Gastroenterol 92: 704–706.
22. Thomson AB, Marshall JK, Hunt RH, Provenza JM, Lanza FL, et al. (2002) 14 day endoscopy study comparing risedronate and alendronate in postmenopausal women stratified by Helicobacter pylori status. J Rheumatol 29: 1965–1974.
23. Zhang J, Yun H, Wright NC, Kilgore M, Saag KG, et al. (2011) Potential and pitfalls of using large administrative claims data to study the safety of osteoporosis therapies. Curr Rheumatol Rep 13: 273–282.
24. Walker AM (2011) Identification of esophageal cancer in the General Practice Research Database. Pharmacoepidemiology and Drug Safety 20: 1159–1167.
25. Vinogradova Y, Coupland C, Hippisley-Cox J (2012) Exposure to bisphosphonates and risk of cancer: a protocol for nested case–control studies using the QResearch primary care database. BMJ Open 2.

Identification of Genes for Complex Diseases Using Integrated Analysis of Multiple Types of Genomic Data

Hongbao Cao[1], Shufeng Lei[2], Hong-Wen Deng[3], Yu-Ping Wang[1,3]*

1 Department of Biomedical Engineering, Tulane University, New Orleans, Louisiana, United States of America, **2** Center for Genetic Epidemiology and Genomics, School of Public Health, Medical College of Soochow University, Suzhou, P. R. China, **3** Department of Biostatistics and Bioinformatics, Tulane University, New Orleans, Louisiana, United States of America

Abstract

Various types of genomic data (e.g., SNPs and mRNA transcripts) have been employed to identify risk genes for complex diseases. However, the analysis of these data has largely been performed in isolation. Combining these multiple data for integrative analysis can take advantage of complementary information and thus can have higher power to identify genes (and/or their functions) that would otherwise be impossible with individual data analysis. Due to the different nature, structure, and format of diverse sets of genomic data, multiple genomic data integration is challenging. Here we address the problem by developing a sparse representation based clustering (SRC) method for integrative data analysis. As an example, we applied the SRC method to the integrative analysis of 376821 SNPs in 200 subjects (100 cases and 100 controls) and expression data for 22283 genes in 80 subjects (40 cases and 40 controls) to identify significant genes for osteoporosis (OP). Comparing our results with previous studies, we identified some genes known related to OP risk (e.g., *'THSD4', 'CRHR1', 'HSD11B1', 'THSD7A', 'BMPR1B' 'ADCY10', 'PRL', 'CA8','ESRRA', 'CALM1', 'CALM1', 'SPARC'*, and *'LRP1'*). Moreover, we uncovered novel osteoporosis susceptible genes (*'DICER1', 'PTMA', etc.*) that were not found previously but play functionally important roles in osteoporosis etiology from existing studies. In addition, the SRC method identified genes can lead to higher accuracy for the diagnosis/classification of osteoporosis subjects when compared with the traditional T-test and Fisher-exact test, which further validates the proposed SRC approach for integrative analysis.

Editor: Qingyang Huang, Central China Normal University, China

Funding: This work was supported by National Institutes of Health grant 1R21LM010042-01 (www.nlm.nih.gov). The funders had no role in study design, data collection and analysis, decision to publish, or preparation of the manuscript.

Competing Interests: The authors have declared that no competing interests exist.

* E-mail: wyp@tulane.edu

Introduction

In genomic data analysis, one of the crucial issues is to identify disease susceptible genes from the vast amount of data [1]–[8]. Some genes are related to the diagnosis task, but many are presumably irrelevant [1]. During the past few years, various clustering techniques have been developed to identify subsets of genes significant for diagnosis or classification of diseases [1]–[7]. Among those gene selection methods, a variety of statistical methods were used. For example, Yang *et al.* [1] used forward sequential feature selection (FSFS) method to remove irrelevant SNP data. Soneson *et al.* [2] used Canonical Correlation Analysis (CCA) for joint analysis of gene expression and copy number variations (CNVs). Berger *et al.* [4] developed a generalized singular value decomposition (GSVD) to locate genes with both high variations and high correlations across samples of gene expression changes and CNVs. These methods demonstrated limited success; there has been continuous demand for the development of efficient data integration technique. In this work, we developed a sparse representation based clustering (SRC) method for gene selection, based on multiple features extracted from genomic data. The features we used here were the statistical measurements of the original genomic data, such as the mean and standard deviation *etc.*. We refer the raw genomic data (SNPs or gene expressions) as variables. The variable selection was performed using the features of the original data instead of using the raw data directly. In this work, we employed 5 features in the analysis of the two data sets (see Section 2.3 'Features selection' for the detailed description). Sparse representation or compressive sensing (CS) is a novel statistical method recently developed in statistics and applied mathematics, which has found many successful applications in diverse disciplines. For example, Wright *et al.* proposed a CS based method for face recognition, which showed better accuracy and resistance to noise [8]. We have developed and applied the SRC method for chromosome image classification and showed improved accuracy [9]. In this work, we apply the SRC algorithm to select genes/variables that are significant for OP using joint analysis of two different types of genomic data: gene expression and SNP data. The description of 'SRC clustering' algorithm is given in **Supporting Material S1**.

To validate our method, we apply it to the study of osteoporosis, which is a major public health problem over the world [10]. Osteoporosis is characterized by the low bone mineral density (BMD) [11], which leads to increased risk to fragility fracture. Genetic factors play an important role in the pathogenesis of osteoporosis, as evidenced by high heritability (≥50%) of BMD [12]–[14]; however, specific genetic factors both influencing BMD and contributing to the development of osteoporosis are largely uncharacterized.

Identifying genetic factors for osteoporosis is challenging because of the nature of complex genetic determinations, including polygenic determinations, multiple gene-gene interactions, and multiple gene-environment interactions. So far, great attempts have been made to identify osteoporosis risk genes; however, most of them focused on DNA, RNA, or protein levels individually, which were rarely combined or integrated in a statistically rigorous manner to ascertain the importance of certain gene(s) for bone phenotypes [15], [16]. For example, current genome-wide association studies established relationship of gene(s) and phenotypes (e.g., BMD) at DNA level [17], [18] without considering RNA or protein expression, thus lacking an immediate insight on the functions of genes or gene expression regulations. Integrating substantial evidences from different levels (i.e., DNA, RNA and protein) can not only improve chances of identifying genetic factors for osteoporosis, but also ascertain the potential functioning mechanisms of genes and their contributions to osteoporosis.

The paper is organized as follows. We first briefly describe the SRC method and the resulting gene shaving algorithm we proposed. Then we apply the method to gene selection with integrative analysis of both gene expression and SNP data from osteoporosis patients. For the purpose of comparison with individual data analysis, we also performed the study on each data type (e.g., SNPs and gene expression data) respectively. To demonstrate the advantage of our proposed integrative approach, we compared the selected genes using the SRC method with the previously reported osteoporosis susceptive genes [5], [19]. To further validate the selected genes, we applied the method to the classification of osteoporosis patients with the selected gene expression and/or SNP data. Results showed that the SRC method is able to better locate genes significant for the diagnosis of osteoporosis patients than those from a single data set. In addition, our proposed SRC method gives better diagnosis results when compared with the T-test and Fisher-exact test. In particular, we identified two new osteoporosis risk genes (e.g., *'DICER1'*, *'PTMA'*) through joint data analysis. These genes cannot be identified with single data set but show significant roles in osteoporosis etiology from studies published in existing literatures, which suggests that an integrated data analysis can lead to better identification of genes, resulting in improved diagnosis.

Methods

In this section, we first describe the genomic data used in our study (Section 2.1). Then we present the SRC model (Sec. 2.2), the feature selection method (Sec. 2.3) and the SRC based gene/variable shaving algorithm (Sec. 2.4). Finally, we describe the method used for validating the selected genes (Sec. 2.5).

2.1 Data

We applied the SRC method to the integrative analysis of two data sets (i.e., gene expression data set and a SNP data set) from our osteoporosis study. We describe the data sets as follows.

The gene expression data were from female osteoporosis subjects with extremely low (N = 40) (cases) vs. high (N = 40) (controls) bone mineral densities (BMDs). In the present study we selected circulating monocytes as our target cells because circulating monocytes serve as progenitors of osteoclasts [21]–[23], and secrete osteoclastogenic cytokines, such as IL-1, IL-6, and TNF-α [24]–[26]. Circulating monocytes were isolated from 50 *ml* whole blood. After RNA extraction, expression levels of 22283 transcripts were quantified by Affymetrix Human Genome U133A 2.0 Array (Affymetrix, Santa Clara, CA). GCOS 1.2 (Gene Chip Operating Software) was used to process the probe-level raw data. We used the RMA (Robust Multi-array Average) algorithm [6] implemented in R package to transform the probe-level raw data into gene expression data.

The SNP data set was from osteoporosis vs. healthy subjects, which were recruited with the purpose of identifying genetic factors underlying osteoporosis via genome-wide association study in a total of 1000 random subjects (age: 50.3+18.3 years) [17]. These subjects were genotyped with Human Mapping 500K Array Set that examined about 500000 SNPs with a relatively even distribution across the entire human genome. Since the gene expression data currently used are from female samples, we first distributed the total 501 female samples according to the hip Z-score of BMD and then selected the bottom 100 and top 100 subjects of the BMD phenotypic distribution as cases and controls, respectively. A total of 376821 eligible SNPs were used in final analysis. In addition, we randomly selected 70 cases and 70 controls as training data for gene selection, and the rest 30 cases and 30 controls were used as an independent testing data set.

To perform joint data analysis, we generate a combined data set from the two single data sets, which are described as follows. For the *i*-th gene, there are n_{t1} gene expressions and n_{t2} SNPs (in the gene expression data set, one gene may have one or more gene expressions; in the SNP data set, one gene usually has more than one SNPs). Thus for the *i*-th gene, we make a cross combination of the n_{t1} expressions and n_{t2} SNPs to obtain the $n_{t1} \times n_{t2}$ vector consisting of these two data (shown in Figure 1), which will be used for the selection of genes. Specifically, with the combination of gene expression (22283 expressions) and SNP data (376821 SNPs), we have a new data vector with 360930 variables (some of the genes do not appear in both data sets, which were not taken into consideration for the combined analysis). For each gene, the feature vector contains two sub-vectors: gene expression and SNP data, which will be used together as the input to our SRC method for joint data analysis.

2.2 SRC clustering algorithm

Figure 2 shows the diagram of the proposed SRC model. The 'Feature extraction' can be the output of a feature extraction method discussed above (*e.g.*, FSFS, CCA, GSVD), or statistical features such as the mean and variance. $\boldsymbol{Y}=\{\boldsymbol{y}_i\}\in R^{m\times p}$ consists of feature vectors extracted from the data, where $\boldsymbol{y}_i\in R^{m\times 1} i=1,2,\ldots,p$ is the feature vector extracted for the *i*th gene/variable; *m* is the number of features (in this work, we employed m = 5 features for each gene in one type of data, as shown in Section 2.3 'Features selection'); and *p* is the number of

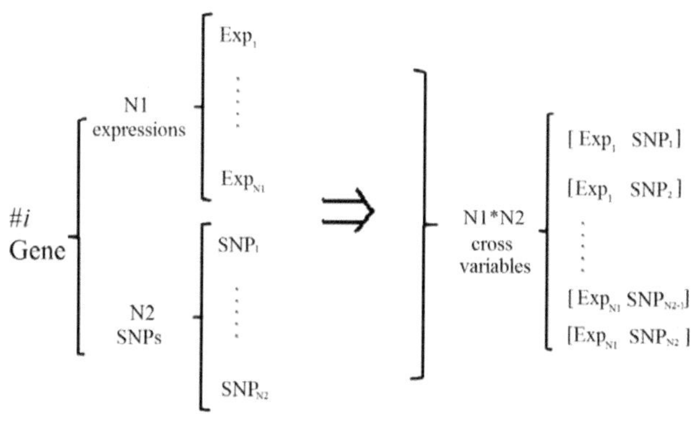

Figure 1. An illustration of the combination of two different types of data for the *i*th gene.

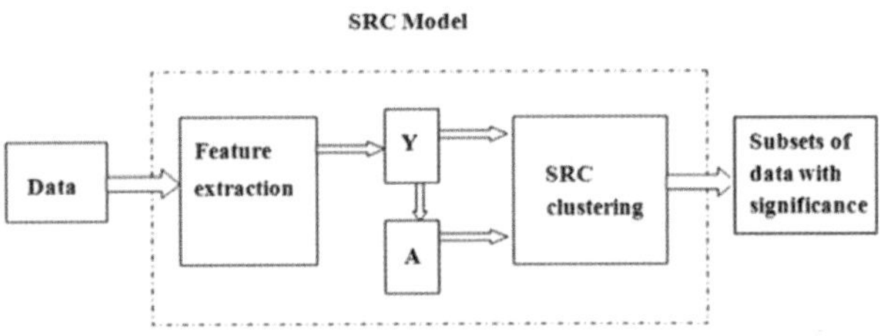

Figure 2. Diagram of SRC model for the data analysis using multi-features.

gene/variables (for the gene expression data used in this work, p = 22283; for the SNP data, p = 376821). $A=[A_1,\ldots,A_c]\in R^{m\times n}$ is the characteristic matrix that we will design to separate the data into c groups. For each group, $A_i\in R^{m\times n_i}$ contains n_i samples, and $n=\sum n_i$. The 'SRC clustering' is to cluster each y_i according to the characteristic matrix $\boldsymbol{A}$ that can be learned from the training data (the column number n is dependent on the number of features m. Detailed description can be seen in **Supporting Material S2**).

The description of the SRC algorithm is given in **Supporting Material S1**. The input of the SRC algorithm is the characteristic matrix $\boldsymbol{A}$, which is designed to cluster the data into different groups. In the previous studies, the characteristic matrix $\boldsymbol{A}$ was formed using the training samples [8]–[9]. In the current work, we design the characteristic matrix $\boldsymbol{A}$ with column vectors $\boldsymbol{v}$ to designate different clusters with specific characteristics extracted from data. The clustering of features is based on both vector angle and amplitude (*e.g.*, measured using the L2 norm of the vector). The vector angle between the two column vectors $\boldsymbol{v}_1$ and $\boldsymbol{v}_2$ is defined by $\theta(\boldsymbol{v}_1,\boldsymbol{v}_2)$, with $\cos(\theta)=(\boldsymbol{v}_1\times\boldsymbol{v}_2)/(\|\boldsymbol{v}_1\|\|\boldsymbol{v}_2\|)$. The design of characteristic matrix $\boldsymbol{A}$, is described in **Supporting Material S2** and the description of extracted feature vectors $\boldsymbol{y}_i$ will be given in Section 2.3.

2.3 Features selection

As shown in Figure 2, we used the extracted features $\boldsymbol{Y}$ from the original data as the input for the variable/gene selection. In this work, we proposed to employ five features. Specifically, for each gene/variable (gene expressions or SNPs), we have a feature vector defined by Eq. (1):

$$\left[std_0,std_1,|\bar{X}_0-\bar{X}_1|,|corr|,1-\|a\|_2\right]^T \qquad (1)$$

where $\bar{X}_0$ and $\bar{X}_1$, std_0 and std_1 are the means and standard deviation of control and case group respectively; *corr* is the Pearson correlation coefficient between each gene expression (or SNP) data and the healthy status ('1' for patients, and '0' for controls); and a is the normalized amplitude of vector $[std_0,std_1,|\bar{X}_0-\bar{X}_1|,|corr|]^{\mathrm{T}}$ Features std_0 and std_1 reflect the difference within each group, mean difference $|\bar{X}_0-\bar{X}_1|$ and the Pearson correlation coefficient $|corr|$ reflect the difference between the control and case groups. Therefore, feature vectors with smaller first two entries while larger last three entries are considered to be significant for discriminating control and case groups.

For a data set, we can extract feature vectors for each variable/gene to construct a feature matrix $\boldsymbol{Y}=[\boldsymbol{Y}_1,\boldsymbol{Y}_2,\cdots\boldsymbol{Y}_p]\in\mathbb{R}^{r\times p}$ where p is the number of variables/genes, and r is the number of features. In this work, r = 5 for the analysis of one type of data and r = 10 for the integrative analysis of two types of data. For the integrative analysis, since each gene has two types of data, features were extracted from both sub-vectors as illustrated in Figure 1. Since different feature has different range, a scale transformation is performed for each row of the feature matrix $\boldsymbol{Y}$ so that all the entries of $\boldsymbol{Y}$ are within the range of [0, 1]. In **Supporting Material S3**, we discuss the significance of these selected features and the relationships between them (see Fig. 1 and Fig. 2 in **Supporting Material S3**).

2.4 The SRC based gene/variable shaving

Once we have the characteristic matrix $\boldsymbol{A}$ and the feature vectors $\boldsymbol{Y}$, the SRC algorithm given by **Supporting Material S1** can be applied for gene shaving or for the selection of significant genes. Figure 3 gives an illustration of the gene/variable shaving process using the SRC based method. As shown in Figure 3, all genes were first grouped into different clusters using the SRC algorithm (Figure 3 (a)). Since each group is designed to have different statistical significances, those genes that fall into the group(s) of a particular significance can be selected for further analysis (Figure 3 (b)), while others will be shaved off. The process will continue until the number of remaining genes meets the threshold set with prior knowledge.

When the data set is very large, which is always the case for genomic data, a sliding window is applied and the gene selection is performed within the window (Figure 4 (a)) in order to account for local variations in the data. We also performed data shuffle with Fisher-Yates Shuffling algorithm [20] to reduce bias. Those genes selected with highest frequencies will be the ones that are most significant, as shown in Figure 4 (b). A description of the SRC based gene shaving algorithm with a sliding window is given as ***Algorithm 2***.

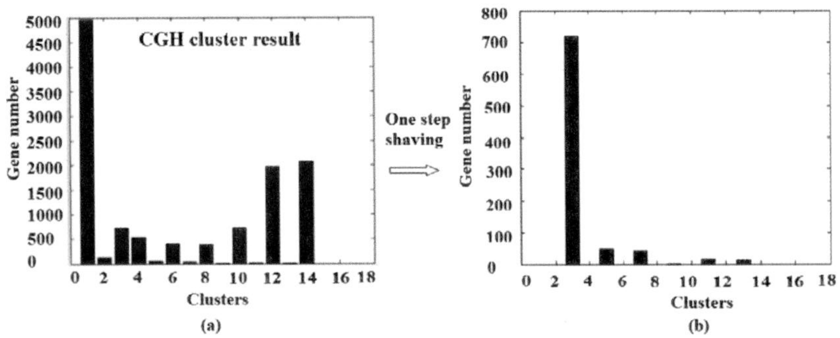

Figure 3. Diagram of gene shaving by SRC. (a) all genes were clustered into different groups; and (b) only clusters of a particular significance were selected for further analysis.

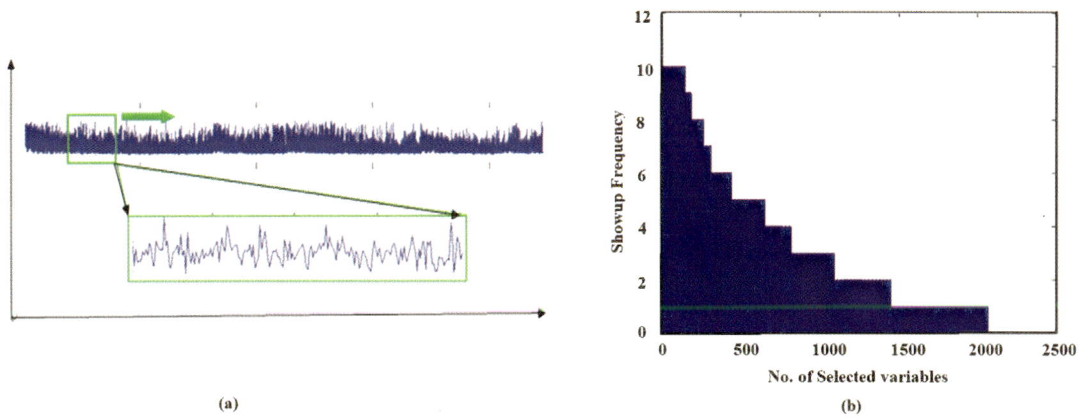

Figure 4. The SRC based gene shaving with a sliding window. (a) Gene selection was performed within each sliding window; (b) Genes selected with Fisher-Yates Shuffling algorithm; the higher the selected frequencies, the more significance of the variable (see the explanation of Algorithm 2).

Algorithm 2: SRC based gene shaving algorithm.

1. Set the window length, the window sliding step length, and the starting point;
2. For the l-th iteration, perform gene selection within a window and record the selected genes;
3. Slide the window from the starting point with the pre-set step length, and repeat Step 2 until the window reaches the ending point of the data sample.
4. Shuffle the data with Fisher-Yates Shuffling algorithm; and repeat Step 2–Step 3.
5. Compare the gene list generated by all l iterations with that generated by previous l-1 iterations; if the gene list percentage similarity (PS) is higher than a pre-set threshold, exit; otherwise, go to Step 4.

In ***Step*** 5, the gene list percentage similarity (PS) between the two different lists is defined by Eq. (2).

$$PS = \frac{(\#\text{variables from list1}) \cap (\#\text{variables from list2})}{\#\text{variables from list1}} \qquad (2)$$

2.5 Validation

Two strategies were taken to validate our method: 1.We test if the osteoporosis susceptive genes selected by our method can be confirmed with previously reported ones, in addition to the identification of new genes. 2. We test if gene expression/SNPs corresponding to selected genes are able to identify osteoporosis patients from healthy controls, which are quantified with classification ratio (CR). We define CR in this work as the ratio between the number of correctly classified samples and total number of samples. We conducted the leave-one-out (LOO) cross validation. We compared our method with current ones for gene selection (e.g., T-test for expression data and Fisher-exact test for SNP data). In addition, we compared the results of using combined data sets (gene expression and SNPs) with those of using each individual data set, in order to demonstrate the advantage of the proposed integration approach.

Results

One goal of our work was to study whether integrative analysis approach with our proposed SRC algorithm can lead to better identification of susceptible genes for the diagnosis of complex diseases such as osteoporosis. We conducted the analysis on two data sets with different structures, ranges and formats: gene expression (40 patients/40 controls, 22283 gene expressions), and SNP association analysis data (70 patients/70 controls, 376821 SNPs) from osteoporosis study. To validate the selected genes, we compared our selected gene lists with those previously reported. In addition, we tested if the selected genes can result in better diagnosis of osteoporosis. We performed the leave-one-out (LOO) cross validation for both data sets and the test using an independent SNP data set (30 patients/30 controls, 376821 SNPs). To demonstrate the performance of our SRC method, the results of our SRC method for gene selection were compared with those from both T-test and Fisher-exact test. In addition, the results of classifying osteoporosis using individual and joint data sets were compared, showing that integrated analysis can give higher diagnosis accuracy.

3.1 Comparison of selected genes using different methods

To show the differences between integrative analysis and individual analysis using both the SRC and conventional feature selection methods (e.g., T-test and Fisher-exact test), we compared the first 500 gene expressions and 1000 SNPs selected by different methods using the Venn diagram, as shown in Figure 5. The intersection between individual analysis using the SRC method and T-test for the gene expression data is about 45% (Figure 5 (a), the intersection between B and C); the intersection between the SRC method and Fisher-exact test for individual analysis of SNPs is about 39% (Figure 5 (b), the intersection between B and C area); and the intersection between combined analysis using SRC method and individual analysis is below 10% (A and B, A and C area for both Figure 5 (a) and (b)).

When compared the results with the previous study, our SRC based variable selection method was able to locate osteoporosis susceptive genes that were reported before [19] such as *'ESRRA', 'CALM1', 'CALM1', 'SPARC','LRP1', 'THSD4', 'CRHR1', 'HSD11B1', 'THSD7A', 'BMPR1B', 'ADCY10', 'PRL', 'CA8', et. al.* **Supporting Material S6** gives the first 50 gene expressions and

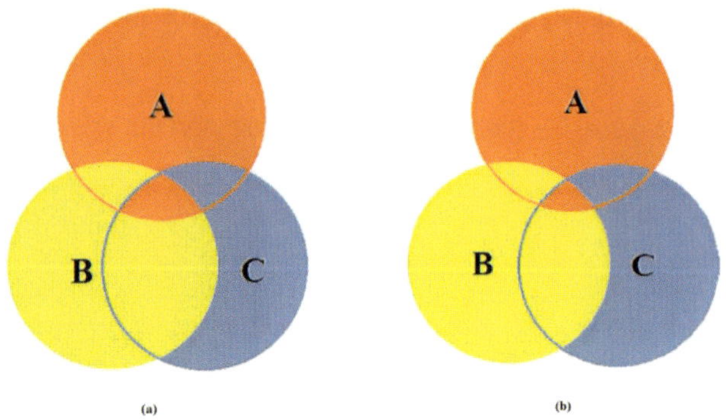

Figure 5. Comparison of the selected variables (expressions/ SNPs) using the Venn diagram. (a) comparison of the first 500 gene expressions selected with integrative analysis by the SRC method (orange area A), individual data analysis using SRC method (yellow area B) and using T-test (blue area C) respectively; (b) comparison of the first 1000 SNPs selected with integrative analysis with the SRC method (orange area A), individual analysis with the SRC method (yellow area B) and Fisher- exact test (blue area C) respectively. **Supporting Materials** S4 and S**5** give the first 50 variables (gene expressions/SNPs) selected using individual analysis. **Supporting Material** S**6** gives the first 50 variables (gene expressions and SNPs) selected using integrative analysis, and Fig. 1 in Supporting Material S6 compares the selected variables in cases and controls.

SNPs selected using joint data sets. In particular, there were some significant genes that were not identified by individual data analysis, such as *'DICER1'*, *'PTMA'* *etc*. However, evidences have existed to show that these genes may be associated with the osteoporosis disease (details in the Section of Discussion).

3.2 Validation of the selected genes on the diagnosis of osteoporosis

We further validated the selected genes for the diagnosis of osteoporosis subjects, whose accuracy was measured with the LOO cross-validation.

First, we showed that using gene expression or SNPs selected with our proposed SRC method can give higher diagnosis accuracy than that of the current methods such as the t-test and Fisher exact test. When using selected gene expression data alone to identify the osteoporosis patients, we got the highest classification ratio (CR) (86.25%) with 73 expression data, while for t-test method we got the highest CR of 90% with 225 gene expressions, as shown in Figure 6 (a). For the SNP data set, we got the highest CR (100%) with 883 SNPs using the SRC, while the highest CR (96.5%) with 1460 SNPs using Fisher-exact test, as shown in Figure 6 (b). Both results indicate that the classification of osteoporosis with the SRC is significantly better than the t-test and Fisher-exact test, which are currently widely used for the study of osteoporosis diseases.

Besides the LOO cross-validation, we also performed a blind test on the selection of OP susceptive genes. We applied the method to the classification of osteoporosis on an independent SNP data set (30 patients/30 controls, 376821 SNPs), and compared the results with the Fisher-exact test analysis, as shown in Figure 7. Using the SRC selected SNPs, the classification ratio reached as high as 98.33%, while using the SNPs selected with Fisher-exact test, the highest CR was only 88.33%, as shown in Figure 7.

Finally, we compared the classification accuracy of using combined data set with that of using individual data. For the combined data set, each selected feature vector contains two sub-vectors (SNP and gene expression sub-vector). Therefore, we calculated the CRs of using the whole feature vector and each sub-vector respectively. Figure 8 demonstrates that higher identification accuracy can be obtained with complementary information from both data sets than using an individual data.

Discussion

Identification of candidate genes from vast amount of genomic data for the diagnosis of complex disease has been a significant challenge. In this study, we address the problem by developing a sparse representation based clustering (SRC) method that can be used for integrative analyses of various types of genomic data. We applied the SRC based gene/variable selection method to the identification of genes associated with osteoporosis diseases. The SRC method demonstrates two advantages: 1. Different from

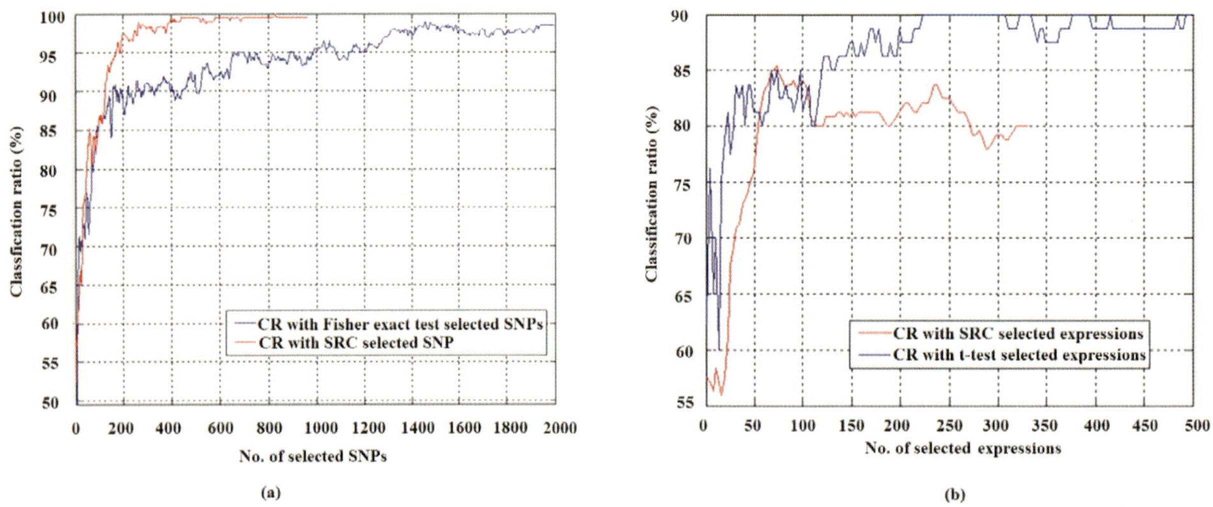

Figure 6. Comparison of classification accuracy with LOO cross-validation using the selected variables. (a)Validation results for the gene expression data by SRC the method and t-test method respectively. (b)Validation results for the SNP data by the SRC method and Fisher-exact test method respectively.

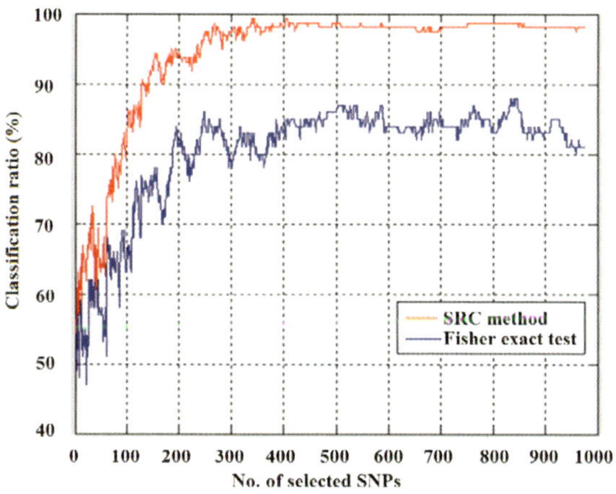

Figure 7. The classification of osteoporosis patients on an independent SNP data set.

other analysis methods, the SRC method employs multi-features extracted from diverse data sets rather than the original raw data, facilitating the integration of data with different formats and structures. 2. The SRC method outperforms several currently used significance test methods such as the T-test and Fisher-exact test, by employing a more sophisticated clustering based approach.

When compared with previously reported osteoporosis susceptible genes, the SRC based gene shaving method not only identified genes that were previously reported [19], such as *'THSD4'*, *'CRHR1'*, *'HSD11B1'*, *'THSD7A'*, *'BMPR1B'* *'ADCY10'*, *'PRL'*, *'CA8'*, *'ESRRA'*, *'CALM1'*, *'CALM1'*, *'SPARC'*, *'LRP1'*, but also new susceptive genes (*'DICER1'*, *'PTMA' et. al.*). Evidences [27–35] have shown that these genes play a significant role in the etiology of osteoporosis, as discussed below. In particular, it should be noticed that these genes cannot be identified with the analysis of an individual data set, demonstrating the advantage of integrative analysis of multiple types of data. In the following, we further elucidate the relevance of the identified new genes to osteoporosis from previous studies.

DICER1 (dicer 1, ribonuclease type III), also known as Dicer, is essential for microRNA (miRNA) processing and the synthesis of small interfering RNAs from long double-stranded RNA [27]. This gene is located at 14q32.13. Some evidences suggested that *DICER1* was closely associated with bone metabolism. For example, Dicer in osteoclasts controls activity of bone resorption in vivo [28]. Gene silencing of Dicer by small interfering RNA revealed global inhibition of osteoclast transcription factor expression and function, decreased osteoclastogenesis, and decreased bone resorption in vitro [29]. Dicer possessed significantly decreased miR-21 levels and increased PDCD4 protein levels so that RANKL-induced osteoclastogenesis was impaired in those cells [30]. Dicer generated miRs are necessary for two periods of bone formation, to promote osteoblast differentiation before birth, and control bone accrual in the adult [31].

PTMA (prothymosin, alpha) may play important roles in osteoporosis. Over-expressed PTMA enhanced p53 transcriptional activity in reporter gene assays for p53 target gene promoters hdm2, p21, and cyclin G, and increased mRNA and protein levels for endogenous p53 target genes, hdm2 and p21 [32]. Some studies reported that p53 regulates osteoblast differentiation, bone formation, and osteoblast-dependent osteoclast differentiation [33]. As p53+/m mice age, they reveal an early onset of phenotypes associated with aging. A recent serendipitously also generated p53 mutant allele resulted in a hypermorphic version of p53 that mediates decreased longevity. The reduced longevity is accompanied by the accelerated onset of a variety of aging phenotypes. These include reduced longevity, osteoporosis, generalized organ atrophy and a diminished stress tolerance [34], [35].

When we compared the selected gene list with that selected by a t-test and Fisher-exact test (see Figure 5(a) and (b)), it can be seen that the variables (SNPs/expressions) selected by the SRC method are quite different (>50% in the number). However, the integrative analysis with the SRC method selects two sub-vectors simultaneously and gives better classification accuracy, because of the use of complementary information. For example, using the SNP data, the SRC based method can give the highest CR of 100% than 97.14% of using Fisher exact test with less number of SNPs (see Figure 6). When using both types of data for the cross validation, the CR of using combined data sets with the SRC

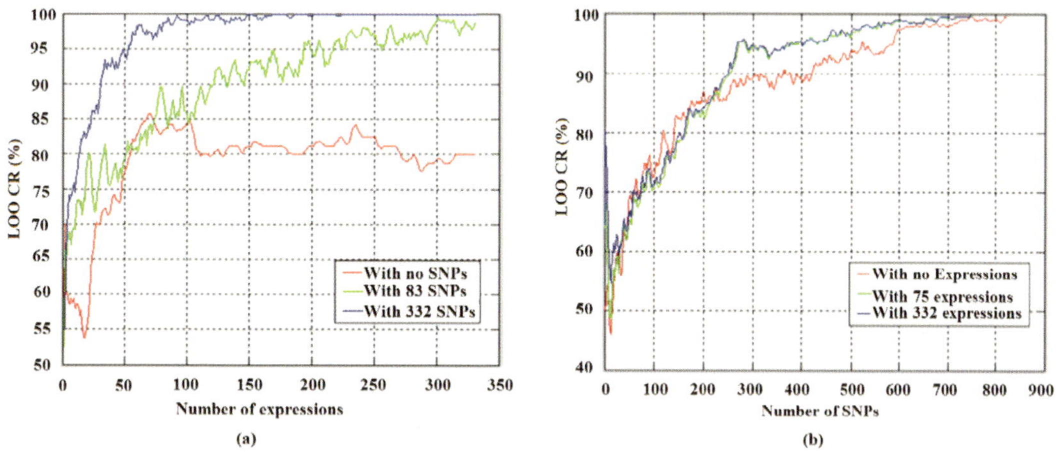

Figure 8. Using selected variables from both data sets for the classification of osteoporosis patients. (a) Classification accuracy using gene expressions along with N = 0, 83, 332 selected SNPs employed for the classification. (b) Classification accuracy using SNPs along with N = 0, 75, 332 selected gene expressions employed for the classification.

method is much higher than that of using one type of data (see Figure 8), demonstrating the significance of integrative data analysis. In addition, when performing a blind test on an independent SNP data set (30 cases 30 controls), the CR can be as high as 98.33% with the SRC method; with Fisher-exact test selected SNPs, the highest classification ratio is only 88.33%, showing the advantage of the SRC method.

In our integrative analysis method, gene expression and SNP data were combined in terms of each gene. Therefore, our method uses joint information from two complementary data rather than from a single type of data, which can lead to the increase of reliability in gene identification. Besides the significance discussed above, the integrative analysis employed in this work can be generalized to include more than two types of data. We are currently testing the method for the integration of multiple genomic data from the TCGA database for improved diagnosis of cancers such as the leukemia. In addition, the sample size in this work is small (100/100 cases/controls for the SNP data set and 40/40 subjects for the gene expression data set). To further validate the proposed method and the significance of the selected genes, larger data sets will be tested.

Supporting Information

Supporting Material S1 Sparse Representation-based clustering (SRC) algorithm.

Supporting Material S2 Design of Characteristic matrix *A*.

Supporting Material S3 Significance of the selected features.

Supporting Material S4 The first 50 selected expressions (with corresponding gene names) by the individual analysis of OP gene expression data.

Supporting Material S5 The first 50 selected SNPs (with corresponding gene names) by the individual analysis of OP SNP data.

Supporting Material S6 The first 50 selected SNPs and gene expressions selected (with corresponding gene names) by the joint analysis of both OP SNP and gene expression data.

Author Contributions

Conceived and designed the experiments: YPW. Performed the experiments: HBC. Analyzed the data: HBC HWD. Contributed reagents/materials/analysis tools: SL. Wrote the paper: HBC HWD YPW.

References

1. Yang HH, Liu JY, Sui J, Pearlson Gand Calhoun VD (2010) A hybrid machine learning method for fusing fMRI and genetic data: combining both improves classification of schizophrenia. Frontiers in Human Neuroscience 4:1–9.
2. Soneson C, Lilljebjörn H, Fioretos T, Fontes M (2010) Integrative analysis of gene expression and copy number alterations using canonical correlation analysis. BMC Bioinformatics 11:191
3. Cao KA L, Martin PG, Robert-Granie C, Besse P (2009) Sparse canonical methods for biological data integration: application to a cross platform study. BMC Bioinformatics 10:34.
4. Berger JA, Hautaniemi S, Mitra SK, Astola J (2006) Jointly Analyzing Genes Expression and Copy Number Data in Breast Cancer using Data Reduction model. IEEE T Comput B I. 3(1):2–16.
5. Liu YJ, Shen H, Xiao P, Xiong DH, Li LH, et al. (2005) Molecular Genetic Studies of Gene Identification for Osteoporosis: A 2004 Update. Journal of Bone and Mineral Research, 21(10): 1551–1535.
6. Wang P, Kim Y, Pollack J, Narasimhan B, Tibshirani R (2005) A Method for Calling Gains and Losses in Array CGH Data. Biostatistics 6: 45–58.
7. Hautaniemi S, Ringner M, Kauraniemi P, Autio R, Edgren H, et al. (2004) A Strategy for Identifying Putative Causes of Gene Expression Variation in Human Cancers. J Franklin Inst. 341: 77–88.
8. Loo LWM, Grove DI, Williams EM, Neal CL, Cousens LA, et al. (2004) Array Comparative Genomic Hybridization Analysis of Genomic Alterations in Breast Cancer Subtypes. Cancer Research 64: 8541–8549.
9. Cao HB, Deng HW, Li M, Wang YP (2012) Classification of Multicolor Fluorescence In-situ Hybridization (M-FISH) Images with Sparse Representation. IEEE Tans Nano Biosciences 11:111–118.
10. Melton LJ, Chrischilles EA, Cooper C, Lane AW, Riggs BL (2005) How many women have osteoporosis? JBMR Anniversary Classic. J Bone Miner Res. 20:886–892.
11. Cummings SR, Nevitt MC, Browner WS, Stone K, Fox KM, et al. (1995) Risk factors for hip fracture in white women. Study of Osteoporotic Fractures Research Group. N Engl J Med. 332:767–773.
12. Deng HW, Mahaney MC, Williams JT, Li J, Conway T, et al. (2002) Relevance of the genes for bone mass variation to susceptibility to osteoporotic fractures and its implications to gene search for complex human diseases. Genet Epidemiol. 22:12–25.
13. Liu PY, Qin YJ, Recker RR, Deng HW (2004) Evidence for a major gene underlying bone size variation in the Chinese. Am J Hum Biol. 16:68–77.
14. Jian WX, Long JR, Li MX, Liu XH, Deng HW (2005) Genetic determination of variation and covariation of bone mineral density at the hip and spine in a Chinese population. J Bone Miner Metab. 23:181–185.
15. Hsu YH, Zillikens MC, Wilson SG, Farber CR, Demissie S, et al. (2010) An integration of genome-wide association study and gene expression profiling to prioritize the discovery of novel susceptibility Loci for osteoporosis-related traits. PLoS Genet. 6(6):1–16.
16. Deng FY, Lei SF, Chen XD, Tan LJ, Zhu XZ, et al. (2011) An integrative study ascertained SOD2 as a susceptibility gene for osteoporosis in Chinese. J Bone Miner Res. 26(11): 2695–2701.
17. Xiong DH, Liu XG, Guo YF, Tan LJ, Wang L, et al. (2009) Genome-wide association and follow-up replication studies identified ADAMTS18 and TGFBR3 as bone mass candidate genes in different ethnic groups. Am J Hum Genet. 84(3): 388–398.
18. Yang TL, Chen XD, Guo Y, Lei SF, Wang JT, et al. (2008) Genome-wide copy-number-variation study identified a susceptibility gene,UGT2B17, for osteoporosis. Am J Hum Genet. 83(6):663–674.
19. Xu XH, Dong SS, Guo Y, Yang TL, Lei SF, et al. (2010) Molecular Genetic Studies of Gene Identification for Osteoporosis: The 2009 Update, Endocr Rev. 31: 447–505.
20. Fisher RA, Yates F (1948) Statistical tables for biological, agricultural and medical research, 3rd ed. London: Oliver and Boyd. pp. 26–27.
21. Udagawa N, Takahashi N, Akatsu T, Tanaka H, Sasaki T, et al. (1990) Origin of osteoclasts: mature monocytes and macrophages are capable of differentiating into osteoclasts under a suitable microenvironment prepared by bone marrow-derived stromal cells. Proc Natl Acad Sci U S A 87(18):7260–7264.
22. Zambonin ZA, Teti A, Primavera MV (1984) Monocytes from circulating blood fuse in vitro with purified osteoclasts in primary culture. J Cell Sci. 66:335–342.
23. Fujikawa Y, Quinn JM, Sabokbar A, McGee J, Athanasou NA (1996) The human osteoclast precursor circulates in the monocyte fraction. Endocrinology 137(9):4058–4060.
24. Cohen-Solal ME, Graulet AM, Denne MA, Gueris J, Baylink D, et al. (1993) Peripheral monocyte culture suppernatants of menopausal women can induce bone resorption: involvement of cytokines. J Clin Endocrinol Metab. 77(6):1648–1653.
25. Eghbali-Fatourechi G, Khosla S, Sanyal A, Boyle WJ, Lacey DL, et al. (2003) Role of RANK ligand in mediating increased bone resorption in early postmenopausal women. J Clin Invest. 111(8):1221–1230.
26. Pacifici R (1996) Estrogen, cytokines, and pathogenesis of postmenopausal osteoporosis. J Bone Miner Res. 11(8):1043–1051.
27. Nagaraja AK, Andreu-Vieyra C, Franco HL, Ma L, Chen R, et al. (2008) Deletion of Dicer in somatic cells of the female reproductive tract causes sterility. Mol Endocrinol. 22(10): 2336–2352.
28. Mizoguchi F, Izu Y, Hayata T, Hemmi H, Nakashima K, et al. (2010) Osteoclast-specific Dicer gene deficiency suppresses osteoclastic bone resorption. J Cell Biochem. 109(5): 866–875.
29. Sugatani T, Hruska KA (2009) Impaired micro-RNA pathways diminish osteoclast differentiation and function. J Biol Chem. 284(7): 4667–4678.
30. Sugatani T, Vacher J, Hruska KA (2011) A microRNA expression signature of osteoclastogenesis. Blood, 117(13): 3648–3657.
31. Gaur T, Hussain S, Mudhasani R, Parulkar I, Colby JL, et al. (2010) Dicer inactivation in osteoprogenitor cells compromises fetal survival and bone

formation, while excision in differentiated osteoblasts increases bone mass in the adult mouse. Dev Biol. 340(1):10–21.

32. Kobayashi T, Wang T, Maezawa M, Kobayashi M, Ohnishi S, et al. (2006) Over expression of the oncoprotein prothymosin alpha triggers a p53 response that involves p53 acetylation. Cancer Res. 66(6): 3137–3144.
33. Wang X, Kua HY, Hu Y, Guo K, Zeng Q, et al. (2006) p53 functions as a negative regulator of osteoblastogenesis, osteoblast-dependent osteoclastogenesis, and bone remodeling. J Cell Biol. 172(1): 115–125.
34. Dumble M, Gatza C, Tyner S, Venkatachalam S, Donehower LA (2004) Insights into aging obtained from p53 mutant mouse models. Ann N Y Acad Sci. 1019:171–177.
35. Tyner SD, Venkatachalam S, Choi J, Jones S, Ghebraniousk N, et al. (2002) p53 mutant mice that display early ageing-associated phenotypes. Nature 415(6867): 45–53.

15

Bone Health History in Breast Cancer Patients on Aromatase Inhibitors

Marilyn L. Kwan[1]*, Joan C. Lo[1], Li Tang[2], Cecile A. Laurent[1], Janise M. Roh[1], Malini Chandra[1], Theresa E. Hahn[2], Chi-Chen Hong[2], Lara Sucheston-Campbell[2], Dawn L. Hershman[3], Charles P. Quesenberry Jr.[1], Christine B. Ambrosone[2], Lawrence H. Kushi[1], Song Yao[2]

1 Division of Research, Kaiser Permanente Northern California, Oakland, California, United States of America, **2** Department of Cancer Prevention and Control, Roswell Park Cancer Institute, Buffalo, New York, United States of America, **3** Department of Medicine and the Herbert Irving Comprehensive Cancer Center, Columbia University, New York, New York, United States of America

Abstract

A cross-sectional study was performed to assess bone health history among aromatase inhibitor (AI) users before breast cancer (BC) diagnosis, which may impact fracture risk after AI therapy and choice of initial hormonal therapy. A total of 2,157 invasive BC patients initially treated with an AI were identified from a prospective cohort study at Kaiser Permanente Northern California (KPNC). Data on demographic and lifestyle factors were obtained from in-person interviews, and bone health history and clinical data from KPNC clinical databases. The prevalence of osteoporosis and fractures in postmenopausal AI users was assessed, compared with 325 postmenopausal TAM users. The associations of bone health history with demographic and lifestyle factors in AI users were also examined. Among all initial AI users, 11.2% had a prior history of osteoporosis, 16.3% had a prior history of any fracture, and 4.6% had a prior history of major fracture. Postmenopausal women who were taking TAM as their initial hormonal therapy had significantly higher prevalence of prior osteoporosis than postmenopausal AI users (21.5% vs. 11.8%, $p<0.0001$). Among initial AI users, the associations of history of osteoporosis and fracture in BC patients with demographic and lifestyle factors were, in general, consistent with those known in healthy older women. This study is one of the first to characterize AI users and risk factors for bone morbidity before BC diagnosis. In the future, this study will examine lifestyle, molecular, and genetic risk factors for AI-induced fractures.

Editor: Debashis Ghosh, SUNY Upstate Medical University, United States of America

Funding: Funded by the U.S. National Institutes of Health, National Cancer Institute (R01 CA166701 to M.L.K. and S.Y. and R01 CA105274 to L.H.K.). The funders had no role in study design, data collection and analysis, decision to publish, or preparation of the manuscript.

Competing Interests: The authors have declared that no competing interests exist.

* Email: Marilyn.L.Kwan@kp.org

Introduction

Aromatase inhibitors (AI) have been replacing tamoxifen (TAM) as adjuvant hormonal therapy for postmenopausal women diagnosed with early stage, hormone receptor (HR)-positive breast cancer. The current third-generation AIs inhibit 96–99% *in vivo* aromatase enzyme activity [1], thereby decreasing endogenous estrogen levels far below levels from natural menopause [2]. This highly efficient estrogen depletion by AIs benefits breast cancer patients by extending recurrence-free survival superior to TAM [3,4,5]. However, AIs put patients at high risk of fractures due to the central role of estrogen in maintaining normal bone metabolism [6]. In contrast, TAM is generally believed to be bone-conserving [2]. Several expert groups have developed guidelines for evaluating fracture risk in breast cancer patients who are planning to start AI therapy [7,8,9,10], so that the benefits and harms of AIs can be carefully assessed to make an educated decision on choice of hormonal therapy.

The aforementioned guidelines vary slightly but usually include bone mineral density (BMD) testing and clinical assessment of risk factors for fracture [7,8,9,10]. Although BMD remains a strong predictor for fracture risk, several studies have shown that a large proportion of patients who experienced fragility fractures had T-scores in the non-osteoporotic range [11,12], which highlights the importance of evaluation of BMD-independent risk factors, such as *a priori* bone health history, age, physical activity, smoking, and alcohol intake [13,14]. However, to our knowledge, only a few small studies have examined bone health history among AI users prior to breast cancer diagnosis [15,16], and no studies have investigated lifestyle factors and prior risk of fracture in this patient population. In a real-world clinical setting, it is unknown how bone health history would affect hormonal therapy choice among postmenopausal women with HR-positive breast cancer. These data will be important to inform treatment and prevention strategies for AI users as a high-risk population for bone morbidity. Furthermore, it is of clinical significance to also examine whether

Table 1. Baseline characteristics of study cohort by initial use of aromatase inhibitor (AI) or tamoxifen (TAM).

	Overall	Postmenopausal Only		
	AI (Initial Use)	AI (Initial Use)	TAM (Initial Use)	p value[1]
	n = 2157	n = 2033	n = 325	
	n (%)	n (%)	n (%)	
Age at Breast Cancer (BC) Diagnosis (years)				**<0.0001**
<50	80 (3.7)	28 (1.4)	47 (14.5)	
50–59	640 (29.7)	581 (28.6)	101 (31.1)	
60–69	891 (41.3)	883 (43.4)	99 (30.5)	
≥70	546 (25.3)	541 (26.6)	78 (24.0)	
Mean (SD)	64.4 (9.1)	65.2 (8.5)	62.0 (11.2)	
Menopausal Status				–
Premenopausal	118 (5.5)	0 (0)	0 (0)	
Postmenopausal	2033 (94.5)	2033 (100)	325 (100)	
AJCC Stage at BC Diagnosis				**0.0003**
I	1165 (54.0)	1120 (55.1)	218 (67.1)	
II	751 (34.8)	693 (34.1)	85 (26.2)	
III	206 (9.6)	187 (9.2)	20 (6.2)	
IV	35 (1.6)	33 (1.6)	2 (0.6)	
Race/Ethnicity				0.62
White	1541 (71.4)	1467 (72.2)	222 (68.3)	
African American	124 (5.8)	115 (5.7)	22 (6.8)	
Asian	221 (10.3)	202 (9.9)	31 (9.5)	
Hispanic	225 (10.4)	205 (10.1)	43 (13.2)	
Other	46 (2.1)	44 (2.2)	7 (2.2)	
BMI (kg/m²)				**<0.0001**
<25	642 (30.0)	595 (29.5)	127 (39.4)	
25–29.9	680 (31.8)	645 (31.9)	108 (33.5)	
≥30	816 (38.2)	780 (38.6)	87 (27.0)	
Mean (SD)	29.0 (6.5)	29.0 (6.5)	27.6 (6.4)	
Mod-Vig Physical Activity (MET-hours/week)				
Mean (SD)	27.6 (28.6)	27.6 (28.9)	33.0 (34.0)	**0.03**
Median (IQR)	19.5 (7.3–39.1)	19.4 (7.1–39.1)	24.4 (9.3–45.4)	
Smoking History				0.28
Never	1118 (52.0)	1046 (51.5)	183 (56.3)	
Former	913 (42.5)	874 (43.0)	129 (39.7)	
Current	118 (5.5)	111 (5.5)	13 (4.0)	
Alcohol Intake (g/day)				0.24
Never	511 (27.9)	477 (27.5)	81 (29.7)	
≤median[2]	665 (36.2)	618 (35.7)	106 (38.8)	
>median	659 (35.9)	637 (36.8)	86 (31.5)	
Vitamin Supplement Use			**0.003**	
None	1263 (62.7)	177 (55.0)		
Calcium	334 (16.6)	61 (18.9)		
Vitamin D	259 (12.9)	43 (13.4)		
Both	158 (7.9)	41 (12.7)		
<0.0001				
No	1792 (88.2)	225 (78.5)		
≤6	165 (8.1)	50 (12.3)		
>6	76 (3.7)	30 (9.2)		
Any Fracture Before BC Diagnosis (years)			0.27	

Table 1. Cont.

	Overall	Postmenopausal Only		
	AI (Initial Use)	**AI (Initial Use)**	**TAM (Initial Use)**	**p value[1]**
	n = 2157	**n = 2033**	**n = 325**	
	n (%)	**n (%)**	**n (%)**	
No	1695 (83.4)	272 (83.7)		
≤6	179 (8.8)	23 (7.1)		
>6	159 (7.8)	30 (9.2)		
0.13				
No	1937 (95.3)	306 (94.2)		
≤6	60 (3.0)	11 (3.4)		
>6	36 (1.8)	8 (2.5)		

NOTE: Pharmacy data through December 31, 2013; Missing data for entire cohort: menopausal status (n = 9), BMI (n = 28), smoking (n = 13), alcohol (n = 552), vitamin supplements (n = 37).

[1] Logistic regression adjusted for age at breast cancer diagnosis as a continuous variable.

[2] Median (overall) = 3.10 g/day, median (postmenopausal women) = 2.90 g/day.

[3] Osteoporosis defined by ICD-9 code (733.00–733.09) or any prior bisphosphonate prescription.

[4] Major fracture includes fracture of spine, humerus, wrist, or hip.

known risk factors for fractures are also relevant in breast cancer patients, considering the paradoxical role of estrogens in promoting carcinogenesis yet maintaining bone health.

In a cross-sectional analysis of one of the largest contemporary cohorts of breast cancer patients, we describe history of osteoporosis and fracture and the prevalence of risk factors for fracture (age, race/ethnicity, body mass index (BMI), physical activity, smoking, alcohol intake, and calcium and vitamin D supplement use) before breast cancer diagnosis among initial AI users. We also compare prevalence of bone health history in postmenopausal AI users with postmenopausal TAM users. Lastly, we examine associations of these fracture risk factors with prior history of osteoporosis and fracture outcomes in AI users.

Materials and Methods

Study Population

The Pathways Study is a prospective study of 4,505 women with newly diagnosed invasive breast cancer who are members of Kaiser Permanente Northern California (KPNC), a large, integrated health care delivery system covering the San Francisco-Oakland Bay Area, Sacramento, and surrounding counties. Recruitment was from January 2006 to April 2013 through rapid case ascertainment procedures designed to enroll women prior to initiation of chemotherapy, as described elsewhere [17]. Eligibility criteria included: KPNC female members at least 21 years of age; had no previous history of malignancy other than non-melanoma skin cancer; spoke English, Spanish, Cantonese, or Mandarin; and resided within a 65-mile radius of a field interviewer. The mean time from diagnosis to enrollment was 2.0 (±0.7) months.

For this bone health sub-study, women were included if they had at least one hormonal therapy prescription of an AI or TAM that was indicated for treatment of their first primary breast cancer. A total of 1,159 women who had no hormonal therapy, 27 women who initiated hormonal therapy after recurrence of their original breast cancer, and 4 women who initiated hormonal therapy after their second primary breast cancer were excluded. The final study population consisted of 3,315 eligible women. Based on complete hormonal therapy prescription data through December 2013, 2,157 (65.1%) were initial AI users, and 1,158 (34.9%) were initial TAM users. For this analysis of baseline bone health history, only the initial AI users were included. In selected analyses, 325 postmenopausal women who received TAM as their initial hormonal therapy drug were also included as a comparison group to postmenopausal AI users (n = 2,033).

Clinicopathologic Characteristics

Clinical and diagnostic tumor characteristics were obtained from the KPNC Cancer Registry approximately four months post-diagnosis [18]. These included: stage at diagnosis, estrogen/progesterone receptor (ER/PR) positivity, HER2/neu (Her2) status, surgery type, and treatment received.

Self-reported Participant Information

The baseline interview was conducted at enrollment into the cohort approximately two months post-diagnosis, and included interviewer and self-administered questionnaires on sociodemographics, diet, physical activity, smoking, established breast cancer risk factors, health history, and use of vitamin/mineral supplements. Anthropometric measures were also obtained at baseline.

Information was collected on hysterectomy and oophorectomy and associated dates of the surgery, and age or date of last period. Menopause was defined as the absence of menses for 12 consecutive months or more relative to the date of the baseline interview, or having a complete hysterectomy or oophorectomy of both ovaries.

Physical activity was assessed using an activity frequency questionnaire based on the validated Arizona Activity Frequency Questionnaire (AAFQ) [19]. Activities in four main domains were asked: household, recreational, transportation, and sedentary. Diet was assessed using a 139-item modified version of the Block 2005 food frequency questionnaire (FFQ) (NutritionQuest, Berkeley, CA). Alcohol consumption (beer, wine, and liquor), including frequency and portion size, was obtained on the FFQ.

Pharmacy Data

Prescription drug data for nearly 100% of KPNC enrollees is recorded in the KPNC pharmacy database, including drug name,

Table 2. Baseline characteristics in relation to osteoporosis[1] before breast cancer diagnosis (BC) in aromatase inhibitor (AI) users.

	Osteoporosis Before BC Diagnosis – Yes	Osteoporosis Before BC Diagnosis – No	OR[2]	95% CI[2]	p for trend
	n = 242	n = 1915			
	n (%)	n (%)			
Age at BC Diagnosis (years)					**<0.0001**
<60	31 (12.8)	689 (36.0)	Ref		
60–69	95 (39.3)	796 (41.6)	**2.43**	**(1.58, 3.72)**	
≥70	116 (47.9)	430 (22.5)	**5.65**	**(3.68, 8.69)**	
Race/Ethnicity					–
White	182 (75.2)	1359 (71.0)	Ref		
African American	5 (2.1)	119 (6.2)	**0.38**	**(0.15, 0.94)**	
Asian	30 (12.4)	191 (10.0)	**1.82**	**(1.17, 2.81)**	
Hispanic	19 (7.9)	206 (10.8)	0.86	(0.52, 1.43)	
Other	6 (2.5)	40 (2.1)	1.46	(0.60, 3.54)	
BMI (kg/m²)					**<0.0001**
<25	114 (47.3)	528 (27.8)	Ref		
25–29.9	77 (32.0)	603 (31.8)	**0.55**	**(0.40, 0.76)**	
≥30	50 (20.8)	766 (40.4)	**0.32**	**(0.22, 0.45)**	
Mod-Vig Physical Activity (MET-hours/week)					–
Never	16 (6.7)	92 (4.8)	Ref		
≤median[3]	102 (42.5)	915 (48.2)	0.92	(0.51, 1.67)	
>median	122 (50.8)	893 (47.0)	1.25	(0.69, 2.27)	
Smoking History					–
Never	134 (55.4)	984 (51.6)	Ref		
Former	101 (41.7)	812 (42.6)	0.86	(0.65, 1.15)	
Current	7 (2.9)	111 (5.8)	0.62	(0.28, 1.39)	
Alcohol Intake (g/day)					–
Never	77 (34.8)	434 (26.9)	Ref		
≤median[3]	73 (33.0)	591 (36.6)	0.73	(0.51, 1.05)	
>median	71 (32.1)	589 (36.5)	0.72	(0.50, 1.04)	
Vitamin Supplement Use					–
None	146 (60.8)	1202 (63.5)	Ref		
Calcium	40 (16.7)	311 (16.4)	1.08	(0.73, 1.58)	
Vitamin D	34 (14.2)	235 (12.4)	1.06	(0.69, 1.63)	
Both	20 (8.3)	145 (7.7)	1.03	(0.61, 1.74)	

NOTE: Pharmacy data through December 31, 2013.
[1] Osteoporosis defined by ICD-9 code (733.00–733.09) or any prior bisphosphonate prescription.
[2] Logistic regression adjusted for age, race/ethnicity, menopausal status, and year of breast cancer diagnosis.
[3] Median (physical activity) = 20.9 metabolic equivalent (MET)-hours/week; median (alcohol intake) = 3.1 g/day.

National Drug Code, dosage and therapeutic class; prescription dates and cost; dispensing and refills; and prescribing physician, thus minimizing recall bias [20]. The pharmacy database was accessed to identify any outpatient prescriptions of AIs (anastrozole, letrozole, and exemestane) and TAM after breast cancer diagnosis. Prescriptions of bisphosphonates (BP) any time before breast cancer diagnosis were also captured. BPs are inhibitors of bone resorption and commonly prescribed to treat osteoporosis and other related conditions.

Prior Bone Outcomes

International Classification of Diseases, 9th edition (ICD-9) outpatient and hospitalization diagnoses of bone outcomes were obtained from the KPNC electronic medical record (EMR). These diagnosis codes include: (1) osteoporosis (733.00–733.09); (2) any prior fracture involving the neck, trunk, upper and lower extremities (805, 807–815, 817–825, 827–829, excluding open fractures, fractures involving spinal cord injury, fractures of the face/skull, fingers and toes, and those associated with major trauma); and (3) any major osteoporotic fracture of the spine, humerus, wrist, or hip (805.0, 805.2, 805.4, 805.8, 812.0, 812.2, 813.4, 813.5, 820.0, 820.2, 820.8, excluding those associated with major trauma) were ascertained as previously described [21].

Considering potential under-diagnosis or documentation of osteoporosis by clinicians [22,23], we assumed that if a woman was prescribed a BP prior to breast cancer diagnosis, and considering

Table 3. Baseline characteristics in relation to any fracture before breast cancer (BC) diagnosis in aromatase inhibitor (AI) users.

	Any Fracture Before BC Diagnosis – Yes	Any fracture Before BC Diagnosis – No	OR[1]	95% CI[1]	p for trend
	n = 352	n = 1805			
	n (%)	n (%)			
Age at BC Diagnosis (years)					**<0.0001**
<60	70 (19.9)	650 (36.0)	Ref		
60–69	143 (40.6)	748 (41.4)	**1.76**	**(1.27, 2.43)**	
≥70	139 (39.5)	407 (22.6)	**3.13**	**(2.24, 4.37)**	
Race/Ethnicity					–
White	268 (76.1)	1273 (70.5)	Ref		
African American	24 (6.8)	100 (5.5)	1.30	(0.81, 2.08)	
Asian	17 (4.8)	204 (11.3)	**0.50**	**(0.30, 0.84)**	
Hispanic	34 (9.7)	191 (10.6)	0.97	(0.66, 1.44)	
Other	9 (2.6)	37 (2.1)	1.37	(0.65, 2.90)	
BMI (kg/m^2)					0.86
<25	93 (26.6)	549 (30.7)	Ref		
25–29.9	135 (38.6)	545 (30.5)	**1.43**	**(1.06, 1.92)**	
≥30	122 (34.9)	694 (38.8)	1.00	(0.74, 1.36)	
Mod-Vig Physical Activity (MET-hours/week)					–
Never	26 (7.5)	82 (4.6)	Ref		
≤median[2]	164 (47.0)	853 (47.6)	0.83	(0.51, 1.35)	
>median	159 (45.6)	856 (47.8)	0.84	(0.51, 1.37)	
Smoking History					–
Never	178 (50.7)	940 (52.3)	Ref		
Former	152 (43.3)	761 (42.3)	0.93	(0.73, 1.19)	
Current	21 (6.0)	97 (5.4)	1.24	(0.75, 2.07)	
Alcohol Intake (g/day)					–
Never	89 (30.4)	422 (27.4)	Ref		
≤median[2]	88 (30.0)	576 (37.4)	0.73	(0.52, 1.01)	
>median	116 (39.6)	544 (35.3)	1.00	(0.73, 1.38)	
Vitamin Supplement Use					–
None	203 (58.8)	1145 (64.0)	Ref		
Calcium	60 (17.4)	291 (16.3)	1.21	(0.88, 1.68)	
Vitamin D	49 (14.2)	220 (12.3)	1.12	(0.78, 1.61)	
Both	33 (9.6)	132 (7.4)	1.21	(0.79, 1.86)	
Osteoporosis Before BC Diagnosis					–
No	267 (75.9)	1648 (91.3)	Ref		
Yes	85 (24.2)	157 (8.7)	**2.86**	**(2.10, 3.89)**	

NOTE: Pharmacy data through December 31, 2013.
[1] Logistic regression adjusted for age, race/ethnicity, menopausal status, and year of breast cancer diagnosis.
[2] Median (physical activity) = 20.9 metabolic equivalent (MET)-hours/week; median (alcohol intake) = 3.1 g/day.

that BPs are usually indicated for clinical treatment of osteoporosis, she was most likely diagnosed with the condition. Therefore, we expanded our definition of osteoporosis to include any prescription of BP before breast cancer diagnosis regardless of whether or not an ICD-9 diagnosis code was present. Thus, osteoporosis was defined as having any relevant ICD-9 diagnosis code or any prior prescription of BP.

Statistical Analysis

Analyses of initial AI or TAM use in postmenopausal breast cancer patients by select characteristics, including prior history of osteoporosis and fracture, were conducted using logistic regression with adjustment for age at breast cancer diagnosis as a continuous variable.

In the overall initial AI user group, we calculated odds ratios (OR) and 95% confidence intervals (CI) using logistic regression to estimate the associations of lifestyle and clinical factors at breast

Table 4. Baseline characteristics in relation to major fracture[1] before breast cancer (BC) diagnosis in aromatase inhibitor (AI) users.

	Major Fracture Before BC Diagnosis – Yes	Major Fracture Before BC Diagnosis – No	OR[2]	95% CI[2]	p for trend
	n = 99	n = 2058			
	n (%)	n (%)			
Age at BC Diagnosis (years)					**<0.0001**
<60	16 (16.2)	704 (34.2)	Ref		
60–69	32 (32.3)	859 (41.7)	1.54	(0.81, 2.93)	
≥70	51 (51.5)	495 (24.1)	**4.23**	**(2.29, 7.83)**	
Race/Ethnicity					–
White	82 (82.8)	1459 (70.9)	Ref		
African American	3 (3.0)	121 (5.9)	0.52	(0.16, 1.70)	
Asian	4 (4.0)	217 (10.5)	0.47	(0.17, 1.30)	
Hispanic	6 (6.1)	219 (10.6)	0.59	(0.25, 1.37)	
Other	4 (4.0)	42 (2.0)	2.20	(0.76, 6.39)	
BMI (kg/m^2)					0.38
<25	28 (28.3)	614 (30.1)	Ref		
25–29.9	39 (39.4)	641 (31.4)	1.33	(0.80, 2.21)	
≥30	32 (32.3)	784 (38.5)	0.93	(0.55, 1.59)	
Mod-Vig Physical Activity (MET-hours/week)					–
Never	15 (15.5)	93 (4.6)	Ref		
≤median[3]	40 (41.2)	977 (47.8)	**0.33**	**(0.17, 0.64)**	
>median	42 (43.3)	973 (47.6)	**0.36**	**(0.18, 0.70)**	
Smoking History					–
Never	49 (49.5)	1069 (52.2)	Ref		
Former	48 (48.5)	865 (42.2)	1.05	(0.69, 1.60)	
Current	2 (2.0)	116 (5.7)	0.44	(0.11, 1.86)	
Alcohol Intake (g/day)					–
Never	24 (28.2)	487 (27.8)	Ref		
≤median[3]	24 (28.2)	640 (36.6)	0.76	(0.43, 1.38)	
>median	37 (43.5)	623 (35.6)	1.16	(0.67, 2.00)	
Vitamin Supplement Use					–
None	61 (63.5)	1287 (63.2)	Ref		
Calcium	13 (13.5)	338 (16.6)	0.82	(0.44, 1.53)	
Vitamin D	12 (12.5)	257 (12.6)	0.89	(0.46, 1.72)	
Both	10 (10.4)	155 (7.6)	1.20	(0.59, 2.45)	
Osteoporosis Before BC Diagnosis					–

Table 4. Cont.

	Major Fracture Before BC Diagnosis – Yes	Major Fracture Before BC Diagnosis – No	OR[2]	95% CI[2]	p for trend
	n = 99	n = 2058			
	n (%)	n (%)			
No	67 (67.7)	1848 (89.8)	Ref		
Yes	32 (32.3)	210 (10.2)	3.15	(1.98, 5.02)	

NOTE: Pharmacy data through December 31, 2013.
[1] Major fracture includes fracture of spine, humerus, wrist, or hip.
[2] Logistic regression adjusted for age, race/ethnicity, menopausal status, and year of breast cancer diagnosis.
[3] Median (physical activity) = 20.9 metabolic equivalent (MET)-hours/week; median (alcohol intake) = 3.1 g/day.

cancer diagnosis with prior history of 1) osteoporosis, 2) any fracture, and 3) any major osteoporotic fracture. All models were adjusted for age, race/ethnicity, menopausal status, and year of breast cancer diagnosis, and all p-values were two-tailed with a significance level of 0.05. Analyses were repeated after excluding those diagnosed with breast cancer before menopause. The results were similar to those from the overall initial AI user group and thus are not presented here.

All analyses were conducted in SAS version 9.3 (Cary, N.C.).

Ethics Statement

The study was approved by the KPNC institutional review board.

Results

As shown in **Table 1**, the mean age at breast cancer diagnosis among AI users was 64.4 years, with 2,033 (94.5%) initially diagnosed after menopause and 118 (5.5%) before menopause. As expected, the majority of the initial AI users were diagnosed with early stage disease (AJCC stage I–III) (98.4%). The study cohort was multi-ethnic, with 71.4% White, 10.4% Hispanic, 10.3% Asian, 5.8% African American, and 2.1% other race/ethnicity. The mean BMI at baseline was 29.0 kg/m^2, with 31.8% being overweight and 38.2% obese. The median (IQR) of moderate-vigorous physical activity at baseline was 19.5 (7.3–39.1) metabolic equivalent (MET)-hours/week. Over half of the patients were never smokers at baseline (52.0%), 42.5% were former smokers, and only 5.5% were current smokers. Alcohol intake was light at baseline, with 27.9% being never drinkers, and among those who drank, the median intake was 3.10 grams/day. Nearly two-thirds of the patients did not take either calcium or vitamin D supplements at baseline (63.2%), 16.5% took calcium, 12.6% took vitamin D, and 7.7% took both supplements.

Among the initial AI users, 11.2% had a prior history of osteoporosis, including 3.5% at 6 years or more before breast cancer diagnosis, and 7.7% within 6 years (**Table 1**). 16.3% of the patients had a prior history of any fracture, including 7.6% at 6 years or more before cancer diagnosis, and 8.7% within 6 years. For major fractures of the spine, humerus, wrist, or hip, 4.6% had a prior history of these fractures, including 1.7% at 6 years or more before cancer diagnosis, and 2.9% within 6 years.

Among postmenopausal patients with HR-positive breast cancer, the majority received AIs as their initial hormonal therapy (n = 2,033, 86.2%), and 325 patients (n = 13.8%) received TAM as their initial hormonal therapy. No apparent secular trend was found in the use of AIs relative to TAM during the study period (2005–2013). To explore whether bone health history or other known risk factors for fractures might affect the choice of hormonal therapy drugs, comparisons were conducted between postmenopausal initial AI users and postmenopausal initial TAM users. As shown among the postmenopausal women in **Table 1**, compared to initial AI users, women on TAM were younger (mean age 62.0 years vs. 65.2 years, $p<0.0001$), more likely to have stage I disease (67.1% vs. 55.1%, $p = 0.0003$), less obese (mean BMI 27.6 kg/m^2 vs. 29.0 kg/m^2, $p = 0.0001$), and more physically active (median 19.4 MET-hours/week vs. 24.4 MET-hours/week, $p = 0.03$). No differences in race/ethnicity, smoking history, or alcohol intake were found between the two groups. For bone health history prior to breast cancer diagnosis, although initial TAM users were younger, they had a significantly higher prevalence of prior osteoporosis than initial AI users (21.5% vs. 11.8%, $p<0.0001$), but a similar prevalence of any prior fracture (16.3% vs. 16.6%, $p = 0.27$) and major prior fracture (5.9% vs.

4.8%, p = 0.13). Consistent with a higher prevalence of prior osteoporosis compared with AI users, TAM users were more likely to take calcium and/or vitamin D than AI users (45.0% vs. 37.3%, p = 0.003).

In Tables 2–4, the associations of selected risk factors with prior history of osteoporosis and fractures among overall initial AI users are presented. In models adjusted for age, race/ethnicity, menopausal status, and year of breast cancer diagnosis, older age (60–69 y OR = 2.43; 95% CI: 1.58, 3.72, ≥70 y OR = 5.65; 95% CI: 3.68, 8.69; p for trend<0.0001) and being Asian (OR = 1.82; 95% CI: 1.17, 2.81) were associated with higher odds of prior osteoporosis, whereas increasing BMI (overweight OR = 0.55; 95% CI: 0.40, 0.76; obese OR = 0.32; 95% CI: 0.22, 0.45; p for trend<0.0001) and being African American (OR = 0.38; 95% CI: 0.15, 0.94) were associated with lower odds (**Table 2**).

Associations of patient characteristics and lifestyle factors with prior history of any fracture are given in **Table 3**. Older age was associated with higher odds of any prior fracture (p for trend< 0.0001), whereas being Asian (OR = 0.50; 95% CI: 0.30, 0.84) was associated with lower odds of any prior fracture. In contrast to associations with prior osteoporosis, no significant increasing BMI trend was found, yet being overweight was associated with increased odds of any prior fracture (OR = 1.43; 95% CI: 1.06, 1.92). Finally, as expected, prior history of osteoporosis was associated with increased odds of prior fracture (OR = 2.86; 95% CI: 2.10, 3.89). Associations of patient characteristics and lifestyle factors with prior major fracture were largely consistent with any prior fracture, but with wider CIs (**Table 4**). Unique to analyses of major fracture, however, any moderate-vigorous physical activity was associated with reduced odds of major fracture in the AI users (≤median 20.9 MET-hours/week OR = 0.33 95% CI: 0.17, 0.64; >median OR = 0.36; 95% CI: 0.18, 0.70).

Discussion

In a large contemporary cohort of breast cancer survivors who were initially treated with AIs, we found that 11.2% had a prior history of osteoporosis, 16.3% any fracture, and 4.6% major fracture before breast cancer diagnosis. Although the majority of postmenopausal women were initially treated with AIs, a sizable proportion (13.8%) was initially treated with TAM. Furthermore, these TAM users had nearly twice the prevalence of prior osteoporosis compared with initial AI users. Finally, the associations of selected risk factors with prior history of bone health outcomes in breast cancer patients initially treated with AIs were largely consistent with those expected from the healthy older population [13,14].

To our knowledge, our observational study is the largest to date to describe the use of AIs as primary hormonal therapy in conjunction with prior bone morbidity. A previous study of 343 women with early-stage breast cancer about to initiate AI therapy reported 22.2% with osteoporosis and 11.4% with any fracture [16]. Another study of 497 breast cancer patients also at the onset of AI therapy found 19.1% with non-vertebral fractures [15]. Compared with our prevalence findings of 11.2% osteoporosis and 16.3% any fracture, Servitja et al. reported a higher rate of osteoporosis but a lower rate of fracture, whereas Bouvard et al. reported a higher rate of fracture. While these studies were limited by small sample size, they did collect baseline bone health measures of BMD, spinal X-rays, and 25-hydroxyvitamin D [25-(OH)D] concentrations. Our current analysis does not consider these data, yet in future prospective analyses of fracture risk, we will be incorporating BMD measures and 25(OH)D concentrations around baseline entry into the cohort.

For postmenopausal women diagnosed with early stage, HR-positive breast cancer, AIs have been shown to have superior efficacy in lowering risk of recurrence compared with TAM, and thus have become the preferable choice for this patient subgroup. However, TAM remains a viable choice for initial hormonal therapy for those who seek to avoid AIs' musculoskeletal effects. This is likely true for women deemed to have low risk of recurrence but are susceptible to fractures, as suggested by our results. In postmenopausal patients in our study, initial TAM users were slightly younger than initial AI users, yet the former had significantly higher prevalence of osteoporosis history. However, initial TAM users were more likely to have stage I disease than initial AI users, suggesting their risk of recurrence was lower. A lower risk of recurrence coupled with a higher risk of fracture might have influenced physicians and patients to favor TAM over AIs as their first choice of initial hormonal therapy. This speculation was further strengthened by the findings of higher usage of calcium and/or vitamin D supplement and higher physical activity in the initial TAM users than in the initial AI users. As supplement use and physical activity were surveyed soon after breast cancer diagnosis, we could not assess whether these data represent exposure status before or after the diagnosis of osteoporosis. Higher usage of supplements and being more physically active might have been in response to being diagnosed with osteoporosis (reverse causality). It is also interesting to note that a small proportion of initial AI users were diagnosed with breast cancer before menopause. Most likely those patients experienced menopause due to chemotherapy or radiation therapy and were subsequently eligible for AI therapy.

Among initial AI users, we identified several risk factors associated with history of osteoporosis, including older age, Asian race, and lower BMI. Older age was also associated with fracture history and being physically active was associated with lower risk of major prior fracture. These associations were in the same direction as expected in a general healthy older population, suggesting common mechanisms for osteoporosis and fracture regardless of later breast cancer diagnosis. Although smoking and alcohol consumption are risk factors for osteoporosis and fracture in non-cancer patients, we did not find such associations in initial AI users, possibly due to the small proportion (5.5%) of current smokers in the study and light alcohol intake in the cohort (median intake of 3.10 grams/day among drinkers). We also found that Asian AI users had a higher risk of osteoporosis but lower risk of prior fracture than Whites. This observation potentially reflects known racial/ethnic differences of lower bone mineral density, yet decreased fracture risk, in healthy Asians compared with Whites [24,25,26].

When comparing our proportion of prior fracture to healthy postmenopausal women at a similar age in the Women's Health Initiative (WHI) [27], initial postmenopausal AI users were approximately two times less likely to have a history of fracture (16.6% vs. 34.4%, p = 0.0039). The lower rate of prevalent osteoporosis and fracture seen among breast cancer patients in our study may be explained by the paradoxical association between high BMD and breast cancer risk [28]. As estrogen plays a central role in bone growth and maintenance, it also drives the development of breast cancer. Therefore, at the time of diagnosis, women with breast cancer may have had higher lifetime estrogen exposure and associated BMD than non-cancer women at a similar age, which may explain the lower prevalence of osteoporosis and fracture among breast cancer patients seen in our study.

Our study was based on a large prospective breast cancer cohort from one of the nation's largest integrated healthcare delivery systems where complete electronic medical records and pharmacy information are available on all patients. This enabled us to accurately assess bone health history through their health insurance membership with Kaiser Permanente. Moreover, the cohort was established in 2005, a time concurrent with the widespread use of AIs. Our study was further strengthened by the availability of extensive demographic and lifestyle information collected at the time of diagnosis through in-person interviews.

Nevertheless, our study is not without limitations. Due to its cross-sectional nature, we could not infer causality of the selected risk factors for prevalent osteoporosis and fracture among breast cancer patients. In addition, osteoporosis was potentially underdiagnosed in our patient population. However, this is not a unique challenge to this study. Clinicians vary in their use and coding of the term osteoporosis such that it may be identified after BMD testing, after a primary care visit, at the time of a specialty visit, at the time of bisphosphonate initiation, or at the time of fracture. Further, a diagnosis may not always mean that the T-score is in the osteoporosis range, and a diagnosis could also be made in the presence of a fragility fracture while BMD is only in the osteopenic range. There have also been temporal changes in the frequency of osteoporosis diagnosis [29], which may explain the greater proportion of AI users with *a priori* osteoporosis diagnosis, as AIs did not become the preferential choice of hormonal therapy for postmenopausal breast cancer patients until the mid-2000's. To overcome this limitation, we classified patients with BP treatment but without an ICD-9 diagnosis of osteoporosis as osteoporotic. The results were similar when we relied only on osteoporosis ICD-9 diagnosis. Furthermore, the prevalence of prior spine fractures could have been underestimated due to asymptomatic fractures not being coded by the physician, but for our analyses, we considered spine fractures as clinically diagnosed. Finally, given our access to electronic medical records on the cohort, we estimate that only 35% had BMD measurements before breast cancer diagnosis based on Current Procedural Terminology (CPT) codes, thus precluding us from classifying osteoporosis status based on BMD data for the entire cohort. To note, the prevalence of prior BMD screening in our cohort is greater than 16% reported in a small study of BMD screening adherence among 342 breast cancer patients on AIs, and these women were also members of an integrated health care system [30].

To conclude, a small proportion of breast cancer patients initially treated with AIs had a positive history of osteoporosis or fracture before their cancer diagnosis. A history of osteoporosis might influence the choice of initial hormonal therapy drug among patients with low risk of recurrence. Risk factors for osteoporosis and fracture before breast cancer diagnosis were similar to those among healthy older women. Given that adverse effects on bone health is a common comorbidity concern for many cancer survivors [31], our findings may have wide clinical applicability beyond breast cancer that emphasize the importance of full consideration of prior bone health history before initiation of cancer treatment.

Author Contributions

Conceived and designed the experiments: MLK SY. Analyzed the data: CAL JMR MC CPQ MLK SY. Contributed reagents/materials/analysis tools: MLK SY. Contributed to the writing of the manuscript: MLK JCL LT JMR TEH CCH LSC DLH CPQ CBA LHK SY.

References

1. Geisler J, Haynes B, Anker G, Dowsett M, Lonning PE (2002) Influence of letrozole and anastrozole on total body aromatization and plasma estrogen levels in postmenopausal breast cancer patients evaluated in a randomized, cross-over study. J Clin Oncol 20: 751–757.
2. Chien AJ, Goss PE (2006) Aromatase inhibitors and bone health in women with breast cancer. J Clin Oncol 24: 5305–5312.
3. Boccardo F (2008) Switching to anastrozole after tamoxifen improves survival in postmenopausal women with breast cancer. Nat Clin Pract Oncol 5: 76–77.
4. Dowsett M, Cuzick J, Ingle J, Coates A, Forbes J, et al. (2010) Meta-analysis of breast cancer outcomes in adjuvant trials of aromatase inhibitors versus tamoxifen. J Clin Oncol 28: 509–518.
5. Burstein HJ, Prestrud AA, Seidenfeld J, Anderson H, Buchholz TA, et al. (2010) American Society of Clinical Oncology clinical practice guideline: update on adjuvant endocrine therapy for women with hormone receptor-positive breast cancer. J Clin Oncol 28: 3784–3796.
6. Hadji P (2009) Aromatase inhibitor-associated bone loss in breast cancer patients is distinct from postmenopausal osteoporosis. Crit Rev Oncol Hematol 69: 73–82.
7. Hillner BE, Ingle JN, Chlebowski RT, Gralow J, Yee GC, et al. (2003) American Society of Clinical Oncology 2003 update on the role of bisphosphonates and bone health issues in women with breast cancer. J Clin Oncol 21: 4042–4057.
8. Body JJ, Bergmann P, Boonen S, Boutsen Y, Devogelaer JP, et al. (2007) Management of cancer treatment-induced bone loss in early breast and prostate cancer – a consensus paper of the Belgian Bone Club. Osteoporos Int 18: 1439–1450.
9. Reid DM, Doughty J, Eastell R, Heys SD, Howell A, et al. (2008) Guidance for the management of breast cancer treatment-induced bone loss: a consensus position statement from a UK Expert Group. Cancer Treat Rev 34 Suppl 1: S3–18.
10. Gralow JR, Biermann JS, Farooki A, Fornier MN, Gagel RF, et al. (2013) NCCN Task Force Report: Bone Health In Cancer Care. J Natl Compr Canc Netw 11 Suppl 3: S1–50; quiz S51.
11. Siris ES, Genant HK, Laster AJ, Chen P, Misurski DA, et al. (2007) Enhanced prediction of fracture risk combining vertebral fracture status and BMD. Osteoporos Int 18: 761–770.
12. Nguyen ND, Eisman JA, Center JR, Nguyen TV (2007) Risk factors for fracture in nonosteoporotic men and women. The Journal of clinical endocrinology and metabolism 92: 955–962.
13. Cummings SR, Nevitt MC, Browner WS, Stone K, Fox KM, et al. (1995) Risk factors for hip fracture in white women. Study of Osteoporotic Fractures Research Group. The New England journal of medicine 332: 767–773.
14. Robbins J, Aragaki AK, Kooperberg C, Watts N, Wactawski-Wende J, et al. (2007) Factors associated with 5-year risk of hip fracture in postmenopausal women. Jama 298: 2389–2398.
15. Bouvard B, Hoppe E, Soulie P, Georgin-Mege M, Jadaud E, et al. (2012) High prevalence of vertebral fractures in women with breast cancer starting aromatase inhibitor therapy. Annals of oncology: official journal of the European Society for Medical Oncology/ESMO 23: 1151–1156.
16. Servitja S, Nogues X, Prieto-Alhambra D, Martinez-Garcia M, Garrigos L, et al. (2012) Bone health in a prospective cohort of postmenopausal women receiving aromatase inhibitors for early breast cancer. Breast 21: 95–101.
17. Kwan ML, Ambrosone CB, Lee MM, Barlow J, Krathwohl SE, et al. (2008) The Pathways Study: a prospective study of breast cancer survivorship within Kaiser Permanente Northern California. Cancer Causes Control 19: 1065–1076.
18. Oehrli MD, Quesenberry CP (2013) 2013 Annual Report on Trends, Incidence, and Outcomes. Kaiser Permanente, Northern California Cancer Registry.
19. Staten LK, Taren DL, Howell WH, Tobar M, Poehlman ET, et al. (2001) Validation of the Arizona Activity Frequency Questionnaire using doubly labeled water. Med Sci Sports Exerc 33: 1959–1967.
20. Selby JV, Smith DH, Johnson ES, Raebel MA, Friedman GD, et al. (2005) Kaiser Permanente Medical Care Program. In: BL S, editor. Pharmacoepidemiology. West Sussex: John Wiley & Sons, Ltd. 241–259.
21. Chau S, Chandra M, Grimsrud CD, Gonzalez JR, Hui RL, et al. (2014) Femur fracture classification in women with a history of breast cancer. Journal of Bone Oncology 3: 49–53.
22. Siris ES, Miller PD, Barrett-Connor E, Faulkner KG, Wehren LE, et al. (2001) Identification and fracture outcomes of undiagnosed low bone mineral density in postmenopausal women: results from the National Osteoporosis Risk Assessment. JAMA: the journal of the American Medical Association 286: 2815–2822.
23. Vestergaard P, Rejnmark L, Mosekilde L (2005) Osteoporosis is markedly underdiagnosed: a nationwide study from Denmark. Osteoporosis international: a journal established as result of cooperation between the European Foundation for Osteoporosis and the National Osteoporosis Foundation of the USA 16: 134–141.
24. Liu XS, Walker MD, McMahon DJ, Udesky J, Liu G, et al. (2011) Better skeletal microstructure confers greater mechanical advantages in Chinese-American

women versus white women. Journal of bone and mineral research: the official journal of the American Society for Bone and Mineral Research 26: 1783–1792.
25. Walker MD, Liu XS, Stein E, Zhou B, Bezati E, et al. (2011) Differences in bone microarchitecture between postmenopausal Chinese-American and white women. Journal of bone and mineral research: the official journal of the American Society for Bone and Mineral Research 26: 1392–1398.
26. Walker MD, Saeed I, McMahon DJ, Udesky J, Liu G, et al. (2012) Volumetric bone mineral density at the spine and hip in Chinese American and White women. Osteoporosis international: a journal established as result of cooperation between the European Foundation for Osteoporosis and the National Osteoporosis Foundation of the USA 23: 2499–2506.
27. Jackson RD, LaCroix AZ, Gass M, Wallace RB, Robbins J, et al. (2006) Calcium plus vitamin D supplementation and the risk of fractures. N Engl J Med 354: 669–683.
28. Eastell R (2007) Breast cancer and the risk of osteoporotic fracture: A paradox. The Journal of clinical endocrinology and metabolism 92: 42–43.
29. National Osteoporosis Foundation (2002) America's Bone Health: The State of Osteoporosis and Low Bone Mass in Our Nation. Available: http://noforg/files/nof/public/content/file/63/upload/49pdf. Accessed 2014 Jun 13.
30. Spangler L, Yu O, Loggers E, Boudreau DM (2013) Bone mineral density screening among women with a history of breast cancer treated with aromatase inhibitors. Journal of women's health 22: 132–140.
31. Lustberg MB, Reinbolt RE, Shapiro CL (2012) Bone health in adult cancer survivorship. Journal of clinical oncology: official journal of the American Society of Clinical Oncology 30: 3665–3674.

16

Effect of Low-Magnitude Whole-Body Vibration Combined with Alendronate in Ovariectomized Rats: A Random Controlled Osteoporosis Prevention Study

Guo-Xian Chen[1,2]¶, Shuai Zheng[1]¶, Shuai Qin[3]¶, Zhao-Ming Zhong[1], Xiu-Hua Wu[1], Zhi-Ping Huang[1], Wei Li[1], Ruo-Ting Ding[1], Hui Yu[1], Jian-Ting Chen[1]*

1 Department of Orthopedic Spinal Surgery, Nanfang Hospital, Southern Medical University, Guangdong Province, Guangzhou, China, **2** Department of Orthopedic, the First Hospital of Putian City, Fujian Province, Putian City, China, **3** Department of ophthalmology, The People's Hospital of Zhuhai, Zhuhai, China

Abstract

Background: Alendronate (ALE) is a conventional drug used to treat osteoporosis. Low-magnitude whole-body vibration (WBV) exercise has been developed as a potential treatment for osteoporosis. The aim of this study was to investigate whether low-magnitude WBV could enhance the protective effect of ALE on bone properties in ovariectomized rats.

Methods: A total of 128 Sprague-Dawley rats were randomly divided into five groups (SHAM, OVX+VEH, OVX+WBV, OVX + ALE, OVX+WBV+ALE). The level of WBV applied was 0.3 g at 45–55 Hz for 20 min/day, 5 day/week and for 3 months. ALE was administered in dose of 1 mg/Kg once a week. Every four weeks eight rats from each group were sacrificed and their blood and both tibiae were harvested. The expression of osteocalcin and CTX in serum was measured by enzyme-linked immunosorbent assay (ELISA) and the tibiae were subjected to metaphyseal three-point bending and μCT analysis.

Results: Osteocalcin rose after ovariectomy and was not appreciably changed by either alendronate or WBV alone or in combination. Alendronate treatment significantly prevented an increase in CTX. WBV alone treatment did not alter this effect. Compared with the OVX+WBV group, nearly all tested indices such as the BV/TV, TV apparent, Tb.N, Tb.Th, and Conn.D were higher in the OVX+ALE group at week 12.Compared with the OVX+WBV group, certain tested indices such as BV/TV, TV apparent, Tb.N, and Con.D, were higher in the OVX+WBV+ALE group at week 12. At week 12, tibiae treated with WBV+ALE exhibited a significantly higher F_{max} compared to the OVX+VEH group, and a significant difference was also found in energy absorption between the OVX+WBV+ALE and OVX+VEH groups.

Conclusions: Compared with the WBV, ALE was more effective at preventing bone loss and improved the trabecular architecture. However, WBV enhanced the effect of alendronate in ovariectomized rats by inducing further improvements in trabecular architecture.

Editor: Luc Malaval, INSERM U1059/LBTO, Université Jean Monnet, France

Funding: This work was supported in part by the National Natural Science Foundation of China (No. 81000785, 81272042), and by the Natural Science Foundation of Guangdong Province (No. S2012040006830, S2012010008875). The funders had no role in study design, data collection and analysis, decision to publish, or preparation of the manuscript.

Competing Interests: The authors have declared that no competing interests exist.

* E-mail: chenjt99@tom.com

¶ These authors contributed equally to this work.

Introduction

With an increasing aging population worldwide, osteoporosis has become a growing public concern [1]. Osteoporosis is characterized by an imbalance between bone formation and absorption. Osteoporosis causes not only osteoporotic fracture and postural deformities, but also causes chronic and acute back pain, which can potentially results in disability and deterioration in the quality of life (QOL) in elderly females [2–3]. In humans, menopause is accompanied by increased bone turnover, which can result in bone loss of approximately 2%/year over five years and an increased susceptibility to fractures [4–5]. Moreover, osteoporotic fractures can increase the financial burden of medical care [6–7]. Thus, there is an urgent need to develop effective and safe approaches to increase bone strength.

Bisphosphonates, such as alendronate (ALE), are potent inhibitors of osteoclast-mediated bone resorption that suppress bone turnover through their ability to prevent the initiation of new erosion sites and to reduce ongoing excavation [8–9]. ALE is therapeutic candidate for preventing bone loss in estrogen-deficient states [10–11]. ALE has been proven effective in rats in preventing bone loss associated with immobilization by reducing bone resorption [12]. Previous evidence suggests that ALE can reduce back pain and increase activities of daily living in elderly females [3]. Furthermore, it is well-known that many drugs, including ALE, have corresponding adverse reactions, which limit certain patients from taking this drug long-term.

Recently, low-magnitude whole-body vibration (WBV) exercise has been developed as a new and effective method for treating osteoporosis [13]. Many studies have shown that mechanical stimulation via WBV is beneficial for maintaining and/or enhancing bone mass [14–16], and improving neuromuscular function [17–18], as well as other physiological benefits. The attractiveness of such a therapy relies on its ability to be applied in a low-impact manner, which is critical for individuals with impaired mobility and attenuated muscle strength [19–20]; for example elderly or diseased people.

However, to the best of our knowledge, there are no published studies investigating the effect of WBV combined with ALE in ovariectomized rats. The aim of this study was to investigate the effect of WBV combined with ALE in ovariectomized rats and to determine whether WBV exercise would enhance the effect of ALE on bone turnover and bone properties in ovariectomized rats.

Materials and Methods

Ethics statement

This study was performed in strict accordance with the guidelines of caring for laboratory animals of the Ministry of Science and Technology of the People's Republic of China. All animal procedures were approved by the Committee on the Ethics of Animal Experiments of Southern Medical University. All surgeries were performed using isoflurane anesthesia, and every effort were made to minimize suffering. At the end of the experiment isoflurane was used for animal euthanasia.

Specimens

A total of 128 (32 in the Sham group, and 24 in each treatment groups) female Sprague-Dawley rats (eight weeks old, purchased from the Laboratory Animals center of Southern Medical University, acclimate to one week in our facility) were used in this experiment. The rats were raised in a 12-h light/dark cycle and fed a standard rodent diet (provided by Laboratory Animals center of Southern Medical University) and water ad libitum. The experimental animals were randomly assigned to five groups (Sham, OVX+VEH, OVX+WBV, OVX+ALE, OVX+WBV+ALE) according to body weight with either skin incision and suture, ovariectomized with VEH (Vehicle, in this study it was PBS which was used to make RSA solution.), ovariectomized with WBV (0.3 g at 45–55 Hz for continuous 20 min/day, 5 day/week, for 3 months), ovariectomized with ALE (intragastric administration 1 mg/Kg, once a week) or ovariectomized with WBV and ALE.

During the experimental period, the body weight of the rats in all groups was measured using electronic scale every four weeks during the experimental period. The rats were sacrificed at four predetermined time points for the Sham group (0, 4, 8 and 12 weeks) and three time points for the remaining four groups (4, 8 and 12 weeks). There were 32 animals in the Sham groups and 24 animals in each treatment groups. At sacrifice, whole blood was collected with a cardiac puncture to determine the serum osteocalcin (OC) and CTX (C-terminal cross-linked telopeptides of type I collagen, CTX) using standard laboratory techniques. The bilateral tibiae were collected, with the soft tissues being thoroughly removed and wrapped in normal saline-soaked gauze and stored at −20°C until further use for biomechanical testing and micro-CT scanning.

Ovariectomy procedure

In this study, surgery was performed on 96 Sprague-Dawley rats to remove the ovaries. Sham surgeries (where the surgery was performed, but the ovaries were not removed) were performed on 36 rats (Sham group). The animals were anesthetized using isoflurane. The lower abdomen was surgically scrubbed and an incision was made to expose the ovaries and uterus. The ovaries were removed, and subsequently, the muscles and skin were sutured. All animals recovered from the surgery without incident. Uterine weight was measured using electronic scale.

Serum markers

Blood was obtained from the rat cardiac puncture prior to their sacrifice, and the specimens were centrifuged to isolate the serum and stored at −80°C, until the samples were further analyzed for osteocalcin (OC bone formation markers) and CTX, bone resorption markers according to the manufacturer's instructions. The two markers were measured using an enzyme-linked immunosorbent assay (ELISA Cusabio, Wu Han, China). The absorbance at 450 nm was measured using a spectrophotometric plate reader.

Micro-CT scanning

The left tibiae were stored in the saline soaked gauze at −20°C. The micro-architecture of the trabecular bone were assessed by using a high-resolution micro-CT system (μCT80, Scanco Medical AG, Bassersdorf, Switzerland) equipped with a 12 μm focal spot microfocus X-ray tube as the source.

The bone morphology and density parameters were measured at one location in the left tibia. The scanning region used for the structural evaluation was defined as a 2-mm region, which started from 2 mm distal to the proximal growth plate (Fig. 1 A and C). The tissue volume (TV) was determined by thresholding the image at 0.50 g/cm^3, and quantifying the enclosed voxels with an additional dilation-erosion step to fill in the occasional small voids in the cortical wall. The bone volume (BV) was a subset of the tissue volume threshold. The ratio of BV/TV represented the normalized bone volume. Low-density foam was used to position the specimen tightly in the sample holder to ensure that there would be no relative movement between the specimen and the sample holder during the scan. The resulting grayscale images obtained had an isotropic voxel size of 12 μm, and the X-ray tube was operated at 55 k V p and 49 μA.

Biomechanical testing

The mechanical properties of the tibiae were investigated using the three-point bending method using a miniature Instron materials testing machine (Electroplus E1000 Test System) with a 2000 N load cell (Fig. 1B). The tibiae were thawed at room temperature for 30 min prior to testing the region of interest, as shown in Fig. 1C. The samples, which were continuously moistened with isotonic saline solution during the test, were placed on a base consisting of an aluminum block with one-rounded edge-free notch on the top (Fig. 1B). The end of the dorsal proximal tibia (the two condyles) was placed in one of the notches (b in Fig. 1B). Because of its curved shape, the posterior distal diaphysis was rested on the other side of base (c in Fig. 1B). During the breaking test, the proximal tibia could not slip due to the notch on the base, but it was able to lengthen along the diaphyseal axis. The tip of the stamp consisted of an axle-led aluminum roller (8 mm high, 8 mm wide, 8 mm in diameter). A 2-mm-wide and 1-mm-deep circular notch with rounded edges was located in the center of the roller (a in Fig. 1B). The speed of the

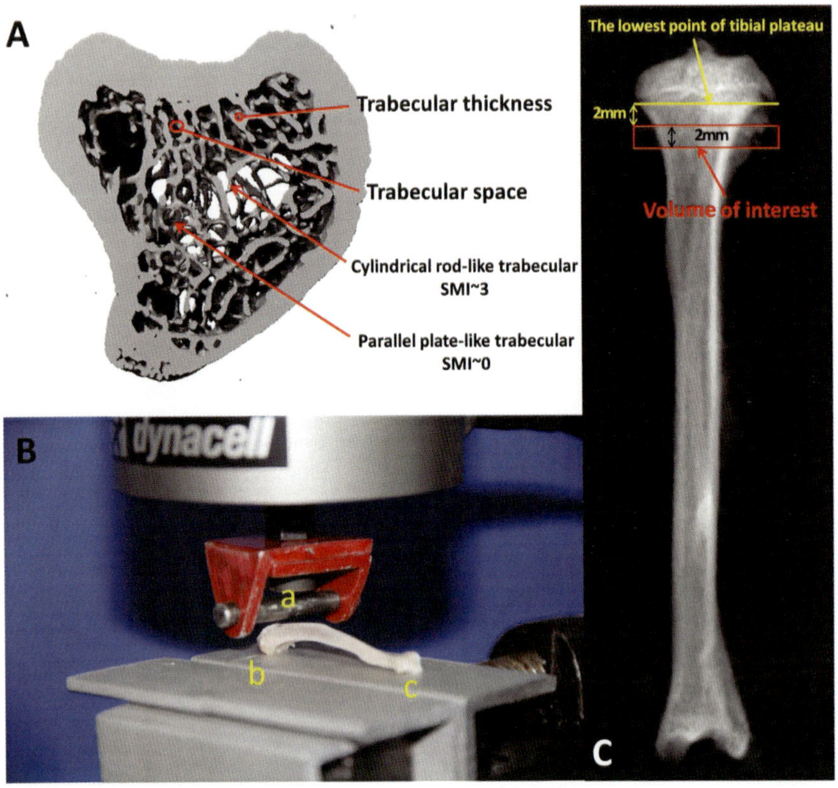

Figure 1. General introduction of the experimental methods of μCT and the three-point bending test. (A) Experimental parameters of the rat tibia scanned using μCT. (B) Details on the experimental design of the three-point bending test consisting of an aluminum block and rounded edge-free notches. (C) The volume of test samples using μCT and the three-point bending test.

feed motion was 5 mm/min with 5% strain rate, and the test was automatically stopped after a loss of strength at >20 N or a linear change of >2 mm to avoid shattering the tibial specimens. The maximum load (Fmax), energy absorption and stiffness (S) were collected using Bluehill 2 (Version 2.28.832, Instron, a Division of Illinois Tool Works Inc). The experiment was blinded with regard to the association between the bones and animal groups.

Statistical analyses

The results were expressed as the means ± standard deviation (SD). Significant differences between the means for different groups were compared using one-way analysis of variance (ANOVA). Multiple comparisons were performed using the LSD method or Dunnett's C method. Comparisons of several treatments with the control group were evaluated using the Dunnett's T3 procedure. All statistical analyses were performed using SPSS 13.0 software. A significance level of $P<0.05$ was used for all comparisons.

Results

Monitoring

The uterus index was represented as the uterus weight divided by body weight. The data were expressed as mean ± SD (Fig. 2). As shown in Fig. 2, at week 0 of ovariectomy surgery, there was no significant difference in average weight among all the testing groups. However, the average weight of sham group was significantly lower than that of the other four study groups at week 4, at week 8, and at week 12. There was a general trend of longitudinal increase in the body weight for all the testing groups. The uterus index of the sham group was significantly higher than that of the other four study groups. However, there were no significant differences among the four study groups in both indices.

Serum markers

The results for osteocalcin and CTX in the different groups at different time points are provided in Table 1. Compared with the Sham group osteocalcin (OC) rose in OVX+VEH group as well as in the other three treatment groups. The OVX+ALE group showed a significantly elevated level of OC at week 4 (+9%, $p=0.036$), and the OVX+WBV group also exhibited a significantly elevated level of OC at week 8 (+13.4%, $P<0.001$) compared with the OVX+VEH group. However, OVX + WBV+ALE group showed no significant difference compared with the OVX+VEH group.

With regard to bone resorption,CTX rose after ovariectomy. ALE treatment significantly prevented an increase in this serum marker. WBV alone treatment did not alter this effect. As shown in the table 1, the OVX+ALE and OVX+WBV+ALE group showed a significantly lower level of CTX compared to the OVX+VEH group at week 4 (−28.2%, $P=0.002$; −29%, $P=0.001$), week 8 (−19.6%, $P=0.002$; −21.1%, $P=0.002$) and week 12 (−29.6%, $P<0.001$; −25.5%, $p<0.001$). Moreover, at no point in the study was a significant difference found between the OVX+VEH and OVX+WBV groups for CTX.

Micro-CT scanning

The alteration of trabecular micro-architecture in the tibial metaphyseal region measured using μ CT is shown in Fig. 3, and

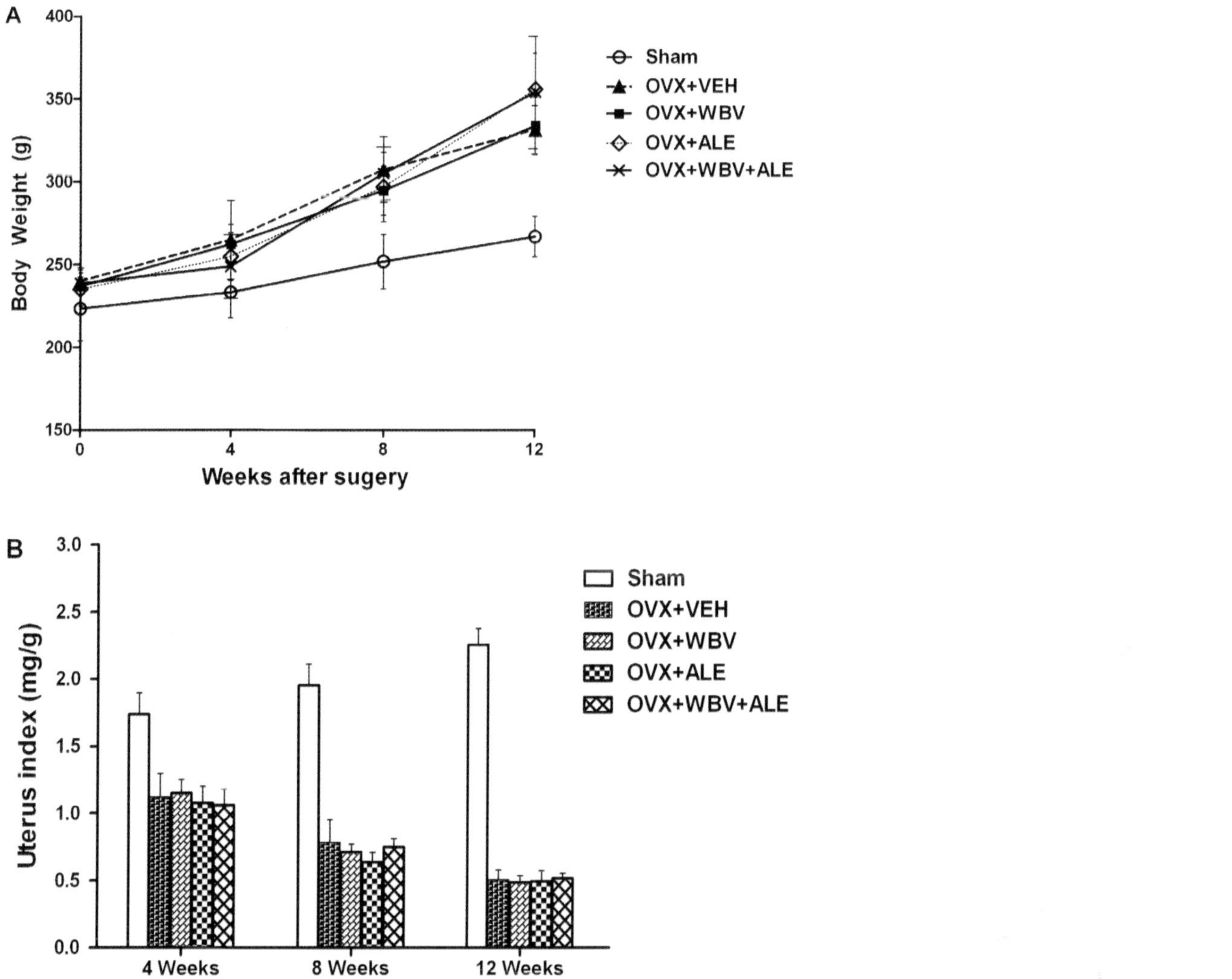

Figure 2. The body weight and uterus index of rats are provided in Fig.2. Body weight (A) and uterus index (B) changes measured using an electronic scale. *P<0.01 compared with the sham group.

the representative three-dimensional micro-CT reconstructions images are illustrated in Fig. 4.

At week 4, all of the morphological parameters [bone volume/ tissue volume (BV/TV), structure model index (SMI), connective density (Conn. D), trabecular number (Tb. N), TV apparent, BV material, trabecular thickness (Tb. T h) and trabecular space (Tb. Sp)] showed no significant difference between the OVX+VEH and OVX+WBV groups, the OVX+VEH and OVX+ALE groups, the OVX+WBV and OVX+ALE groups, and the OVX+WBV and OVX+WBV+ALE groups (P>0.05). Furthermore, the OVX+ALE group elevated the BV/TV (+20%, p = 0.037) and Tb. T h (+23.6%, P = 0.006) compared with the OVX+VEH group at week 8.

Compared with the OVX+VEH group, nearly all tested indices were higher in the OVX+ALE group at week 12, such as the BV/ TV (+73%, P<0.001), TV apparent (+89.9%, P<0.001), Tb. N (+ 29.9%, P<0.001), Tb. T h (+56.3%, P<0.001), and Conn. D (+ 53.6%, P = 0.012), and the SMI (−31.3%, P<0.001) and Tb. Sp (−38.7%, P = 0.027) were lower in the OVX+ALE group. Moreover, compared with the OVX+VEH group, the BV/TV (+38.1%, P<0.001), Tb. N (+12.3%, P = 0.015), Tb. Th (+33.7%, P = 0.001), and Conn. D (+47.5%, P = 0.029) were higher, and the SMI (−17.9%, P = 0.003) was lower in the OVX+WBV group.

Compared with the OVX+WBV group, the BV/TV (+25.3%, p = 0.004), TV apparent (+60.3%, P<0.001), BV material (+ 28.4%, P = 0.044), Tb. N (+15.6%, P = 0.001), and Tb. T h (+ 16.9%, p = 0.037) were higher, and the SMI (−16.4%, p = 0.013) was lower in the OVX+ALE group at week 12. At week 12, significant differences were found for some tested indices between the OVX+ALE and OVX+WBV+ALE groups. Compared with the OVX+ ALE group, the BV/TV (+25%, p = 0.001), TV apparent (+30.4%, P = 0.032), Tb. N (+10%, P = 0.015), and Con. D (+44.5%, p = 0.042) were higher, and the SMI (−18.4%, p = 0.042) was lower in the OVX+WBV+ALE group.

Biomechanical testing

The mean maximum load (F_{max}), energy absorption and stiffness for all five groups at different time points are shown in Fig. 5. As the rats become older, the F_{max} of the sham group increased from 85.55±10.67 N at week 4 to 106.78±12.17 N at week 12 (+24.8%). Furthermore, the bone biomechanical parameters in the right tibiae were unchanged in all five groups at week 4. Moreover, the F_{max} in the right tibia showed no significant

Table 1. Quantitative analysis of bone formation (osteocalcin) and resorption (CTX) markers of the serum levels in rats.

Groups		Weeks after surgery			
		0	4	8	12
Osteocalcin (ng/mL)	SHAM	30.13±1.04	30.52±1.35	28.78±1.04	28.10±1.69
		(3.45%)	(4.41%)	(3.61%)	(6.03%)
	OVX+VEH	——	36.92±1.54[a]	33.21±1.15[a]	35.29±2.38[a]
			(4.17%)	(3.45%)	(6.75%)
	OVX+WBV	——	35.49±1.00a	37.66±0.82[a+b]	34.45±1.40[a]
			(2.82%)	(2.19%)	(4.07%)
	OVX +ALE	——	39.87±0.82[a+b]	37.89±3.43[a]	37.48±2.12[a]
			(2.05%)	(9.05%)	(5.66%)
	OVX+WBV+ALE	——	35.61±1.27[a]	37.07±2.99[a]	36.85±2.78[a]
			(3.56%)	(8.06%)	(7.53%)
CTX (ng/mL)	SHAM	21.52±1.98	31.02±3.95	34.21±1.56	33.71±4.06
		(9.20%)	(12.74%)	(4.55%)	(12.04%)
	OVX+VEH	——	43.05±4.34[a]	44.09±3.14[a]	51.61±3.86[a]
			(10.07%)	(7.12%)	(7.47%)
	OVX+WBV	——	48.70±2.55[a]	42.15±4.13[a]	49.24±4.03[a]
			(5.24%)	(9.79%)	(8.18%)
	OVX +ALE	——	30.90±2.15[b] (6.96%)	35.47±1.96[b] (5.52%)	36.31±2.37[b] (6.53%)
	OVX+WBV+ALE	——	30.56±2.86[b]	34.78±1.15[b]	38.45±2.27[b]
			(9.38%)	(3.32%)	(5.91%)

Values were the mean ± SD. The coefficient of variation of each bone biomarkers were presented under the data.
[a]: Significant difference from the SHAM group ($p<0.05$);
[b]: Significant difference from the OVX+VEH group ($p<0.05$).

difference between the OVX+VEH and OVX+WBV groups (P = 1.000), the OVX+WBV and OVX+ALE groups (P = 1.000), and the OVX+ALE and OVX+WBV+ALE groups (P = 1.000) at week 8 or week 12. However, compared with the OVX+ VEH (69.80±9.23 N) group, the F_{max} were higher in the OVX+ALE group (89.07±4.96 N, +27.6%, P = 0.009) or in the OVX+WBV+ ALE group (89.86±6.21 N, +28.7%, P = 0.008) at week 12.

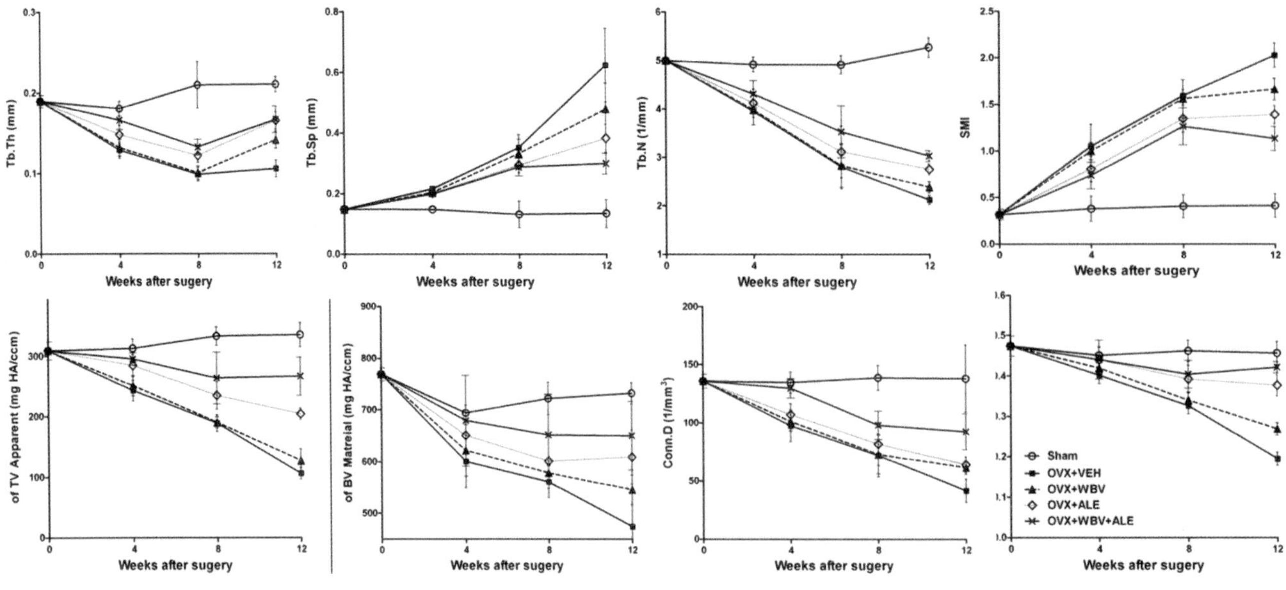

Figure 3. Morphological parameters of trabecular changes throughout the experiment as measured using μCT. Each value was derived from a single serial cross-section obtained from the left tibia of the rats. Data were presented as the mean ± SD.

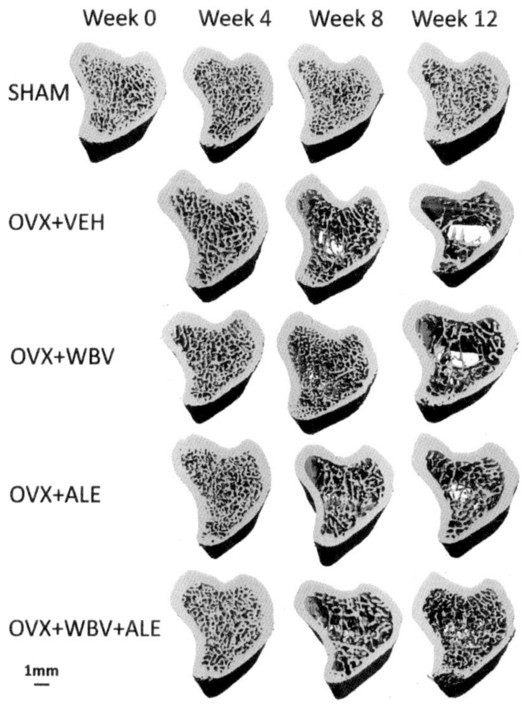

Figure 4. Three-dimensional μCT images of the metaphyseal tibia of the SHAM, OVX+VEH, OVX+WBV, OVX+ALE, and OVX+WBV+ALE-treated Sprague Dawley rats at the time of operation and follow-up measurements after four, eight and 12 weeks. Images were selected from animals with median cancellous BV/TV values.

As shown in Fig. 5, the bone energy absorption and bone stiffness in the tibia gradually decreased from four weeks to 12 weeks in the four study groups. At week 8, there were no significant differences for energy absorption in the four groups examined. At week 12, compared with the OVX+ VEH group (52.03±1.58 N), bone energy absorption were higher in both the OVX+ALE group (66.27±2.64 N, +27.4%, P = 0.040) and the OVX+WBV+ALE group (76.81±3.23 N, +47.6%, P = 0.003), but no significant differences were detected between the OVX+VEH and OVX+WBV groups (p = 0.815). As well, there were no significant differences for stiffness at any point in the four study groups examined.

Discussion

This study investigated the effects of ALE, low-magnitude WBV and the combination of ALE and low-magnitude WBV on the ovariectomy-induced osteoporosis. In our study, the changes in bone quality were assessed through biomarkers, micro-CT, and three-point bending tests.

The SHAM group served as a negative control to illustrate normal bone growth over the course of the experiment. The OVX+VEH group was a positive control group to study changes occurring during the development of osteoporotic condition following the ovariectomy. Our results showed similar differences between the OVX+VEH and SHAM groups as have been previously characterized by micro-CT [21–25] and three point bending tests [26]. In our study, the OVX+VEH group had significantly higher levels of OC and CTX compared to the SHAM group. The uterus index of the sham group in our experiment was significantly higher than that of the other four groups. The effects of individual treatments such as ALE or low-magnitude WBV have also been extensively studied. However, to the best of our knowledge, there are no published studies investigating the effect of WBV combined with ALE on ovariectomized rats. Here we have shown the addition of low-magnitude WBV to ALE therapy improves trabecular architecture.

Bisphosphonates, such as ALE, have demonstrated compelling effects in the treatment of osteoporosis [27]. ALE has been shown to increase lumbar bone mineral density (BMD) and prevent vertebral fractures in post-menopausal females with osteoporosis [28–29]. Bisphosphonates are potent inhibitors of bone turnover [30]. These inhibitors act directly on osteoclasts to reduce bone resorption [31] and have been shown to reduce bone loss in established osteoporosis [32–33] and prevent bone loss in early menopause [34] or after surgical oophorectomy [35]. As shown in the table 1, vehicle-treated ALE significantly reduced the CTX serum level (−28.2%, at week 4; −19.6%, at week 8; −29.6%, at week 12) and increased the OC serum level (+9%, at week 4) compared with the OVX+VEH group. Osteocalcin, a non-collagenous protein synthesized by mature osteoblasts, is generally regarded as a specific marker of bone formation [36–37]. Furthermore, CTX, a collagen degradation product released by osteoclasts, is considered as a marker of bone resorption [38–39]. This study demonstrated that ALE inhibited osteoclast-mediated bone resorption and improved osteoblast-mediated bone formation.

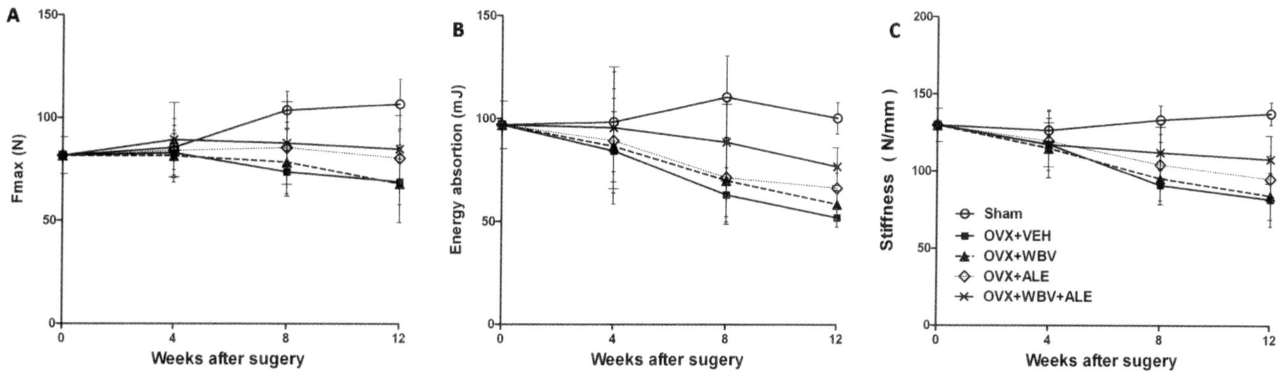

Figure 5. Change in the mechanical property at the metaphyseal tibia as measured using the three-point bending test. Each value was obtained from the right tibia of the rats. Data were presented as the mean ± SD.

Compared with histological analyses, micro-CT, can directly measure bone micro-architecture without relying on stereological models and is now regarded as the "gold standard" for the evaluation of bone morphology and micro-architecture in rats and other small animal models [40]. Micro-CT has provided evidence of a slight, local beneficial effect of ALE on trabecular bone. Our data fromμCT revealed that the micro-architectural bone parameters in the OVX+ALE group were significantly higher than that in the OVX+VEH group in nearly all tested indices at week 12. Thus, on the basis of these results ALE improve trabecular architecture.

The three-point bending test was utilized in this study to evaluate bone strength. The tibia samples were placed on a base that consisted of an aluminum block with one rounded edge-free notch on the top, and this design prevented slipping or tipping of the tibia with increasing punctual strength (Fig. 1B). At week 12, tibia treated with OVX+ALE had a significantly higher F_{max} and bone energy absorption compared to the OVX+VEH group. As such, ALE improved trabecular architecture and bone strength.

Therapeutic low-magnitude high-frequency whole-body vibration (WBV) has been shown to mitigate bone loss and improve neuromuscular function in specific studies [41–42]. It has been well-established that mechanical stimulation of bone formation is largely affected by the magnitude of the applied bone strain [43–47]. Many present studies show that WBV can subtly affect aging bone characteristics, depending on the region and vibrated parameters. For example, one study [48] showed that an acceleration of 0.5 g was favorable for bone density throughout most of the femur, whereas 1.5 g was largely ineffective in the femur, although it enhanced bone strength and stiffness in the radius. There was also a significant increase in the mineralizing surface in the distal femur for both vibration magnitudes. Another study showed [49] that WBV applied at increasing accelerations (0.1, 0.3, and 1.0 g) enhanced trabecular bone volume >30% in a non-dose-dependent fashion as assessed by histomorphometry in the proximal tibia of adult rats while no effect was observed at other bone sites such as vertebrae or femur. Thus the frequency and the amplitude of the sinusoidal vibration may have variable effects at different sites. The physical condition of the patient might also contribute to the efficacy of WBV [50–51]. Current literature [52–53] suggests a provisional consensus is building toward low-amplitude, high-frequency vibration as an effective and safe form of vibration. In contrast, high-amplitude vibration has unwanted consequences when chronically applied, as noted by a generation of studies correlating low back pain and other ailments to occupational vibration [54]. In animal models, bone formation rate has been shown to be retained in a model of disuse osteopenia when treated with 0.25 g WBV [55]. Similarly, in an oophorectomized rat model, 3.0 g WBV have a good effective on promoting the bone formation, as well as retention of muscle strength otherwise lost to the hormonal deficiency [42]. Garman et al. [56] reported that trabecular bone formation rate to bone surface ratio (BFR/BS) and mineralizing surface to bone surface ratio (MS/BS) were enhanced in female mice following 3 weeks of vibration. These enhancements in BFR/BS and MS/BS were acceleration-dependent with higher BFR/BS and MS/BS with the 0.3 g treatment vs. 0.6 g treatment.

In our study, we used the low-magnitude, low-amplitude high-frequency stimulus. WBV significantly increased the OC serum level (+13.4%, at week 8) compared with the OVX+VEH group. As shown in Fig. 3 and Fig. 4 the micro-architectural bone parameters (BV/TV, Tb. N, Tb. T h, Conn. D) in OVX+WBV group were significantly higher than that of the OVX+VEH group at week 12. This finding was similar to several published studies [57–58]. In conclusion, our results supported that WBV could improve bone formation and trabecular architecture.

To compare the different effect of the ALE drug and low-magnitude whole-body vibration on the bone parameters of ovariectomized rats was one aim of the study. Compared with the OVX+WBV group, nearly all of the tested indices (BV/TV, TV apparent, BV material, Tb. N, Tb. Th) were higher in the OVX+ ALE group at week 12. Our result showed that the effect of alendronate on preventing bone loss and improving trabecular architecture was better than that of WBV.

Another aim of this study was to investigate the effect of WBV combined with ALE in ovariectomized rats. As shown in the table 1, WBV combined with ALE significantly reduced the CTX serum level (−29%, at week 4; −21.1%, at week 8; −25.5%, at week 12). In the OVX+ALE+WBV group, the trabecular BV/TV, Tb. N and Tb. T h were higher in the tibia compared to the OVX+VEH group (Fig. 3). At week 12, tibia treated with WBV+ ALE had significantly higher F_{max} compared to the OVX+VEH group, and a significant difference was also found at week 12 for energy absorption between the OVX+WBV+ALE and OVX+ VEH groups. As such, our study showed that WBV provide an additive effect to alendronate treatment which resulted in further reduction in bone mass and improvement in both trabecular architecture and bone strength.

The serum markers of bone turnover and bone biomechanical testing were not significant different between the OVX+ALE and OVX+WBV+ALE groups. However, in the OVX+ALE+WBV group, the trabecular BV/TV, TV apparent, Tb. N and Con. D were higher in the tibia compared to the OVX+ ALE group. This study demonstrated that WBV exercise enhanced the effect of ALE on the trabecular architecture in ovariectomized rats.

Conclusion

Compared with WBV, ALE was more effective at preventing bone loss and to improve the trabecular architecture. However, WBV enhanced the effect of ALE in ovariectomized rats by inducing further improvements in trabecular architecture.

Author Contributions

Conceived and designed the experiments: JTC. Performed the experiments: GXC SZ SQ XHW. Analyzed the data: WL ZPH. Contributed reagents/materials/analysis tools: ZMZ RTD HY. Wrote the paper: GXC.

References

1. Kannus P, Parkkari J, Niemi S. (1995) Age-adjusted incidence of hip fracture. Lancet 346:50–51.
2. Miyakoshi N, Itoi E, Kobayashi M, Kodama H. (2003) Impact of postural deformities and spinal mobility on quality of life in postmenopausal osteoporosis. Osteoporos Int 14: 1007–1012.
3. Iwamoto J, Takeda T, Ichimura S, Uzawa M. (2003) Comarative effects of treatment with etidronate and alendronate on bone resorption, back pain, and activities of daily living in elderly females with symptomatic vertebral fracture. Keio J Med 52:230–235.
4. Raisz LG, Smith JA. (1989) Pathogenesis, prevention, and treatment of osteoporosis. Annu Rev Med 40:251–267.
5. Cummings SR. Kelsey JL, Nevitt MC. O'Dowd KJ (1985) Epidemiology of osteoporosis and osteoporotic fracturs. Epidemiol Rev 7:178–208.
6. Cummings SR, Melton LJ (2002) Epidemiology and outcomes of osteoporotic fractures. Lancet 359: 1761–1767.
7. Woolf AD, Akesson K, Hazes JMW. (2002) The bone and joint decade monitor project: The burden of musculoskeletal conditions at the start of the new millennium. Osteoporosis Int 13: S84–S85.

8. Schenk R, Eqqli P, Fleisch H, Rosini S. (1986) Quantitative morphometric evaluation of the inhibitory activity of new aminobisphosphonates on bone resorption in the rat. Calcif Tissue Int 38: 342–349.
9. Boonekamp PM, van der Wee-Pals LJ, van Wijk-van Lennep MM, Thesing CW, Bijvoet O. (1986) Two modes of action of bisphosphonates on osteoclastic resorption of mineralized matrix. Bone Miner 1:27–39.
10. Schenk R, Merz WA, Muhlbauer R, Russell RGG, Fleisch H. (1973) Effect of ethane-1-hydroxy-1,l-diphosphonate (EHDP) and dichloromethylene diphosphonate (Cl2MDP) on the calcification and resorption of cartilage and bone in the tibial epiphysis and metaphysis of rats. Calcif Tissue Res 11:196–214.
11. Marie PJ, Hott M, Garba MT. (1985) Inhibition of bone matrix apposition by (3-amino-l-hydroxypropylidene)-l, l-bisphosphonate (AHPrBP) in mouse. Bone 6:193–200.
12. Thompson DD, Seedor JG, Weinreb M, Rosini S, Rodan GA. (1990) Aminohydroxybutane bisphosphonate inhibits bone loss due to immobilization in rats. J Bone Miner Res 5: 279–286.
13. Ward K, Alsop C, Caulton J, Rubin C, Adams J, et al. (2004) Low magnitude mechanical loading is osteogenic in children with disabling conditions. J Bone Miner Res 19: 360–369.
14. Rubin C, Judex S, Qin YX. (2006) Low-level mechanical signals and their potential as a non-pharmacological intervention for osteoporosis. Age Ageing 35:ii32–ii36.
15. Rubin C, Recker R, Cullen D, Ryaby J, McCabe J, et al. (2004) Prevention of postmenopausal bone loss by a low-magnitude, high-frequency mechanical stimuli: A clinical trial assessing compliance, efficacy, and safety. J Bone Miner Res 19: 343–351.
16. Gilsanz V, Wren TA, Sanchez M, Dorey F, Judex S, et al. (2006) Low-level, high-frequency mechanical signals enhance musculoskeletal development of young females with low BMD.J Bone Miner Res 21: 1464–1474.
17. Roelants M, Verschueren SM, Delecluse C, Levin O, Stijnen V. (2006) Whole-body-vibration-induced increase in leg muscle activity during different squat exercises. J Strength Cond Res 20: 124–129.
18. Marin PJ, Rhea MR. (2010) Effects of vibration training on muscle strength: A meta-analysis. J Strength Cond Res 24:548–556.
19. Leung KS, Shi HF, Cheung WH, Qin L, Ng WK, et al. (2009) Low-magnitude high-frequency vibration accelerates callus formation, mineralization, and fracture healing in rats. J Orthop Res 27: 458–465.
20. Shi HF, Cheung WH, Qin L, Leung AH, Leung KS. (2010) Low-magnitude high-frequency vibration treatment augments fracture healing in ovariectomy-induced osteoporotic bone. Bone 46: 1299–1305.
21. Boyd SK, Davison P, Müller R, Gasser JA. (2006) Monitoring individual morphological changes over time in ovariectomized rats by in vivo micro-computed tomography. Bone 39: 854–62.
22. Barbier A, Martel C, Vernejoul MC, Tirode F, Nys M, et al. (1990) The visualization and evaluation of bone architecture in the rat using three-dimensional X-ray microcomputed tomography. J Bone Miner Metab 17: 37–44.
23. Bauss F, Lalla S, Endele R, Hothorn LA. (2002) Effects of treatment with ibandronate on bone mass, architecture, biomechanical properties, and bone concentration of ibandronate in ovariectomized aged rats. J Rheumatol 2002; 29: 2200–2208.
24. Kharode YP, Sharp MC, Bodine PV. (2008) Utility of the ovariectomized rat as a model for human osteoporosis in drug discovery. Methods Mol Biol 455: 111–124.
25. Stuermer EK, Sehmisch S, Rack T, Wenda E, Seidlova-Wuttke D, et al. (2010) Estrogen and raloxifene improve metaphyseal fracture healing in the early phase of osteoporosis. A new fracture-healing model at the tibia in rat. Langenbecks Arch Surg 395: 163–172.
26. Stuermer EK, Seidlová-Wuttke D, Sehmisch S, Rack T, Wille J, et al. (2006) Standardized bending and breaking test for the normal and osteoporotic metaphyseal tibias of the rat: effect of estradiol, testosterone, and raloxifene. J Bone Miner Res 21: 89–96.
27. Masud T, Giannini S. (2003) Preventing osteoporotic fractures with bisphosphonates: a review of the efficacy and tolerability. Aging Clin Exp Res 15: 89–98.
28. Shiraki M, Kushida K, Fukunaga M, Kishimoto H, Taga M, et al. (1990) A double-masked multicenter comparative study between alendronate and alfacalcidol in Japannese patients with osteoporosis. Osteoporos Int 10: 183–192.
29. Kushida K, Shiraki M, Nakamura T, Kishimoto H, Morii H, et al. (2002) The efficacy of alendronate in reducing the risk for vertebral fracture in Japanese patients with osteoporosis:a ramdomized, double-blind, active-controlled, double-dummy trial. Curr Ther Res 63: 606–620.
30. Fleisch H. (1987) Bisphosphonates - history and experimental basis. Bone 8: 523–528.
31. Schenk R, Eggli P, Fleisch H, Rosini S (1986) Quantitative morphometric evaluation of the inhibitory activity of new aminobisphosphonates on bone resorption in the rat. Calcif Tissue Int 38: 342–239.
32. Storm T, Thamsborg G, Steiniche T, Rosini S. (1990) Effect of intermittent cyclical etidronate therapy on bone mass and fracture rate in women with postmenopausal osteoporosis. N Engl J Med 322:1265–1271.
33. Watts NB. Harris ST, Genant HK, Wasnich RD, Miller PD, et al. (1990) Intermittent cyclical etidronate treatment of postmenopausal osteoporosis. N Engl J Med 323:73–79.
34. JY. Reginster, R. Deroisy, D. Denis, J. Collette, MP. Lecart, et al. (1989) Prevention of post-menopausal bone loss by tiludronate. Lancet 2: 1469–1471.
35. Smith ML. Fogelman I. Hart DM, Scott E, Bevan J, et al. (1989) Effect of etidronate disodium on bone turnover following surgical menopause. Calcif Tissue Int 44: 74–79.
36. Akesson K, Ljunghall S, Jonsson B, Sernbo I, Johnell O, et al. (1995) Assessment of biochemical markers of bone metabolism in relation to the occurrence of fracture: a retrospective and prospective population-based study of females. J Bone Miner Res 10: 1823–1829.
37. Valimaki MJ, Farrerons-Minguella J, Halse J, Kroger H, Maroni M, et al. (2007) Effects of risedronate 5 mg/d on bone mineral density and bone turnover markers in late-postmenopausal women with osteopenia: a multinational, 24-month, randomized, double-blind, placebo-controlled, parallel-group, phase III trial. Clin Ther 29: 1937–1949.
38. Calvo MS, Eyre DR, Gundberg CM. (1996) Molecular basis and clinical application of biological markers of bone turnover. Endocr Rev 17: 333–368.
39. Rosen HN, Moses AC, Garber J, Iloputaife ID, Ross DS, et al. (2000) Serum CTX: a new marker of bone resorption that shows treatment effect more often than other markers because of low coefficient of variability and large changes with bisphosphonate therapy. Calcif Tissue Int 66: 100–103.
40. Bouxsein ML, Boyd SK, Christiansen BA, Guldberg RE, Jepsen KJ, et al. (2010) Guidelines for assessment of bone microstructure in rodents using micro-computed tomography. J Bone Miner Res 25: 1468–1486.
41. Verschueren SM, Roelants M, Delecluse C, Swinnen S, Vanderschueren D, et al. (2004) Effect of 6-month whole body vibration training on hip density,muscle strength,and postural control in postmenopausal females:a randomized controlled pilot study. J Bone Miner Res 19(3):352–359.
42. Oxlund BS, Ortoft G, Andreassen TT, Oxlund H. (2003) Low-intensity, high-frequency vibration appear to prevent the decrease in strength of the femur and tibia associated with ovariectomy of adult rats. Bone 32: 69–77.
43. Rubin CT, Lanyon LE. (1985) Regulation of bone mass by mechanical strain magnitude. Calcif Tissue Int 37: 411–417.
44. Frost HM. (1982) Mechanical determinants of bone modeling. Metab Bone Dis Relat Res 4: 217–229.
45. Lanyon LE. (1984) Functional strain as a determinant for bone remodeling. Calcif Tissue Int 36: S56–61.
46. Goodship AE, Lanyon LE, McFie H. (1979) Functional adaptation of bone to increased stress. An experimental study. J Bone Joint Surg Am 61:539–546.
47. Hsieh YF, Robling AG, Ambrosius WT, Burr DB, Turner CH. (2001) Mechanical loading of diaphyseal bone in vivo: the strain threshold for an osteogenic response varies with location. J Bone Miner Res 16: 2291–2297.
48. Wenger KH, Freeman JD, Fulzele S, Immel DM, Powell BD, et al. (2010) Effect of whole-body vibration on bone properties in aging mice. Bone 47: 746–755.
49. Christiansen BA, Silva MJ. (2006) The effect of varying magnitudes of whole-body vibration on several skeletal sites in mice. Ann Biomed Eng 34: 1149–1156.
50. Cardinale M, Wakeling J. (2005) Whole body vibration exercises: are vibrations good for you? Br J Sports Med 39:585–589
51. Santos-Filho SD, Meyer PF, Ronzio OA, Bonelli L, Fonseca AS, et al. (2010) Whole body vibration exercise: what do you know about scientific interest? Fiep Bull 80:875–878.
52. Bovenzi M. (2005) Health effects of mechanical vibration. G Ital Med Lav Ergon 27: 58–64.
53. Nelson CM, Brereton PF. (2005) The European vibration directive. Ind Health 43: 472–479.
54. Abercromby AF, Amonette WE, Layne CS, McFarlin BK, Hinman MR, et al. (2007) Vibration exposure and biodynamic responses during whole-body vibration training. Med Sci Sports Exerc 39: 1794–1800.
55. Rubin C, Xu G, Judex S. (2001) The anabolic activity of bone tissue, suppressed by disuse, is normalized by brief exposure to extremely low-magnitude mechanical stimuli. FASEB J 15: 2225–2229.
56. Garman R, Gaudette G, Donahue LR, Rubin C, Judex S. (2007) Low-level accelerations applied in the absence of weight bearing can enhance trabecular bone formation. J Orthop Res 25 (6), 732–740.
57. Xie L, Rubin C, Judex S. (2008) Enhancement of the adolescent murine musculoskeletal system using low-level mechanical vibrations. J Appl Physiol 104:1056–1062.
58. Xie L, Jacobson JM, Choi ES, Busa B, Donahue LR, et al. (2006) Low-level mechanical vibrations can influence bone resorption and bone formation in the growing skeleton. Bone 39:1059–1066.

Multidetector Computed Tomography-Based Microstructural Analysis Reveals Reduced Bone Mineral Content and Trabecular Bone Changes in the Lumbar Spine after Transarterial Chemoembolization Therapy for Hepatocellular Carcinoma

Miyuki Takasu*, Takuji Yamagami, Yuko Nakamura, Daisuke Komoto, Yoko Kaichi, Chihiro Tani, Shuji Date, Masao Kiguchi, Kazuo Awai

Department of Diagnostic Radiology, Graduate School of Biomedical Sciences, Hiroshima University, Hiroshima, Japan

Abstract

Purpose: It is well recognized that therapeutic irradiation can result in bone damage. However, long-term bone toxicity associated with computed tomography (CT) performed during interventional angiography has received little attention. The purpose of this study was to determine the prevalence of osteoporosis and trabecular microstructural changes in patients after transarterial chemoembolization (TACE) for hepatocellular carcinoma therapy using an interventional-CT system.

Materials and Methods: Spinal microarchitecture was examined by 64-detector CT in 81 patients who underwent TACE, 35 patients with chronic hepatitis, and 79 controls. For each patient, the volumetric CT dose index (CTDIv) during TACE (CTDIv (TACE)), the dose-length product (DLP) during TACE (DLP (TACE)), and CTDIv and DLP of routine dynamic CT scans (CTDIv (CT) and DLP (CT), respectively), were calculated as the sum since 2008. Using a three dimensional (3D) image analysis system, the tissue bone mineral density (tBMD) and trabecular parameters of the 12th thoracic vertebra were calculated. Using tBMD at a reported cutoff value of 68 mg/cm^3, the prevalence of osteoporosis was assessed.

Results: The prevalence of osteoporosis was significantly greater in the TACE vs. the control group (39.6% vs. 18.2% for males, $P<0.05$ and 60.6% vs. 34.8% for females, $P<0.01$). Multivariate regression analysis demonstrated that sex, age, and CTDIv (CT) significantly affected the risk of osteoporosis. Of these indices, CTDIv (CT) had the highest area under the curve (AUC) (0.735). Correlation analyses of tBMD with cumulative radiation dose revealed weak correlations between tBMD and CTDIv (CT) ($r^2=0.194$, $P<0.001$).

Conclusion: The prevalence of osteoporosis was significantly higher in post TACE patients than in control subjects. The cumulative radiation dose related to routine dynamic CT studies was a significant contributor to the prevalence of osteoporosis.

Editor: Joseph P. R. O. Orgel, Illinois Institute of Technology, United States of America

Funding: MT was supported by Grant-in-Aid for Scientific Research (KAKENHI) (C) [23591768] in Japan. The funder had no role in study design, data collection and analysis, decision to publish, or preparation of the manuscript.

Competing Interests: The authors have declared that no competing interests exist.

* Email: my-takasu@syd.odn.ne.jp

Introduction

The number of computed tomography (CT)-guided interventional procedures has increased because they are less invasive and more cost-effective than open surgery [1–3]. Transarterial embolization therapies involve the transcatheter delivery of solid particles into an artery feeding a target tumor for the purpose of blocking its blood supply. These therapies include bland embolization, transarterial chemoembolization (TACE), and chemoembolization using drug-eluting beads. TACE is a method in which chemotherapeutic drugs are combined with embolization particles and then injected into the artery that supplies the tumor. TACE via the hepatic artery has been used as treatment for hepatocellular carcinoma (HCC) in cases where surgical resection is not a viable option or as a means of downstaging HCC to fit within Milan criteria for the possibility of further management with orthotopic liver transplantation. Trials performed by Hong Kong [4] and Barcelona [5] researchers showed a significant increase in survival rates of subjects compared to controls. In some institutions, CT arterial portography and CT during hepatic arteriography are performed to confirm the existence or to evaluate the characteristics of liver tumors during TACE [6]. Additionally, two-dimensional or three-dimensional CT images are acquired to generate a road map of the targets and their positions relative to the interventional instruments. This valuable information provides guidance for the operator to locate the target, plan an interventional path, adjust the interventional instruments, and evaluate the efficacy of the procedure. A priori knowledge of the distribution of contrast material in the tumor from performance of CT arteriography through the selected arterial branch ensures that anticancer drugs and embolic agents are infused effectively.

A concern regarding the use of CT during angiography may be the radiation exposure to the patients, because the number of CT scans performed during TACE with the interventional-CT system is high; around ten times per procedure. It is well recognized that therapeutic irradiation can result in bone damage and may increase fracture risk. The main evidence for the effect of irradiation on fracture risk comes from a long-term follow-up study of two European randomized trials (Stockholm I and II) [7,8] evaluating the effect of short-course irradiation on patients with operable rectal cancer [9]. Pathologically, vascular injury and decrease of osteoblast cells following irradiation have been reported [10–14].

Recently, a case of 12th thoracic vertebral fracture that occurred after multiple TACE procedures to treat multiple hepatocellular carcinomas was seen. Fluorodeoxyglucose (FDG)-positron-emission tomography (FDG-PET)-CT performed to screen for pathologic fractures revealed diffusely decreased FDG uptake within the lower thoracic to lumbar spine (Figure 1). This finding gave us the impression that this area might have corresponded to the radiation field during the TACE procedures because the liver and vessels such as hepatic arteries, their branches, superior mesenteric artery, and portal vein, which are repeatedly imaged during TACE procedures, are all located around the same spinal level. Therefore, we hypothesized that radiation exposure from CT scans during angiographies led to decreased bone density and bone strength associated with secondary osteoporosis.

Bone strength and fracture susceptibility are governed in large part by the amount of bone, which can be assessed by dual-energy X-ray absorptiometry measurements of areal bone mineral density. However, many other structural and material properties of bone, including microarchitecture, contribute considerably and independently to fragility [15–17]. Recently, high-resolution peripheral quantitative CT [18,19] and multidetector CT (MDCT) [20,21] have been used noninvasively to visualize the details of trabecular microarchitecture.

The long-term bone toxicity associated with CT during interventional angiography has received little attention. The purpose of this study was to determine the prevalence of osteoporosis and trabecular microstructural changes using clinical MDCT-based microstructural analysis in patients after TACE with the interventional-CT system to treat hepatocellular carcinoma.

Materials and Methods

Ethics Statement

This retrospective, single-institution study was approved by the Institutional Review Board of Hiroshima University Hospital, with a waiver of informed consent. Patient records and information were anonymized and de-identified prior to analyses.

Subjects

First, consecutive patients who underwent unenhanced abdominal CT performed with a specific CT unit in our institution from September 2010 to January 2014 were selected. Next, a total of 195 of these patients were enrolled in the study after exclusion of subjects with a history of chemotherapy (n = 4), total or partial gastrectomy (n = 4), esophagectomy (n = 1), radiation therapy to the pelvis (n = 1), vertebral fracture (n = 1), chronic steroid use

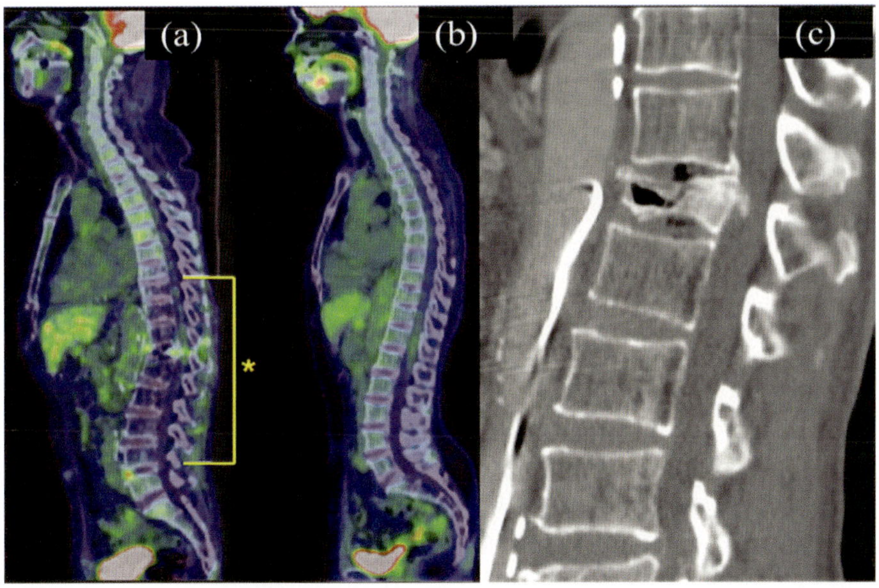

Figure 1. Sagittal reconstructed fluorodeoxyglucose-positron-emission tomography (FDG-PET)-CT image (a) and MDCT image (c) of the spine obtained from a 62-year-old man after eight transarterial chemoembolization procedures for hepatocellular carcinomas. FDG-PET-CT reveals diffusely decreased FDG uptake within the lower thoracic to lumbar spine (*). Sagittal reconstructed FDG-PET-CT image is accompanied by that of a 72-year old woman performed five years after resection of a uterine cervical cancer, in which there is normal spinal FDG uptake, for comparison (b). Sagittal reconstructed CT shows a vertebral fracture of the 12th thoracic vertebra.

(n = 1), and patients with a gait disturbance caused by cerebrovascular disease (n = 4) or myopathy (n = 1). There were no patients with a history of rheumatoid arthritis, inflammatory bowel disease, chronic obstructive pulmonary disease, or organ transplantation. Patients in the TACE group (n = 81) had HCC with a history of TACE and a diagnosis of either type B or type C hepatitis. Patients in the chronic hepatitis (CH) group (n = 35) had a diagnosis of either type B or type C hepatitis and had no history of any angiographic or CT-guided fluoroscopic procedures. The majority of HCC patients had persistent infection from hepatitis B virus or hepatitis C virus. Therefore, we established the CH group to determine whether there were radiation effects from TACE procedures only. Subjects in the control group (n = 79) were randomly selected from our hospital's radiology information system; they had undergone MDCT of the body to screen for tumor recurrences other than liver tumors, to rule out internal malignancy, and to diagnose abdominal or back pain. We did not recruit healthy control subjects from the local community for ethical reason.

Tables 1 and 2 summarize the characteristics of these patients.

TACE Procedure

All patients in the TACE group had adequate hepatic function to undergo TACE. The interventional procedures were performed using an interventional-CT system consisting of a unified CT and angiography unit (Aquilion LB combined with Infinix Celeve-i INFX-8000V, Toshiba Medical Systems, Tokyo, Japan). In addition to angiographic examinations, CT scans were performed during common or proper hepatic arteriography to evaluate hemodynamics in the HCC, map the arterial anatomy, and assess portal flow. Further selective hepatic arteriograms were also performed using CT scanning to confirm the distribution of contrast material in the HCC from the selected arterial branch just before infusing anti-cancer drugs and embolic agents.

The X-ray tube was equipped with a built-in kerma area product (KAP) meter at the collimator exit with capability to display the cumulative KAP for fluoroscopic and radiographic examinations. The KAP is the integral of air kerma (the energy extracted from an X-ray beam per unit mass of air in a small irradiated air volume; for diagnostic X-rays, the dose delivered to that volume of air) across the entire X-ray beam emitted from the X-ray tube. It is a surrogate measure of the amount of energy delivered to the patient [22]. Entrance skin dose was calculated from KAP, beam area, and the calibration coefficient of the KAP meter at the calibrated distance for the focal-to-skin distance. It is important to estimate entrance skin dose during and after fluoroscopically guided interventions because a skin dose that exceeds 15 Gy is thought to be a sentinel event [23]. The volumetric CT dose index during TACE (CTDIv (TACE)) and dose-length product during TACE (DLP (TACE)) were obtained directly from the scanner console. The computed tomography dose index (CTDI) is a measure of the radiation output of the CT slice comprising the quality of the X-rays produced, the type of filtration and the geometry of the X-ray beam including focus size and collimation [24]. CTDIv, which was introduced for modern CT scanners, is obtained from the average CTDI in an irradiated

Table 1. Comparison of clinical characteristics and cumulative radiation doses.

Men	TACE	CH	Control
Background data	n=48	n=17	n=33
Age (years)	67.1±9.0	66.3±7.6	66.5±7.1
BMI (kg/m^2)	23.2±2.8	21.8±2.4	23.8±3.9
Radiation exposure			
CTDIv (CT) (mGy)	350†† [50, 1950]	200** [50, 950]	50 [0, 700]
CTDIv (TACE) (mGy)	148 [15, 528]		
DLP (CT) (mGy×cm)	14350††,+ [2000, 78000]	7600 [0, 22900]	4500 [0, 22200]
DLP (TACE) (mGy×cm)	2818 [305, 17985]		
Entrance skin dose (mGy)	790.9 [36, 5911]		
Women	**TACE**	**CH**	**Control**
Background data	n=33	n=18	n=46
Age (years)	67.4±7.8	61.7±6.9	62.5±9.3
BMI (kg/m^2)	23.0±3.4	22.9±4.4	22.5±3.4
Radiation exposure			
CTDIv (CT) (mGy)	374††, ** [100, 1650]	250 [0, 1150]	0 [0, 200]
CTDIv (TACE) (mGy)	101 [26, 1723]		
DLP (CT) (mGy×cm)	9450†, ** [2800, 33000]	6900 [0, 36000]	1900 [0, 13000]
DLP (TACE) (mGy×cm)	1880 [489, 6599]		
Entrance skin dose (mGy)	817 [76, 4465]		

Note. Values represent the means ± standard deviation or medians [range].
BMI, body mass index; CTDIv (CT): CTDIv of routine dynamic CT scan; CTDIv (TACE): CTDIv during TACE; DLP (CT): DLP of routine dynamic CT scan; DLP (TACE): DLP during TACE.
** $P<0.01$, control vs. CH group.
†† $P<0.01$, † $P<0.05$ control vs. TACE group.
+ $P<0.05$, TACE group vs. CH group.

slice divided by a helical pitch. To obtain a dose quantity describing the radiation exposure for a full scan, the DLP was introduced [25,26]. DLP can be obtained by CTDIv divided by the scan length, which means it depends on the patient's height.

For each patient, cumulative radiation doses obtained from each index were calculated as the sum of all TACE procedures performed since 2008.

Imaging by MDCT

All patients were scanned with a 64-section MDCT (LightSpeed VCT; GE Healthcare, Little Chalfont, UK) with spatial resolution equivalent to 16.4 line pair per centimeter at a 2% setting for the modulation transfer function. The collimation was 64×0.625 mm, and table translation speed was 23.4 cm/sec. The tube parameters were 300 mA and 120 kV, with a pitch of 0.586. Unenhanced and three-phase contrast-enhanced helical scans of the entire liver were obtained.

For each patient, the cumulative radiation doses obtained from each of two indices (e.g., CTDIv (CT) and DLP (CT)) were calculated as the sum from all dynamic CT scans since 2008.

Bone mineral density measurement and MDCT-based microstructural analysis

To obtain tissue bone mineral density (tBMD) data by MDCT, the patients were scanned simultaneously with a bone mineral reference phantom (B-MAS2000; Kyotokagaku Co., Kyoto, Japan) containing calibration objects with equivalent densities of 0, 50, 100, 150, and 200 mg/cm^3 calcium hydroxyapatite.

Images of the whole lumbar spine obtained by unenhanced scanning were reconstructed using an acquisition matrix of 512×512 and a field of view of 100 mm, resulting in a voxel size of 0.20×0.20×0.16 mm^3. An edge-enhancing reconstruction kernel (Bone Plus; GE Healthcare, Little Chalfont, UK) was used. The 12th thoracic vertebra (T12) was chosen for the analysis in this study because vertebral fractures typically occur at the thoracolumbar junction (T12 and the first lumbar vertebra) [26,27].

For microstructural analysis, the volume of interest (VOI) was defined manually as a 10-mm thickness of the central part of the T12 vertebral body to avoid the cortex, the basivertebral foramen, and both endplates.

Microstructural parameters were calculated using a computer program for a three dimensional (3D) image analysis system (TRI/3D-BON; RATOC System Engineering, Tokyo, Japan), as described elsewhere [20]. Briefly, using a volumetric bone mineral density value for trabecular bone, >150 mg/cm^3 within the bone marrow was extracted. We used a global threshold method. A standardized method of image threshold levels based on the attenuation histogram of a selected region of interest was used to ensure consistency in the image threshold levels across all subjects studied.

The following trabecular microstructural parameters were obtained: apparent trabecular bone volume fraction (app BV/TV), apparent trabecular number (app Tb.N), apparent trabecular separation (app Tb.S), Euler's number (E), degree of anisotropy (DA), and the structure model index (SMI). Details of these methods are described elsewhere [20,21] but briefly, bone volume (BV) was calculated using tetrahedrons corresponding to the enclosed volume of the triangulated surface. Total tissue volume (TV) analyzed was the entire marrow area volume including trabecular bone. Apparent BV/TV was calculated from these values. App Tb.S was determined by filling maximal spheres into the structure according to the method described by Hildebrand and Rügsegger [28]. App Tb.N was estimated as a trabecular bone number crossing the line perpendicular to the growing direction of vertebrae based on the plate model [29]. Euler's number was calculated by using the Euler method of Odgaard and Gundersen [30]. Degree of anisotropy was determined from the ratio between the maximal and minimal radii of the mean intercept length ellipsoid [31]. By displaying the surface of the structure to an infinitesimal amount, SMI was calculated according to the method described by Hildebrand and Rügsegger [28]. The SMI quantifies the plate vs. rod characteristics of trabecular bone. An SMI of 0 reflects a purely plate-shaped bone and an SMI of 3 indicates a purely rod-like bone.

A cutoff value of 68 mg/cm^3 was determined from a previous study that evaluated tBMD (bone mineral content/tissue volume (BMC/TV)) in 67 patients with osteoporosis using the 64-section MDCT and the same 3D image analysis system [32].

One author (M.T.) performed microstructural analysis, and precision was confirmed as described elsewhere [20].

Statistical Analysis

The characteristics, cumulative radiation doses, trabecular microstructural parameters, and tBMD of the three groups were compared by the Kruskal-Wallis test followed by the Steel-Dwass test because some indices were non-normally distributed. The Kolmogorov-Smirnov test was used to determine whether values were normally distributed. The prevalence of osteoporosis in the three groups was calculated. For patients in the TACE group, a multivariate general linear model with binomial distribution and logit-link was constructed to identify the predictors of osteoporosis. We calculated the odds ratios for osteoporosis associated with risk factors. To evaluate the diagnostic performance of contributors to osteoporosis, comparisons of the receiver operating characteristic (ROC) curves were performed, and the areas under the curves (AUCs) were calculated. Correlations of tBMD with cumulative radiation dose were determined. The raw datasets of tBMD and CTDIv (CT) showed significant heteroscedasticity and data were transformed to a log scale. Since log-transformed tBMD and CTDIv (CT) were non-normally distributed, the Spearman rank correlation test was used for simple regression analysis. All analyses were performed with a spreadsheet application (Microsoft Office Excel 2010, Redmond, WA, USA) and ROC analysis software (ROCKIT 0.9.1; Charles E. Metz, University of Chicago, Chicago, IL, USA).

Results

Table 1 summarizes the patients' characteristics and cumulative radiation doses. In male subjects, CTDIv (CT) and DLP (CT) were significantly greater in the TACE group than in the control group ($P<0.01$). CTDIv (CT) was significantly greater in the CH group than in the control group ($P<0.01$), and DLP (CT) was significantly greater in the TACE group than in the CH group ($P<0.05$). Patients' age and BMI were similar among the three groups. In female subjects, CTDIv (CT) and DLP (CT) were significantly greater in the TACE group and the CH group than in the control group ($P<0.01$). Patients' age and BMI were similar among the three groups.

The prevalence of osteoporosis in the three groups was calculated (Table 2). The prevalence of osteoporosis was significantly greater in the TACE compared to the control group (39.6% vs. 18.2%, $P<0.05$ for males and 60.6% vs. 34.8%, $P<0.01$ for females, respectively). The prevalence of osteoporosis in the CH group was less than in the TACE group and greater than in the control group, but these results were not statistically significant.

Table 2. Comparison of bone mineral density of the lumbar spine among the three groups.

Male	TACE	CH	Control
tBMD (mg/cm^3)	78.6±35.4†	82.0±26.5	91.6±24.9
<68 mg/cm^3 (osteoporosis)	19	6	6
≥68 mg/cm^3	29	11	27
Prevalence of osteoporosis (%)	39.6	35.3	18.2
Female	**TACE**	**CH**	**Control**
tBMD (mg/cm^3)	60.3±31.0††	76.4±30.6	84.6±29.2
<68 mg/cm^3 (osteoporosis)	20	9	16
≥68 mg/cm^3	13	9	30
Prevalence of osteoporosis (%)	60.6	50.0	34.8

$^{\dagger\dagger}P<0.01$, $^{\dagger}P<0.05$, control vs. post TACE.

Results of comparison of microstructural parameters among the three groups are shown in Table 3. Among the microstructural indexes, app Tb.N was significantly lower in the TACE group than in the control group ($P<0.05$). Apparent Tb.S ($P<0.05$ for males, $P<0.01$ for females), structure model index ($P<0.05$ for males, $P<0.01$ for females), and Euler number ($P<0.01$) were significantly higher in the TACE group than in the control group. In female patients, app BV/TV was significantly lower in the TACE group than in the control group ($P<0.01$). These findings indicate that trabecular bones in the patients of the TACE group were fewer, less dense, and more rod-like than in the controls.

Multivariate regression analysis demonstrated that sex, age, and CTDIv (CT) significantly affected the risk of osteoporosis (Table 4). The AUC having the highest discriminatory power to distinguish osteoporotic patients from controls was that for CTDIv (CT) (AUC = 0.735; 95% confidence intervals (CIs), 0.557, 0.732), with an optimal cutoff value of 400 mGy; the sensitivity and specificity were 63.2% (CIs, 0.367, 0.642) and 73.2% (CIs, 0.557, 0.922), respectively. Regarding the same distribution, the AUC for age was 0.692 (CIs, 0.622, 0.771), with an optimal cutoff value of 64 years old; the sensitivity and specificity were 88.6% (CIs, 0.817, 0.972) and 58.8% (CIs, 0.377, 0.811), respectively. Analysis of CTDIv (TACE) revealed no contribution to the risk of osteoporosis.

Correlation analyses of tBMD with cumulative radiation dose showed a weak correlation between tBMD and CTDIv (CT) ($rs = -0.441$, $r^2 = 0.194$, $P<0.001$, Figure 2).

Representative images are shown in Figures 3 and 4.

Discussion

In early 2010, the U.S. Food and Drug Administration introduced the "Initiative to Reduce Unnecessary Radiation Exposure from Medical Imaging" [33]. In this report, CT and associated CT-guided interventions were identified as contributors to increasing the radiation dose to patients, and- the authors pointed out that a lack of awareness of radiation-induced injuries to patients among the users of medical radiation may be contributing to an increase of radiation exposure.

In the current study, weak correlations were found between tBMD and the cumulative radiation dose of patients in the TACE group. Bone loss due to high doses of irradiation therapy has been identified in diagnostic radiographic images [34]. However, to the best of our knowledge, no study has demonstrated an association between bone mass and radiation dose from diagnostic imaging procedures such as CT scans.

The primary effect of irradiation on bone is atrophy. Several pathological findings regarding blood vessels were identified in the radiation-induced changes in bone. They included loss of vasculature [10], sub-intimal fibrosis, and hyaline thickening of the media [12], followed by the later replacement of smooth

Table 3. Comparison of microstructural parameters among the three groups.

	Male			Female		
	TACE	CH	Control	TACE	CH	Control
App BV/TV (%)	27.8±13.5	28.6±8.7	31.9±7.8	21.2±10.5**	27.8±10.8	29.8±9.6
App Tb.N (1/mm^3)	0.34±0.08*	0.36±0.06	0.38±0.05	0.30±0.10*	0.35±0.06	0.36±0.07
App Tb.S (μm)	842±281*	775±147	710±109	1003±392**	811±171	770±195
SMI	1.76±0.53*	1.74±0.39	1.61±0.36	2.00±0.44**	1.75±0.48	1.69±0.40
Euler's number	−1426±1149**	−1792±1105	−2185±977	−665±879**	−1074±681	−1402±825
Degree of anisotropy	1.41±0.11	1.43±0.12	1.41±0.09	1.48±0.10	1.52±0.20	1.45±0.11

**$P<0.01$, *$P<0.05$, control vs. post TACE.
app BV/TV, apparent trabecular bone volume fraction; app Tb.N, apparent trabecular number; app Tb.S, apparent trabecular separation; SMI, structure model index.

Table 4. Multivariate regression analysis examining the effects of patients' characteristics and cumulative radiation dose on osteoporosis in the TACE group.

Variable	*β ± Standard error	*P* Value	Odds ratio (CI)
Sex	0.38±0.62	0.001	1.25 (1.65, 7.43)
Age	0.88±0.02	<0.001	1.11 (1.06, 1.17)
CTDIv (CT)	0.85±0.00	<0.001	1.03 (1.00, 1.01)

*β, Standardized partial regression coefficient.

muscle cells [35]. Other investigators have reported a reduction in the number of osteoblast cells following irradiation, which was associated with decreased collagen production and alkaline phosphatase activity [13]. Since both collagen and alkaline phosphatase play a role in mineralization, it has been proposed that this is a pathway to osteopenia [14].

A radiation dose-effect relationship was also demonstrated by several animal experiments. Bone atrophy was detected after irradiation of the femur of rats with doses of 20–25 Gy, and there was also a significant reduction in the relative amounts of calcium and phosphorus in bone, suggesting that atrophy was associated with bone mineral loss [36]. Although the results from animal studies cannot be applied to patients in clinical settings, they could partly explain the relationship between the cumulative radiation dose and tBMD in this study.

On the basis of the multivariate regression analysis, the greatest contributor to the prevalence of osteoporosis among the indices for radiation exposure was the CTDIv (CT) from routine CT examinations to assess or screen for hepatocellular carcinoma. The cumulative radiation dose from angiographic procedures (e.g., the CTDIv (TACE)) did not significantly contribute to the prevalence of osteoporosis.The cumulative radiation dose from routine CT examinations can be up to four times higher than that of angiographic procedures, as shown in Table 1. Thus, a

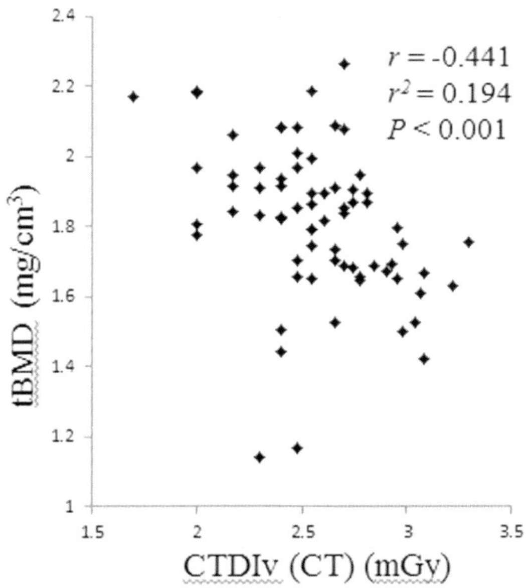

Figure 2. Correlation analysis of tBMD with cumulative radiation dose shows a significant correlation between tBMD and CTDIv (CT).

reduction in radiation dose for patients who have to undergo repeat TACE treatments will be best achieved by minimizing the dose from routine CT examinations.The most practical methods to achieve this will be to avoid unnecessary CT scans, to use a lower tube current (mA) or peak beam energy (peak kV), and increase the noise settings for tube current modulation [37,38].

Among the microstructural indices in this study, app Tb.N and app BV/TV were significantly lower and app Tb.S and SMI were significantly higher in the TACE group compared to the control group.

There have been several reports of results regarding radiation effects on trabecular morphology that are consistent with those of our study. In 2009, Willey et al. [39] investigated the effect on mice of whole-body irradiation of 2 Gy X-rays. They demonstrated that the trabecular microarchitectural properties of L5 included decreased volumetric BMD, BV/TV, and Tb.N and elevated SMI and Tb.S. In 2014, Xu. et al. [40] reported similar results with X-ray radiation of Wistar rats, which had significantly reduced BMD, BV/TV, and Tb.N, but increased SMI.

We did not include trabecular thickness for microstructural analysis in this study. In 2007, correlation analysis of morphological parameters findings of high-resolution peripheral quantitative CT vs. micro-CT was performed by MacNeil et al. [41]. They showed that, among trabecular parameters, trabecular thickness had the lowest correlation coefficient ($r^2 = 0.59$), whereas other high-resolution peripheral quantitative CT-indices, such as trabecular bone volume fraction, trabecular number and trabecular separation, correlated well with the gold-standards methods results ($r^2 > 0.83$). In addition, regarding changes in trabecular thickness after radiation exposure, several previous studies have had contradictory findings even using micro-CT. For example, Hamilton et al. [42] reported an insignificant increase in trabecular thickness after radiation exposure of 2-Gy to tibiae and femurs of mice. More recently, Chandra et al. [43] demonstrated a slight but significant increase in trabecular thickness after irradiation with a clinically relevant dose of the proximal tibiae of rats. We used clinical MDCT with spatial resolution of 200 μm×200 μm×160 μm to investigate trabecular bones that are known to have about the same size as the imaging spatial resolution. In the previous study [20] performed by using the same CT scanner and 3D image analysis system, the apparent trabecular thickness was around 700 μm, when many studies using micro-CT report an average Tb.Th of 150–200 μm. We speculate that the actual Tb.Th is overestimated by clinical MDCT due to the combined effects of limited spatial resolution and missing thin trabeculae during the thresholding step. Thus, we think that an evaluation of Tb.Th using clinical CT is inappropriate.

There were several limitations to this study. First, there are several other factors that could cause osteoporosis in the CH- and TACE groups. Risk factors for osteoporosis include advanced age, low body mass index, underlying disease (rheumatoid arthritis,

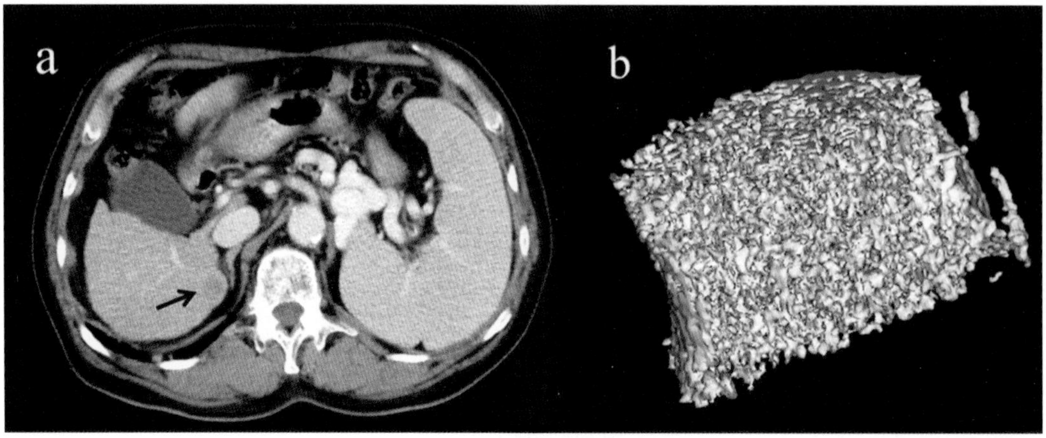

Figure 3. Representative 3D MDCT images of the L3 vertebra obtained from a 71-year-old man after five dynamic CT scans and two transarterial chemoembolization procedures for hepatocellular carcinomas. An axial CT image of the liver shows a recurrence of hepatocellular carcinoma in S7 as a low density area compared to adjacent liver parenchyma(a), (black arrow). The 3D image of the L3 vertebra is shown (b). Tissue bone mineral density (76.8 mg/cm^3) is normal for age. The image is cut in half along the longitudinal midline.

inflammatory bowel disease, chronic obstructive pulmonary disease, history of organ transplantation), smoking, excessive alcohol consumption, and high glucocorticoid dose [44]. Glucocorticoid-induced osteoporosis is the most common and severe form of iatrogenic osteoporosis [44–47]. In patients with glucocorticoid-induced osteoporosis, the loss of bone mineral density occurs at the rate of approximately 3% yearly after the first year [44]. In an animal study [48], peripheral quantitative CT analysis revealed glucocorticoid-induced BMD loss of approximately 7% in wild-type mice. On the other hand, in a rat study [43], radiation from micro-CT scans following the irradiation generated in a clinically relevant range led to more reductions in BMD (26% in BMD and 37% in BV/TV). In fact, we excluded patients with a history of chronic steroid use; in addition, patients' characteristics including age and BMI were similar among the three groups in this study. Thus, we attribute the reduced tBMD in the present study mainly to radiation exposure. Second, there might be some error in the results of this study due to the low spatial resolution of clinical MDCT, although the results of several previous reports regarding radiation effects on trabecular morphology are consistent with those of our study. Validation of microstructural parameters obtained using clinical MDCT by comparing with results using the gold-standard method, micro-CT, is needed during future studies. Third, the radiation dose per each single CT scan or TACE was not identical, and the intervals between these procedures varied across individuals in this study. One clinical study showed the effects of changes in the dose per fraction on the radiation response of mature bone of post mastectomy patients [49]. Spontaneous rib fracture was significantly higher in the group treated with a larger dose/fraction than in the more standard lower dose/fraction group. The patients who underwent repeat TACE in this study tended to have shorter between-scan intervals than control subjects. Such interindividual variability could have affected our results.

In conclusion, the prevalence of osteoporosis detected with MDCT was significantly higher in post TACE patients than in

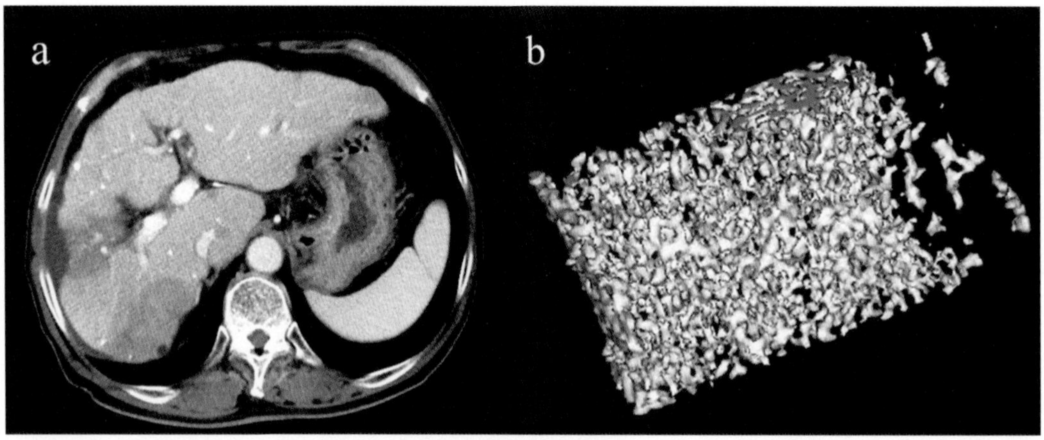

Figure 4. Representative 3D MDCT images of the L3 vertebra obtained from a 71-year-old man after 24 dynamic CT scans and seven transarterial chemoembolization (TACE) procedures for hepatocellular carcinomas. An axial CT image of the liver shows segmental low density areas in the S5 and S7 areas due to previous TACE procedures(a). The 3D image shows sparse trabecular bones (b) compared to those of the patient in Figure 3. Tissue bone mineral density (36.2 mg/cm^3) is lower than the mean value of control subjects. The image is cut in half along the longitudinal midline.

control subjects. The cumulative radiation dose related to routine dynamic CT studies was a significant contributor to the prevalence of osteoporosis. There is a weak relationship between local irradiation to bone and reduced bone density. Based on our study, reduction of the radiation dose for HCC patients might be achieved by minimizing the dose from routine CT examinations; unnecessary CT scans should be avoided.

Author Contributions

Conceived and designed the experiments: MT TY. Performed the experiments: MT YN DK YK CT SD MK. Analyzed the data: MT TY KA. Contributed reagents/materials/analysis tools: MT MK. Wrote the paper: MT.

References

1. Carlson SK, Bender CE, Classic KL, Zink FE, Quam JP, et al. (2001) Benefits and safety of CT fluoroscopy in interventional radiologic procedures. Radiology 219: 515–520.
2. Silverman SG, Deuson TE, Kane N, Adams DF, Seltzer SE, et al. (1998) Percutaneous abdominal biopsy: cost-identification analysis. Radiology 206: 429–435.
3. Fraser-Hill MA, Renfrew DL, Hilsenrath PE (1992) Percutaneous needle biopsy of musculoskeletal lesions. Part 2. Cost-effectiveness. AJR 158: 813–818.
4. Lo CM, Ngan H, Tso WK, Liu CL, Lam CM, et al. (2002) Randomized controlled trial of transarterial lipiodol chemoembolization for unresectable hepatocellular carcinoma. Hepatology 35: 1164–1171.
5. Llovet JM, Real MI, Montaña X, Planas R, Coll S, et al. (2002) Arterial embolisation or chemoembolisation versus symptomatic treatment in patients with unresectable hepatocellular carcinoma: a randomized controlled trial. Lancet 359: 1734–1739.
6. Ishikawa M, Yamagami T, Kakizawa H, Hieda M, Toyota N, et al. (2014) Transarterial therapy of hepatocellular carcinoma fed by the right renal capsular artery. J Vasc Interv Radiol. 25: 389–395.7. Stockholm Colorectal Cancer Study Group. (1995) The Stockholm I trial of preoperative short term radiotherapy in operable rectal carcinoma: a prospective randomized trial. Cancer 75: 2269–2275.
7. Stockholm Colorectal Cancer Study Group (1996) Randomized study on preoperative radiotherapy in rectal carcinoma. Ann Surg Oncol 3: 423–430.
8. Holm T, Singnomklao T, Rutqvist LE, Cedermark B (1996) Adjuvant preoperative radiotherapy in patients with rectal carcinoma: adverse effects during long term follow- up of two randomized trials. Cancer 78: 968–976.
9. Ewing J (1926) Radiation osteitis. Acta Radiol 6: 399–412.
10. Warren S (1994) Histopathology of radiation lesions. Physiol Rev 24: 225–245.
11. Gyorkey Z, Pollock FJ (1940) Radiation necrosis of the ossicles. Arch Otolaryngol 71: 793–799.
12. Sams A (1966) The effects of 2000r of X-rays on the acid and alkaline phosphatase of mouse tibiae. Int J Radiat Biol 10: 123–140.
13. Ergun H, Howland WJ (1980) Post-irradiation atrophy of mature bone. CRC Crit Rev Diagn Imag 12: 225–243.
14. Laib A, Hauselmann HJ, Ruegsegger P (1998) In vivo high resolution 3D-QCT of the human forearm. Technol Health Care 6: 329–337.
15. Laib A, Ruegsegger P (1999) Comparison of structure extraction methods for in vivo trabecular bone measurements. Comput Med Imaging Graph 23: 69–74.
16. Cheung AM, Detsky AS (2008) Osteoporosis and fractures: missing the bridge? JAMA 299: 1468–1470.
17. Stein EM, Liu XS, Nickolas TL, Cohen A, McMahon DJ, et al. (2012) Microarchitectural abnormalities are more severe in postmenopausal women with vertebral compared to nonvertebral fractures. J Clin Endocrinol Metab 97: E1918–E1926.
18. Boutroy S, Bouxsein ML, Munoz F, Delmas PD (2005) In vivo assessment of trabecular bone microarchitecture by high-resolution peripheral quantitative computed tomography. J Clin Endocrinol Metab 90: 6508–6515.
19. Takasu M, Tani C, Ishikawa M, Date S, Horiguchi J, et al. (2011) Multiple myeloma: microstructural analysis of lumbar trabecular bones in patients without visible bone lesions-preliminary results. Radiology 260: 472–479.
20. Ito M, Ikeda K, Nishiguchi M, Shindo H, Uetani M, et al. (2005) Multi-Detector Row CT Imaging of Vertebral Microstructure for Evaluation of Fracture Risk. J Bone Miner Res 20: 1828–1836.
21. Miller DL, Balter S, Cole PE, Lu HT, Schueler BA, et al. (2003) Radiation doses in interventional radiology procedures: the RAD-IR study. I. Overall measures of dose. J Vasc Interv Radiol 14: 711–727.
22. The Joint Commission (2006) Radiation Overdose as a Reviewable Sentinel Event, Update March 7, 2006. Available: http://www.jointcommission.org/assets/1/18/Radiation_Overdose.pdf. Accessed 2014 July 18.
23. Shope TB, Gagne RM, Johnson GC (1981) A method for describing the doses delivered by transmission X-ray computed tomography. Med. Phys 8: 488–495.
24. European commission (1999) European Guidelines on Quality Criteria for Computed Tomography. Report EUR 16262 EN. Luxembourg: Office for Official Publications of the European Communities.
25. Carberry GA, Pooler BD, Binkley N, Lauder TB, Bruce RJ, et al. (2013).
26. Unreported vertebral body compression fractures at abdominal multidetector CT. Radiology 268: 120–126.
27. Cooper C, Atkinson EJ, O'Fallon WM, Melton LJ 3rd (1992) Incidence of clinically diagnosed vertebral fractures: a population-based study in Rochester, Minnesota, 1985–1989. J Bone Miner Res 7: 221–227.
28. Hildebrand T, Ruegsegger P (1997) A new method for the model-independent assessment of thickness in threedimensional images. J Microsc 185: 67–75.
29. Parfitt AM, Drezner MK, Glorieux FH, Kanis JA, Malluche H, et al. (1987) Bone histomorphometry: Standardization of nomenclature, symbols, and units. Report of the ASBMR Histomorphometry Nomenclature Committee. J Bone Miner Res 2: 595–610.
30. Odgaard A, Gundersen HJ (1993) Quantification of connectivity in cancellous bone, with special emphasis on 3-D reconstructions. Bone 14: 173–182.
31. Harrigan TP, Mann RW (1984) Characterization of microstructural anisotropy in orthotropic materials using a second rank tensor. J Mater Sci 19: 761–767.
32. Matsuzaki K, Ito M, Kaneko H, Kato M, Hikata T, et al (2013) Efficacy of osteoporotic agents in trabecular microstructure. Osteoporosis Japan 21: 102–105.
33. U.S. Food and Drug Administration Website, Center for Devices and Radiological Health (2010) Initiative to reduce unnecessary radiation exposure from medical imaging. Available: http://www.fda.gov/Radiation-emittingProducts/RadiationSafety/RadiationDoseReduction/default.htm. Accessed 2014 September 29.
34. Howland WJ, Loeffler RK, Starchman DE, Johnson RG (1975) Postirradiation atrophic changes of bone and related complications. Radiology 117: 677–685.
35. Hopewell JW, Calvo W, Reinhold HS (1989) Radiation effects on blood vessels: Role in normal tissue damage. In: Steel GG, Adams G, Horwich A, editors. Biological basis of radiotherapy. 2nd edition. Amsterdam: Elsevier Scientific; 1989. 101–113.
36. Pitkanen MA, Hopewell JW (1983) Functional changes in the vascularity of the irradiated rat femur: Implications for late effects. Acta Radiol Oncol 22: 253–256.
37. McCollough CH (2008) CT dose: how to measure, how to reduce. Health Phys 95: 508–517.
38. Bankier AA, Tack D (2010) Dose reduction strategies for thoracic multidetector computed tomography: background, current issues, and recommendations. J Thorac Imaging 25: 278–288.
39. Willey JS, Livingston EW, Robbins ME, Bourland JD, Tirado-Lee L, et al. (2010) Risedronate prevents early radiation-induced osteoporosis in mice at multiple skeletal locations. Bone 46: 101–111.
40. Xu D, Zhao X, Li Y, Ji Y, Zhang J, et al. (2014) The combined effects of X-ray radiation and hindlimb suspension on bone loss. J Radiat Res Apr 3. [Epub ahead of print].
41. MacNeil JA, Boyd SK (2007) Accuracy of high-resolution peripheral quantitative computed tomography for measurement of bone quality. Med Eng Phys 29: 1096–1105.
42. Hamilton SA, Pecaut MJ, Gridley DS, Travis ND, Bandstra ER, et al. (2006) A murine model for bone loss from therapeutic and space-relevant sources of radiation. J Appl Physiol (1985) 101: 789–793.
43. Chandra A, Lan S, Zhu J, Lin T, Zhang X, et al. (2013) PTH prevents the adverse effects of focal radiation on bone architecture in young rats. Bone 55: 449–457.
44. Weinstein RS (2011) Clinical practice. Glucocorticoid-induced bone disease. N Engl J Med 365: 62–70.
45. Compston J (2010) Management of glucocorticoid-induced osteoporosis. Nat Rev Rheumatol 6: 82–8.
46. Hofbauer LC, Hamann C, Ebeling PR (2010) Approach to the patient with secondary osteoporosis. Eur J Endocrinol 162: 1009–1020.
47. Maricic M (2011) Update on glucocorticoid-induced osteoporosis. Rheum Dis Clin North Am 37: 415–431.
48. Hofbauer LC, Zeitz U, Schoppet M, Skalicky M, Schüler C, et al. (2009) Prevention of glucocorticoid-induced bone loss in mice by inhibition of RANKL. Arthritis Rheum. 60: 1427–1437.
49. Overgaard M (1998) Spontaneous radiation-induced rib fractures in breast cancer patients treated with post-mastectomy irradiation. Acta Oncol 27: 117–122.

18

Recombinant Human Parathyroid Hormone Related Protein 1-34 and 1-84 and Their Roles in Osteoporosis Treatment

Hua Wang[1,2], Jingning Liu[1,3], Ying Yin[1,2], Jun Wu[1], Zilu Wang[2], Dengshun Miao[1], Wen Sun[1]*

1 The Research Center for Bone and Stem Cells, Department of Anatomy, Histology and Embryology, Nanjing Medical University, Nanjing, P.R. of China, **2** Institute of Dental Research, Stomatological College, Nanjing Medical University, Nanjing, P.R. of China, **3** Department of Geriatrics, The Second Affiliated Hospital of Nanjing Medical University, Nanjing, P.R. of China

Abstract

Osteoporosis is a common disorder characterized by compromised bone strength that predisposes patients to increased fracture risk. Parathyroid hormone related protein (PTHrP) is one of the candidates for clinical osteoporosis treatment. In this study, GST Gene Fusion System was used to express recombinant human PTHrP (hPTHrP) 1-34 and 1-84. To determine whether the recombinant hPTHrP1-34 and 1-84 can enhance renal calcium reabsorption and promote bone formation, we examined effects of recombinant hPTHrP1-34 and 1-84 on osteogenic lineage commitment in a primary bone marrow cell culture system and on osteoporosis treatment. Results revealed that both of recombinant hPTHrP1-34 and 1-84 increased colony formation and osteogenic cell differentiation and mineralization in vitro; however, the effect of recombinant hPTHrP1-84 is a little stronger than that of hPTHrP1-34. Next, ovariectomy was used to construct osteoporosis animal model (OVX) to test activities of these two recombinants in vivo. HPTHrP1-84 administration elevated serum calcium by up-regulating the expression of renal calcium transporters, which resulted in stimulation of osteoblastic bone formation. These factors contributed to augmented bone mass in hPTHrP1-84 treated OVX mice but did not affect bone resorption. There was no obvious bone mass alteration in hPTHrP1-34 treated OVX mice, which may be, at least partly, associated with shorter half-life of hPTHrP1-34 compared to hPTHrP1-84 in vivo. This study implies that recombinant hPTHrP1-84 is more effective than hPTHrP1-34 to enhance renal calcium reabsorption and to stimulate bone formation in vivo.

Editor: Jan Peter Tuckermann, University of Ulm, Germany

Funding: This work was supported by Project grants from the National Natural Science Foundation of China (No. 81200755) and by Natural Science Foundation of Jiangsu Province, China (BK2012440) and by Research Fund for the Doctoral Program of Higher Education of China (20123234120007). The funders had no role in study design, data collection and analysis, decision to publish, or preparation of the manuscript.

Competing Interests: The authors have declared that no competing interests exist.

* E-mail: wensun@njmu.edu.cn

Introduction

Osteoporosis is a common disorder characterized by compromised bone strength that predisposes patients to increased fracture risk. It arises, in part, as a consequence of bone loss secondary to an imbalance between the processes of bone resorption and formation during the normal bone remodeling cycle [1]. Clinical practice revealed that postmenopausal osteoporosis and age-related osteoporosis are the most common primary forms of bone loss.

A variety of drugs are now available for osteoporosis treatment, including antiresorptive and anabolic agents. Antiresorptive drugs treating osteoporosis, act by inhibiting osteoclast activity and consequently slowing the rate of bone remodeling, rather than by rebuilding bone. Antiresorptive drugs including estrogens, the selective estrogen receptor modulator, raloxifene, bisphosphonates and calcitonin [2]. Besides antiresorptive agents, the usage of anabolic agents is an important new advancement in osteoporosis treatment. Anabolic agents reduce fracture incidence by directly stimulating bone formation in addition to increasing bone mass. The only anabolic agent currently being approved in the United States for osteoporosis treatment, parathyroid hormone 1-34 (PTH1-34, teriparatide), has emerged as a major therapeutic approach to treat osteoporosis. PTH normally regulates serum calcium levels by binding and activating the type 1 PTH receptor (PTHR1) in bone and kidney [3]. As long as the dose and pattern of administration are carefully selected, exogenous PTH can stimulate bone formation in animals and in humans [2,4]. However, PTH has its side effect, which stimulates cortical bone loss [5]. Besides PTH, there are also some other potential anabolic agents for osteoporosis treatment, including parathyroid hormone related protein (PTHrP), growth hormone, insulin-like growth factor-1 (IGF-1), and so on [6–7]. Among these drugs, PTHrP has gained more and more attention in recent years [8].

PTHrP, a factor isolated from tumors associated with the paraneoplastic syndrome of humoral hypercalcemia of malignancy, shares homology with PTH1-34 [9–10]. Mice heterozygous for the *PTHrP*-null allele (*PTHrP*$^{+/-}$ mice) exhibit a form of skeletal haploinsufficiency characterized by decreased bone volume and bony structural alterations consistent with premature, advanced osteoporosis, which means PTHrP is necessary for bone remodeling [11]. Our previous studies have demonstrated that PTHrP is a key factor in bone formation [12–13]. PTHrP is a poly-hormone which can be translated and processed into many smaller bioactive forms, including an N-terminal peptide, midregion, nuclear localization sequence (NLS) and C-terminal region. The N-terminal PTHrP1-34 is structurally and functionally similar to PTH. The mid-region PTHrP35-84 or 86 exhibits a major role in placental calcium transport. The amino acids 88-107 region of NLS, targets PTHrP to the nucleus, where it regulates cell differentiation and apoptosis through an intracrine pathway. The C-terminal PTHrP108-141 acts as osteoclast activity inhibition [14–17].

Consistent with this concept, recombinant PTHrP1 84 treatment caused an increase in placental calcium transfer, whereas synthetic PTHrP1-34 had no such effect [18]. It supports the concept that the mid-molecule region of PTHrP is functionally important in placental calcium transport. Our previous studies also demonstrated that PTHrP1-86 can enhanced renal calcium reabsorption by promoting calcium transporters expression in kidney [19]. However, it is unclear whether there are some differences between PTHrP1-34 and 1-84 on renal calcium reabsorption and on bone formation. To answer this question, GST Gene Fusion System was used to express recombinant human PTHrP1-34 (hPTHrP1-34) and 1-84 (hPTHrP1-84). We tested the hypothesis that the recombinant hPTHrP1-84 is more effective than hPTHrP1-34 to enhance renal calcium reabsorption and to stimulate bone formation. We used the bilateral ovariectomized mice as osteoporosis animal model to test this hypothesis. We also explored the mechanism of the effect of recombinant N-terminal domain of PTHrP (hPTHrP1-34 and 1-84) on bone and kidney in this setting.

Materials and Methods

The use of animals in this study was approved by the Institutional Animal Care and Use Committee of Nanjing Medical University (Approval ID 2008-00318).

Cloning and expression of *hPTHrP1-34* and *1-84* in *pGEX-2TK*

The *hPTHrP1-34* and *1-84* fragments were amplified by RT-PCR from human bony complementary DNA using P1 (5′- TTTCCGGGATCCATGGCTGTGTCTGAACATCAGCT)/P2 (5′-TTTCCGGAATTCTCAAGCTGTGTGGATTTCTGCG) and P3 (5′- TTTCCGGGATCCATGGCTGTGTCTGAACATCAGCT)/P4 (5′- TTTCCGGAATTCTCACTTGAGCGGCTGCTCTTTG) primers, and the resulting product was digested with BamHI and EcoRI (sites underlined) and ligated into the GST fusion vector *pGEX-2TK* vector (Amersham). The recombinant DNA was used to transform competent E. coli BL21 (DE3) strains. Ampicillin resistance colonies were grown overnight in agar plate containing 50 μg/ml ampicillin, diluted ten times in the same medium, and grown to a concentration of 1 absorbance U/ml (at 600 nm). Expression of hPTHrP1-34 and 1-84 were induced with 1 mM isopropyl-beta-D-thiogalactopyranoside (IPTG) for 0h, 1h, 2h, 3h or 4h, and the bacterial suspension were harvested. The cells were pelleted, resuspended at 1/20 volume in cold 1×PBS, and sonicated on ice. Total protein from soluble fractions was dissolved in 2×SDS-PAGE buffer (2% SDS, 20% glycerol, 0.001% Bromphenol blue, and 0.125 M Tris-HCl pH 6.8) with subsequent boiling and fractionated by SDS-PAGE.

Purification of hPTHrP1-34 and 1-84

Purification of soluble hPTHrP1-34 and 1-84 separately from 1 liter culture of E. coli BL21 were performed on Glutathione Sepharose 4B columns (Amersham) using the recommended procedure. The fusion protein was digested 4h on the column with 20 U thrombin (Amersham) and eluted with 1 ml 1×PBS. Binding and elution steps were carried out in the cold to decrease proteolytic degradation of hPTHrP1-34 and 1-84. Purified hPTHrP1-34 and 1-84 were quantitated by a kit (Bio-Rad, Mississauga, Ontario, Canada) and prepared for Western blotting, in vitro and in vivo experiments as described below.

Primary bone marrow cell cultures

Tibiae and femurs of 200-g male Wistar rats were removed under aseptic conditions, and bone marrow cells (BMC) were flushed out with Dulbecco's modified Eagle's minimal essential medium containing 10% fetal calf serum, 50 μg/ml ascorbic acid, 10 mM β-glycerophosphate, and 10^{-8} M dexamethasone. Cells were dispersed by repeated pipetting, and a single-cell suspension was achieved by forcefully expelling the cells through a 22-gauge syringe needle. 10^6 total bone marrow cells were cultured in 36-cm^2 Petri dishes in 5 ml of the above-mentioned medium. All the dishes were assigned to three different groups. Each of the group treated with vehicle (Control), 10^{-7} M hPTHrP1-34 or 10^{-7} M hPTHrP1-84. The medium was changed every 4 days. The non-adherent cells containing hematopoietic elements were removed by pipetting gently when the medium was changed for the first time [20]. Only monocytic cells remained. Cultures were maintained for 12–18 days. At the end of the culture period cells were stained cytochemically or RNA was extracted from these cells for RT-PCR as described below.

Cytochemical staining

The cells from 18-day primary BMC cultures were washed with PBS and fixed by the addition of cold ethanol. After fixation, the cultures were stained sequentially for alkaline phosphatase (ALP)-positive colonies, calcified colonies, collagen-positive colonies, and total colonies as described previously [21]. After each staining procedure, the culture dishes were photographed, destained, and then restained as required. The numbers of colonies were counted macroscopically by hand. Total fibroblastic colonies, *i.e.* colonies predominantly containing cells with a mesenchymal morphology, were considered to represent colony forming units fibroblastic (CFU-f). Colonies that also stained positive for ALP, calcium, and/or collagen were considered to be derived from CFU-f with the ability to express ALP, calcium, and/or synthesize collagen and were termed CFU-f_{ALP}, CFU-f_{Ca}, and CFU-f_{Col}.

In vivo experiments

Twenty four female C57BL/6J mice, 8 weeks age, were assigned to four different groups, with six mice per group. All mice were anesthetized with chloral hydrate (0.4 ml/100 g body weight) and subjected to surgery on day 0. Sham surgery was performed on the Sham group (Sham) by identifying the bilateral ovaries and ovariectomy (OVX) was performed on the other groups by removing the bilateral ovaries. After surgery, all mice were maintained in a virus- and parasite-free barrier facility and exposed to a 12-h/12-h light/dark cycle under standard conditions in the Medical Experimental Animal Center of Nanjing Medical University for 9 weeks. HPTHrP1–34 was subcutaneously administered at a dose of 10 nmol/kg (40 μg/kg) body weight everyday for the last 4 weeks. HPTHrP1–84 was subcutaneously administered at a dose of 10 nmol/kg (100 μg/kg) body weight everyday for the last 4 weeks. Each of the mice received vehicle (vehicle-treated sham-operated mice and vehicle-treated OVX mice), hPTHrP1-34 (hPTHrP1-34-treated OVX mice) or hPTHrP1-84 (hPTHrP1-84-treated OVX mice). At the end of experiments, all mice were sacrificed by exsanguination under chloral hydrate anesthesia and blood were collected for serum calcium, phosphorus and ALP analyses, bones and kidneys were then removed for the analyses described below.

Serum PTHrP analyses

The OVX mice were injected with vehicle or 10 nmol/kg hPTHrP1-34 or 10 nmol/kg hPTHrP1-84 subcutaneously. Subsequently, blood samples were drawn at 15 and 30 minutes, 1, 2, 4 and 6 hours after the injections. Serum concentrations of hPTHrP1-34 or hPTHrP1-84 were measured by enzyme linked immunosorbent assay (ELISA) that used Phoenix Pharmaceuticals PTHrP(1-34)- EIA Kit (Phoenix Pharmaceuticals, USA). Procedures were performed according to the instructions of the kit.

Serum calcium, phosphorus and ALP analyses

Serum calcium, phosphorus and ALP were determined at 4 weeks after the administration of drugs by autoanalyzer (Beckman Synchron 67; Beckman Instruments).

Radiography

Thoracic vertebrae were removed and dissected free of soft tissue. Contact radiographs were taken using a Faxitron model 805 radiographic inspection system (Faxitron Contact, Faxitron, Germany) (22 kV voltage and 4 mins exposure time). X-Omat TL film (Eastman Kodak Co., Rochester, NY, USA) was used and processed routinely.

Micro-computed tomography (micro-CT)

Thoracic vertebrae were fixed overnight in 70% ethanol and analyzed by micro-CT with a SkyScan 1072 scanner and associated analysis software (SkyScan, Antwerp, Belgium) as described [22]. Briefly, image acquisition was performed at 100 kV and 98 μA with a 0.9° rotation between frames. During scanning, the samples were enclosed in tightly fitting plastic wrap to prevent movement and dehydration. Thresholding was applied to the images to segment the bone from the background. Two-dimensional images were used to generate three-dimensional renderings using the 3D Creator software supplied with the instrument. The resolution of the micro-CT images is 18.2 μm.

Histology

Lumbar vertebrae or tibiae were removed and fixed in PLP fixative (2% paraformaldehyde containing 0.075 M lysine and 0.01 M sodium periodate solution) overnight at 4°C and processed histologically as described [23]. Lumbar vertebrae were decalcified in ethylene-diamine tetraacetic acid (EDTA) glycerol solution for 5–7 days at 4°C. Decalcified samples were dehydrated and embedded in paraffin after which 5 μm sections were cut on a rotary microtome. The sections were stained with hematoxylin and eosin (H&E) or histochemically for total collagen, ALP and tartrate-resistant acid phosphatase (TRAP) as described below. Undecalcified bones were embedded in LR White acrylic resin (London Resin Co. Ltd., Theale, UK). Sections of 1 μm were cut on an ultramicrotome and stained for mineral with the von Kossa staining procedure and using toluidine blue as counter stain.

Histochemical staining for collagen, ALP and TRAP

Total collagen was detected in paraffin sections using a modified method of Lopez-De Leon and Rojkind [24]. Dewaxed sections were exposed to 1% sirius red in saturated picric acid for 1h. After washing with distilled water, the sections were counterstained with hematoxylin and mounted with Biomount medium.

Enzyme histochemistry for ALP activity was performed as described [25]. Briefly, following preincubation overnight in 100 mM $MgCl_2$ in 100 mM Tris-maleate buffer (pH 9.2), dewaxed sections were incubated for 2 hours at room temperature in 100 mM Tris-maleate buffer containing naphthol AS-MX phosphate (0.2 mg/ml, Sigma) dissolved in ethylene glycol monomethyl ether (Sigma) as substrate and fast red TR (0.4 mg/ml, Sigma) as a stain for the reaction product. After washing with distilled water, the sections were counterstained with Vector methyl green nuclear counterstain (Vector laboratories) and mounted with Kaiser's glycerol jelly.

Enzyme histochemistry for TRAP was performed using a modification of a previously described protocol [26]. Dewaxed sections were preincubated for 20 min in buffer containing 50 mM sodium acetate and 40 mM sodium tartrate at pH 5.0. Sections were then incubated for 15 min at room temperature in the same buffer containing 2.5 mg/ml naphthol AS-MX phosphate (Sigma) in dimethylformamide as substrate and 0.5 mg/ml fast garnet GBC (Sigma) as a color indicator for the reaction product. After washing with distilled water, the sections were counterstained with methyl green and mounted in Kaiser's glycerol jelly.

Double calcein labeling

Double calcein labeling was performed by intraperitoneal injection of mice with 10 μg calcein/g body weight (C-0875, Sigma-Aldrich Corp., St. Louis, MO) at 10 and 3 day before death. Bones were harvested and embedded in LR White acrylic resin. Serial sections were cut, and the freshly cut surface of each section was viewed and imaged using fluorescence microscopy. The double calcein-labeled width of bone was measured using Northern Eclipse image analysis software version 6.0 (Empix Imaging, Inc., Mississauga, Canada), and the mineral apposition rate (MAR) was calculated as the interlabel width/labeling period.

RNA isolation and Quantitative real-time PCR

RNA was isolated from 14-day cultured cells using Trizol reagent (Invitrogen) according to the manufacturer's protocol. Femurs were isolated and weighted. Homogenize tissue samples in 1 ml of TRIzol reagent per 50–100 mg of tissue using mortar and pestle with liquid nitrogen. After homogenization, remove insoluble material from the homogenate by centrifuging at 12,000 RPM for 10 min at 4°C. Transfer the top layer solution into a new tube. RNA of this solution was precipitated with isopropanol, washed with 75% ethanol and dissolved with DEPC water [27]. Reverse transcription reactions were performed using the SuperScript First-Strand Synthesis System (Invitrogen) as previously described [22]. To determine the number of cDNA molecules in the reverse transcribed samples, real-time PCR analyses were performed using the LightCycler system (Roche, Indianapolis, IN) as previously described [19].

Western blot analysis

Purified hPTHrP1-34 and 1-84 and proteins extracted from kidney were quantitated by a kit (Bio-Rad, Mississauga, Ontario, Canada). Thirty μg protein samples were fractionated by SDS-PAGE and transferred to nitrocellulose membranes. Immunoblotting was carried out as described [22] using antibodies against PTHrP1-34, TRPV5 (ECaC1), calbindin-D_{9K} and calbindin-D_{28K}, Na^+/Ca^{2+} exchanger 1 (NCX1), and β-tubulin (Santa Cruz, CA, USA). Bands were visualized using ECL chemiluminescence (Amersham) and quantitated by Scion Image Beta 4.02 (Scion Corporation, NIH).

Computer-assisted image analysis

After HE staining or histochemical staining of sections from six mice of each genotype, images of fields were photographed with a Sony digital camera. All images were digitally recorded using a rectangular template, and recordings were processed and analyzed using Northern Eclipse image analysis software as described [23,26,28].

Statistical analysis

Data from image analysis are presented as means ± SEM. Statistical comparisons were made using Student's t-test, with $P<0.05$ being considered significant.

Results

Construction and expression of *hPTHrP1-34* and *1-84* in *pGEX-2TK*

The recombinant expression vectors *pGEX-2TK/hPTHrP1-34* were used to transform competent E. coli BL21 (DE3) and five randomly picked ampicillin resistant colonies were grown. Plasmids were extracted and identified by PCR, and confirmed by double restriction enzyme digestion and sequencing (Fig. 1a). All of the selected transformants expressed an IPTG inducible protein which located in the expected site on SDS-PAGE. The optimal concentration of IPTG determined for protein induction is 1 mM (results not shown). Among the selected colonies, the one exhibited highest level of soluble expression was chosen for subsequent optimization studies and scale-up. Construction of *hPTHrP1-84* in *pGEX-2TK* followed the same procedures as described above.

The GST-hPTHrP1-34 and GST-hPTHrP1-84 fusion protein were both expressed mostly as soluble forms. Upon induction with IPTG, the fusion protein expression levels were continuously increased until reached a maximum concentration 3 hours later. The expression levels were increased with time of cultures after the induction (Figs. 1b and d). Therefore, we harvested the culturing engineered bacteria at 3 hours after the induction for more soluble fusion protein production.

Purification and characterisation of recombinant hPTHrP1-34 and 1-84

Scale up production was carried out in 1 liter medium using the optimal conditions identified by small scale production (3-hour-induction with 1 mM IPTG). The 30-kDa GST-hPTHrP1-34 and 36-kDa GST-hPTHrP1-84 fusion protein were bound to Glutathione Sepharose 4B columns as described in Materials and Methods. After thrombin cleavage, 4-kDa hPTHrP1-34 and 10-kDa hPTHrP1-84 were released from the matrix (Figs. 1c and e). The total amount of purified soluble hPTHrP1-34 and 1-84 productions were varied from 100 to 200 μg/liter of cultures. Western blotting of the purified protein using N-terminal hPTHrP antibody revealed that purified hPTHrP1-34 and 1-84 both had immunologic activities (Fig. 1f).

Recombinant hPTHrP1-34 and 1-84 promotes osteoprogenitor commitment to osteogenic lineage

To determine actions of recombinant hPTHrP1-34 and 1-84 on osteoprogenitor commitment, the primary bone marrow cultures were performed. The cells resulting cultures were examined for colony formation, and for markers of osteogenic differentiation including ALP activity, total collagen content, and mineralization of extracellular matrix. The results showed that treatment with hPTHrP1-34 and 1-84 at day 0 caused a significant increase in colony formation and osteogenic cell differentiation and mineralization compared with control cultures (Figs. 2a-h). Whereas it is noteworthy that the number of total colony forming units fibroblastic (CFU-f) and ALP-positive CFU-f were increased in hPTHrP1-84 treated cultures compared to hPTHrP1-34 treated cultures (Figs. 2a–h). We also examined the alterations of expression levels of genes related to osteogenic differentiation and mineralization. RNA was isolated from 14-day primary bone marrow cells (BMC) cultures and real time RT-PCR was performed. Results showed that gene expression levels of *Cbfa-1*, *ALP*, *type I collagen (Col I)* and *osteocalcin (OCN)* were upregulated significantly in hPTHrP1-34 and 1-84 treated primary BMC cultures compared with control cultures (Fig. 2i). These alterations were consistent with the osteogenic differentiation and mineralization observed by morphocytological analyses.

Effects of recombinant hPTHrP1-34 and 1-84 on serum chemistry and on expression levels of calcium transporters in kidney

To determine whether the administrations of recombinant hPTHrP1-34 and 1-84 altered serum mineral ion levels and osteoblast activity in OVX mice, serum calcium (Fig. 3a) and phosphorus (Fig. 3b) and bone specific ALP (Fig. 3c) were examined at 4 weeks after the drug administration. Serum ALP levels, most likely reflect osteoblast stimulation. The vehicle-treated OVX mice displayed hypocalcemia, hyperphosphatemia, and increased serum ALP levels compared with vehicle-treated sham-operated mice. Serum mineral ion and ALP levels had no significant differences between vehicle-treated and hPTHrP1-34-treated OVX mice. Whereas recombinant hPTHrP1-84-treated OVX mice displayed normocalcemia, normophosphatemia, and more obviously ALP elevations compared with vehicle-treated sham-operated mice (Figs. 3a–c).

To determine whether the raised serum calcium levels induced by recombinant hPTHrP1-84 were due to increased renal reabsorption of calcium, we examined the protein expression levels of the renal calcium transporters by Western blot (Fig. 3d). The results revealed that the protein levels of calbindin-D_{28K}, calbindin-D_{9K}, NCX1, and TRPV5 were down-regulated in the kidney of vehicle-treated and hPTHrP1-34-treated OVX mice relative to vehicle-treated sham-operated mice,however, they were up-regulated dramatically by hPTHrP1-84 treatment (Figs. 3d and 3e).

Effects of recombinant hPTHrP1-34 and 1-84 on bone volume

To assess whether the administrations of recombinant hPTHrP1-34 and 1-84 could prevent estrogen deficiency induced bone loss, bone mineral density and bone volume were analyzed in vertebrae by radiography (Fig. 4a), micro-CT (Figs. 4b and 4c), histology (Fig. 4d) and histochemistry for total collagen (Fig. 4f). The results revealed that the radiolucency was increased in vertebrae in vehicle-treated and hPTHrP1-34-treated OVX mice, was normalized in hPTHrP1-84-treated OVX mice compared to vehicle-treated sham-operated mice (Fig. 4a). This was further verified by 3D micro-CT scanning and histological analysis, which demonstrated that trabecular bone volume and cortical thickness were decreased dramatically in vehicle-treated OVX mice compared to vehicle-treated sham-operated mice. Both parameters were not altered significantly in hPTHrP1-34-treated OVX mice, but were increased significantly in hPTHrP1-84-treated OVX mice compared to vehicle-treated and hPTHrP1-34-treated OVX mice (Figs. 4b–g). We also examined the alterations of bone volume in tibiae, which were consistent with the results observed in vertebrae (Figs. S1a and S1c).

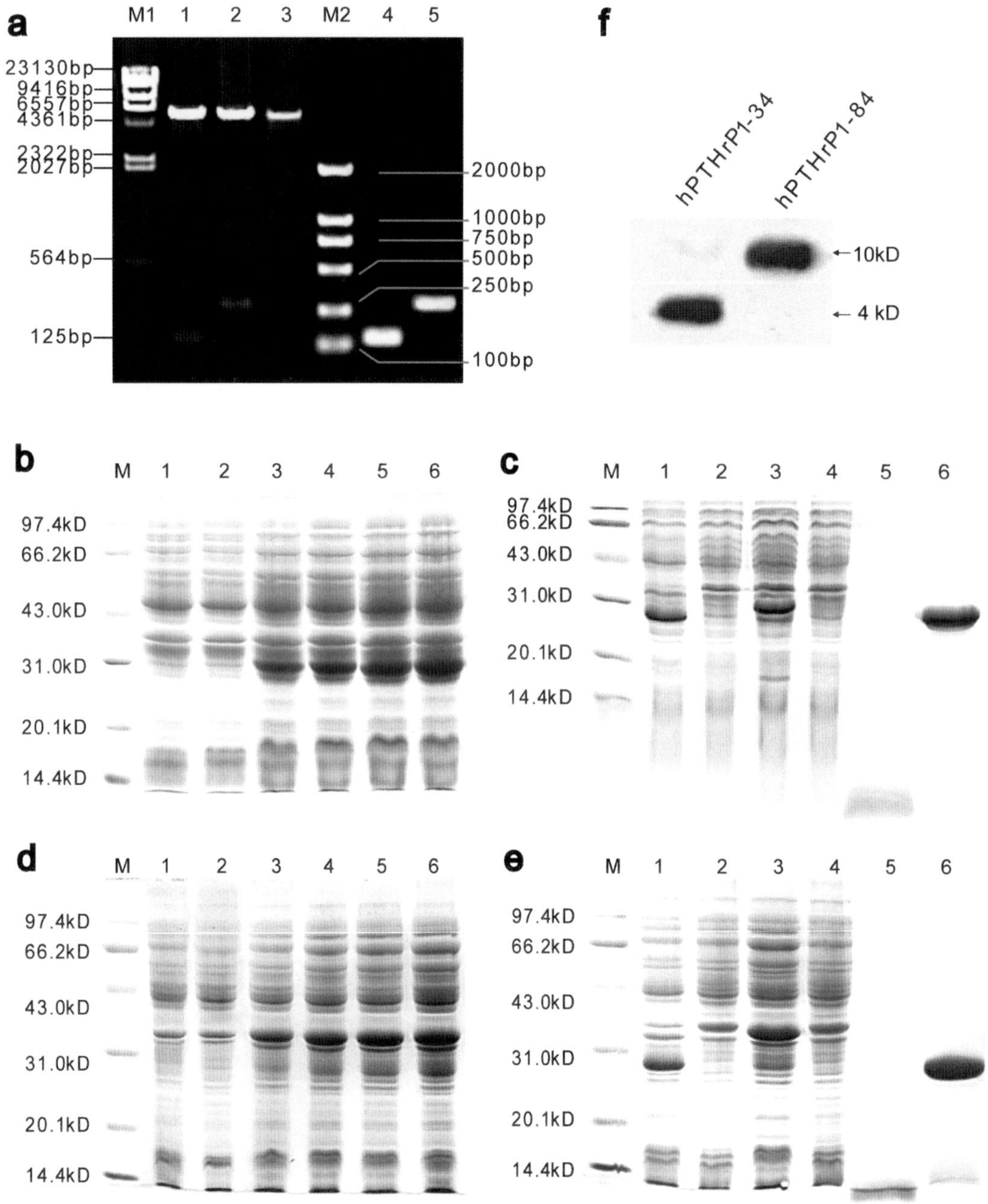

Figure 1. Preparation of Recombinant hPTHrP1-34 and 1-84. (a) Determination of the recombinants by PCR and double-enzyme (EcoR I+ BamH I) digestion. LaneM1, I-Hind III digest DNA marker; Lane1-3, double-enzyme digestion patterns of recombinant *hPTHrP1-34*, *hPTHrP1-84* and *pGEX-2TK*; LaneM2, DL2000 DNA marker; Lane4-5, PCR band patterns of recombinant hPTHrP1-34 and hPTHrP1-84. SDS-PAGE analysis of the GST-hPTHrP1-34 (b) or GST-hPTHrP1-84 (d) fusion protein under inducing condition and stained with coomassie blue. LaneM, molecular weight marker; Lane1, total cell soluble protein of BL21, control; Lanes2–6, cells with *pGEX-2TK/hPTHrP1-34* or *pGEX-2TK/hPTHrP1-84* after inducing with IPTG 0 h, 1 h, 2 h, 3 h, 4 h respectively. SDS-PAGE analyses of hPTHrP1-34 (c) or hPTHrP1-84 (e) peptide expression and purification. LaneM, molecular weight marker; Lane1, IPTG induction of BL21 transformed with *pGEX-2TK* without insert (expression control); Lane2, BL21 transformed with *pGEX-2TK/hPTHrP1-34* or *pGEX-2TK/hPTHrP1-84* without IPTG induction (induction control); Lane3, IPTG induction of BL21 transformed with *pGEX-2TK/hPTHrP1-34* or *pGEX-2TK/hPTHrP1-84*; Lane4, The proteins not bound to GSTrap FF column; Lane5, Purified hPTHrP1-34 or hPTHrP1-84 obtained after binding to GSTrap FF column and cleaved by thrombin; Lane6, GST-tag eluted from GSTrap FF column. (f) Western blot analysis of purified recombinant hPTHrP1-34 and hPTHrP1-84 with N-terminal hPTHrP antibody.

Effects of recombinant hPTHrP1-34 and 1-84 on osteoblastic bone formation

To determine whether the alterations of bone volume were associated with those of osteoblastic bone formation, MAR (Fig. 5a), histomorphometric analysis for osteoid volume (Fig. 5c), osteoblast number (Fig. 5e), and ALP activity (Fig. 5g) were examined in vertebrae at 4 weeks after the drug administration. Results showed that the MAR was decreased, osteoid volume was not altered significantly, whereas osteoblast number and ALP

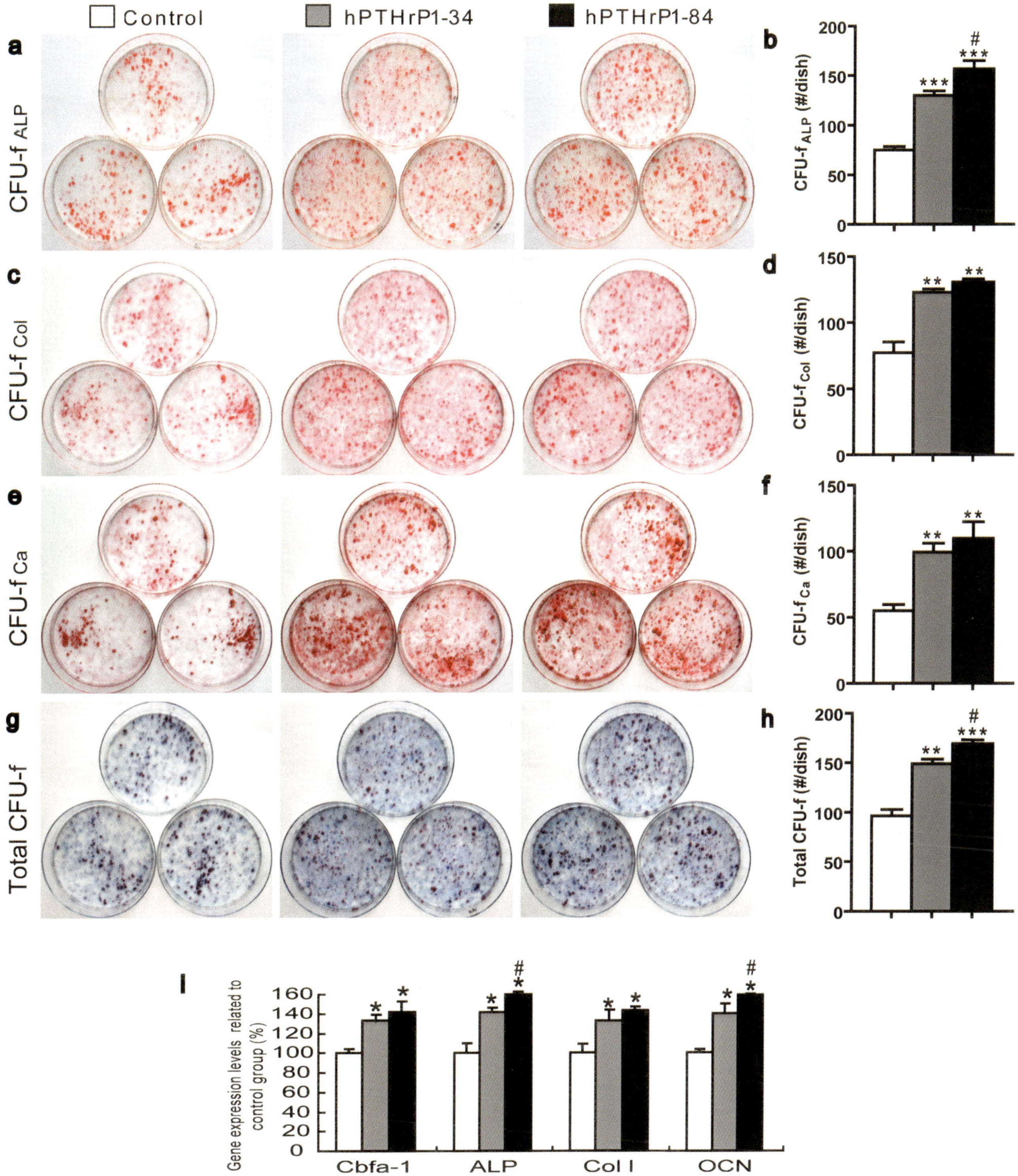

Figure 2. Effects of recombinant hPTHrP1-34 and 1-84 on BMCs. Cells from 18-day primary BMC cultures incubated in the absence (Control) or presence of 10^{-7} M hPTHrP1-34 (hPTHrP1-34) or presence of 10^{-7} M hPTHrP1-84 (hPTHrP1-84) on day 0 were stained cytochemically for ALP (a. CFU-f $_{ALP}$) and with sirius red for total collagen(c. CFU-f $_{Col}$) and with the von Kossa method for calcified colonies(e. CFU-f $_{Ca}$) and with methylene blue to show total CFU-f (g. Total CFU-f) as described in Materials and Methods. The positive number of CFU-f $_{ALP}$ (b), CFU-f $_{Col}$ (d), CFU-f $_{Ca}$ (f) and Total CFU-f number (h) per dish are the mean±SEM of triplicate determinations from three replicate experiments, respectively. (i) Real-time RT-PCR of cells extracts from 14-day primary BMC cultures for the expression of Cbfa I, ALP, Col I and OCN. Messenger RNA expression assessed by real-time RT-PCR is calculated as a ratio to the GAPDH mRNA level and expressed relative to levels of Control group. Each value is the mean ± SEM of three trials. *, $P<0.05$; **, $P<0.01$; ***, $P<0.001$ compared with Control group; #, $P<0.05$ compared with hPTHrP1-34 group.

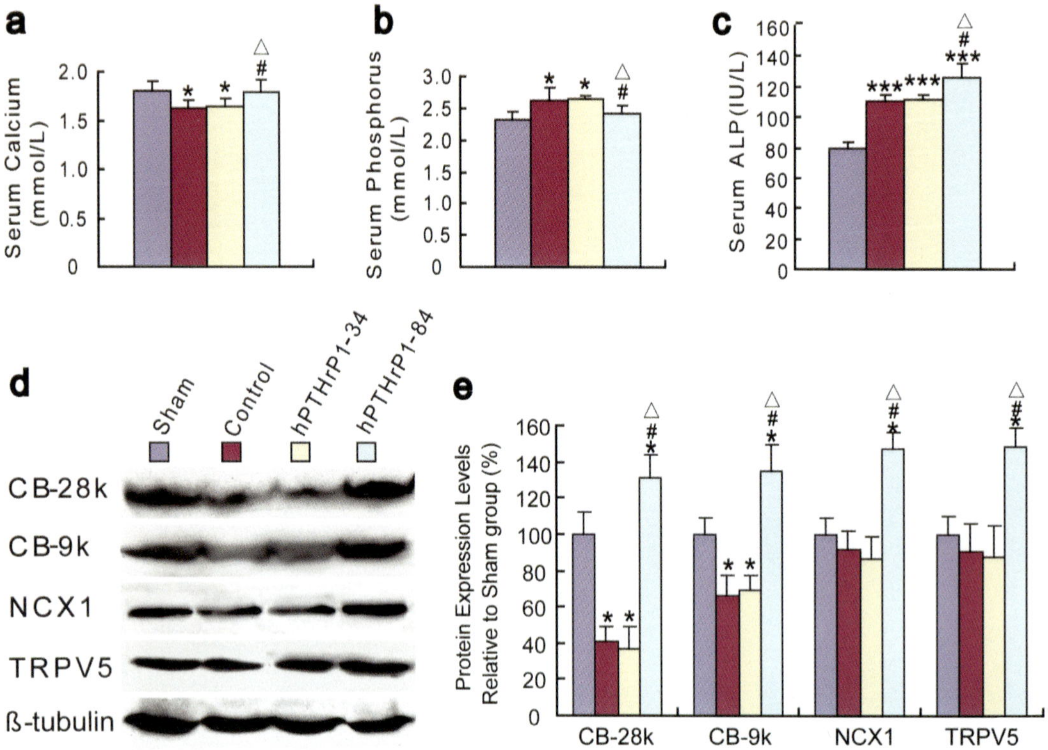

Figure 3. Effects of recombinant hPTHrP1-34 and 1-84 on serum chemistry and on expression of calcium transporters in kidney. (a) Serum calcium, (b) phosphorus and (c) ALP ratio were determined after 4-week administration in vehicle-treated sham-operated mice (Sham), vehicle-treated OVX mice (Control), hPTHrP1-34-treated OVX mice (hPTHrP1-34) and hPTHrP1-84-treated OVX mice (hPTHrP1-84). (d) Western blots of renal extracts for expression of CB_{28K}, CB_{9K}, NCX1 and TRPV5. β-tubulin was used as loading control for Western blots. (e) CB_{28K}, CB_{9K}, NCX1 and TRPV5 protein levels relative to β-tubulin protein level and expressed relative to levels of Sham group. Each value is the mean ± SEM of determinations in six mice of each group.*, $P<0.05$; ***, $P<0.001$ compared with Sham group; #, $P<0.05$ compared with Control group; △, $p<0.05$ compared with hPTHrP1-34 group.

positive area were increased in vehicle-treated and hPTHrP1-34-treated OVX mice compared to vehicle-treated sham-operated mice (Figs. 5a–h). All parameters for osteoblastic bone formation including MAR, osteoid volume, osteoblast number and ALP positive area (Figs. 5a–h) were increased dramatically in hPTHrP1-84-treated OVX mice compared with the other groups. Consistent with these observations, osteoblastic gene expression levels of *Cbfa1*, *ALP* were slightly up-regulated in vehicle-treated and hPTHrP1-34-treated OVX mice compared to vehicle-treated sham-operated mice; however, *Cbfa1*, *ALP*, *Col I*, and *OCN* were all up-regulated significantly in hPTHrP1-84-treated OVX mice compared to the other groups as demonstrated by real-time RT-PCR (Fig. 5i). We also examined the alterations of osteoblast number in tibiae, which were consistent with the results observed in vertebrae (Figs. S1b and S1d).

Effects of recombinant hPTHrP1-34 and 1-84 on osteoclastic bone resorption

To determine whether hPTHrP1-34 and 1-84 exerted catabolic effects on bone in OVX mice, histochemical staining for TRAP (Fig. 6a) were performed and osteoclast number and surface (Figs. 6b and 6c) were determined by image analysis. The results revealed that TRAP positive osteoclast number and surface were increased significantly in vehicle-treated OVX mice compared to vehicle-treated sham-operated mice. Whereas hPTHrP1-34 and 1-84 administration did not further increase TRAP positive osteoclast number and surface in OVX mice compared with vehicle-treated OVX mice (Figs. 6a–c). The ratios of *RANKL/OPG* mRNA levels were increased significantly in vehicle-treated, hPTHrP1-34-treated and hPTHrP 1-84-treated OVX mice compared to vehicle-treated sham-operated mice, however, they had no significant differences among vehicle-treated, hPTHrP1-34-treated and hPTHrP 1-84-treated OVX mice as demonstrated by real-time RT-PCR (Fig. 6d).

Half-life of recombinant hPTHrP1-34 and 1-84 in vivo

To assess whether the different effects of recombinant hPTHrP1-34 and 1-84 in vivo were associated with the differences of their half-life ($t_{1/2}$) in vivo, serum concentrations of hPTHrP1-34 and hPTHrP1-84 were measured at different time points after their administration. Results showed that plasma PTHrP levels were lower than 0.5 pM at all observed time points in vehicle-treated OVX mice, and rose to 9±0.7 and 8.5±0.7 pM at 15 min after the administration in hPTHrP1-34 and hPTHrP1-84-treated OVX mice, respectively. Then plasma PTHrP levels declined gradually until baseline levels at 2 hours in hPTHrP1-34-treated OVX mice, and 4 hours in hPTHrP1-84-treated OVX mice (Fig. 6e). From the figure, it can be seen that the circulating $t_{1/2}$ of hPTHrP1-34 was approximately 45 mins, whereas the $t_{1/2}$ of hPTHrP1-84 was approximately 2 hours.

Discussion

Recombinant hPTHrP1-34 and 1-84 were expressed using the GST Gene Fusion System, allowing purification of free

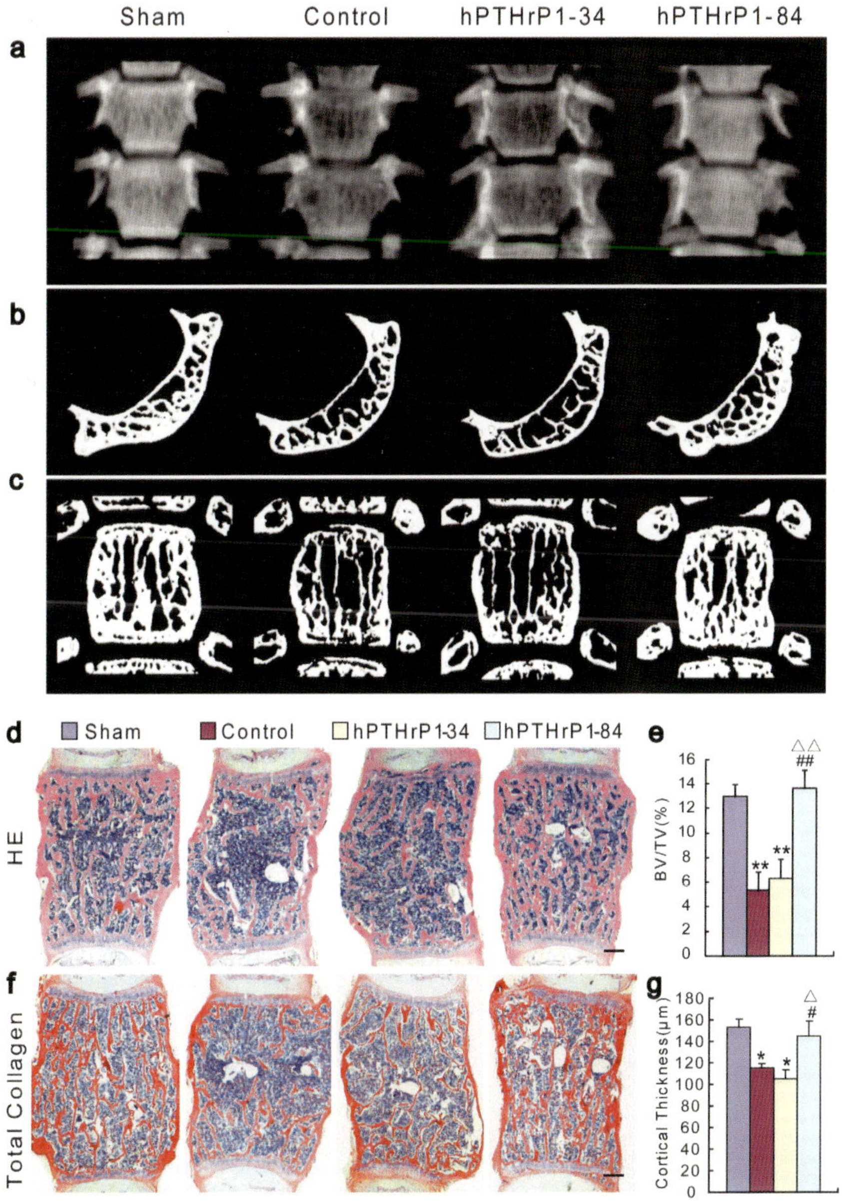

Figure 4. Effects of recombinant hPTHrP1-34 and 1-84 on bone volume. (a) Representative contact radiographs of thoracic vertebrae. Representative (b) cross-sections and (c) longitudinal sections of 3D reconstructed thoracic vertebrae. Micrographs of decalcified paraffin sections of lumbar vertebrae stained with H&E (d) and total collagen (f). Scale bars represent 200 μm in d and f. Trabecular bone volume relative to the tissue volume [BV/TV (%), e] and the cortical thickness (g) of vertebrae were determined by histomorphometric analysis as described in Materials and Methods. Each value is the mean ± SEM of determinations in six mice of each group. *, $P<0.05$; **, $P<0.01$ compared with Sham group; #, $P<0.05$; ##, $P<0.01$ compared with Control group; △, $P<0.05$; △△, $P<0.01$ compared with hPTHrP1-34 group.

recombinant peptide in a single affinity chromatographic step. The results of DNA sequence analysis showed that the gene sequences constructed for the recombinant hPTHrP1-34 and 1-84 were correct templates for expressing them. The molecular weights obtained by SDS-PAGE were the same as the theoretical value calculated from the atomic weight sum of atoms which consists the peptide according to the amino acid sequence. The results of the Western blotting revealed that the recombinant hPTHrP1-34 and 1-84 had immunological activities. Then, we employed them to investigate their actions in promoting BMC commitment to osteogenic lineage and stimulating bone formation.

PTHrP is a ubiquitously produced local paracrine, autocrine and intracrine factor, the role of which is to regulate cellular differentiation, proliferation, cell death, and epithelial calcium transport, both during development as well as in adult life [29–30]. Osteoblasts are also target cells for locally produced PTHrP and circulating PTH, as these cells express PTHR1 [31–33]. Our previous results demonstrated that PTHrP stimulates osteogenic cell proliferation in rat marrow mesenchymal progenitor cells through protein kinase C-dependent activation of the Ras and MAPK signaling pathway [34]. Several groups have demonstrated that PTHrP can influence osteoblast proliferation, differentiation and function [35]. Consistent with these results, our data also

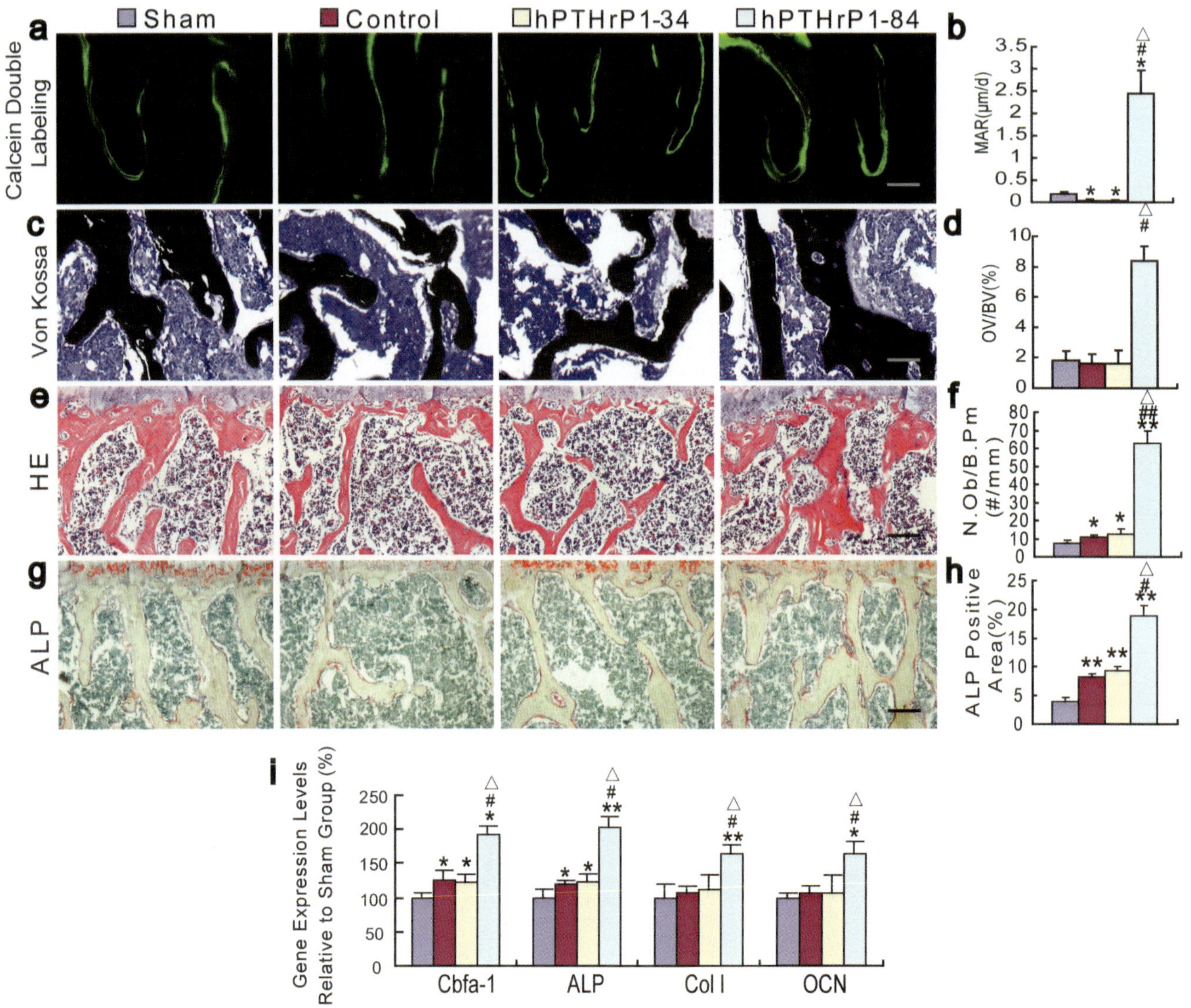

Figure 5. Effects of recombinant hPTHrP1-34 and 1-84 on osteoblastic bone formation parameters. (a) Representative micrographs of calcein double labeling and (c) sections stained with the von Kossa procedure in the trabeculae were imaged from ethanol fixed and undecalcified LR white resin embedded sections of vertebrae. (b) MAR of trabeculae was determined. (d) Osteoid volume was determined in undecalcified von Kossa-stained sections and is presented as a percent of bone volume (OV/BV, %) of trabeculae. Micrographs of decalcified paraffin sections of vertebrae stained with H&E (e) and histochemically for ALP (g). (f) Number of osteoblasts per mm bone parameter (N.Ob/B.Pm, #/mm) and (h) ALP positive area as a percent of the tissue area were determined in the vertebrae. Scale bars represent 25 μm in a and c and 50 μm in e and g. (i) Real-time RT-PCR of long bone extracts for the expression of *Cbfa I*, *ALP*, *Col I* and *OCN*. Messenger RNA expression assessed by real-time RT-PCR is calculated as a ratio to the *GAPDH* mRNA level and expressed relative to levels of Sham group. Each value is the mean ± SEM of determinations in six mice of each group. *, P<0.05; **, P<0.01 compared with Sham group; #, P<0.05; ##, P<0.01 compared with Control group; △, P<0.05 compared with hPTHrP1-34 group.

showed that treatment with hPTHrP1-34 and 1-84 caused a significant increase in colony formation and osteogenic cell differentiation and mineralization in primary bone marrow cultures compared with control cultures. We also found that treatment with PTHrP1-84 resulted in a slightly increase in total CFU-f number and ALP-positive CFU-f number compared with PTHrP1-34 treated cultures. Our findings indicate that both of recombinant hPTHrP1-34 and 1-84 enhance BMC commitment to osteogenic lineage, and the effect of recombinant hPTHrP1-84 is a little stronger than hPTHrP1-34. We have mentioned that Mid-region of PTHrP interact with a yet unidentified receptor to maintain matemo-foetal gradients of calcium [29,36]. So we presume that the Mid-region of PTHrP probably exerts a major influence on calcium transport in hPTHrP1-84-treated primary bone marrow cultures. However, exact mechanism remains to be determined.

In previous work, we have shown that 3-month-old mice heterozygous for the *Pthrp*-null allele exhibit a form of skeletal haploinsufficiency characterized by decreased bone volume and bony structural alterations consistent with premature, advanced osteoporosis [37]. Our previous studies in mice with osteoblast-specific targeted disruption of PTHrP showed that osteoblast-derived PTHrP is a potent endogenous bone anabolic factor which potentiates bone formation by altering osteoblast recruitment and survival [37]. All these evidences support that PTHrP is a potent endogenous bone anabolic agent. With regard to the action of

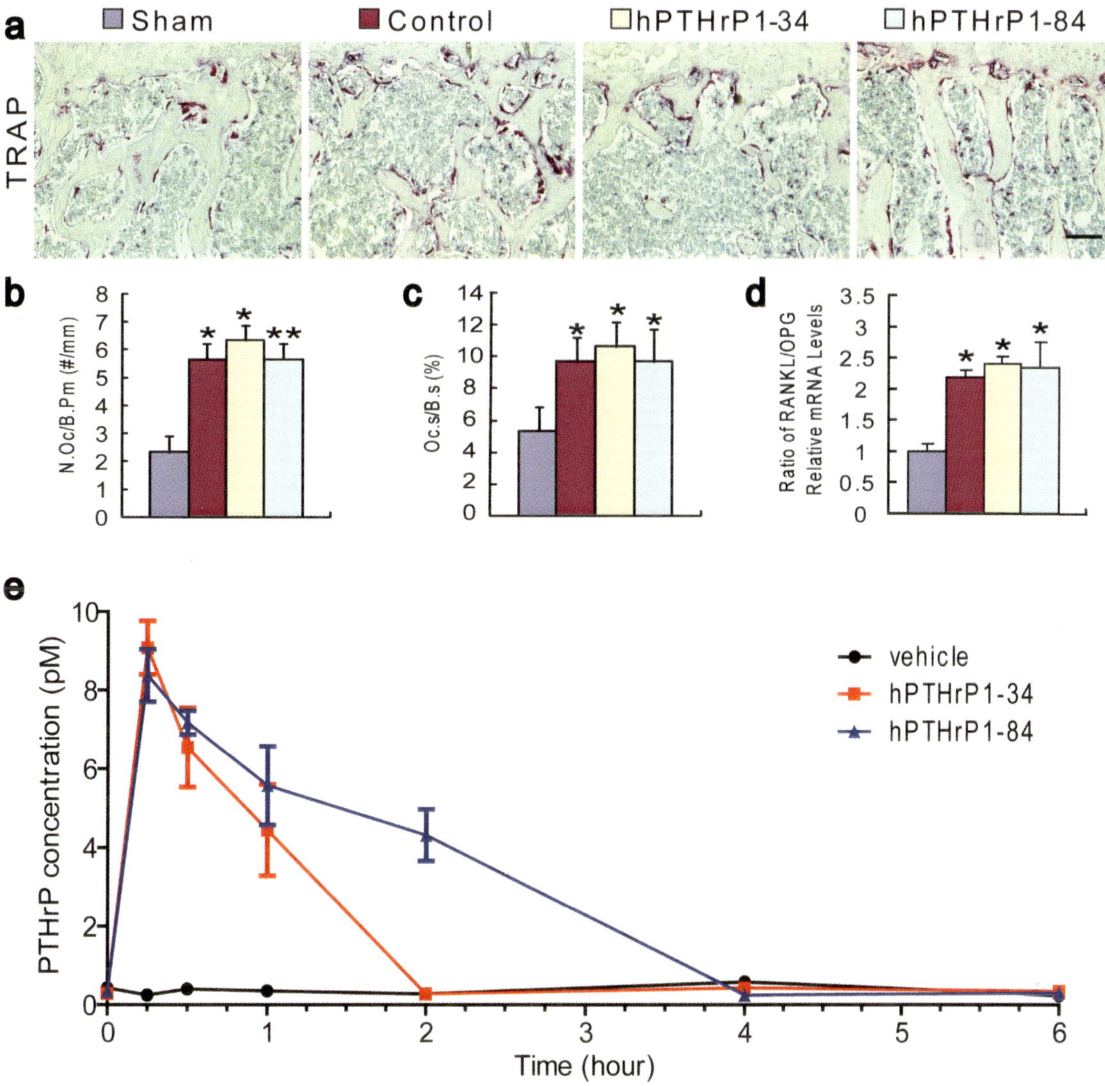

Figure 6. Effects of recombinant hPTHrP1-34 and 1-84 on osteoclastic bone resorption parameters and half-life analyses of recombinant hPTHrP1-34 and 1-84 in vivo. (a) Representative micrographs of paraffin embedded sections of vertebrae stained histochemically for TRAP and photographed at a magnification of 200. Scale bars in a represents 50 μm. (b) Number of TRAP positive osteoclasts per mm bone parameter (N.Oc/B.Pm, #/mm) and (c) the surface of osteoclasts relative to the bone surface (Oc.S/B.S, %) were determined in the trabeculae of TRAP-stained vertebrae. Each value is the mean ± SEM of determinations in 6 animals of each group. (d) Real-time RT-PCR was performed on long bone extracts for *RANKL* and *OPG* mRNA as described in Materials and Methods. Messenger RNA expression assessed by real-time RT-PCR analysis is calculated as a ratio to the *GAPDH* mRNA level and expressed relative to levels of Sham group. Ratio of *RANKL/OPG* relative mRNA levels was calculated and was presented as the mean ± SEM of determinations in six animals of each group. (e) Plasma immunoreactive PTHrP determined using ELISA after subcutaneous injection of vehicle or hPTHrP1-34 or hPTHrP1-84. Blood samples were drawn at the following time points after injection of study drugs: 15 and 30 minutes, then 1, 2, 4, 6 hours. Each value is the mean ± SEM of determinations in 6 animals of each group. *, $P<0.05$; **, $P<0.01$ compared with Sham group.

exogenous PTHrP1-86 on skeletal alteration, we have shown that PTHrP increased cortical and trabecular bone mass with augmented osteoblast number and activity; however, bone resorption was not increased [19]. Consistent with these results, our data also demonstrated that recombinant hPTHrP1-84 administration increased bone mass in osteoporosis mice by stimulating osteoblastic bone formation. After subcutaneously injected hPTHrP1-84 into osteoporosis animal models for 4 weeks, all osteoblastic bone formation parameters including MAR, osteoid volume, osteoblast number, ALP positive area and osteoblastic gene expression levels were increased dramatically in hPTHrP1-84-treated OVX mice compared with the vehicle-treated OVX mice. These results suggest that recombinant hPTHrP1-84 is an effective agent to stimulate bone formation.

Unexpectedly, unlike recombinant hPTHrP1-84, the recombinant hPTHrP1-34 administration did not increased bone mass and osteoblastic bone formation parameters in OVX mice in vivo. We also found that serum calcium and renal calcium transporters were not alterd by hPTHrP1-34 administration, but were increased significantly by hPTHrP1-84 administration in OVX mice. The transcellular calcium transport involves many molecules, including TRPV5 as the apical entry gate for Ca^{2+}, calbindin-D_{9K} and calbindin-D_{28K} as intracellular ferry proteins for Ca^{2+}, and NCX1 as Ca^{2+} extrusion systems across the basolateral membrane to the blood compartment [38]. Our results revealed that the protein levels of renal calcium transporters, including calbindin-D_{9K}, calbindin-D_{28K}, NCX1, and TRPV5 were all down-regulated in the kidney of vehicle-treated and hPTHrP1-34-treated OVX mice compared with vehicle-treated sham-operated mice, however their levels were up-regulated significantly by hPTHrP1-84 administration. These data suggest that raised serum calcium levels induced by recombinant hPTHrP1-84 were due to increased renal reabsorption of calcium. In previous studies, $1,25(OH)_2D_3$ and the vitamin D receptor have been reported to modulate calcium transporters in vivo [39-40]. Our previous study has demonstrated that, similar to PTH1-34, PTHrP1-86 administration up-regulated renal calcium transporters in vivo [19]. Our results indicate that hPTHrP1-84 could modulate renal calcium transporters. In view of the fact that bone resorption was not altered by hPTHrP1-84 administraion, the major mechanism of raised serum calcium levels were mediated by stimulating renal calcium reabsorption. Our previous studies suggest that increased extracellular calcium by endogenous PTH [41] or $1,25(OH)_2D_3$ [42] can increase bone mass and stimulate osteoblastic bone formation mediated by calcium sensing receptor (CaSR). In tissue culture models, elevations in extracellular free ionized calcium concentrations increase osteoblast chemotaxis and proliferation [43-44], and alter the levels of expression of some differentiation markers [45]. Furthermore, deletion of both alleles of the Casr gene in osteoblasts profoundly blocked postnatal growth and skeletal development, a finding that was evident by 3 days of age [46]. These results support that hPTHrP1-84, at least partly, can stimulate osteoblastic bone formation and increase bone mass by increasing extracellular calcium levels mediated by CaSR.

In order to explore possible reason why recombinant hPTHrP1-34 and 1-84 displayed different response in vivo, we examined whether their different effects were associated with the differences of their half-life in vivo. By measured serum concentrations of hPTHrP1-34 and hPTHrP1-84 at different time points after their administration, we found that the circulating lifetime of hPTHrP1-34 is much shorter than hPTHrP1-84, suggesting that hPTHrP1-34 may be degraded more rapidly than hPTHrP1-84 in vivo. On the other hand, it is also possible that hPTHrP1-34 has less affinity with PTHR, which remains to be investigated.

In summary, in this study, GST Gene Fusion System was used to express recombinant hPTHrP1-34 and 1-84. *HPTHrP1-34* and *1-84* gene fragments were cloned into the *pGEX-2TK* vector, the host cells used for the cloning steps were transformed, and the presences of the insert were verified. After scale up production, recombinant hPTHrP1-34 and 1-84 were obtained by means of cell disruption, Glutathione Sepharose 4B column purification and thrombin digestion. Examined activities of recombinants in vitro, we found that treatment of hPTHrP1-34 and 1-84 caused a significant increase in colony formation and osteogenic cell differentiation and mineralization in primary bone marrow cultures; however, the effect of recombinant hPTHrP1-84 is a little stronger than hPTHrP1-34. Next, ovariectomy was used to construct osteoporosis animal model to test activities of recombinants in vivo. HPTHrP1-84 administration elevated extracellular calcium levels by increasing renal calcium transport, which resulted in stimulation of osteoblastic bone formation. These factors contributed to augmented bone mass in hPTHrP1-84-treated OVX mice but did not affect bone resorption. There was no obviously bone volume alteration in hPTHrP1-34 treated OVX mice. For this explanation, we found that the circulating lifetime of hPTHrP1-34 is much shorter than hPTHrP1-84, suggesting that hPTHrP1-34 may be degraded more rapidly than hPTHrP1-84 in vivo. This study implies that recombinant hPTHrP1-84 is more effective than hPTHrP1-34 to enhance renal calcium reabsorption and to stimulate osteoblastic bone formation.

Supporting Information

Figure S1 Effects of recombinant hPTHrP1-34 and 1-84 on the phenotype of tibiae. Micrographs of decalcified paraffin sections of tibiae stained with total collagen (a) and H&E (b). (c) Trabecular bone volume relative to the tissue volume [BV/TV (%)] and (d) number of osteoblasts per mm bone parameter (N.Ob/B.Pm, #/mm) were determined by histomorphometric analysis as described in Materials and Methods. Each value is the mean ± SEM of determinations in six mice of each group. *, $P<0.05$; **, $P<0.01$ compared with Sham group; #, $P<0.05$; ##, $P<0.01$ compared with Control group; △, $P<0.05$; △△, $P<0.01$ compared with hPTHrP1-34 group.

Author Contributions

Conceived and designed the experiments: WS. Performed the experiments: HW JL YY JW. Analyzed the data: WS HW. Contributed reagents/materials/analysis tools: WS ZW. Wrote the paper: WS DM.

References

1. Sobieszczanska M, Jonkisz J, Tabin M, Laszki-Szczachor K (2013) Osteoporosis: genetic determinants and relationship with cardiovascular disease. Adv Clin Exp Med 22: 119–124.
2. Girotra M, Rubin MR, Bilezikian JP (2006) The use of parathyroid hormone in the treatment of osteoporosis. Rev Endocr Metab Disord 7: 113–121.
3. Juppner H, Abou-Samra AB, Freeman M, Kong XF, Schipani E, et al. (1991) A G protein-linked receptor for parathyroid hormone and parathyroid hormone-related peptide. Science 254: 1024–1026.
4. Baron R, Hesse E (2012) Update on bone anabolics in osteoporosis treatment: rationale, current status, and perspectives. J Clin Endocrinol Metab 97: 311–325.
5. Borba VZ, Manas NC (2010) The use of PTH in the treatment of osteoporosis. Arq Bras Endocrinol Metabol 54: 213–219.
6. Girotra M, Rubin MR, Bilezikian JP (2006) Anabolic skeletal therapy for osteoporosis. Arq Bras Endocrinol Metabol 50: 745–754.
7. Khan AW, Khan A (2006) Anabolic agents: a new chapter in the management of osteoporosis. J Obstet Gynaecol Can 28: 136–141.
8. Augustine M, Horwitz MJ (2013) Parathyroid Hormone and Parathyroid Hormone-Related Protein Analogs as Therapies for Osteoporosis. Curr Osteoporos Rep.
9. Strewler GJ, Nissenson RA (1990) Hypercalcemia in malignancy. West J Med 153: 635–640.
10. Grill V, Rankin W, Martin TJ (1998) Parathyroid hormone-related protein (PTHrP) and hypercalcaemia. Eur J Cancer 34: 222–229.
11. Amizuka N, Karaplis AC, Henderson JE, Warshawsky H, Lipman ML, et al. (1996) Haploinsufficiency of parathyroid hormone-related peptide (PTHrP) results in abnormal postnatal bone development. Dev Biol 175: 166–176.
12. Sun W, Liu J, Zhou X, Xiao Y, Karaplis A, et al. (2010) Alterations in phosphorus, calcium and PTHrP contribute to defects in dental and dental alveolar bone formation in calcium-sensing receptor-deficient mice. Development 137: 985–992.
13. Liu J, Lv F, Sun W, Tao C, Ding G, et al. (2011) The abnormal phenotypes of cartilage and bone in calcium-sensing receptor deficient mice are dependent on the actions of calcium, phosphorus, and PTH. PLoS Genet 7: e1002294.
14. Kovacs CS, Lanske B, Hunzelman JL, Guo J, Karaplis AC, et al. (1996) Parathyroid hormone-related peptide (PTHrP) regulates fetal-placental calcium transport through a receptor distinct from the PTH/PTHrP receptor. Proc Natl Acad Sci U S A 93: 15233–15238.
15. Clemens TL, Cormier S, Eichinger A, Endlich K, Fiaschi-Taesch N, et al. (2001) Parathyroid hormone-related protein and its receptors: nuclear functions and roles in the renal and cardiovascular systems, the placental trophoblasts and the pancreatic islets. Br J Pharmacol 134: 1113–1136.
16. Miao D, Su H, He B, Gao J, Xia Q, et al. (2008) Severe growth retardation and early lethality in mice lacking the nuclear localization sequence and C-terminus of PTH-related protein. Proc Natl Acad Sci U S A 105: 20309–20314.

17. Fenton AJ, Martin TJ, Nicholson GC (1993) Long-term culture of disaggregated rat osteoclasts: inhibition of bone resorption and reduction of osteoclast-like cell number by calcitonin and PTHrP[107-139]. J Cell Physiol 155: 1–7.
18. Abbas SK, Pickard DW, Rodda CP, Heath JA, Hammonds RG, et al. (1989) Stimulation of ovine placental calcium transport by purified natural and recombinant parathyroid hormone-related protein (PTHrP) preparations. Q J Exp Physiol 74: 549–552.
19. Xue Y, Zhang Z, Karaplis AC, Hendy GN, Goltzman D, et al. (2005) Exogenous PTH-related protein and PTH improve mineral and skeletal status in 25-hydroxyvitamin D-1alpha-hydroxylase and PTH double knockout mice. J Bone Miner Res 20: 1766–1777.
20. Conget PA, Minguell JJ (1999) Phenotypical and functional properties of human bone marrow mesenchymal progenitor cells. J Cell Physiol 181: 67–73.
21. Erben RG, Scutt AM, Miao D, Kollenkirchen U, Haberey M (1997) Short-term treatment of rats with high dose 1,25-dihydroxyvitamin D3 stimulates bone formation and increases the number of osteoblast precursor cells in bone marrow. Endocrinology 138: 4629–4635.
22. Xue Y, Karaplis AC, Hendy GN, Goltzman D, Miao D (2005) Genetic models show that parathyroid hormone and 1,25-dihydroxyvitamin D3 play distinct and synergistic roles in postnatal mineral ion homeostasis and skeletal development. Hum Mol Genet 14: 1515–1528.
23. Miao D, Bai X, Panda D, McKee M, Karaplis A, et al. (2001) Osteomalacia in hyp mice is associated with abnormal phex expression and with altered bone matrix protein expression and deposition. Endocrinology 142: 926–939.
24. Panda DK, Miao D, Bolivar I, Li J, Huo R, et al. (2004) Inactivation of the 25-hydroxyvitamin D 1alpha-hydroxylase and vitamin D receptor demonstrates independent and interdependent effects of calcium and vitamin D on skeletal and mineral homeostasis. J Biol Chem 279: 16754–16766.
25. Miao D, Scutt A (2002) Histochemical localization of alkaline phosphatase activity in decalcified bone and cartilage. J Histochem Cytochem 50: 333–340.
26. Miao D, Scutt A (2002) Recruitment, augmentation and apoptosis of rat osteoclasts in 1,25-(OH)2D3 response to short-term treatment with 1,25-dihydroxyvitamin D3 in vivo. BMC Musculoskelet Disord 3: 16.
27. Chomczynski P, Sacchi N (1987) Single-step method of RNA isolation by acid guanidinium thiocyanate-phenol-chloroform extraction. Anal Biochem 162: 156–159.
28. Miao D, He B, Karaplis AC, Goltzman D (2002) Parathyroid hormone is essential for normal fetal bone formation. J Clin Invest 109: 1173–1182.
29. Wysolmerski JJ (2012) Parathyroid hormone-related protein: an update. J Clin Endocrinol Metab 97: 2947–2956.
30. Bisello A, Horwitz MJ, Stewart AF (2004) Parathyroid hormone-related protein: an essential physiological regulator of adult bone mass. Endocrinology 145: 3551–3553.
31. Abou-Samra AB, Juppner H, Force T, Freeman MW, Kong XF, et al. (1992) Expression cloning of a common receptor for parathyroid hormone and parathyroid hormone-related peptide from rat osteoblast-like cells: a single receptor stimulates intracellular accumulation of both cAMP and inositol trisphosphates and increases intracellular free calcium. Proc Natl Acad Sci U S A 89: 2732–2736.
32. Walsh CA, Birch MA, Fraser WD, Lawton R, Dorgan J, et al. (1995) Expression and secretion of parathyroid hormone-related protein by human bone-derived cells in vitro: effects of glucocorticoids. J Bone Miner Res 10: 17–25.
33. Wealthall RJ (2009) In vitro regulation of proliferation and differentiation within a postnatal growth plate of the cranial base by parathyroid hormone-related peptide (PTHrP). J Cell Physiol 219: 688–697.
34. Miao D, Tong XK, Chan GK, Panda D, McPherson PS, et al. (2001) Parathyroid hormone-related peptide stimulates osteogenic cell proliferation through protein kinase C activation of the Ras/mitogen-activated protein kinase signaling pathway. J Biol Chem 276: 32204–32213.
35. Datta NS, Abou-Samra AB (2009) PTH and PTHrP signaling in osteoblasts. Cell Signal 21: 1245–1254.
36. Kovacs CS, Kronenberg HM (1997) Maternal-fetal calcium and bone metabolism during pregnancy, puerperium, and lactation. Endocr Rev 18: 832–872.
37. Miao D, He B, Jiang Y, Kobayashi T, Soroceanu MA, et al. (2005) Osteoblast-derived PTHrP is a potent endogenous bone anabolic agent that modifies the therapeutic efficacy of administered PTH 1-34. J Clin Invest 115: 2402–2411.
38. Choi KC, An BS, Yang H, Jeung EB (2011) Regulation and molecular mechanisms of calcium transport genes: do they play a role in calcium transport in the uterine endometrium? J Physiol Pharmacol 62: 499–504.
39. Kumar R, Tebben PJ, Thompson JR (2012) Vitamin D and the kidney. Arch Biochem Biophys 523: 77–86.
40. Walters JR, Balesaria S, Khair U, Sangha S, Banks L, et al. (2007) The effects of Vitamin D metabolites on expression of genes for calcium transporters in human duodenum. J Steroid Biochem Mol Biol 103: 509–512.
41. Cao G, Gu Z, Ren Y, Shu L, Tao C, et al. (2009) Parathyroid hormone contributes to regulating milk calcium content and modulates neonatal bone formation cooperatively with calcium. Endocrinology 150: 561–569.
42. Ji J, Lu R, Zhou X, Xue Y, Shi C, et al. (2011) 1,25-Dihydroxyvitamin D(3) contributes to regulating mammary calcium transport and modulates neonatal skeletal growth and turnover cooperatively with calcium. Am J Physiol Endocrinol Metab 301: E889–900.
43. Godwin SL, Soltoff SP (1997) Extracellular calcium and platelet-derived growth factor promote receptor-mediated chemotaxis in osteoblasts through different signaling pathways. J Biol Chem 272: 11307–11312.
44. Yamaguchi T, Chattopadhyay N, Kifor O, Butters RR Jr, Sugimoto T, et al. (1998) Mouse osteoblastic cell line (MC3T3-E1) expresses extracellular calcium (Ca2+o)-sensing receptor and its agonists stimulate chemotaxis and proliferation of MC3T3-E1 cells. J Bone Miner Res 13: 1530–1538.
45. Dvorak MM, Siddiqua A, Ward DT, Carter DH, Dallas SL, et al. (2004) Physiological changes in extracellular calcium concentration directly control osteoblast function in the absence of calciotropic hormones. Proc Natl Acad Sci U S A 101: 5140–5145.
46. Chang W, Tu C, Chen TH, Bikle D, Shoback D (2008) The extracellular calcium-sensing receptor (CaSR) is a critical modulator of skeletal development. Sci Signal 1: ra1.

The Vitamin D Analogue ED71 but Not $1,25(OH)_2D_3$ Targets HIF1α Protein in Osteoclasts

Yuiko Sato[1,2]ⁿ, Yoshiteru Miyauchi[1]ⁿ, Shigeyuki Yoshida[3]ⁿ, Mayu Morita[3], Tami Kobayashi[1,4], Hiroya Kanagawa[1], Eri Katsuyama[1], Atsuhiro Fujie[1], Wu Hao[1], Toshimi Tando[1], Ryuichi Watanabe[1], Kana Miyamoto[1], Hideo Morioka[1], Morio Matsumoto[1], Yoshiaki Toyama[1], Takeshi Miyamoto[1,4]*

1 Department of Orthopedic Surgery, Keio University School of Medicine, Shinjuku-ku, Tokyo, Japan, **2** Department of Musculoskeletal Reconstruction and Regeneration Surgery, Keio University School of Medicine, Shinjuku-ku, Tokyo, Japan, **3** Department of Dentistry and Oral Surgery, Keio University School of Medicine, Shinjuku-ku, Tokyo, Japan, **4** Department of Integrated Bone Metabolism and Immunology, Keio University School of Medicine, Shinjuku-ku, Tokyo, Japan

Abstract

Although both an active form of the vitamin D metabolite, $1,25(OH)_2D_3$, and the vitamin D analogue, ED71 have been used to treat osteoporosis, anti-bone resorbing activity is reportedly seen only in ED71- but not in $1,25(OH)_2D_3$ -treated patients. In addition, how ED71 inhibits osteoclast activity in patients has not been fully characterized. Recently, HIF1α expression in osteoclasts was demonstrated to be required for development of post-menopausal osteoporosis. Here we show that ED71 but not $1,25(OH)_2D_3$, suppress HIF1α protein expression in osteoclasts *in vitro*. We found that $1,25(OH)_2D_3$ or ED71 function in osteoclasts requires the vitamin D receptor (VDR). ED71 was significantly less effective in inhibiting M-CSF and RANKL-stimulated osteoclastogenesis than was $1,25(OH)_2D_3$ *in vitro*. Downregulation of c-Fos protein and induction of *Ifnβ* mRNA in osteoclasts, both of which reportedly block osteoclastogenesis induced by $1,25(OH)_2D_3$ *in vitro*, were both significantly higher following treatment with $1,25(OH)_2D_3$ than with ED71. Thus, suppression of HIF1α protein activity in osteoclasts *in vitro*, which is more efficiently achieved by ED71 rather than by $1,25(OH)_2D_3$, could be a reliable read-out in either developing or screening reagents targeting osteoporosis.

Editor: Brenda Smith, Oklahoma State University, United States of America

Funding: This work was supported by a grant-in-aid for Scientific Research. The funders had no role in study design, data collection and analysis, decision to publish, or preparation of the manuscript.

Competing Interests: The authors have declared that no competing interests exist.

* Email: miyamoto@z5.keio.jp

ⁿ These authors contributed equally to this work.

Introduction

A cause for concern in developed countries is the increasing number of osteoporosis patients and individuals suffering fragility fractures due to osteoporosis [1]. Estrogen-deficiency due to menopause is a risk factor for both [2]. Vitamin D insufficiency is also reportedly observed in osteoporosis patients with fragility fractures and considered a cause of osteoporotic fractures [3]. Indeed, vitamin D is known to play a crucial role in skeletal development, and lack of the vitamin D receptor (VDR) or low vitamin D intake results in Rickets [4] [5].

Currently, active vitamin D analogues are used in several countries to treat patients with bone and mineral disorders associated with chronic renal disease or osteoporosis [6]. Interestingly, $1,25(OH)_2D_3$ has been demonstrated to promote osteoclastogenesis in co-cultures of osteoclast progenitor cells and osteoblastic cells [7]; in addition, $1,25(OH)_2D_3$ elevated receptor activator of nuclear factor kappa B ligand (RANKL), an essential cytokine for osteoclastogenesis, but inhibited expression of OPG, a decoy receptor of RANKL, in osteoblastic cells to promote osteoclast differentiation [8] [9]. In contrast, $1,25(OH)_2D_3$ was shown to inhibit osteoclast differentiation in osteoblastic cell-free culture systems: osteoclast formation induced by macrophage colony stimulating factor (M-CSF) and RANKL was inhibited in the presence of $1,25(OH)_2D_3$ [10] [11]. c-Fos protein, an essential transcription factor for osteoclast differentiation, or interferon beta (Ifnβ), an inhibitor of osteoclastogenesis, was downregulated or elevated by $1,25(OH)_2D_3$, respectively, in osteoclast progenitor cells [10] [11]. However, patients treated with a $1,25(OH)_2D_3$ pro-drug, alfacalcidol, did not show inhibition of osteoclastic activity or increased bone mass, while patients treated with the vitamin D analogue ED71 exhibited significantly reduced osteoclast activities and increased bone mass [12].

Since postmenopausal osteoporosis is caused in part by estrogen-deficiency, treating of patients with estrogen is one option. However, continuous estrogen administration is associated with adverse effects such as uterine or mammary gland tumors or cardio-vascular disease [13]. Recently, we reported that hypoxia inducible factor 1 alpha (HIF1α) is required for osteoclast activation following estrogen-deficiency and for development of postmenopausal osteoporosis in animal models [14]. We found that in pre-menopausal mice, HIF1α activity in osteoclasts is continuously suppressed by estrogen but then HIF1α accumulate in osteoclasts following estrogen deficiency due to menopause, which in turn activates osteoclastic activity and promotes bone loss. Osteoclast specific HIF1α knockout or administration of a HIF1α inhibitor completely abrogated ovariectomy (OVX)-induced osteoclast activation and bone loss [14]. This study suggests that HIF1α could be a therapeutic target for postmenopausal osteoporosis.

Here, we show that HIF1α is a target of ED71 *in vitro*. HIF1α in osteoclasts was suppressed by ED71 but not by $1,25(OH)_2D_3$. Since inhibition of osteoclast activity was seen in the patients treated with ED71 but not with $1,25(OH)_2D_3$, this work confirms that HIF1α could be a target to treat postmenopausal osteoporosis patients.

Materials and Methods

Mice

C57BL/6 background wild-type mice were purchased from Sankyo Labo Service (Tokyo, Japan). VDR-deficient mice were established previously [4]. Animals were maintained under specific pathogen-free conditions in animal facilities certified by the Keio University School of Medicine animal care committee. All animal procedures were approved by the Keio University School of Medicine animal care committee.

Cell culture

To assess *in vitro* osteoclast formation, bone marrow cells isolated from $Hif^{flox/flox}$ or Ctsk Cre/$Hif^{flox/flox}$ mouse femurs and tibias were cultured for 72 hours in αMEM (Sigma-Aldrich Co., St. Louis, MO, USA) containing 10% heat-inactivated fetal bovine serum (FBS, JRH Biosciences Lenexa, KS, USA) and GlutaMax (Invitrogen Corp., Carlsbad, CA, USA) supplemented with M-CSF (50 ng/ml, Kyowa Hakko Kirin Co. Tokyo, Japan). Subsequently, adherent cells were collected and cultured under indicated conditions containing M-CSF (50 ng/ml), recombinant soluble RANKL (25 ng/ml, PeproTech Ltd., Rocky Hill, NJ, USA) using 1×10^5 cells per well in 96-well plates. Osteoclastogenesis was evaluated by TRAP staining [15] [16]. Raw264.7 cells were maintained in DMEM (Sigma-Aldrich Co.) containing 10% heat-inactivated FBS (JRH Biosciences) and GlutaMax (Invitrogen

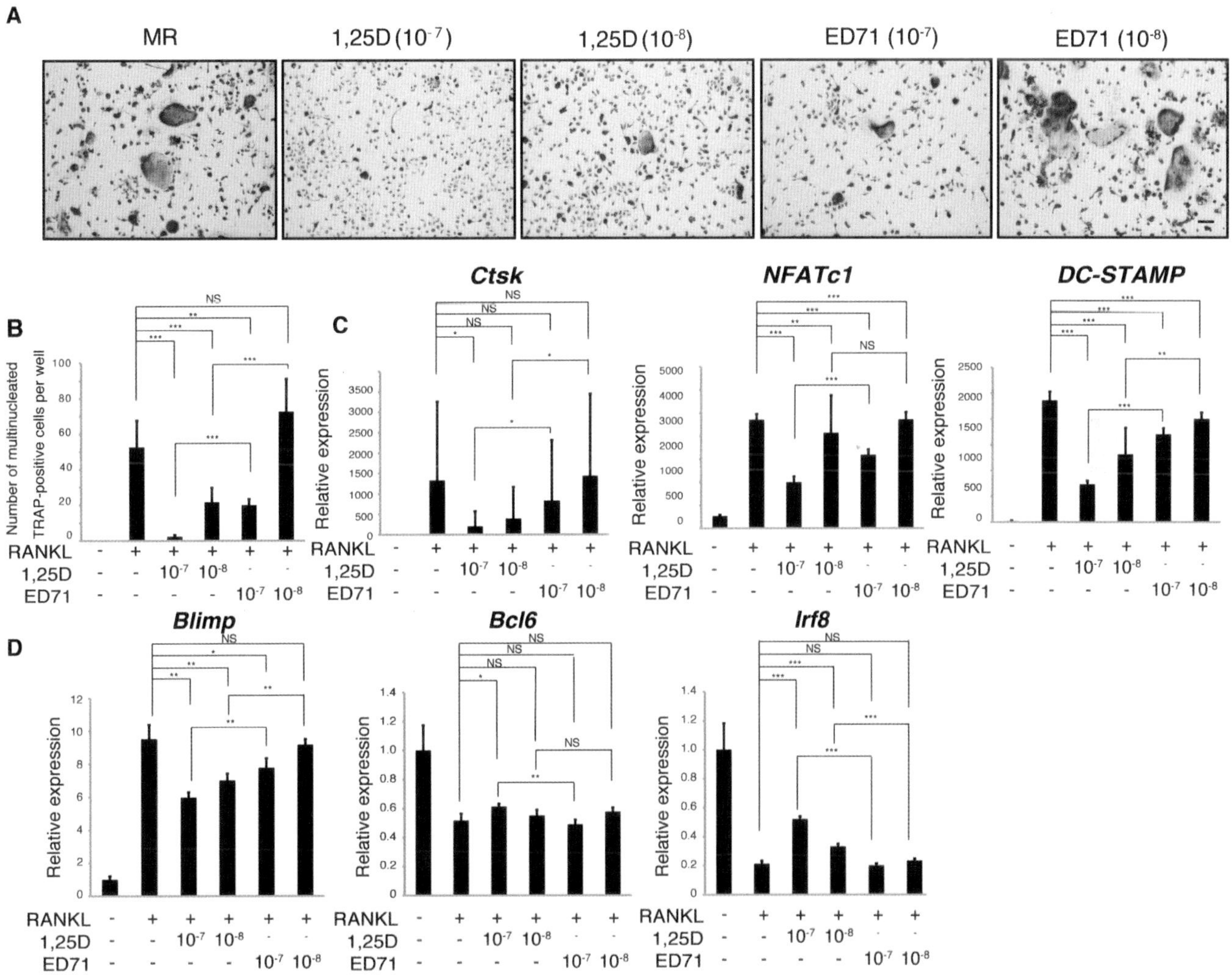

Figure 1. $1,25(OH)_2D_3$ is a more potent inhibitor of osteoclastogenesis *in vitro* than is ED71. (**A, B** and **C**) M-CSF-dependent osteoclast progenitor cells were isolated from wild-type mice and cultured in the presence of M-CSF (M, 50 ng/ml) + RANKL (R, 25 ng/ml) with or without indicated concentrations of ED71 or $1,25(OH)_2D_3$ (1,25D) for 5 days. Cells were then stained with TRAP (**A**) and the number of multi-nuclear TRAP-positive cells was counted (**B**). Expression of *Ctsk*, *NFATc1* and *DC-STAMP*, all of which are osteoclastic genes, was analyzed by realtime PCR (**C**). Expression of *Blimp1*, *Bcl6* and *Irf8* was analyzed by realtime PCR (**D**). Data represent mean expression of each relative to *Actb* ± SD ($n=5$). *$P<0.05$; **$P<0.01$; ***$P<0.001$; NS, not significant.

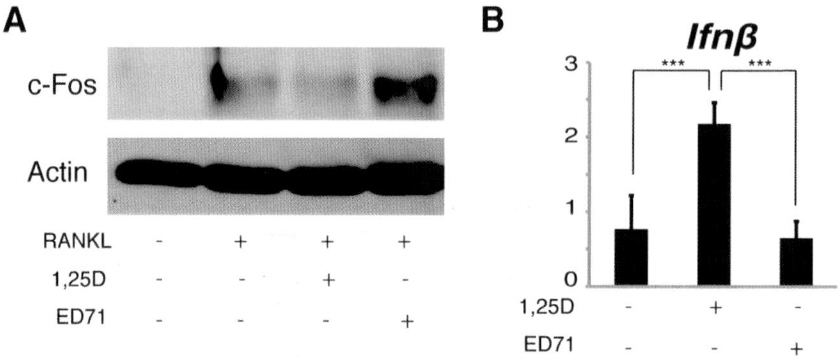

Figure 2. 1,25(OH)$_2$D$_3$ is more active in promoting c-Fos protein inhibition and *Ifnβ*-induction in osteoclasts compared with ED71. (A and B) M-CSF-dependent osteoclast progenitor cells were isolated from wild-type mice and cultured in the presence of M-CSF alone (50 ng/ml) or M-CSF + RANKL (25 ng/ml) with or without 10^{-7} M ED71 or 1,25(OH)$_2$D$_3$ (1,25D) for 5 days. c-Fos protein was then assessed by western blot (A). *Ifnβ* expression was analyzed by realtime PCR (B). Data represent mean *Ifnβ* expression relative to that of *Actb* ± SD ($n = 5$). ***$P < 0.001$.

Corp.). For chemical treatment, cells were cultured in phenol red-free media containing 10% charcoal-stripped FBS (Thermo Fisher Scientific K.K., Yokohama, Japan), and treated with 1,25(OH)$_2$D$_3$ (Wako Pure Chemicals Industries, Osaka, Japan, 10^{-7} M) or ED71 (provided by Chugai Pharmaceutical Co., Ltd, Tokyo, Japan, 10^{-7} M). Hypoxic cultures was performed at 5% O_2/5% CO_2 using an INVIVO2 hypoxia workstation (Ruskin Technology Ltd., Bridgend, UK) according to manufacturer's instruction.

Quantitative PCR analysis

Total RNA was isolated from bone marrow cultures using an RNeasy mini kit (Qiagen), and cDNA synthesis was done by using oligo (dT) primers and reverse transcriptase (Wako Pure Chemicals Industries). Quantitative PCR was performed using SYBR Premix ExTaq II reagent and a DICE Thermal cycler (Takara Bio Inc., Shiga, Japan), according to the manufacturer's instructions. *β-actin* (*Actb*) expression served as an internal control. Primers for *Nfatc1*, *Ctsk*, *DC-STAMP*, *Ifnβ* and *Actb* were as follows.

Ctsk-forward: 5′-ACGGAGGCATTGACTCTGAAGATG-3′

Ctsk-reverse: 5′-GGAAGCACCAACGAGAGGAGAAAT-3′

NFATc1-forward: 5′-CAAGTCTCACCACAGGGCTCACT-A-3′

NFATc1-reverse: 5′-GCGTGAGAGGTTCATTCTCCAAG-T-3′

DC-STAMP-forward: 5′-TCCTCCATGAACAAACAGTTC-CAA-3′

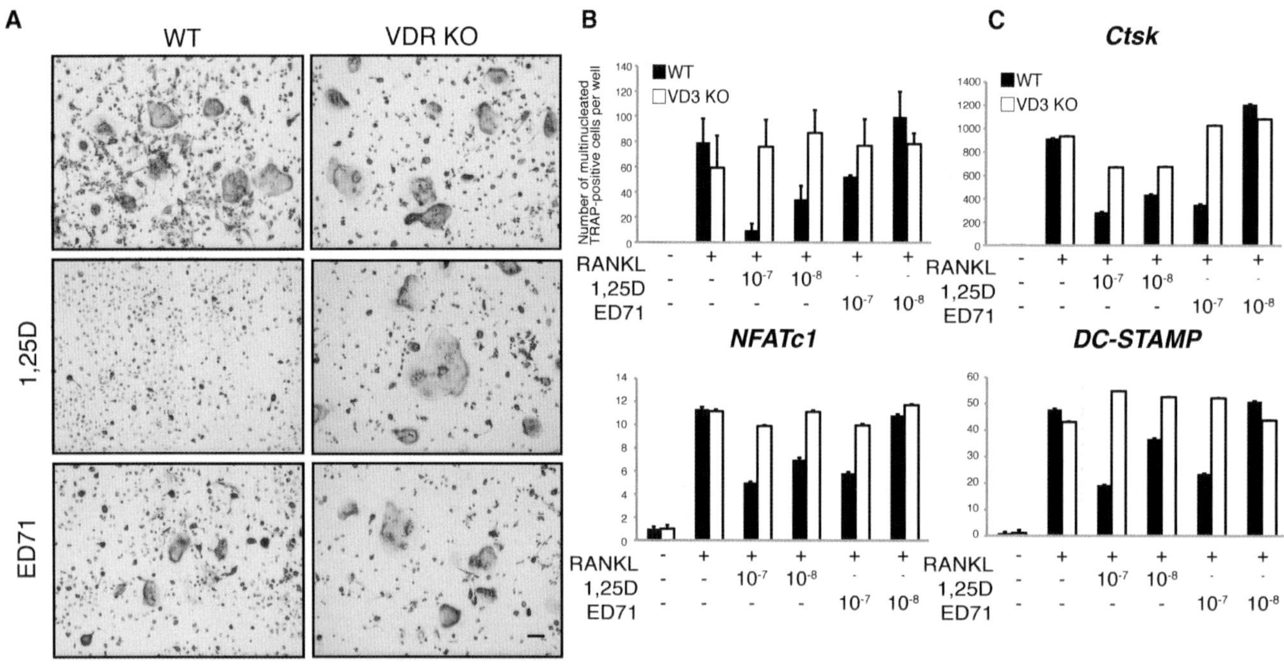

Figure 3. ED71 or 1,25(OH)$_2$D$_3$ activity requires the VDR. (**A, B** and **C**) M-CSF-dependent osteoclast progenitor cells were isolated from wild-type (WT) or VDR-deficient (VDR KO) mice and cultured in the presence of M-CSF alone (50 ng/ml) or M-CSF + RANKL (25 ng/ml) with or without indicated concentrations of ED71 or 1,25(OH)$_2$D$_3$ for 5 days. Cells were then stained with TRAP (**A**), and multi-nuclear TRAP-positive cells were counted (**B**). Expression of *Ctsk*, *NFATc1* and *DC-STAMP* was assessed by realtime PCR (**C**). Data represent mean *Ctsk*, *NFATc1* or *DC-STAMP* expression relative to that of *Actb* ± SD ($n = 5$).

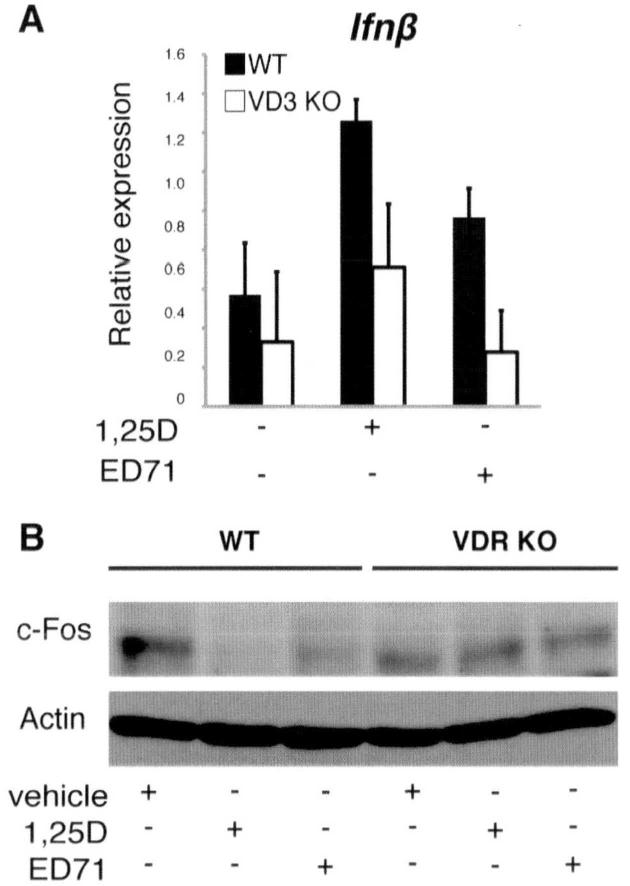

Figure 4. ED71 or 1,25(OH)$_2$D$_3$ induce *Ifnβ* and suppress c-Fos protein through the VDR. (**A** and **B**) M-CSF-dependent osteoclast progenitor cells were isolated from wild-type or VDR-deficient mice and cultured in the presence of M-CSF alone (50 ng/ml) or M−CSF + RANKL (25 ng/ml) with or without 10^{-7} M of ED71 or 1,25(OH)$_2$D$_3$ (1,25D) for 5 days. *Ifnβ* expression was then analyzed by realtime PCR (**A**). Data represent mean *Ifnβ* expression relative to that of *Actb* ± SD ($n = 5$). c-Fos protein was analyzed by western blot (**B**).

DC-STAMP-reverse: 5′-AGACGTGGTTTAGGAATGCAG-CTC-3′

Ifnβ-forward: 5′– AAAGCAAGAGGAAAGATTGACGTG -3′

Ifnβ-reverse: 5′– ATCCAGGCGTAGCTGTTGTACTTC -3′

Blimp1-forward: 5′-TTCTTGTGTGGTATTGTCGGGAC-TT-3′

Blimp1-reverse: 5′-TTGGGGACACTCTTTGGGTAGAGT-T-3′

Irf8-forward: 5′-CAGGATTACAATCAGGAGGTGGA-3′

Irf8-reverse: 5′-TCAAAATCTGGGCTCTTGTTCAG-3′

β-actin-forward: 5′-TGAGAGGGAAATCGTGCGTGAC-3′

β-actin-reverse: 5′-AAGAAGGAAGGCTGGAAAAGAG-3′

Immunoblotting

Whole cell lysates were prepared using RIPA buffer (1% Triton X-100, 1% sodium deoxycholate, 0.1% SDS, 150 mM NaCl, 5 mM EDTA, 1 mM dithiothreitol, 10 mM Tris-HCl, pH 7.5) supplemented with a protease inhibitor cocktail (Sigma-Aldrich Co.) and MG-132 (EMD Millipore Corporation). The insoluble fraction was removed by centrifugation followed. Equivalent amounts of protein were separated by SDS-PAGE and transferred to a PVDF membrane (EMD Millipore Corporation). Proteins were detected using the following antibodies: anti-Fos (Santa Cruz Biotechnology, Santa Cruz, CA, USA), anti-HIF1α (Novus Biologicals, Littleton, CO, USA), anti-Actin(Sigma-Aldrich Co.), and anti-Vinculin (Sigma-Aldrich Co.) as previously described [14].

VDR knockdown

Raw264.7 cells transduced with MISSION shRNA lentiviruses targeting the VDR or with lentiviruses harboring non-target control constructs (Sigma-Aldrich Co.) were generated according to the manufacturer's instructions.

Statistical analyses

Statistical analyses were performed using an unpaired two-tailed Student's *t*-test (*$P<0.05$; **$P<0.01$; ***$P<0.005$; NS, not significant, throughout the paper). All data are expressed as the mean ± SD.

Results

1,25(OH)$_2$D$_3$ inhibits osteoclastogenesis more potently than does ED71 *in vitro*

Since treatment with ED71, a vitamin D3 analogue, inhibits osteoclast activity and increases bone mineral density more effectively than does the pro-1,25(OH)$_2$D$_3$ agent, alfacalcidol [12], we asked whether ED71 inhibited osteoclastogenesis more effectively than 1,25(OH)$_2$D$_3$ (1,25D) *in vitro* (Fig. 1). To do so, we isolated osteoclast progenitor cells from wild-type mice and cultured them in the presence of M-CSF and RANKL with or without ED71 or 1,25(OH)$_2$D$_3$. We then evaluated osteoclastogenesis by counting multi-nuclear TRAP-positive osteoclasts and examining expression of osteoclastic genes (Fig. 1A-D). Indeed ED71 significantly inhibited osteoclast differentiation based on both TRAP and gene expression analysis, while 1,25(OH)$_2$D$_3$ was more effective in inhibiting osteoclastogenesis than was ED71 *in vitro* (Fig. 1A and B). Expression of osteoclast differentiation markers such as *Cathepsin K* (*Ctsk*), *nuclear factor of activated T cells 1* (*NFATc1*) and *dendritic cell specific transmembrane protein* (*DC-STAMP*) was more significantly inhibited by 1,25(OH)$_2$D$_3$ than by ED71 treatment (Fig. 1C). Induction of B lymphocyte-induced maturation protein 1 (Blimp1) followed by suppression of B cell lymphoma 6 and interferon regulatory factor 8 (Irf8) is reportedly required for osteoclastogenesis [14,17,18]. We found that treatment of osteoclast progenitors with 1,25(OH)$_2$D$_3$ elicited more robust inhibition of *Blimp1* and activation of *Bcl6* and *Irf8* than did treatment with ED71 (Fig. 1D), suggesting that 1,25(OH)$_2$D$_3$ is more potent in inhibiting osteoclastogenesis induced by M-CSF and RANKL than ED71.

1,25(OH)$_2$D$_3$ reportedly inhibits osteoclast differentiation induced by M-CSF and RANKL by inhibiting c-Fos protein expression *in vitro* [10]. We found that, by western blot, c-Fos protein was induced by RANKL, and ED71 did not suppress c-Fos protein in osteoclasts as effectively as did 1,25(OH)$_2$D$_3$ (Fig. 2A). Although 1,25(OH)$_2$D$_3$ reportedly inhibits osteoclastogenesis induced by M-CSF and RANKL via *Ifnβ* induction *in vitro* [11], we found that, unlike 1,25(OH)$_2$D$_3$, ED71 did not induce *Ifnβ* expression in osteoclasts (Fig. 2B).

The VDR is required for both 1,25(OH)$_2$D$_3$ and ED71 activity on osteoclasts

Since 1,25(OH)$_2$D$_3$ and ED71 activities differ in osteoclasts, we utilized vitamin D receptor (VDR)-deficient mice to test whether

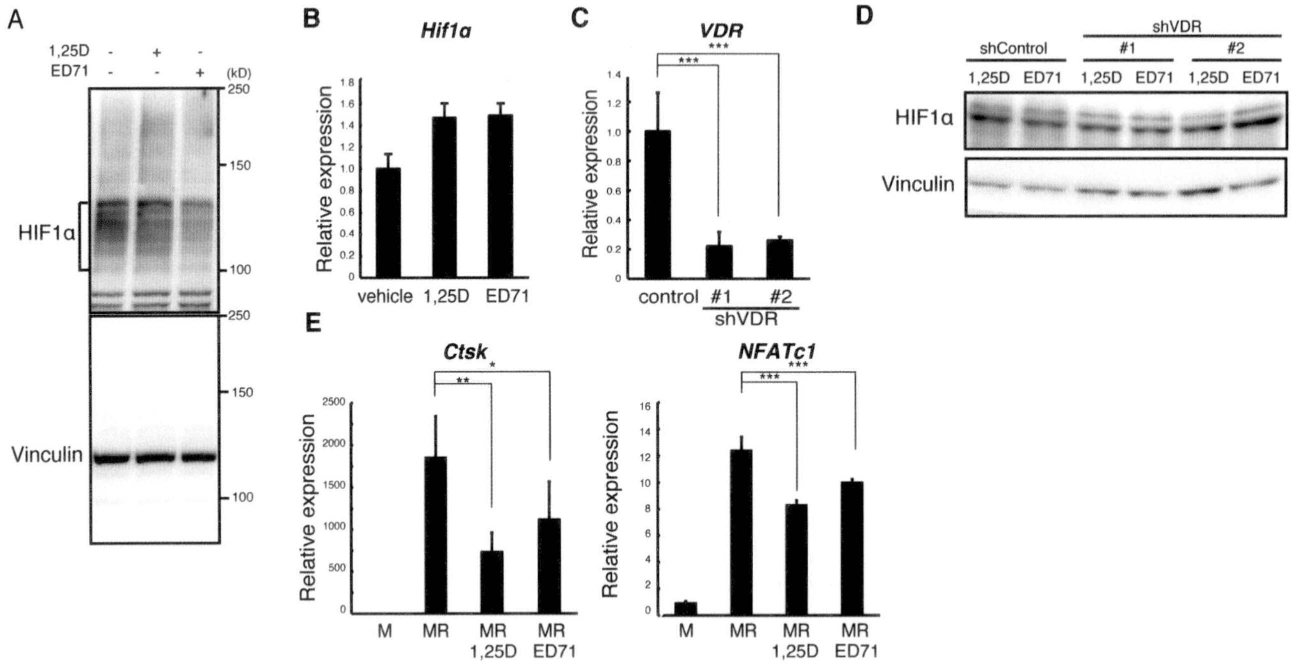

Figure 5. HIF1α protein is suppressed by ED71 but not by $1{,}25(OH)_2D_3$. (**A**) Western analysis of Raw264.7 cells cultured in hypoxic conditions with or without 10^{-7} M of ED71 or $1{,}25(OH)_2D_3$ (1,25D). (**B**) *Hif1α* mRNA levels in Raw264.7 cells cultured in hypoxic conditions were analyzed by realtime PCR in the presence or absence of 10^{-7} M ED71 or $1{,}25(OH)_2D_3$. Data represent mean *Hif1α* expression relative to that of *Actb* ± SD ($n=5$). (**C**) Levels of *VDR* transcripts in Raw264.7 cells transfected with shRNA targeting the VDR (shVDR) or control shRNA (Control) were determined by realtime PCR. Data represent mean *VDR* expression relative to that of *Actb* ± SD ($n=5$). (**D**) Western analysis of control (shControl) or VDR-suppressed (shVDR#1 or shVDR#2) Raw264.7 transformants cultured in hypoxic conditions with ED71 or $1{,}25(OH)_2D_3$ (1,25D), both at 10^{-7} M. (**E**) M-CSF-dependent Ctsk Cre/*Hif*$^{flox/flox}$ cells were cultured in normoxic conditions to suppress HIF1α in the presence of M-CSF (50 ng/ml) plus RANKL (25 ng/ml) with either ED71 or $1{,}25(OH)_2D_3$ (1,25D) both at 10^{-7}M for 4 days. Expression of *Ctsk* and *NFATc1* was then assessed by realtime PCR. Data represent mean *Ctsk* or *NFATc1* expression relative to that of *Actb* ± SD ($n=5$). *$P<0.05$; **$P<0.01$; ***$P<0.001$.

both compounds act on osteoclasts via the VDR (Fig. 3). Osteoclast progenitors were isolated from wild-type and VDR-deficient mice and cultured in the presence of M-CSF and RANKL with or without $1{,}25(OH)_2D_3$ or ED71 (Fig. 3). Inhibitory effects of either $1{,}25(OH)_2D_3$ or ED71 on osteoclast differentiation were not seen in VDR-deficient osteoclasts (Fig. 3A and B). Similarly, inhibition of the expression of osteoclastic genes *Ctsk*, *NFATc1* and *DC-STAMP* seen following $1{,}25(OH)_2D_3$ or ED71 treatment was absent in osteoclasts lacking the VDR (Fig. 3C).

Moreover, decreased c-Fos protein and elevated *Ifnβ* expression seen following treatment with $1{,}25(OH)_2D_3$ or ED71 were abrogated in VDR-deficient osteoclasts (Fig. 4A and B), supporting the idea that both compounds act on osteoclasts via the VDR.

HIF1α is a target of ED71 but not $1{,}25(OH)_2D_3$ in osteoclasts

Next, we asked whether HIF1α is a target of ED71 in osteoclasts (Fig. 5). Interestingly, we found that in cultured osteoclasts, HIF1α protein levels were suppressed by ED71 but not by $1{,}25(OH)_2D_3$ (Fig. 5A). In contrast, *Hif1α* mRNA expression in osteoclasts was not inhibited by either treatment (Fig. 5B), suggesting that ED71 suppresses HIF1α at the protein level as demonstrated by estrogen treatment [14]. To determine if the VDR is required for ED71-mediated HIF1α protein suppression in osteoclasts, we generated two independent VDR knockdown Raw264.7 lines using shVDR#1 and shVDR#2 as well as a control (shControl) line (Fig. 5C) and then treated cells with ED71 or $1{,}25(OH)_2D_3$ (Fig. 5D). HIF1α protein suppression by ED71 seen in control cells was abrogated in both VDR knockdown lines, suggesting that HIF1α protein suppression by ED71 is VDR-dependent. We then isolated osteoclast progenitors from Ctsk Cre/*Hif1α*$^{flox/flox}$ mice, cultured them in normoxic conditions to suppress HIF1α protein, and treated cells with or without ED71 or $1{,}25(OH)_2D_3$ (Fig. 5E). ED71 treatment effectively inhibited osteoclast differentiation, even in HIF1α-suppressed cells, suggesting that ED71 likely targets factors other than HIF1α protein in osteoclasts (Fig. 5E). However, ED71 was less effective than $1{,}25(OH)_2D_3$ in inhibiting osteoclastogenesis in HIF1α-suppressed cells (Fig. 5E).

Discussion

Postmenopausal osteoporosis treatment is required to prevent disruption of daily activity or adverse outcomes due to fragile fractures. Among anti-osteoporosis agents, anti-bone resorptive or bone-forming agents include bisphosphonates, selective estrogen receptor modulator (SERM), ED71 and denosumab, or teriparaide, respectively. Strong inhibition of osteoclastic activity beyond physiological levels by bisphosphonates frequently causes adverse effects such as osteonecrosis of the jaw or severely suppressed bone turnover (SSBT) [19] [20]. Meanwhile, teriparatide treatment is limited to less than two years in order to prevent development of tumors, particularly osteosarcoma.

Recently, we showed that HIF1α protein accumulation in osteoclasts following estrogen-deficiency was accompanied by osteoclast activation and bone loss in mice [14]. Either osteoclast-specific HIF1α conditional knockout or wild-type mice administered a HIF1α inhibitor were protected from

OVX-induced osteoclast activation and bone loss. Moreover, HIF1α inhibition did not interfere with physiological osteoclast activities [14]. Thus, blocking HIF1α pharmacologically could represent an ideal treatment for postmenopausal osteoporosis, as it could target pathologically-activated osteoclasts without altering physiological osteoclastogenesis required for bone turnover. In this study, we found that both ED71, which is used as therapeutic agents for postmenopausal osteoporosis therapy, inhibits HIF1α protein expression. Indeed, patients treated with ED71 exhibit reduced osteoclastic activity and increased bone mass without adverse effects such as osteopetrosis [12], jaw osteonecrosis or SSBT, as seen in treated bisphosphonate-treated patients [19] [20].

Bone is a target tissue of vitamin D, and indeed, VDR was identified in osteoblasts [21–24]. In contrast, it is controversial whether the VDR is expressed in osteoclasts, with some authors reporting expression [25–28] and others not [21,23,29,30]. Recently, Wang et al. demonstrated that the VDR is not expressed in multi-nuclear osteoclasts using immunohistochemistry of EGTA-decalcified adult mouse bones [21]. In addition, direct effects of 1,25(OH)$_2$D$_3$ have been demonstrated in osteoclasts and osteoclast progenitors [10] [11], and here we report that these effects are VDR-dependent (Fig. 3). Taken together, these studies suggest that extremely low levels of the VDR in osteoclasts may be sufficient to transduce vitamin D signals.

ED71 and 1,25(OH)$_2$D$_3$ have been demonstrated to inhibit osteoclast-bone resorption activity by reducing expression of the sphigosine-1-phosphate receptor 2 (S1PR2) in circulating osteoclast precursor cells and blocking the migration of these cells to the bone surface by S1P; although differences in pharmacological action between ED71 and 1,25(OH)$_2$D$_3$ were not demonstrated [31]. Here, we observed that, although 1,25(OH)$_2$D$_3$ was more potent than ED71 in inhibiting osteoclastogenesis induced by M-CSF and RANKL *in vitro*, HIF1α inhibition in osteoclasts was specific to ED71. We also found that ED71 inhibited osteoclastogenesis even in HIF1α-suppressed cells, suggesting that ED71 likely targets factors other than HIF1α protein in osteoclasts. However, ED71 was less effective than 1,25(OH)$_2$D$_3$ in inhibiting osteoclastogenesis in HIF1α-suppressed cells, which contrasts with observations seen in patients where the effect of ED71 on osteoclastogenesis is superior to that of 1,25(OH)$_2$D$_3$ [12]. The cause of this difference remains to be elucidated, but the difference of potential activity to target HIF1α-protein in osteoclasts explains, at least in part, this difference. In addition, it is possible that ED71 inhibits osteoclastogenesis through effects on different cell types. Further investigations are needed to define molecular actions of vitamin D3 analogues on bone metabolism. Nonetheless, HIF1α inhibition could serve as an index to assess osteoclastogenesis *in vitro* when developing anti-osteoporosis agents. Moreover, our study indicates that targeting HIFα could constitute an effective treatment for osteoporosis, one that would not interfere with physiological bone turnover.

Acknowledgments

This work was supported by a grant-in-aid for Scientific Research. We thank Prof. M. Suematsu and Dr. Y.A. Minamishima for technical support in performing hypoxic culture. We also thank Dr. Shigeaki Kato for providing VDR-deficient mice.

Author Contributions

Conceived and designed the experiments: HM M. Matsumoto YT TM. Performed the experiments: YS YM SY M. Morita. Analyzed the data: HK EK AF WH TT RW KM. Contributed reagents/materials/analysis tools: TK. Wrote the paper: TM.

References

1. Report of a WHO Study Group (1994) Assessment of fracture risk and its application to screening for postmenopausal osteoporosis. World Health Organ Tech Rep Ser 10: 1–129.
2. Ettinger B, Pressman A, Sklarin P, Bauer DC, Cauley JA, et al. (1998) Associations between low levels of serum estradiol, bone density, and fractures among elderly women: the study of osteoporotic fractures. J Clin Endocrinol Metab 83: 2239–2243.
3. Sakuma M, Endo N, Hagino H, Harada A, Matsui Y, et al. (2011) Serum 25-hydroxyvitamin D status in hip and spine-fracture patients in Japan. J Orthop Sci 16: 418–423.
4. Yoshizawa T, Handa Y, Uematsu Y, Takeda S, Sekine K, et al. (1997) Mice lacking the vitamin D receptor exhibit impaired bone formation, uterine hypoplasia and growth retardation after weaning. Nat Genet 16: 391–396.
5. Winzenberg T, Jones G (2013) Vitamin D and bone health in childhood and adolescence. Calcif Tissue Int 92: 140–150.
6. Plum LA, DeLuca HF (2010) Vitamin D, disease and therapeutic opportunities. Nat Rev Drug Discov 9: 941–955.
7. Takahashi N, Akatsu T, Udagawa N, Sasaki T, Yamaguchi A, et al. (1988) Osteoblastic cells are involved in osteoclast formation. Endocrinology 123: 2600–2602.
8. Yasuda H, Shima N, Nakagawa N, Yamaguchi K, Kinosaki M, et al. (1998) Osteoclast differentiation factor is a ligand for osteoprotegerin/osteoclastogenesis-inhibitory factor and is identical to TRANCE/RANKL. Proc Natl Acad Sci U S A 95: 3597–3602.
9. Miyamoto T, Suda T (2003) Differentiation and function of osteoclasts. Keio J Med 52: 1–7.
10. Takasu H, Sugita A, Uchiyama Y, Katagiri N, Okazaki M, et al. (2006) c-Fos protein as a target of anti-osteoclastogenic action of vitamin D, and synthesis of new analogs. J Clin Invest 116: 528–535.
11. Sakai S, Takaishi H, Matsuzaki K, Kaneko H, Furukawa M, et al. (2009) 1-Alpha, 25-dihydroxy vitamin D3 inhibits osteoclastogenesis through IFN-beta-dependent NFATc1 suppression. J Bone Miner Metab 27: 643–652.
12. Matsumoto T, Ito M, Hayashi Y, Hirota T, Tanigawara Y, et al. (2011) A new active vitamin D3 analog, eldecalcitol, prevents the risk of osteoporotic fractures—a randomized, active comparator, double-blind study. Bone 49: 605–612.
13. Nelson ER, Wardell SE, McDonnell DP (2013) The molecular mechanisms underlying the pharmacological actions of estrogens, SERMs and oxysterols: implications for the treatment and prevention of osteoporosis. Bone 53: 42–50.
14. Miyauchi Y, Sato Y, Kobayashi T, Yoshida S, Mori T, et al. (2013) HIF1alpha is required for osteoclast activation by estrogen deficiency in postmenopausal osteoporosis. Proc Natl Acad Sci U S A 110: 16568–16573.
15. Yagi M, Miyamoto T, Sawatani Y, Iwamoto K, Hosogane N, et al. (2005) DC-STAMP is essential for cell-cell fusion in osteoclasts and foreign body giant cells. J Exp Med 202: 345–351.
16. Miyamoto H, Suzuki T, Miyauchi Y, Iwasaki R, Kobayashi T, et al. (2012) DC-STAMP is essential for cell-cell fusion in osteoclasts and foreign body giant cells. J Bone Miner Res 27: 1289–1297.
17. Zhao B, Takami M, Yamada A, Wang X, Koga T, et al. (2009) Interferon regulatory factor-8 regulates bone metabolism by suppressing osteoclastogenesis. Nat Med. 15: 1066–1071.
18. Nishikawa K, Nakashima T, Hayashi M, Fukunaga T, Kato S, et al. (2010) Blimp1-mediated repression of negative regulators is required for osteoclast differentiation. Proc Natl Acad Sci U S A. 107: 3117–3122.
19. Migliorati CA (2003) Bisphosphanates and oral cavity avascular bone necrosis. J Clin Oncol 21: 4253–4254.
20. Visekruna M, Wilson D, McKiernan FE (2008) Severely suppressed bone turnover and atypical skeletal fragility. J Clin Endocrinol Metab 93: 2948–2952.
21. Wang Y, Zhu J, Deluca HF (2014) Identification of the vitamin d receptor in osteoblasts and chondrocytes but not osteoclasts in mouse bone. J Bone Miner Res 29: 685–692.
22. Berger U, Wilson P, McClelland RA, Colston K, Haussler MR, et al. (1988) Immunocytochemical detection of 1,25-dihydroxyvitamin D receptors in normal human tissues. J Clin Endocrinol Metab 67: 607–613.
23. Clemens TL, Garrett KP, Zhou XY, Pike JW, Haussler MR, et al. (1988) Immunocytochemical localization of the 1,25-dihydroxyvitamin D3 receptor in target cells. Endocrinology 122: 1224–1230.
24. Narbaitz R, Stumpf WE, Sar M (1981) The role of autoradiographic and immunocytochemical techniques in the clarification of sites of metabolism and action of vitamin D. J Histochem Cytochem 29: 91–100.
25. Johnson JA, Grande JP, Roche PC, Kumar R (1996) Ontogeny of the 1,25-dihydroxyvitamin D3 receptor in fetal rat bone. J Bone Miner Res 11: 56–61.

26. Mee AP, Hoyland JA, Braidman IP, Freemont AJ, Davies M, et al. (1996) Demonstration of vitamin D receptor transcripts in actively resorbing osteoclasts in bone sections. Bone 18: 295–299.
27. Menaa C, Barsony J, Reddy SV, Cornish J, Cundy T, et al. (2000) 1,25-Dihydroxyvitamin D3 hypersensitivity of osteoclast precursors from patients with Paget's disease. J Bone Miner Res 15: 228–236.
28. Langub MC, Reinhardt TA, Horst RL, Malluche HH, Koszewski NJ (2000) Characterization of vitamin D receptor immunoreactivity in human bone cells. Bone 27: 383–387.
29. Boivin G, Mesguich P, Pike JW, Bouillon R, Meunier PJ, et al. (1987) Ultrastructural immunocytochemical localization of endogenous 1,25-dihydroxyvitamin D3 and its receptors in osteoblasts and osteocytes from neonatal mouse and rat calvaria. Bone Miner 3: 125–136.
30. Merke J, Klaus G, Hugel U, Waldherr R, Ritz E (1986) No 1,25-dihydroxyvitamin D3 receptors on osteoclasts of calcium-deficient chicken despite demonstrable receptors on circulating monocytes. J Clin Invest 77: 312–314.
31. Kikuta J, Kawamura S, Okiji F, Shirazaki M, Sakai S, et al. (2013) Sphingosine-1-phosphate-mediated osteoclast precursor monocyte migration is a critical point of control in antibone-resorptive action of active vitamin D. Proc Natl Acad Sci U S A 110: 7009–7013.

Insignificant Medium-Term Vitamin D Status Change after 25-Hydroxyvitamin D Testing in a Large Managed Care Population

Meng Wei[1], Run Yu[2]*, Stephen C. Deutsch[1]

1 Cedars-Sinai Medical Care Foundation, Beverly Hills, California, United States of America, **2** Division of Endocrinology, Cedars-Sinai Medical Center, Los Angeles, California, United States of America

Abstract

Objectives: To examine the clinical utility of 25-hydroxyvitamin D (25(OH)D) testing in achieving medium-term vitamin D (VD) sufficiency in a managed care population.

Methods: Retrospective study of a continuously-enrolled patient population in a 3-year period between 2011 and 2013. Primary outcome was VD status at ~1 year after 25(OH)D testing. Patient demographics, comorbidities, medications, and 25(OH)D test results were gathered from relevant databases and multivariate logistic regression analysis used to study the risk factors of persistent VD deficiency or insufficiency.

Results: Of 22,784 patients, 7533 (females 69.3%) did 14,563 25(OH)D tests, with an estimated cost of $582,520. Of the 7533 patients, 1126 had another 25(OH)D test at 300–400 days after the first one. Based on the two test results, 234 patients (20.8%) maintained sufficient 25(OH)D levels; 132 (11.7%) turned from VD-sufficient into VD-insufficient or -deficient; 538 (47.8%) remained VD-insufficient or -deficient, and only 222 (19.7%) improved to be VD-sufficient. Overall, only 8.0% more patients were VD-sufficient at ~1 year after 25(OH)D testing. Only younger age and higher BMI were independent risk factors for persistent low 25(OH)D levels and high-dose VD use was not associated with achieving VD sufficiency.

Conclusions: 25(OH)D testing only benefits a small portion of patients thus lacks clinical utility in achieving VD sufficiency in the medium term but incurs a significant cost. A practical strategy to treat VD deficiency or insufficiency is needed; without it, 25(OH)D testing adds little value to most patients' health and should be used with discretion.

Editor: Andrzej T. Slominski, University of Tennessee, United States of America

Funding: The authors have no support or funding to report.

Competing Interests: The authors have declared that no competing interests exist.

* Email: run.yu@cshs.org

Introduction

Extremely low levels of vitamin D (VD), measured by serum 25-hydroxyvitamin D (25(OH)D) levels, are detrimental to bone health and VD supplementation in patients with very low 25(OH)D levels is beneficial in correcting osteomalacia or osteoporosis [1,2]. There have been many studies suggesting that higher 25(OH)D levels are associated with better outcomes of numerous non-skeletal diseases such as cardiovascular diseases and cancers [3,4]. Although there is no consensus on who should undergo 25(OH)D testing and routine screening for VD status is not recommended due to lack of evidence on feasibility, cost-effectiveness, or benefits of such screening [1,2], some physicians may be convinced that it is worthwhile to screen for VD deficiency and to treat patients with VD if they do have it. In developed countries, 25(OH)D testing and the associated cost, mostly for screening purpose, have been dramatically increased over the last decade [5,6]. To justify a screening test, the discovered condition has to be treatable if found earlier in its course. In the case of 25(OH)D testing, the discovered condition, VD deficiency (or insufficiency), is theoretically very treatable by sun exposure and VD supplements. Our clinical experience suggests that treatment of VD deficiency or insufficiency, however, is challenging in current clinical practice, especially if the VD status is followed in longer term [7]. The few prospective randomized clinical trials on VD supplementation, on the other hand, have not demonstrated consistent benefits in fracture risk reduction in community-dwelling individuals [1,2,8–11].

To test our hypothesis that most patients with VD deficiency (or insufficiency) remain VD-deficient (or -insufficient), we did a retrospective review of 25(OH)D testing and its clinical utility in achieving medium-term VD sufficiency in a managed care population in the 3 years between 2011 and 2013. The results of our study demonstrate that 25(OH)D testing lacks clinical utility in achieving VD sufficiency and should not be routinely performed in managed care populations or in other contemporary clinical practice.

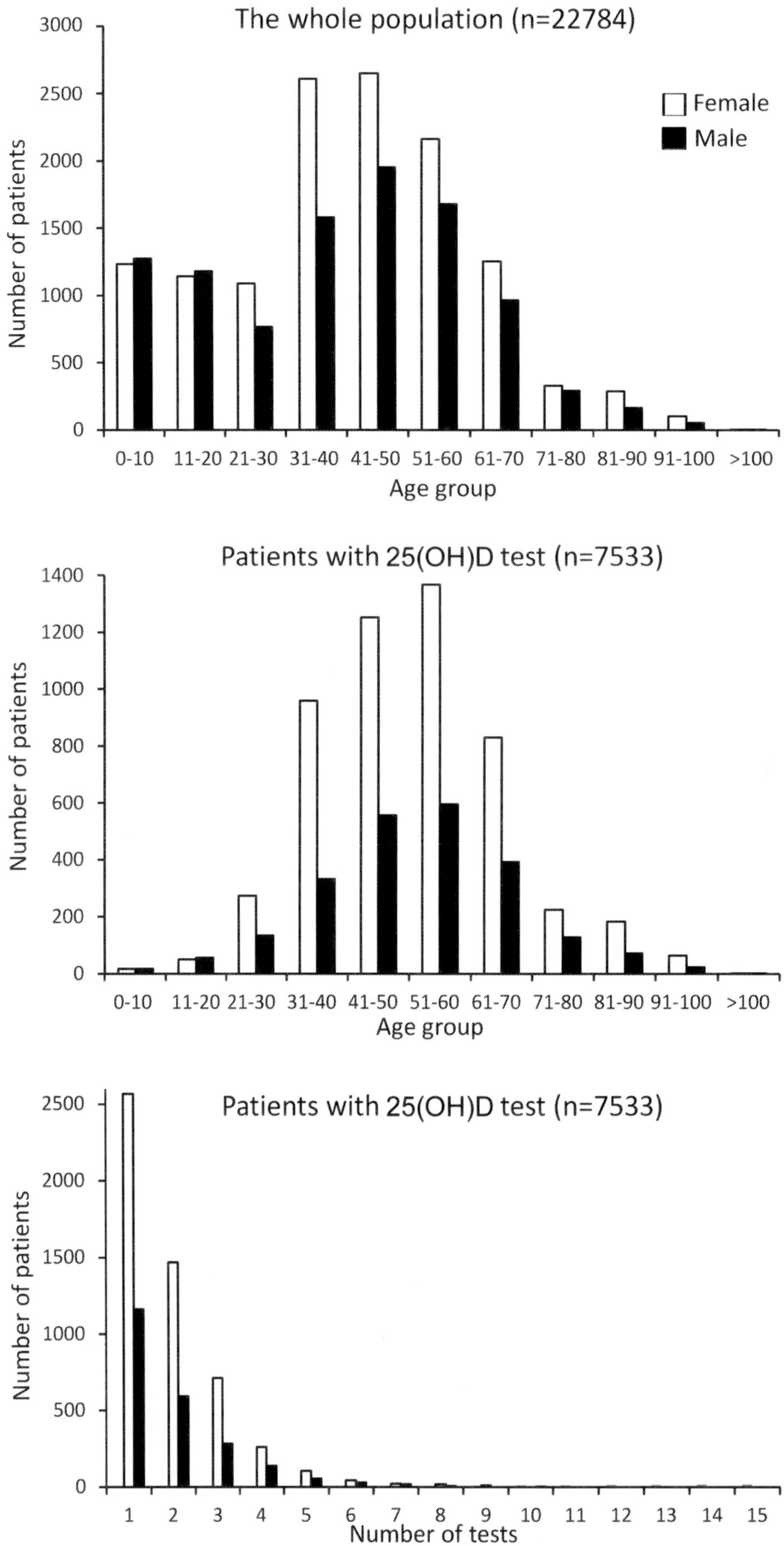
The whole population (n=22784)
Number of patients
3000
2500
2000
1500
1000
500
0
Female
Male
0-10 11-20 21-30 31-40 41-50 51-60 61-70 71-80 81-90 91-100 >100
Age group
Patients with 25(OH)D test (n=7533)
Number of patients
1400
1200
1000
800
600
400
200
0
0-10 11-20 21-30 31-40 41-50 51-60 61-70 71-80 81-90 91-100 >100
Age group
Patients with 25(OH)D test (n=7533)
Number of patients
2500
2000
1500
1000
500
0
1 2 3 4 5 6 7 8 9 10 11 12 13 14 15
Number of tests

Figure 1. Demographics of the managed care population (Top) and the patients who underwent 25(OH)D testing (Middle) over a 3-year period. The numbers of patients who did multiple tests were also shown (Bottom).

Methods

Patients and 25(OH)D tests

This study has been approved by the Cedars-Sinai Institutional Review Board. Requirement of written or verbal consent was waived by the Review Board for this retrospective study. Health records were de-identified prior to use. All managed care patients who were continuously enrolled at a large medical group and an independent physician association from January 1, 2011 to December 31, 2013 were eligible. There were no exclusion criteria for this population-based study. The list of patients was obtained from the managed care enrollment database, race and body mass index (BMI) from the electronic medical records database, and 25(OH)D testing data from the laboratory encounter database. VD status was defined as follows: deficiency (25(OH)D≤20 ng/ml), insufficiency (>20 but <30 ng/ml), and sufficiency (≥30 ng/ml) [2]. The economic burden of 25(OH)D testing was calculated as the total cost of 25(OH)D testing within the study patient population in the 3 years of study period, based on the Medicare rate.

Co-morbidities, procedures, and medications

Data on osteoporosis, pathologic fractures, obesity, fat malabsorption (including Crohn's disease, ulcerative colitis, celiac disease, cystic fibrosis, and history of pancreatectomy, gastrectomy, or small bowel resection), chronic kidney disease, HIV, dual-energy X-ray absorptiometry (DEXA), and bariatric surgery were based on ICD-9 and CPT codes and obtained from encounter database. Medication records and high-dose VD dispensing (50,000 international units or 1.25 mg) data were obtained from pharmacy claim database. To study the risk factors for repeated 25(OH)D testing and failure to improve VD status after testing, the co-morbidities, procedures, and medications for osteoporosis and seizure recorded 6 months before and after the only or the first 25(OH)D test were used as variables. To study the risk factors for failure to improve VD status after testing, high-dose VD dispensed within 350 days after the only or the first 25(OH)D test was used.

Statistics

Student t test was used to compare of the means of continuous data between two groups. Chi square or Fisher's exact test was used to compare the rates of categorical data between groups. Multivariate logistic regression analysis was used to discover independent risk factors associated with a change of VD status [3,12]. All statistical analyses were performed using the JMP Statistical Discovery software (Cary, NC).

Results

Of the 22,784 managed care patients continuously enrolled in the 3-year study period (Fig. 1), 7533 patients did 14,563 25(OH)D tests with valid results, corresponding to an annual test

Table 1. Comparison of patients who did only 1 25(OH)D test and those who did 2 or more 25(OH)D tests in the study period.

	Only 1 25(OH)D test	>=2 25(OH)D tests
n	3,731	3,802
Age (range), yr	48.9 (3–105)***	53.5 (8–100)
Female, %	68.8	69.9
African American, %	22.1	21.5
Results of the only or first test (range), ng/ml	23.8 (0–115)***	26.0 (0–154.9)
Sufficiency/insufficiency/deficiency at the only or first test, %	33.4/29.3/37.3***	31.8/34.3/33.9
Osteoporosis diagnosis, %	5.2***	9.3
Pathologic fractures, %	0.5	0.4
Osteoporosis medications, %	5.2***	8.9
DEXA, %	5.8***	11.1
Obesity diagnosis, %	14.3	15.8
BMI (range)	27.1 (13.4–66.6)***	27.6 (13.4–62.3)
BMI≥30, %	24.8	26.5
History of bariatric surgery, %	1.1**	1.9
Fat malabsorption, %	1.4	1.5
Chronic kidney disease, %	2.0*	2.8
HIV, %	0.9***	2.4
Anti-epileptics, %	0.3	0.2
High-dose VD prescription, %	3.2***	8.2

Statistical analysis was performed to assess the significance of the differences between the two groups.
*$p<0.05$,
**$p<0.01$,
***$p<0.001$.

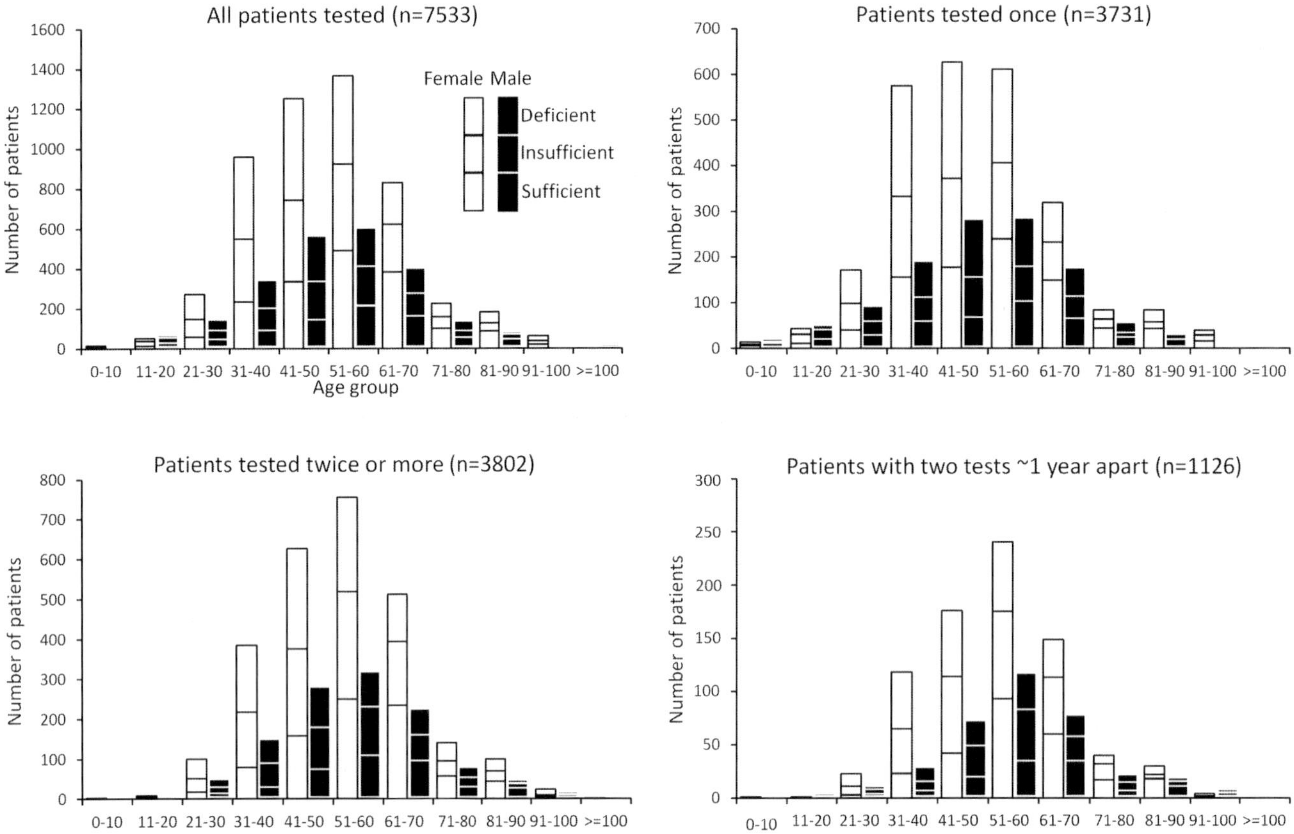

Figure 2. 25(OH)D test results. The results of the only or the first 25(OH)D test were classified into 3 groups: deficiency (≤20 ng/ml), insufficiency (>20 but <30 ng/ml), or sufficiency (≥30 ng/ml). Upper left, results from all patients who underwent 25(OH)D testing. Upper right, results from the patients who had only been tested once. Lower left, results from the patients who had 2 or more 25(OH)D tests. Lower right, results from the patients who had another test at 300–400 days after the first one.

rate of 11.0% of the managed care population and 0.21 25(OH)D test per patient per year. Based on Medicare rates, the total cost of the 25(OH)D tests for the 7533 patients was $582,520. Most tested patients were between 31 and 70 years old (83.4%), and those between 41 and 60 years old made up 50.0%. Females (n = 5224, 69.3%) were tested much more frequently than males (n = 2309, 30.7%) across all age groups. Of the 7533 patients, 3731 (49.5%) had only one 25(OH)D test but 3802 (50.5%) had two or more tests (Fig. 1). Compared with those with only 1 25(OH)D test, patients with more than one 25(OH)D test were 4.6 years older and had slightly higher 25(OH)D levels and BMI; they also had more osteoporosis diagnoses, underwent more DEXA scans, and were more likely on osteoporosis medications (Table 1). Overall, <3% of patients had history of bariatric surgery, fat malabsorption, chronic kidney disease, and HIV, or anti-epileptic use. More patients with more than one 25(OH)D test were dispensed with high-dose VD after the first 25(OH)D test than those with only one test (8.2% V 3.2%, $p<0.001$). Between the two groups, there were no significant differences in patients' sex, race, rates of pathologic fractures, or obesity diagnosis.

Based on the results of the first (or the only) 25(OH)D test, 32.6% of the 7533 patients were VD-sufficient while 31.6% VD-insufficient and 35.7% VD-deficient. Similar results were seen in both sexes across age groups (Fig. 2). Interestingly patients between 21 and 50 years old were less VD-sufficient (25.0% v. 39.2%, $p<0.0001$) but also less frequently tested than people of other ages (45.0% v. 55.2%, $p<0.0001$). There were small seasonal variations in 25(OH)D levels which were highest in July and lowest in December (mean levels 27.7 and 22.7 ng/ml, respectively). In the 21–50-year group, those who were VD-insufficient or -deficient were slightly more likely to be tested again than those who were VD-sufficient (46.3% v. 41.1%, $p = 0.0077$). In other age groups, the repeat test rates were not significantly different between those who were VD-insufficient or -deficient and those who were VD-sufficient (56.2% v. 53.7%, $p = 0.1271$).

To study the impact of 25(OH)D testing on future VD status, we identified 1126 patients who had done another 25(OH)D test at 300–400 days after the first one. The distribution of the results of the first 25(OH)D test of the 1126 patients and that of the 3802 patients were grossly similar to that of the 7533 patients (Fig. 2), suggesting that the 1126 patients were representative of all the patients tested more than once. We also compared the demographics and VD status of the 1126 patients with the rest of the 7533 (6507 patients, the difference of 7533 and 1026) over each decade between 21 and 90 years old. If the 25(OH)D results were divided into the 3 categories of sufficiency, insufficiency, and deficiency, the result distribution was not significantly different in most decades except for in the decades of 41–50 and 71–80 years old ($p = 0.0196$ and 0.0468, respectively). If the 25(OH)D results were divided into 2 groups, sufficiency and abnormally low levels (including insufficiency and deficiency), the 25(OH)D result distribution was not significantly different among any decades ($p = 0.1272$–0.9563).

We compared the second and the first 25(OH)D test results of the 1126 patients and identified 4 patterns of VD status change. As the difference between VD deficiency and insufficiency is

Table 2. Comparison of 4 groups of patients who did another 25(OH)D test at ~1 year after the first one.

Characteristics	Sufficient-to-sufficient	Sufficient-to-low	Low-to-sufficient	Low-to-low	All
n (%)	234 (20.8)	132 (11.7)	222 (19.7)	538 (47.8)	1126 (100)
Age (range), yr	59.2 (30–98)*	55.5 (8–91)	55.4 (21–95)***	51.4 (12–98)	54.3 (8–98)
Female, %	72.6	66.7	70.3	68.4	69.4
African American, %	16.9	18.1	12.6***	26.4	22.1
1st result (range), ng/ml	43.1 (30.0–154.9)***	37.0 (30–87.2)	20.9 (0–29.8)***	19.4 (0–29.9)	26.7 (0–154.9)
Difference between 2nd and 1st results (range), ng/ml	−0.57 (−110.2–38.1)***	−23.4 (−69.8–−0.9)	17.6 (0.5–81)***	−2.7 (−29.7–28.0)	−0.7 (−110.2–81)
Osteoporosis diagnosis, %	17.1*	9.1	5.4	5.8	9.2
Pathologic fractures, %	0.9	0	0	0.2	0.3
Osteoporosis medications, %	17.1	9.8	5.9	6.1	9.5
DEXA, %	20.9*	10.6	6.8	9.3	12.3
Obesity diagnosis, %	10.7	15.9	7.2***	19.1	16.1
BMI (range)	25.1 (14.9–43.5)**	26.8 (14.9–49.0)	26.7 (16.9–47.6)***	28.7 (16.5–62.3)	27.3 (14.9–62.3)
BMI≥30, %	10.2**	21.6	15.2***	32.3	24.6
History of bariatric surgery, %	2.6	3.0	0.9	1.7	2.4
Fat malabsorption, %	3.0	3.0	0.5	1.1	1.6
Chronic kidney disease, %	3.4	3.8	2.3	3.3	3.5
HIV, %	6.4	2.3	2.3	1.1	2.9
Anti-epileptics, %	0	0.8	0	0.2	0.2
High-dose VD prescription, %	1.7*	6.1	5.0**	11.9	8.3

Sufficient-to-sufficient, patients with sufficient VD results from both tests; sufficient-to-low, patients with sufficient results from the first test but abnormally low results (VD-insufficient or deficient) from the second; low-to-sufficient, patients with abnormally low results from the first test but sufficient results from the second one; low-to-low, patients with abnormally low results from both tests. Statistical analysis was performed to assess the significance of the differences between the sufficient-to-sufficient and sufficient-to-low groups, and between the low-to-sufficient and low-to-low groups.
*$p<0.05$,
**$p<0.01$,
***$p<0.001$.

controversial and somewhat arbitrary [13], they were collectively labeled as abnormally low VD levels. Only 234 of the 1126 patients (20.8%) exhibited sufficient VD levels on both tests (sufficient-to-sufficient), indicating maintained VD sufficiency, while 132 (11.7%) who were originally VD-sufficient became VD insufficient or deficient (sufficient-to-low) (Table 2). Interestingly, after the first test, 538 patients (47.8%) remained VD-insufficient or -deficient (low-to-low) and only 222 patients (19.7%) improved to be VD-sufficient (low-to-sufficient). Overall, 67.5% of patients were VD-insufficient or -deficient at the first test and 59.5% were so at the second test. Thus only 8.0% patients benefited from the testing by converting from low to sufficient VD levels at approximately a year after the test. To derive risk factors for inability to maintain VD sufficiency and for persistent low VD levels, we compared the characteristics of the 4 groups of patients (Table 2 and Fig. 3). By univariate analysis, compared with those in the sufficient-to-sufficient group, the patients in the sufficient-to-low group were a few years younger, more obese, and with lower 25(OH)D levels from the first test; they also had fewer osteoporosis diagnoses and underwent fewer DEXA scans. Ironically, a small fraction of both groups of patients were dispensed with high-dose VD but those in the sufficient-to-low group were dispensed with relatively more frequently (6.1% v. 1.7%). Multivariate logistic regression analysis showed that only younger age and lower rate of HIV infection were independent risk factors for inability to maintain VD sufficiency. If only the significant variables identified by univariate analysis ($p<0.05$) were used, younger age remained the sole risk factor for inability to maintain VD sufficiency. Compared with those in the low-to-sufficient group, the patients in the low-to-low group were again a few years younger, more obese, and with lower 25(OH)D levels from the first test; more patients were African Americans. More patients in these two groups were dispensed with high-dose VD than those in the sufficient-to-sufficient and sufficient-to-low groups; however, patients in the low-to-low group were dispensed with relatively more high-dose VD than those in the low-to-sufficient group. Multivariate analysis showed that only younger age, higher BMI, history of bariatric surgery, and lower rate of HIV infection were independent risk factors for persistent low VD levels. If only the significant variables identified by univariate analysis ($p<0.05$) were used, younger age and higher BMI remained risk factors for persistent low VD levels.

Discussion

25(OH)D testing to detect VD deficiency has become a fad in recent years, probably driven by numerous correlational studies connecting low 25(OH)D levels and many human diseases [3–6]. As the literature on benefits of VD sufficiency appears somewhat plausible [1–4], one may presumptively accept that VD sufficiency is beneficial to health in general. The key question then becomes

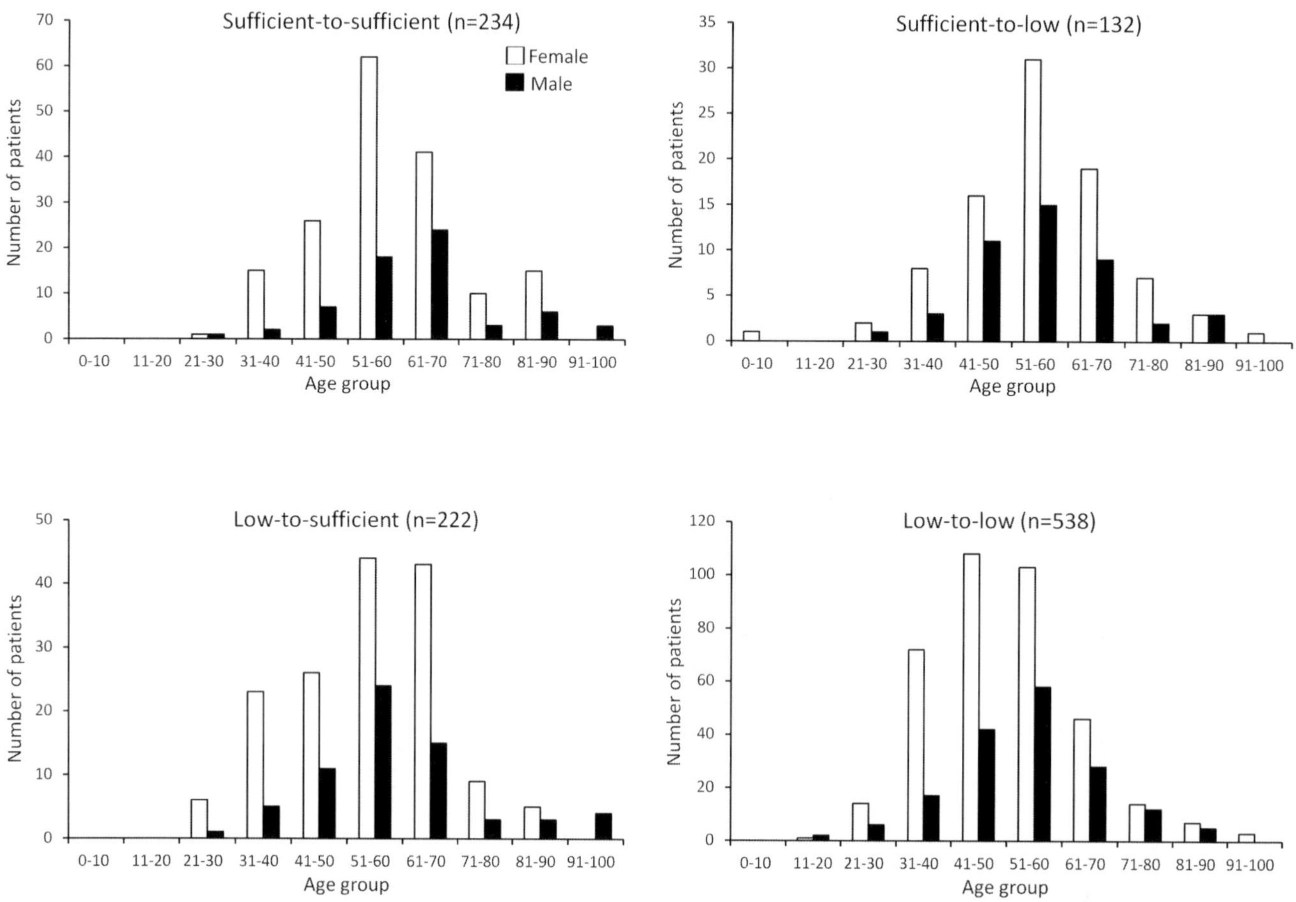

Figure 3. Demographics of the patients who had another 25(OH)D test at about 1 year after the first one. Upper left, the patients with sufficient 25(OH)D results from both tests (sufficient-to-sufficient). Upper right, the patients with sufficient 25(OH)D results from the first test but abnormally low results (VD-insufficient or deficient) from the second (sufficient-to-low). Lower left, the patients with abnormally low results from the first test but sufficient results from the second one (low-to-sufficient). Lower right, the patients with abnormally low results from both tests (low-to-low).

how to effectively help people achieve VD sufficiency. There is no doubt that high-dose VD treatment improves VD status in a few months [2,3,7] (and in years if given every 2 weeks [14]). As VD deficiency or insufficiency is a chronic condition, the key question is whether VD status improves in longer terms after 25(OH)D testing or high-dose VD treatment. Thus in this article, we take a novel approach studying the practical clinical utility of 25(OH)D testing and examine whether 25(OH)D testing helps achieve VD sufficiency in the medium term in a large managed care population.

First of all, the study confirms that VD sufficiency is uncommon (only ~1/3) in the mostly adult managed care population [15]. The most striking finding, however, is that most patients with VD deficiency or insufficiency (~70%) do not achieve VD sufficiency and a portion of patients with VD sufficiency (~40%) lose it at 300–400 days after the first 25(OH)D test. Overall only 8% of the tested patients improve their VD status from deficiency or insufficiency to sufficiency. The true cost of 25(OH)D testing is thus more expensive than the apparent cost because to benefit one patient (to achieve or maintain VD sufficiency after 25(OH)D testing), 12.5 patients (the inverse of 8%) have to be tested. As 1/3 of the entire study population underwent 25(OH)D testing at least once and only <10% of tested patients had osteoporosis diagnosis or history of pathologic fractures, the purpose of the 25(OH)D tests was most likely for screening for VD deficiency. Our results seriously challenge the clinical utility of 25(OH)D testing for screening purpose. First, there does not seem to be a need for screening for VD deficiency or insufficiency if the majority of the population has the condition. Second, the lack of practical and effective treatment of VD deficiency or insufficiency makes VD status screening not worthwhile. Although chronic use of high-dose VD can achieve VD sufficiency for years, this method has not been adopted in clinical practice [14]. Indeed, routine screening for vitamin D status is not recommended by guidelines but the reason for not recommending screening is due to lack of evidence on feasibility, cost-effectiveness, or benefits of such screening [1,2]. Our results provide direct evidence for recommending *against* routine screening for vitamin D status.

Although VD deficiency or insufficiency can be treated in a theoretically straightforward manner by sun exposure and VD supplement, our study clearly shows that it is challenging to be treated in practice. The failure to effectively treat VD deficiency or insufficiency may be either due to lack of counseling on importance and ways to achieve VD sufficiency or due to patients' incompliance. Concern of skin cancer is a known barrier to achieve VD sufficiency [16,17]. Adherence to VD supplementation is an important factor in achieving benefits of VD supplementation on fracture prevention [7,11]. Adherence is satisfactory (60–90%) in elderly populations but unclear in younger populations. If VD sufficiency is indeed critical to health, a practical and effective method is needed to achieve VD sufficiency.

Our study provides novel insights into the potential causes of VD deficiency and failure to improve VD status. In our study, the patients who maintain VD sufficiency are not necessarily healthier than others. They are older and thinner, and tend to have osteoporosis and HIV infection. As most of them do not take high-dose VD supplement, their VD sufficiency is presumably achieved by sun exposure and over-the-counter VD supplement [2,3]. As these measures are dependent on life style, it can be assumed that these patients are highly motivated to achieve VD sufficiency. Although we don't have data on their motivations, their older age and the age-associated osteoporosis in this mostly female population may motivate them to achieve and maintain VD sufficiency. On the other hand, the patients who remain VD-deficient or -insufficient are younger and heavier but fewer of them have osteoporosis or HIV infection. Even though slightly more than 10% of them fill high-dose VD prescriptions, the high-dose VD does not help them achieve VD sufficiency in the medium term. Thus the cause of their persistent VD deficiency or insufficiency is also unconducive life style for VD sufficiency. Their perceived low risk for osteoporosis may give them a disincentive to make life style modifications to achieve VD sufficiency. Compared with other chronic life-style diseases such as obesity, diabetes, and hypertension, VD deficiency can be much more easily treated by simply taking daily 2000–4000 international units of VD without sun exposure [1,2]. The lack of clear evidence that mild VD deficiency or insufficiency indeed causes clear and severe complications is likely the main reason for physicians and patients not to invest in life style modifications to improve VD status. On the other hand, for motivated patients, the physicians should consider the patients' risk factors for persistent low VD levels during counseling; for example, higher doses of VD are likely needed for young and obese patients to achieve VD sufficiency [18–20].

Our study has its strengths and limitations. Because it is based on a population without exclusion criteria, its results more realistically reflect the true characteristics of the population. The defined and stable managed care patient population has several distinct advantages for population studies [21]. As the patients received all their care within the managed care system and their 25(OH)D tests and results, comorbidities, procedures, and medications were all recorded, our study results are accurate and unlikely prone to misinterpretation due to incomplete data. Most importantly, we have followed a cohort of the same patients with 2 25(OH)D tests approximately a year apart so that we can derive specific risk factors for failure to achieve or maintain VD sufficiency. One major limitation is that we do not have data on sun exposure and over-the-counter VD supplement, the main treatments for VD deficiency or insufficiency. Another limitation is that although the cohort of patients we followed appeared to be similar to all patients with 25(OH)D testing, the former has much fewer patients than, and may not represent a random sample of, the latter. The small seasonal variation of 25(OH)D levels should not affect our analysis on medium-term VD status because the second 25(OH)D test was carried out 1 year later, in the same season in which the first test was done.

In summary, this retrospective study of a continuously enrolled managed care population in a 3-year period demonstrates that 25(OH)D testing only benefits a small portion of patients thus lacks clinical utility in achieving VD sufficiency in the medium term but incurs a significant cost. Our data implies that a practical and effective strategy to treat VD deficiency or insufficiency is needed in contemporary managed care practice; without such as strategy, 25(OH)D testing adds little value to most patients' health and should be used with discretion.

Author Contributions

Conceived and designed the experiments: RY SCD. Performed the experiments: MW SCD. Analyzed the data: MW RY. Contributed reagents/materials/analysis tools: MW RY SCD. Contributed to the writing of the manuscript: MW RY SCD.

References

1. IOM (Institute of Medicine) (2011) Dietary reference intakes for calcium and vitamin D. Washington, DC: The National Academies Press; 2011.
2. Holick MF, Binkley NC, Bischoff-Ferrari HA, Gordon CM, Hanley DA, et al. (2011) Evaluation, treatment, and prevention of vitamin D deficiency: an Endocrine Society clinical practice guideline. J Clin Endocrinol Metab 96: 1911–1930.
3. Holick MF (2007) Vitamin D deficiency. N Engl J Med 357: 266–281.
4. Basit S (2013) Vitamin D in health and disease: a literature review. Br J Biomed Sci 70: 161–72.
5. Sattar N1, Welsh P, Panarelli M, Forouhi NG (2012) Increasing requests for vitamin D measurement: costly, confusing, and without credibility. Lancet 379: 95–96.
6. Bilinski KL, Boyages SC (2012) The rising cost of vitamin D testing in Australia: time to establish guidelines for testing. Med J Aust 197: 90.
7. Yu R (2014) Commentary on "Surge in US Outpatient Vitamin D Deficiency Diagnoses: National Ambulatory Medical Care Survey Analysis". South Med J 107: 218–219.
8. Jackson RD1, LaCroix AZ, Gass M, Wallace RB, Robbins J, et al. (2006) Calcium plus vitamin D supplementation and the risk of fractures. N Engl J Med 354: 669–683.
9. Sanders KM1, Stuart AL, Williamson EJ, Simpson JA, Kotowicz MA, et al. (2010) Annual high-dose oral vitamin D and falls and fractures in older women: a randomized controlled trial. JAMA 303: 1815–1822.
10. Bischoff-Ferrari HA1, Willett WC, Orav EJ, Lips P, Meunier PJ, et al. (2012) A pooled analysis of vitamin D dose requirements for fracture prevention. N Engl J Med 367: 40–49.
11. Reid IR, Bolland MJ, Grey A (2014) Effects of vitamin D supplements on bone mineral density: a systematic review and meta-analysis. Lancet 383: 146–155.
12. Looker AC, Pfeiffer CM, Lacher DA, Schleicher RL, Picciano MF, et al. (2008) Serum 25-hydroxyvitamin D status of the US population: 1988–1994 compared with 2000–2004. Am J Clin Nutr 88: 1519–1527.
13. Rosen CJ (2011) Clinical practice. Vitamin D insufficiency. N Engl J Med 364: 248–254.
14. Pietras SM, Obayan BK, Cai MH, Holick MF (2009) Vitamin D2 treatment for vitamin D deficiency and insufficiency for up to 6 years. Arch Intern Med 26: 1806–8.
15. Forrest KY, Stuhldreher WL (2011) Prevalence and correlates of vitamin D deficiency in US adults. Nutr Res 31: 48–54.
16. Reeder AI1, Jopson JA, Gray AR (2012) "Prescribing sunshine": a national, cross-sectional survey of 1,089 New Zealand general practitioners regarding their sun exposure and vitamin D perceptions, and advice provided to patients. BMC Fam Pract 13: 85.
17. Bonevski B, Girgis A, Magin P, Horton G, Brozek I, et al. (2012) Prescribing sunshine: a cross-sectional survey of 500 Australian general practitioners' practices and attitudes about vitamin D. Int J Cancer 130: 2138–2145.
18. Lee P, Greenfield JR, Seibel MJ, Eisman JA, Center JR (2009) Adequacy of vitamin D replacement in severe deficiency is dependent on body mass index. Am J Med 122: 1056–1060.
19. Stratton-Loeffler MJ, Lo JC, Hui RL, Coates A, Minkoff JR, et al. (2012) Treatment of vitamin D deficiency within a large integrated health care delivery system. J Manag Care Pharm 18: 497–505.
20. Drincic A, Fuller E, Heaney RP, Armas LA (2013) 25-hydroxyvitamin D response to graded vitamin D3 supplementation among obese adults. J Clin Endocrinol Metab 98: 4845–4851.
21. Vogt TM1, Elston-Lafata J, Tolsma D, Greene SM (2004) The role of research in integrated healthcare systems: the HMO Research Network. Am J Manag Care 10: 643–648.

21

Dimethyloxalylglycine Prevents Bone Loss in Ovariectomized C57BL/6J Mice through Enhanced Angiogenesis and Osteogenesis

Jia Peng[1]❡, Zuo Gui Lai[1,2]❡, Zhang Lian Fang[1,3], Shen Xing[1], Kang Hui[1], Chen Hao[1], Qi Jin[1], Zhou Qi[1], Wang Jin Shen[1], Qian Nian Dong[1], Zhou Han Bing[1], Deng Lian Fu[1]*

1 Shanghai Institute of Traumatology and Orthopaedics, Shanghai Key Laboratory for Prevention and Treatment of Bone and Joint Diseases with Integrated Chinese-Western Medicine, Ruijin Hospital, Jiao Tong University School of Medicine, Shanghai, China, **2** Department of Orthopaedics, Qian Fo Shan Hospital, Shang Dong University, Ji Nan, China, **3** Department of Orthopaedics, The First Affiliated Hospital of Soochow University, Suzhou, China

Abstract

Hypoxia-inducible factor 1-α (HIF-1α) plays a critical role in angiogenesis-osteogenesis coupling during bone development and bone regeneration. Previous studies have shown that 17β-estradiol activates the HIF-1α signaling pathway and that mice with conditional activation of the HIF-1α signaling pathway in osteoblasts are protected from ovariectomy (OVX)-induced bone loss. In addition, it has been shown that hypoxia facilitates the osteogenic differentiation of mesenchymal stem cells (MSCs) and modulates Wnt/β-catenin signaling. Therefore, we hypothesized that activation of the HIF-1α signaling pathway by hypoxia-mimicking agents would prevent bone loss due to estrogen deficiency. In this study, we confirmed the effect of dimethyloxalylglycine (DMOG), a hypoxia-mimicking agent, on the HIF-1α signaling pathway and investigated the effect of DMOG on MSC osteogenic differentiation and the Wnt/β-catenin signaling pathway. We then investigated the effect of DMOG treatment on OVX-induced bone loss. Female C57BL/6J mice were divided into sham, OVX, OVX+L-DMOG (5 mg/kg/day), and OVX+H-DMOG (20 mg/kg/day) groups. At sacrifice, static and dynamic bone histomorphometry were performed with micro computed tomography (micro-CT) and undecalcified sections, respectively. Bone strength was assessed with the three-point bending test, and femur vessels were reconstructed and analyzed by micro-CT. Serum vascular endothelial growth factor (VEGF), osteocalcin, and C-terminal telopeptides of collagen type(CTX) were measured by ELISA. Tartrate-resistant acid phosphatase staining was used to assess osteoclast formation. Alterations in the HIF-1α and Wnt/β-catenin signaling pathways in the bone were detected by western blot. Our results showed that DMOG activated the HIF-1α signaling pathway, which further activated the Wnt/β-catenin signaling pathway and enhanced MSC osteogenic differentiation. The micro-CT results showed that DMOG treatment improved trabecular bone density and restored the bone microarchitecture and blood vessels in OVX mice. Bone strength was also partly restored in DMOG-treated OVX mice. Dynamic bone histomorphometric analysis of the femur metaphysic revealed that DMOG increased the mineralizing surface, mineral apposition rate, and bone formation rate. The serum levels of VEGF and osteocalcin were higher in DMOG-treated OVX mice. However, there were no significant differences in serum CTX or in the number of tartrate-resistant acid phosphatase-stained cells between DMOG-treated OVX mice and OVX mice. Western blot results showed that DMOG administration partly rescued the decrease in HIF-1α and β-catenin expression following ovariectomy. Collectively, these results indicate that DMOG prevents bone loss due to ovariectomy in C57BL/6J mice by enhancing angiogenesis and osteogenesis, which are associated with activated HIF-1α and Wnt/β-catenin signaling pathways.

Editor: Rajeev Samant, University of Alabama at Birmingham, United States of America

Funding: Deng Lian Fu received funds from Natural Science Foundation of China (No. 81371958, 81061160510), the Basic Key Project of Science and Technology Commission of Shanghai Municipality (12JC1408200), and the Scientific and Technological Support Program in Biological Medicine of Science and Technology Commission of Shanghai Municipality (13431900702) http://www.nsfc.gov.cn/ http://www.stcsm.gov.cn/. The funders had no role in study design, data collection and analysis, decision to publish, or preparation of the manuscript.

Competing Interests: The authors have declared that no competing interests exist.

* Email: china_boneres@163.com

❡ These authors contributed equally to this work.

Introduction

Osteoporosis is a disorder characterized by increased bone fragility, low bone mass, and a consequent increase in fracture risk [1]. Fragility fractures resulting from osteoporosis are the main cause of disablement and death among elderly women. These events lead to the consumption of enormous amounts of medical resources and produce heavy economic burdens [2]. Therefore, using current understanding of disease pathogenesis to develop effective drugs for the prevention and treatment of postmenopausal osteoporosis is vital.

The skeleton is a highly vascularized tissue in which bone remodeling is tightly coupled with angiogenesis. The vasculature supplies nutrients, oxygen, and mesenchymal stem cells (MSCs), which are necessary elements for bone formation, and may direct new bone formation by providing a scaffold for bone-forming cells [3]. Although the main cause of postmenopausal osteoporosis is estrogen deficiency, accumulating evidence from studies in cells, animals, and patients suggests that the local blood supply or decreased angiogenesis contributes to estrogen deficiency-induced osteoporosis [4–11].

Angiogenesis depends on hypoxic stimuli and vascular endothelial growth factor (VEGF) production. The hypoxia-inducible factor-α (HIF-α) pathway is the central regulator of the adaptive response to low oxygen levels. The pathway regulates angiogenic genes (e.g.,*VEGF, angiopoietins*). The HIF family comprises three α subunits, HIF-1α, HIF-2α, and HIF-3α. HIF-α is an oxygen-labile protein that forms a heterodimeric complex with the HIF-β subunit, which is constitutively expressed [12]. Under normoxic conditions, HIF-α is hydroxylated at a proline residue by prolyl hydroxylases (PHDs), which need oxygen, iron, and 2-oxyglutarate as cofactors. When hydroxylated, HIF-α is bound by von Hippel-Lindau protein (pVHL), an E3 ubiquitin ligase, and is then degraded by the proteasome. Under hypoxic conditions, prolyl hydroxylation of HIF-α is inhibited, and HIF-α accumulates in the nucleus, where it heterodimerizes with the HIF-β subunit and transactivates HIF responsive genes [13–15]. The HIF pathway can be activated under normoxic conditions by small molecule inhibitors of PHDs that interfere with the required PHD cofactors by acting as iron chelators (e.g., desferrioxamine (DFO)) or 2-oxyglutarate analogues (e.g., dimethyloxalylglycine (DMOG)) [14,16].

Importantly, the HIF-α pathway plays a critical role in angiogenesis-osteogenesis coupling. Clemens *et al.* showed that activation of the HIF-α pathway in mature osteoblasts in developing bone increased bone modeling and the effect was largely attributed to enhanced VEGF-mediated bone vessel formation [17]. Similar results were reported by Giaccia *et al.*, who generated mice in which HIF-α was overstabilized in osteoprogenitor cells. The mice exhibited excessive accumulation of trabecular bone in the long bone and increased vascularization [18]. Striking and progressive accumulation of cancellous bone with increased microvascular density and bone formation was also observed in mice lacking *Vhl* in osteochondral progenitor cells [19]. Moreover, the HIF-1α pathway was activated during bone repair and could be manipulated genetically and pharmacologically to accelerate bone regeneration [16,20]. Consistent with the "promoting osteogenesis by enhancing angiogenesis" theory, HIF-1α pathway activators (DMOG, DFO) or mesenchymal stem cells overexpressing HIF-1α have been shown to improve fracture and bone defect healing [21–31].

The HIF-α signaling pathway might be involved in the pathogenesis of estrogen deficiency-induced osteoporosis. Our group reported that bone density, bone vessels, and bone formation were lower in *Hif1a* conditional knockout (KO) ovariectomized(OVX) mice than in wild-type OVX mice [32]. Moreover, the expression of HIF-α and VEGF decreased in OVX mice but not in *Vhl* KO OVX mice. In addition, *Vhl* KO OVX mice, which showed increased angiogenesis and osteogenesis due to activation of the HIF-α pathway, were protected from OVX-induced bone loss [33]. It has been suggested that 17β-estradiol increases HIF-1α and VEGF protein levels and partially stimulates human mesenchymal stem cell (hMSC) proliferation via HIF-1α activation [34]. These data are consistent with the findings of Yen *et al.*, who demonstrated that diosgenin, which has estrogenic effects, induces HIF-1 activation and angiogenesis through the src kinase, p38 MAPK, and Akt signaling pathways in osteoblasts [35]. Hence, decreased stimulation of the HIF-1α pathway and angiogenesis might be important factors contributing to estrogen deficiency-induced bone loss. Therefore, activation of the HIF-1α pathway might be a new approach to osteoporosis treatment.

In addition to affecting angiogenesis, hypoxia and hypoxia-mimicking agents increase osteogenesis and modulate Wnt/β-catenin signaling [36]. Hypoxia promotes the proliferation of MSCs and accelerates their differentiation [37,38]. Similarly, overexpression of HIF-1α in MSCs upregulates the mRNA and protein expression of osteogenic markers *in vitro* [24,25,39]. *In vivo* studies using transgenic mice have provided strong evidence that activation of HIF-1α signaling in osteochondral progenitor cells or osteoprogenitor cells increases osteoblast proliferation and differentiation [18,19]. Treatment of MSCs/osteoblasts with DFO also increases osteogenic marker expression, the effect was attributed to activation of the Wnt/β-catenin signaling pathways [40,41]. Two different groups have proposed that DMOG not only improves the angiogenic capacity of MSCs, but also enhances their osteogenic differentiation, though the exact mechanism has not been fully elucidated [21,30]. Considering that reduced osteogenesis of MSCs in postmenopausal women is a causative mechanism for osteoporosis, it is reasonable to promote osteogenesis by activation of the Wnt/β-catenin pathway [42]. Therefore, Wnt/β-catenin pathway stimulation might be a useful approach to osteoporosis treatment [43,44].

In light of their dual role in angiogenesis and osteogenesis, hypoxia-mimicking agents have tremendous potential for inhibiting bone loss. Supporting this notion, two recent studies have shown that activation of HIF-1α signaling by DFO or inactivation of *Vhl* in osteochondral progenitor cells in a tamoxifen-inducible manner prevented age-induced bone loss [19,45]. However, iron overload has been regarded as a risk factor for postmenopausal osteoporosis [46,47]. To exclude the effect of "iron chelation" on the skeleton, we treated OVX mice with DMOG, a cell-permeable prolyl-4-hydroxylase inhibitor that stabilizes HIF-1α under normal oxygen tension by suppressing PHD-mediated HIF-1α degradation [14,16]. DMOG has shown promise as a therapeutic agent for bone defect healing, neuronal protection, diabetic wound healing, renal protection, and prevention of flap necrosis [21,30,48–55].

The present study was designed to assess the effect of DMOG on the skeleton of OVX mice by evaluating bone mass, bone microarchitecture, bone biomechanics, and bone turnover. Furthermore, the mechanism by which DMOG alters the HIF-1α and Wnt/β-catenin pathways was investigated.

Materials and Methods

Reagents and chemicals

All fine chemicals, including DMOG, tetracycline, dexamethasone, ascorbic acid, β-glycerophosphate, alizarin red S (ARS), 17β-estradiol, L-glutamine, paraformaldehyde, ethylenediaminetetraacetic acid (EDTA), 3-(5′-hydroxymethyl-2′-furyl)-1-benzyl indazole (YC-1),and the tartrate-resistant acid phosphatase staining kit (Leukocyte Acid Phosphatase Assay kit), were purchased from Sigma-Aldrich (St. Louis, MO, USA). Dulbecco's modified Eagle's medium (DMEM), fetal bovine serum (FBS), trypsin, penicillin-streptomycin, and TRIzol were purchased from Life Technologies (Gaithersburg, MD, USA). The mouse monoclonal antibodies for HIF-1α and VEGF were purchased from Novus Biologicals (Littleton, CO, USA). The mouse monoclonal antibody for β-catenin was obtained from R&D Systems (Minneapolis, MN, USA), and the mouse monoclonal antibody for β-actin was purchased from Anbo Biotechnology (San Francisco, CA, USA). The rabbit monoclonal antibody for T-cell factor 1 (TCF-1) was from Bioworld Technology, Inc. (St. Louis Park, MN, USA). The lymphoid enhancer-binding factor 1 (LEF-1) polyclonal antibody was obtained from Proteintech Group, Inc. (Chicago, IL, USA). The mouse monoclonal antibody for TATA-binding protein (TBP) was purchased from Abcam (Cambridge, UK). The goat anti-mouse and goat anti-rabbit secondary antibodies conjugated with horseradish peroxidase were purchased from Santa Cruz Biotechnology (Santa Cruz, CA, USA). The VEGF ELISA kit was purchased from R&D Systems (Minneapolis, MN, USA), the osteocalcin ELISA kit was from Biomedical Technologies, Inc. (Ward Hill, MA, USA), and the C-terminal telopeptides of collagen type(CTX) ELISA kit was from Immunodiagnostic Systems (Tyne&Wear, UK). The silicon rubber solution was purchased from Flow Tech (Microfil MV-122; Carver, MA, USA). The primers were synthesized by Invitrogen (Shanghai, China). The RevertAid First Strand cDNA Synthesis Kit was purchased from Thermo Fisher Scientific (Ottawa, Canada). SYBR Premix Ex Taq was purchased from TaKaRa Biotechnology (Dalian, China). The alkaline phosphatase staining (ALP) staining kit was purchased from Shanghai Rainbow Biotechnology (Shanghai, China). The BCA protein assay kit was purchased from Beyotime (Nantong, China). The eECL Western blot kit was obtained from CWBIO (Beijing, China).

Cell culture and treatment

Murine mesenchymal C3H10T1/2 clone 8 cells were obtained from the American Type Culture Collection (Rockville, MD, USA). The cells were cultured in DMEM supplemented with 10% FBS, 50 U/ml penicillin, 50 mg/ml streptomycin, and 4 mM L-glutamine. Cultures were incubated in a humidified incubator at 37°C and 5% CO_2. The cells were passaged every 3–4 days. The cells were then plated in 6-well plates at 1×10^5 cells per well. After 24 hours, the cells were treated with the indicated concentrations of 17β-estradiol, DMOG, or DMOG+YC-1. For the hypoxia experiments, the cells were transferred into humidified incubators at 37°C with 5% CO_2, and the oxygen tension was reduced to 1% using supplemental N_2. In order to confirm the effect of DMOG on HIF-1α signaling pathway, the indicated treatment lasted 24 hours. For the experiment about exploration of DMOG on the differentiation of MSCs, the cells were cultured in osteogenic differentiation medium for 7 days. When treatment finished, the cells were collected for western blotting and quantitative real-time PCR analysis. The culture medium was collected for the measurement of VEGF by ELISA.

Quantitative real-time PCR for mRNA analysis

Total RNA from cells or bone samples were extracted using TRIzol reagent. In order to extract RNA from tibias, the tibias were grounded into pellets after the treatment with liquid nitrogen. cDNA was synthesized using 1 μg of RNA and a RevertAid First Strand cDNA Synthesis Kit. Gene expression was detected with real-time PCR using a SYBR Green qPCR kit and an ABI Step One Plus Real-Time PCR System. The primers used were listed in Table 1.

Western blot analysis

After cells or bone samples were lysed, the protein concentrations were measured using a BCA protein assay kit. Each protein sample (40 g) was subjected to SDS electrophoresis and electroblotted onto a polyvinylidene difluoride membrane (0.45 μm; Millipore, Bedford, MA, USA). Afterwards, the membranes were blocked with 5% non-fat dry milk in Tris-buffered saline with Tween 20 (TBST) for 1 hour. The membranes were probed with primary anti-HIF-1α (1:500), anti-TCF-1 (1:500), anti-LEF-1 (1:1000), anti-β-catenin (1:500), anti-TBP (1:2000), or anti-β-actin (1:5000) antibodies at 4°C overnight. The membranes were then washed three times with TBST and incubated for 1 hour with HRP-conjugated secondary antibodies (1:5000). The antigen-antibody complexes were visualized using the enhanced chemiluminescence detection system as recommended by the manufacturer.

Alkaline phosphatase staining and alizarin red staining

C3H10T1/2 cells were seeded onto 6-well plates at 1×10^5 cells per well. After the cells reached confluence, the medium was changed to osteogenesis differentiation medium containing 10^{-7} M dexamethasone, 0.15 mM ascorbate-2-phosphate, and 2 mM β-glycerophosphate. The cells were cultured for 14 or 21 days and then subjected to ALP or ARS staining. The procedures were conducted according to established protocols. Briefly, the cells were washed with PBS (pH 7.4) three times and fixed with 4% paraformaldehyde (pH 7.4, dissolved in PBS) for 15 min. The cells were then stained with ALP reagent or 0.2% ARS solution for 30 min at 37°C, after which the cells were washed with deionized water three times. The ALP reagent was prepared according to the manufacturer's instructions.

Animal models

All animal care and experimental procedures were approved by the Institutional Animal Ethics Committee of Shanghai Ruijin Hospital (ethical approval number: 138). Two-month-old female C57BL/6J mice were obtained from Shanghai SLAC Laboratory Animal Co., Ltd (Shanghai, China). The mice were housed five per cage and were maintained under a strict 12-h light:12-h dark cycle at 22°C with standard food pellets and free access to tap water. After a 2-week adaptation, ten-weeks-old mice were randomly divided into four groups as follows: sham group (ovary intact+vehicle (normal saline) i.p.), OVX group (OVX+vehicle), OVX+L-DMOG group (OVX+5 mg/kg/day DMOG i.p.), and OVX+H-DMOG group (OVX+20 mg/kg/day DMOG i.p.). The ovariectomy was performed in a surgery room exposed to ultraviolet radiation overnight. After anesthetization, the bilateral ovaries were exposed and removed from OVX animals; in the sham animals, the ovaries were exposed but left intact. After surgery, each mouse received an i.p. injection of gentamicin (1000 U) for three successive days. In order to confirm the successful establishment of OVX model, the femoral BMD of 8 mice were measured by *in vitro* micro computed tomography (micro-CT) before the surgery, and the BMD of another 8 mice were assessed one month later. The mice were sacrificed by anesthetic overdose. The uterus of each mouse was isolated and weighed. The body weight of each mouse was recorded. The femurs were collected for micro-CT, histological analyses and mechanical test. The left tibia of each mouse was used for PCR analysis, and the right tibia was used for western blot analysis.

Analysis of micro-CT scans

The distal metaphysic right femur were scanned with a high-resolution (8 μm) micro-CT scanner (GE eXplore Locus SP) to evaluate bone mass, geometry, and trabecular microarchitecture. The parameters computed from these data included bone mineral density (BMD), bone volume/tissue volume (BV/TV), trabecular thickness (Tb.Th), trabecular number (Tb.N), and trabecular separation (Tb.Sp).

Table 1. Premiers for Real-time PCR analysis.

Gene	Forward Premier	Reverse Premier
VEGF	5′-GGCTCTGAAACCATGAACTTTCT-3′	5′-GCAGTAGCTGCGCTGGTAGAC-3′
β-catenin	5′-GGAAAGCAAGCTCATCATTCT-3′	5′-AGTGCCTGCATCCACCCA-3′
Runx-2	5′-GTGTCACTGCGCTGAAGAGG-3′	5′-GACCAACCGAGTCATTTAAGGC-3′
Osterix	5′-ACCAGGTCCAGGCAACAC-3′	5′-GCAGTCGCAGGTAGAACG-3′
ALP	5′-ACGAGATGCCACCAGAGG-3′	5′-AGTTCAGTVCGGTTCCAG-3′
Osteocalcin	5′-TGCTCACTCTGCTGACCCTG-3′	5′-TTATTGCCCTCCTGCTTG-3′
RANKL	5′-CGTACCTGCGGACTATCTTCA-3′	5′-CTTGGACACCTGGACGCTAA-3′
OPG	5′-CATCGAAAGCACCCTGTA-3′	5′-CACTCAGCCAATTCGGTAT-3′
β-actin	5′-CCCTGTATGCCTCTGGTC-3′	5′-GTCTTTACGGATGTCAACG-3′

Mechanical testing

The femora from the mice were wrapped in medical gauze saturated with normal saline and stored at 4°C for use the next day. Before testing, the samples were brought to room temperature for 1 hour. The three-point bending test of the left femur was carried out using an Instron 5569 materials testing machine (Instron Inc., Norwood, MA, USA). The femur was placed posterior side down between two supports, which were 6 mm apart. A load was applied at the mid-span, which bent the bone about the anteroposterior axis. Load-displacement curves were recorded at a crosshead speed of 1 mm/s.

Imaging of femoral blood vessels

Specimens were prepared as previously reported [33]. Briefly, after the mice were euthanized, the thoracic cavity was opened, and the inferior vena cava was dissected and flushed with 0.9% normal saline containing heparin sodium (100 U/ml) to remove the blood from the vessels. Afterwards, the vasculature was perfused with 10% neutral buffered formalin. The vasculature was then injected with 5 ml of silicone rubber compound. Sufficient perfusion was defined as a yellow color change in the lower limbs and liver. The specimens were stored at 4°C overnight, after which the femora were dissected and fixed in 4% paraformaldehyde for an additional 48 hours. The femora were then decalcified in 10% EDTA for four weeks. Images were obtained with a high-resolution (isotropic voxel size of 16 μm) micro-CT imaging system. A threshold of 100 was chosen, and the vessel volume within a region of 5 mm beginning from the distal end of the femur was evaluated.

Histological preparation and tartrate-resistant acid phosphatase staining

The specimens were decalcified in 10% EDTA for four weeks, and the EDTA solution was changed twice a week. The bones were then dehydrated in a graded series of ethanol washes from 70%–100% before embedding the samples in paraffin. Five-micron-thick longitudinal serial sections were cut and mounted on poly-lysine-coated slides. The deparaffinized slides were washed with PBS three times. The slides were then incubated at 37°C for 60 min in the dark in a solution containing sodium nitrite, fast garnet, naphthol AS-BI phosphoric acid, acetate, and tartrate from the Leukocyte Acid Phosphatase Assay kit, according to the manufacturer's instructions. Finally, the nuclei were counterstained with methyl green. Multinucleated cells with three or more nuclei were scored as osteoclasts. The average number of osteoclasts per mm of bone surface was then calculated for each femur.

Fluorochrome labeling and bone histomorphometry

A double tetracycline (25 mg/kg) label was injected subcutaneously at 10 and 3 days before necropsy. At necropsy, the femora were cleaned of soft tissue and fixed in 70% ethanol. The bones were dehydrated and embedded in methyl methacrylate. Thin frontal sections of the femur (5μm) were cut using a microtome (Leica RM2255). Bone histomorphometric parameters were determined according to the report of the American Society of Bone and Mineral Research Nomenclature Committee [56]. Histomorphometric measurements included single-labeled surface (sLS), double-labeled surface (dLS), and interlabel thickness (IrLTh). These data were used to calculate the mineralizing surface/bone surface ratio (MS/BS), mineral apposition rate (MAR), and bone formation rate (BFR) as follows: MS/BS = (1/2sLS+dLS)/BS(%), MAR = Ir.L.Th/Ir.L.t, and BFR/BS = MAR×MS/BS (m^3/m^2/day).

Enzyme-linked immunosorbent assay

Blood from the mice was collected, and the serum was separated by centrifugation at 3000 rpm for 30 min. Serum VEGF, osteocalcin, and CTX levels were measured by ELISA, following the manufacturers' protocols.

Statistical analysis

The results were expressed as the mean ± SD. All experimental data were analyzed with one-way analysis of variance (ANOVA) followed by Duncan's test. $P<0.05$ was considered statistically significant.

Results

Effect of 17β-estradiol and DMOG on the HIF-1α signaling pathway

Consistent with previous reports, our western blot analysis showed that 17β-estradiol stabilized HIF-1α under normal oxygen tension (Fig. 1A). Furthermore, 17β-estradiol increased the expression of VEGF protein (control vs. $10^{-9}E_2$ $P = 0.001 < 0.05$, control vs. $10^{-7}E_2$ $P = 0.000 < 0.05$, control vs. $10^{-5}E_2$ $P = 0.000 < 0.05$), the main downstream angiogenic target of the HIF-1α pathway, in a dose-dependent manner (Fig. 1B). Similarly, DMOG enhanced HIF-1α protein expression under normal

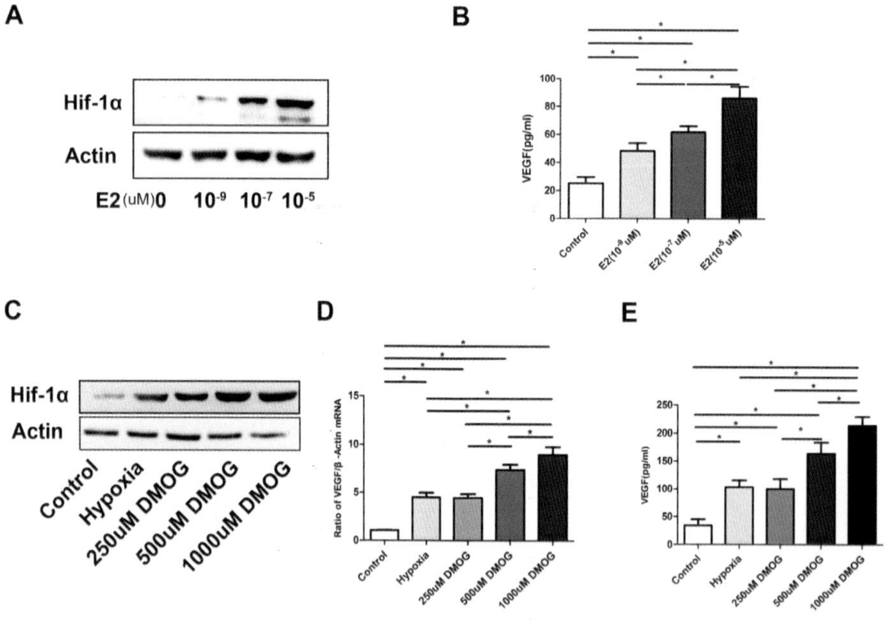

Figure 1. Effect of 17β-estradiol and DMOG on HIF-1α signaling pathway. (A) 17β-estradiol stabilized HIF-1α under normal oxygen pressure. (B) 17β-estradiol upregulated VEGF protein expression. (C) DMOG enhanced HIF-1α protein expression. (D–E) DMOG upregulated VEGF expression at the mRNA and protein levels. $P<0.05$ for comparisons among the groups designated with an asterisk.

oxygen tension and upregulated VEGF expression at the mRNA and protein levels (Fig. 1C–E).

Effect of DMOG on MSC osteogenic differentiation and the Wnt/β-catenin signaling pathway

ALP and ARS staining showed that DMOG treatment enhanced osteogenic differentiation and calcium deposition (Fig. 2A). Consistent with osteogenesis, RUNX-2 and osterix mRNA levels were increased (RUNX-2 $P = 0.000<0.05$, osterix $P = 0.000<0.05$) (Fig. 2B). Investigation into the underlying mechanism revealed that DMOG upregulated the levels of β-catenin mRNA and protein ($P = 0.000<0.05$) (Fig. 2C). To determine whether the effect of DMOG on Wnt/β-catenin signaling was mediated by HIF-1α signaling, we treated MSCs withYC-1, a widely used HIF-1α inhibitor, along with DMOG and assessed the nuclear expression of β-catenin and the downstream effectors LEF-1 and TCF-1. DMOG stimulated HIF-1α protein expression, and YC-1 inhibited the effect of DMOG on HIF-1α. Furthermore, YC-1 attenuated the DMOG-induced increase in nuclear β-catenin, LEF-1, and TCF-1 protein expression (Fig. 2D).

Confirmation of the OVX model

OVX increased body weight by approximately 6% when compared to sham treatment (Sham vs. OVX $P = 0.049<0.05$). However, DMOG treatment did not affect the OVX-induced body weight gain (OVX+L-DMOG vs. OVX $P=0.868>0.05$, OVX+H-DMOG vs. OVX $P=1.000>0.05$) (Fig. S1A). The efficacy of OVX was confirmed by changes in uterine and BMD. The average uterine weights in each group were 0.11137±0.0120 g (sham), 0.0319±0.0079 g (OVX), 0.0337±0.079 g (OVX+L-DMOG), and 0.0326±0.0078 g (OVX+H-DMOG) ($P<0.0001$) (Fig. S1B,C). Before ovariectomy, the BMD of mice was 365.41±18.43 mg/cm^3, and OVX made the BMD of mice decrease to 281.26±29.61 mg/cm^3 ($P<0.0001$) (Fig. S1D).

The effect of DMOG on BMD, bone microarchitecture, and vessels

To characterize the effects of treatment on the trabecular bone compartments, the distal metaphysic of the femoral bone was evaluated with micro-CT imaging (Table. 2). With regard to trabecular bone alterations, OVX mice showed remarkable reductions in BMD, BV/TV, Tb.N, and Tb.Th, as well as increased Tb.Sp (OVX vs. Sham: BMD $P=0.000<0.05$, BV/TV $P=0.000<0.05$, Tb.N $P=0.000<0.05$, Tb.Th $P=0.005<0.05$, Tb.Sp $P=0.000<0.05$). DMOG treatment, especially at high doses, improved the trabecular microarchitecture and increased BMD (OVX vs. OVX+L-DMOG: BMD $P=0.025<0.05$, BV/TV $P=0.184>0.05$, Tb.N $P=0.019<0.05$, Tb.Th $P=0.94>0.05$, Tb.Sp $P=0.191>0.05$; OVX vs. OVX+H-DMOG: BMD $P=0.000<0.05$, BV/TV $P=0.000<0.05$, Tb.N $P=0.000<0.05$, Tb.Th $P=0.047<0.05$, Tb.Sp $P=0.016<0.05$) (Fig. 3A). Microfil-perfused femora were analyzed with micro-CT to assess vascularity. The number of blood vessels in the femur was lower 4 weeks after OVX ($P=0.000<0.05$). However, DMOG treatment led to a dose-dependent increase in femur vessel volume relative to that in the OVX group (OVX vs. OVX+L-DMOG $P=0.045<0.05$, OVX vs. OVX+H-DMOG $P=0.000<0.05$), although differences among the DMOG-treated groups and the sham group were evident (Sham vs. OVX+L-DMOG $P=0.000<0.05$, Sham vs. OVX+H-DMOG $P=0.009<0.05$) (Fig. 3B).

Bone mechanical strength examination

The three-point bending test was used to evaluate bone strength (Table. 3). The femurs of the OVX mice exhibited decreases in ultimate stress, ultimate load, energy to failure, and modulus, all of which reflected a decline in bone strength following OVX (Sham vs. OVX: ultimate stress $P=0.000<0.05$, ultimate load $P=0.000<0.05$, energy to failure $P=0.000<0.05$, modulus $P=0.000<0.05$). DMOG treatment improved ultimate stress, ultimate load, energy to failure, and modulus (OVX vs. OVX+L-DMOG: ultimate stress $P=0.010<0.05$, ultimate load

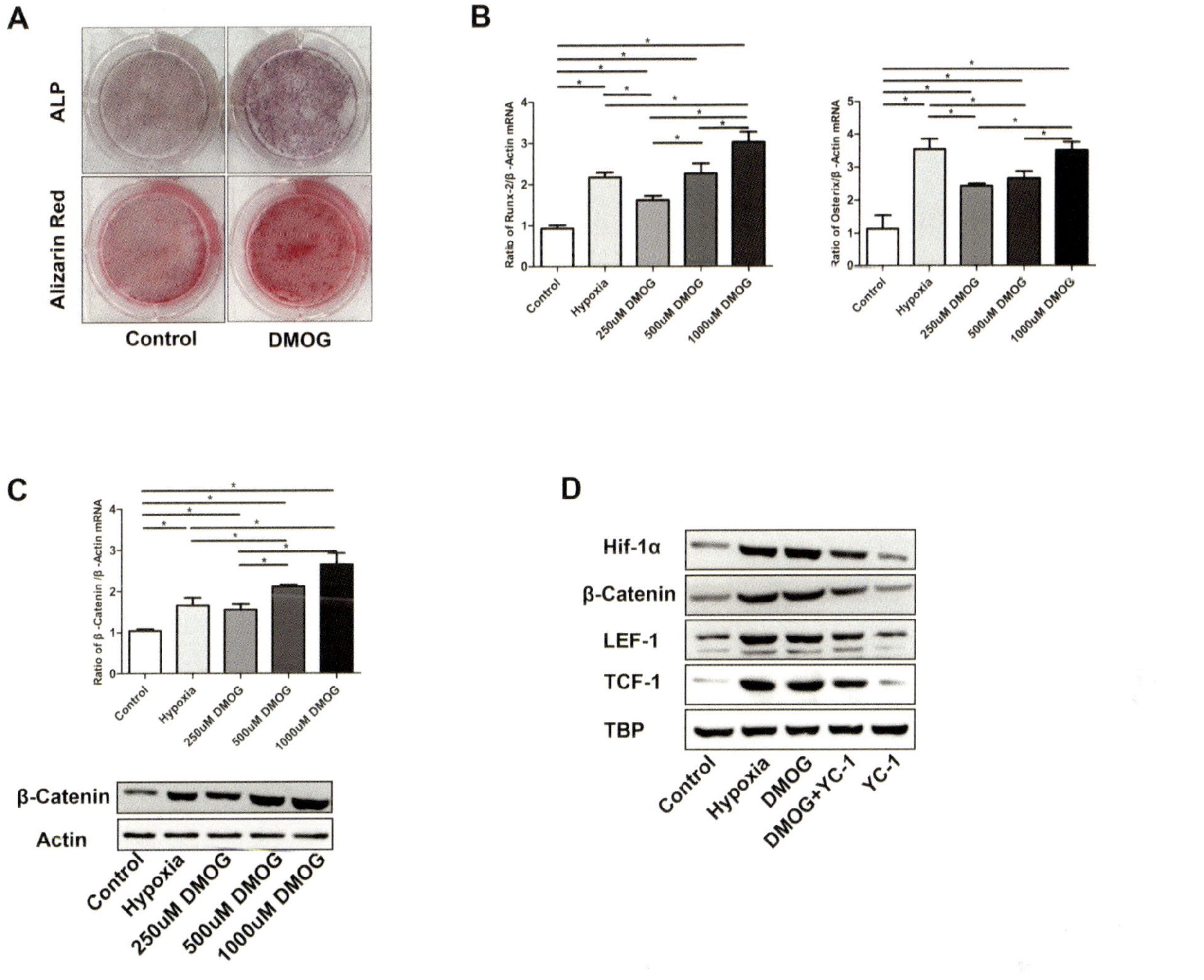

Figure 2. Effect of DMOG on MSC osteogenic differentiation and Wnt/β-catenin signaling. (A) ALP and alizarin red S staining. (B) DMOG promoted RUNX-2 and osterix mRNA expression. (C) DMOG increased β-catenin mRNA and protein expression. (D) DMOG increased nuclear β-catenin, LEF-1, TCF-1, and HIF-1α protein expression. These effects were attenuated by YC-1. $P<0.05$ for comparisons among the groups designated with an asterisk.

$P=0.005<0.05$, energy to failure $P=0.024<0.05$, modulus $P=0.051>0.05$; OVX vs. OVX+H-DMOG ultimate stress $P=0.000<0.05$, ultimate load $P=0.000<0.05$, energy to failure $P=0.001<0.05$, modulus $P=0.009<0.05$).

Serum VEGF, osteocalcin, and CTX levels

The serum level of VEGF, the main angiogenic cytokine upregulated by HIF-1α, was markedly reduced in OVX mice ($P=0.000<0.05$), and DMOG treatment improved VEGF levels in a dose-dependent manner (OVX vs. OVX+L-DMOG $P=0.003<0.05$, OVX vs. OVX+H-DMOG $P=0.000<0.05$).

Table 2. Micro-CT analysis of trabecular BMD, bone microarchitecture and vasculature in the distal femur.

	Sham	OVX	OVX+L-DMOG	OVX+H-DMOG
BMD(mg/cm^3)	379.69±24.61#	284.46±17.49*	309.10±19.03*#	335.62±30.94*#
BV/TV(%)	0.1331±0.0061#	0.0947±0.0139*	0.1013±0.0105*	0.1143±0.0119*#
Tb.N(1/mm)	3.7268±0.2478#	2.5724±0.4024*	2.9317±0.2273*#	3.3250±0.3884*#
Tb.Th(um)	0.0345±0.0013#	0.0322±0.0014*	0.0323±0.0109*	0.0339±0.0025#
Tb.Sp(um)	0.2351±0.0211#	0.3033±0.0379*	0.2854±0.0183*	0.2693±0.0371*#
Vessel volume(mm^3)	0.4441±0.0396#	0.2189±0.0419*	0.2766±0.0243*#	0.3529±0.0315*#

The groups designated with an asterisk shown significant differences with Sham group ($P<0.05$), the groups designated with a pound sign shown significant differences with OVX group ($P<0.05$).

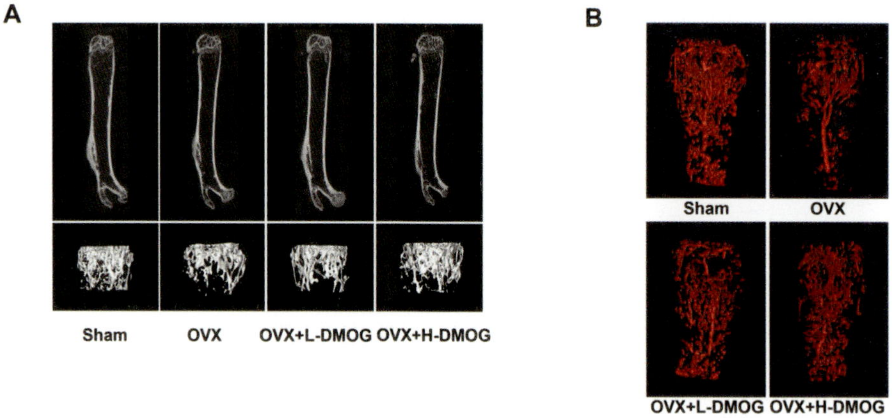

Figure 3. BMD and bone microarchitecture of the trabecular bone in the distal femur. (A) DMOG abrogated the decrease in BMD and the deterioration in bone microarchitecture induced by OVX, as measured by micro-CT. **Morphological analysis of the vasculature within the distal femur from Microfil-perfused mice.** (B) OVX decreased the vessel volume at the distal metaphysic of the femur, while DMOG treatment partly restored vessel volumes.

Serum osteocalcin, a marker for bone formation, was higher in OVX mice than in sham mice, but the difference was not significant ($P = 0.053 > 0.05$). The osteocalcin levels in the DMOG-treated group were significantly higher than those in the OVX group (OVX vs. OVX+L-DMOG $P = 0.008 < 0.05$, OVX vs. OVX+H-DMOG $P = 0.000 < 0.05$). Serum CTX, a marker of bone resorption, was approximately two-fold higher in OVX mice than in sham mice ($P = 0.000 < 0.05$), while DMOG treatment did not affect serum CTX levels (OVX vs. OVX+L-DMOG $P = 0.714 > 0.05$, OVX vs. OVX+H-DMOG $P = 0.770 > 0.05$). All the data were listed in Table 4.

Osteoclast number

Consistent with the results of the serum CTX analysis, the TRAP assay revealed a striking increase in osteoclast number following OVX (5.200±0.836 and 13.200±1.303 in the sham group and OVX group, respectively ($P = 0.000 < 0.05$)). DMOG administration did not noticeably prevent OVX-induced osteoclast formation (12.800±1.643 in the OVX+L-DMOG group and 12.600±2.673 in OVX+H-DMOG group; OVX+L-DMOG vs. the OVX group $P = 1.000 > 0.05$, OVX+H-DMOG vs. the OVX group $P = 0.637 > 0.05$) (Fig. 4A).

Dynamic bone histomorphometry

The dynamic histology of the trabecular bone in the distal femur was compared among the various groups. OVX resulted in significant increases in MS/BS and BFR/BS (Sham vs. OVX: MS/BS $P = 0.000 < 0.05$, BFR/BS $P = 0.004 < 0.05$) and increased MAR though without statistical difference ($P = 0.057 > 0.05$). H-DMOG treatment further increased MS/BS, MAR, and BFR/BS compared with OVX group (MS/BS $P = 0.000 < 0.05$, MAR $P = 0.001 < 0.05$, BFR/BS $P = 0.000 < 0.05$); and L-DMOG administration increased MAR and BFR/BS (MAR $P = 0.035 < 0.05$, BFR/BS $P = 0.000 < 0.05$) but not MS/BS ($P = 0.061 > 0.05$) compared to OVX group (Fig. 4B).

Alterations in HIF-1α and Wnt/β-catenin signaling in DMOG-treated mice

To illustrate the enhanced angiogenesis and osteogenesis in DMOG-treated mice, we used western blot to detect alterations in HIF-1α and Wnt/β-catenin signaling pathways in collected bone samples (Fig. 5A). As previously highlighted, OVX substantially reduced HIF-1α expression; the reduction in HIF-1α was accompanied by a decrease in VEGF expression. However, in the DMOG-treated group, the expression of HIF-1α and VEGF increased significantly. Moreover, DMOG administration enhanced β-catenin expression relative to expression in the OVX group.

Bone formation and bone resorption markers in DMOG-treated mice

Real-time PCR results for ALP, osteocalcin, RUNX-2, RANKL, OPG, and β-actin expression in each group are shown in Fig. 5B. OVX increased ALP, osteocalcin, and RUNX-2 mRNA levels over those in the sham group, but the difference was not statistically significant (ALP $P = 0.262 > 0.05$, osteocalcin

Table 3. Bone quality of the femur as measured by the three-point bending test.

	Sham	OVX	OVX+L-DMOG	OVX+H-DMOG
Ultimate load(N)	15.31±0.85#	11.85±0.30*	13.14±0.42*#	14.11±0.37*#
Ultimate stress(Mpa)	99.41±7.10#	69.56±4.88*	80.98±5.59*#	90.13±2.37*#
Energy to failure(MJ)	8.69±0.50#	6.75±0.24*	7.39±0.30*#	7.92±0.31*#
Modulus(Mpa)	4162.65±377.13#	2910.93±355.07*	3407.78±291.51*	3624.83±255.12*#

The groups designated with an asterisk shown significant differences with Sham group (*P*<*0.05*), the groups designated with a pound sign shown significant differences with OVX group (*P*<*0.05*).

Table 4. Biochemical markers of bone in serum as measured by ELISA.

	Sham	OVX	OVX+L-DMOG	OVX+H-DMOG
VEGF(pg/ml)	116.37±6.21#	82.37±8.90*	93.13±5.51*#	100.75±5.31*#
Osteoclacin(ng/ml)	68.33±14.22	80.80±18.87	98.32±9.95*#	107.60±10.91*#
CTX(ng/ml)	16.21±1.61	28.01±1.95*	28.46±4.35*	27.65±2.10*

The groups designated with an asterisk shown significant differences with Sham group (*P<0.05*), the groups designated with a pound sign shown significant differences with OVX group (*P<0.05*).

$P = 0.089 > 0.05$, RUNX-2 $P = 0.346 > 0.05$). The osteocalcin mRNA level was higher in the DMOG-treated OVX groups than in the OVX groups (OVX vs. OVX+L-DMOG $P = 0.030 < 0.05$, OVX vs. OVX+H-DMOG $P = 0.000 < 0.05$), and ALP and RUNX-2 mRNA levels were markedly higher in the H-DMOG treated group than in the OVX group (ALP $P = 0.001 < 0.05$, RUNX-2 $P = 0.004 < 0.05$). In OVX mice, RANKL/OPG expression was markedly increased when compared with expression in the sham group ($P = 0.006 < 0.05$). However, DMOG administration did not significantly attenuate the OVX-induced increase in RANKL/OPG expression (OVX vs. OVX+L-DMOG $P = 0.733 > 0.05$, OVX vs. OVX+H-DMOG $P = 0.984 > 0.05$).

Discussion

In the present study, DMOG improved angiogenesis and osteogenesis *in vitro*. The effects were attributed to activation of the HIF-1α and Wnt/β-catenin signaling pathways, respectively. We investigated whether DMOG ameliorated OVX-induced osteoporosis in mice. Our results showed that DMOG improved BMD, trabecular microarchitecture, and bone strength in OVX mice. In addition, DMOG treatment partly restored the blood

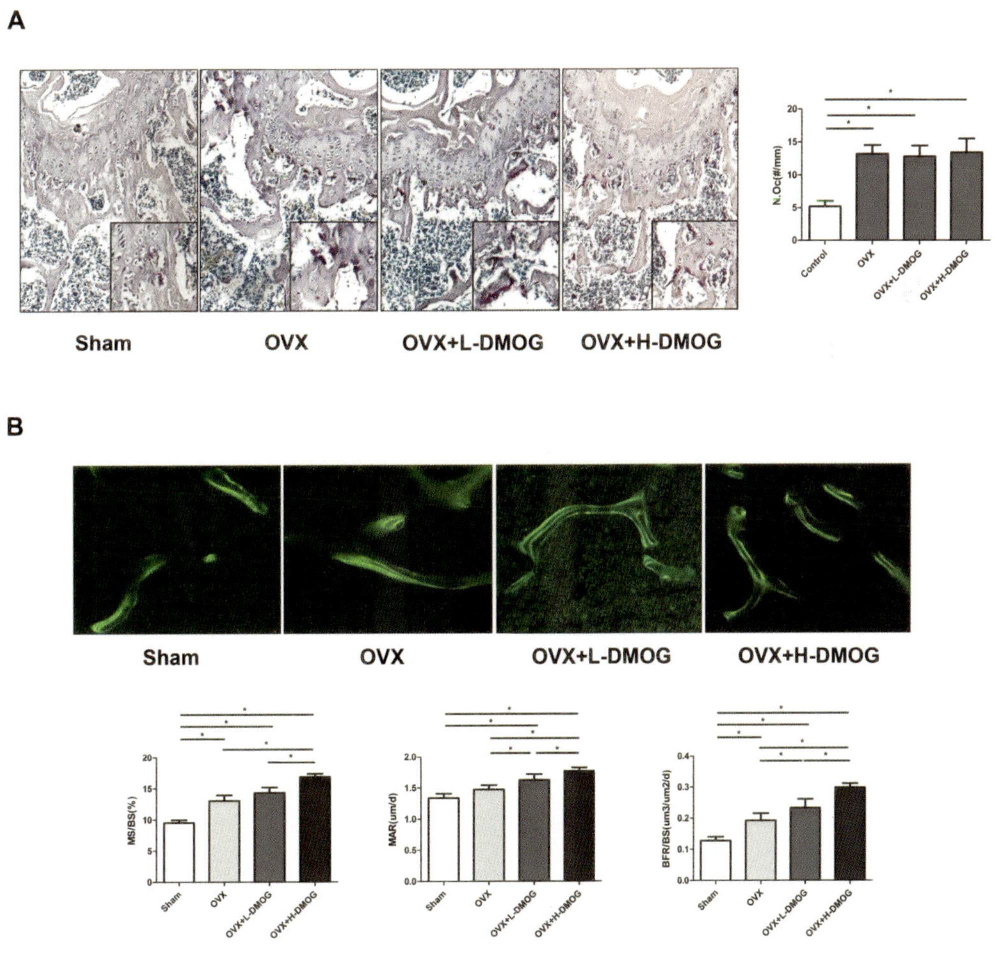

Figure 4. Osteoclast numbers assayed by tartrate-resistant acid phosphatase staining of femoral sections. (A)Osteoclast counting results showed that DMOG treatment had no obvious effect on OVX-enhanced osteoclast formation. Original magnification, ×100. **Dynamic bone formation illustrated by double tetracycline labeling.** (B) DMOG administration promoted bone formation, as evidenced by improved MS/BS, MAR, and BFR/BS. Original magnification, ×200. $P<0.05$ for comparisons among the groups designated with an asterisk.

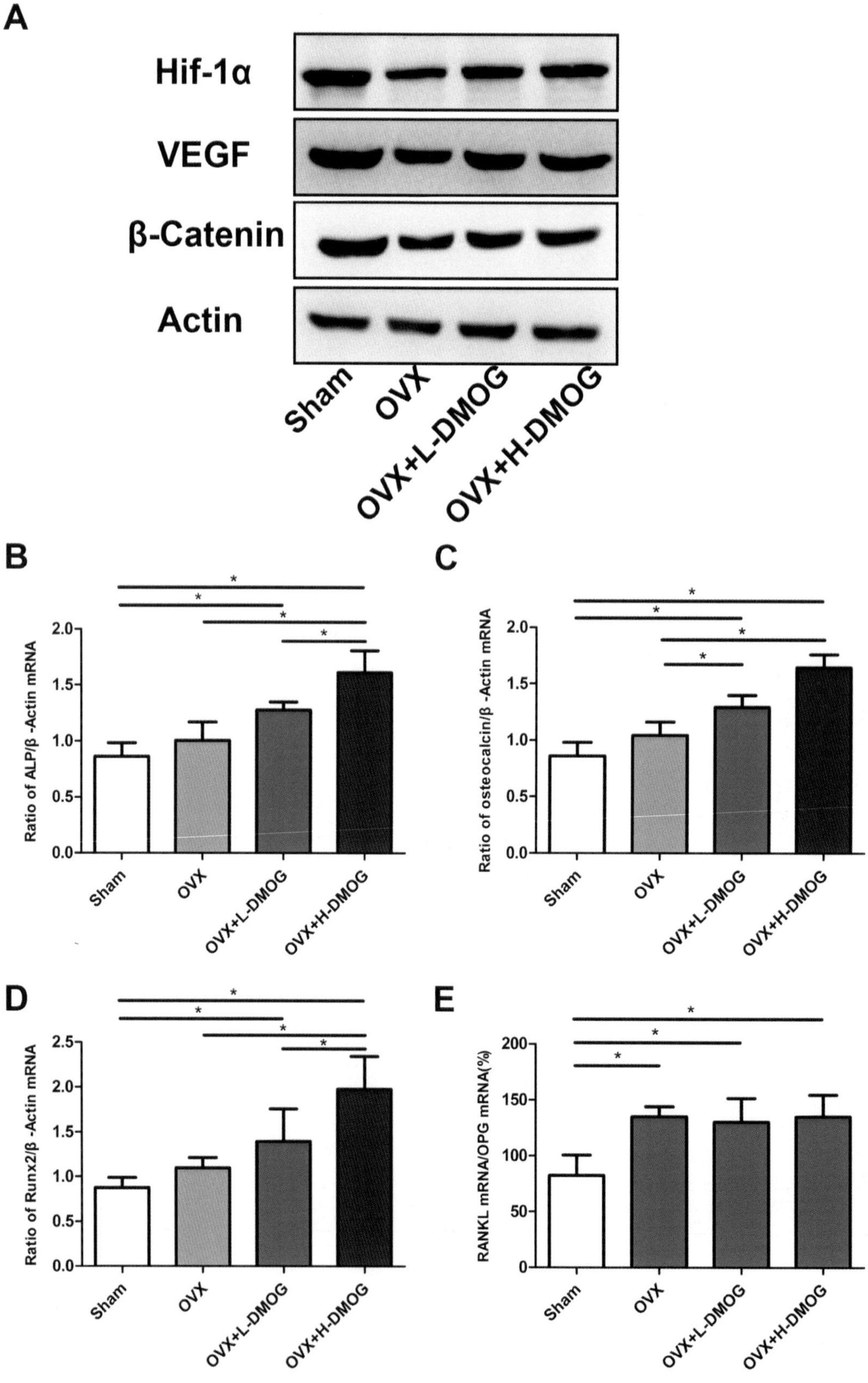

Figure 5. HIF-1α, VEGF, and β-catenin expression in bone samples detected by western blot. (A) HIF-1α, VEGF, and β-catenin expression was lower in OVX mice than in sham mice. However, DMOG treatment increased HIF-1α, VEGF, and β-catenin expression relative to expression in the OVX group. **Effects of DMOG administration on tibial ALP, osteocalcin, RUNX-2, and RANKL/OPG mRNA expression in OVX mice assessed by real-time PCR.** (B) ALP/β-actin ratio. (C) Osteocalcin/β-actin ratio. (D) RUNX-2/β-actin ratio. (E) RANKL/OPG/β-actin ratio. $P<0.05$ for comparisons among the groups designated with an asterisk.

vessels of OVX mice. Enhanced osteogenesis might underlie these improvements, as indicated by the acceleration in MS/BS, BFR/BS, and MAR; the increase in serum osteocalcin; and the upregulation of tibial ALP, osteocalcin, and RUNX-2 mRNA. In addition, significant remediation of angiogenesis resulting from increases in VEGF also led to improved bone health in OVX mice.

Stimuli other than hypoxia also cause HIF-1α to accumulate in normoxic cells. For example, growth factors such as insulin-like growth factor can induce HIF-1α synthesis through activation of the PI3 K/Akt/mTOR signal transduction pathway [57,58]. Here, we found that 17β-estradiol stabilized HIF-1α under normal oxygen tension and increased VEGF protein expression, consistent with previous reports [34,35]. This phenomenon explains our previous finding that OVX decreased HIF-1α and VEGF expression in osteoblasts [33]. Impaired regulation of HIF-1α is also observed in other pathological processes, such as the development of diabetic wounds, and stabilization of HIF-1α is pivotal for reversing these pathological processes [59]. Mice in which HIF-1α signaling was activated developed extremely dense, heavily vascularized bones, and these mice were protected from OVX or age-induced bone loss [19,33]. More importantly, age-related bone loss has been prevented by administration of DFO, a hypoxia-mimicking agent [45]. Therefore, stabilization of HIF-1α by a hypoxia-mimicking agent might also help prevent estrogen deficiency-induced bone loss. Another widely used hypoxia-mimicking agent, DMOG, modulated VEGF mRNA and protein levels, which were mainly associated with activated HIF-1α under normal oxygen pressure [14,16,20].

In addition to its angiogenic effects, DMOG also has potent osteogenic effects. Enhanced osteogenic differentiation of DMOG-treated MSCs was demonstrated by ALP staining and calcium deposition, which are early and late stage osteogenic markers, respectively. To characterize the underlying molecular mechanism, alterations in the mRNA levels of RUNX-2 and osterix, essential transcription factors for the differentiation of osteoblasts from MSCs [60], were assessed. Our results and those of two recent studies indicate that DMOG upregulates RUNX-2 and osterix mRNA expression [21,30]. These results were supported by the finding that osteogenesis was enhanced in MSCs expressing a constitutively active form of HIF-1α [24,25,39]. Osteoblastic differentiation is predominantly regulated by the Wnt/β-catenin signaling pathway. Wnt binds to Frizzled receptors and their co-receptors, low-density lipoprotein receptor-related proteins (LRP5/6), to stabilize cytosolic β-catenin. β-Catenin then enters the nucleus and stimulates the transcription of Wnt target genes [61]. A reduction in serum β-catenin might contribute to the pathogenesis of postmenopausal osteoporosis [62]. In our studies, DMOG upregulated β-catenin mRNA and protein expression in a dose-dependent manner. Our findings are consistent with those of other groups, which showed that hypoxia and hypoxia mimetics, such as DFO, increase Wnt/β-catenin signaling in MSCs and osteoblasts [40,41]. As for the relationship between HIF-1α signaling and Wnt/β-catenin signaling, a previous study showed that HIF-1α modulated Wnt/β-catenin signaling in embryonic stem cells [36]. Our studies showed that this phenomenon occurs in MSCs. DMOG increased the expression of nuclear β-catenin and the downstream effectors LEF-1 and TCF-1. The effects were abrogated by the HIF-1α signaling inhibitor YC-1 [63–66]. These results suggest that the effect of DMOG on Wnt/β-catenin signaling is mediated by HIF-1α signaling.

In view of the dual role of DMOG in angiogenesis and osteogenesis, we hypothesized that DMOG would attenuate bone loss in OVX mice. As expected, DMOG administration increased the BMD of the trabecular bone. In addition to the BMD, the bone microarchitecture is a critical factor commonly associated with bone quality. Our results showed that BV/TV, Tb.N, Tb.Th, and Tb.Sp, the four fundamental indices of trabecular architecture as determined by the American Society for Bone and Mineral Research, were partly restored to differing extents by DMOG treatment, especially in the H-DMOG-treated group [67]. Because both bone mineral density and microarchitecture, two important factors that determine bone quality, improved significantly, we tested bone strength using the three-point bending test, which showed that DMOG treatment partly rescued the decline in bone mechanical strength due to OVX. These findings strongly suggest that DMOG prevents bone loss and improves bone quality in OVX mice.

Given that angiogenesis and osteogenesis are closely coupled, multiple studies have investigated the role of angiogenesis in the pathogenesis of osteoporosis. Accumulating evidence from studies in cells, animals, and patients indicates that low estrogen levels contribute to fewer vessels or decreases in angiogenic factors, resulting in the progression of osteoporosis [4–11]. Our current study supports this idea. OVX decreased the femoral vessel volumes of OVX mice, but femoral vessel volumes were partly restored in the DMOG-treated groups. The alteration in bone vessel volumes was in accordance with that of bone parameters. Furthermore, the restoration of bone vessel volume was coincident with the increased expression of HIF-1α and VEGF in bone samples. VEGF, the best known and most critical angiogenic factor, induces vessel formation and regulates the balance between osteogenic and adipogenic differentiation in MSCs. Mice with VEGF deficiency in osteoblastic precursor cells exhibited an osteoporosis-like phenotype characterized by reduced bone mass and increased bone marrow fat content [68]. Hence, normalization of low VEGF levels in postmenopausal women might be of critical significance.

Compared with antiresorptive drugs, which excessively reduce bone turnover and result in inadequate microdamage repair, drugs targeted towards impaired bone formation might be better suited to the rehabilitation of osteoporotic bone [69]. Our *in vivo* data, including serum osteocalcin, real-time PCR, and dynamic bone histomorphometry results, indicated that DMOG administration further increased osteogenesis in OVX mice [60]. These results are consistent with findings that inactivation of *Vhl* in osteochondral progenitor cells or osteoprogenitor cells increases the proliferation and differentiation of osteoblast lineage cells *in vivo* [18,19]. Furthermore, the expression of osteoprogenitor and osteoblast markers, including osterix, bone γ-carboxyglutamate protein, and integrin-binding sialoprotein, increased in the long bone of DFO-treated aged mice [45]. The enhanced differentiation of osteoblasts was probably attributed to elevated β-catenin protein expression, which was confirmed by westernblot. In addition to the regulation of the Wnt/β-catenin pathway by HIF-1α signaling, demonstrated *in vitro* in this study, the increased level of VEGF might be another pivotal factor for β-catenin accumulation [70]. Although it has been suggested that activation of the Wnt/β-catenin pathway decreases bone resorption, we did not detect a significant alteration in bone resorption following DMOG treatment, as shown by the serum CTX levels and the osteoclast numbers in the femur [71,72].

There were several limitations to this study: 1) the BMD and microarchitecture of the lumbar vertebra were not assessed; 2) it would be better if the treatment lasts longer time.

Conclusions

The results of present study demonstrate that DMOG treatment prevents bone loss, rescues bone microarchitecture deterioration, and restores bone strength in OVX mice. The effects might result from enhanced angiogenesis and osteogenesis. Following DMOG administration, new vessel formation, induced by angiogenic factors, would supply the bone with oxygen, nutrients, and a variety of cells, especially MSCs. Activation of the Wnt/β-catenin signaling pathway would enhance the osteogenic differentiation of MSCs and promote bone formation. To the best of our knowledge, this is the first report to describe the use and dual role of DMOG in the treatment of OVX-induced osteoporosis. DMOG may be a new strategy for the treatment of postmenopausal osteoporosis.

Supporting Information

Figure S1 Body weight, uterus weight, representative picture of uterus in each group and BMD alterations before and after OVX. (A) OVX significantly increased body weight of mice in OVX, OVX+L-DMOG and OVX+H-DMOG groups compared to Sham group. (B) OVX significantly decreased the uterus weight. (C) Representative picture of uterus in each group. (D) OVX obviously decreased the BMD of mice. $P<0.05$ for comparisons among the groups designated with an asterisk.

Acknowledgments

This work was supported by the Natural Science Foundation of China (No. 81371958, 81061160510), the Basic Key Project of Science and Technology Commission of Shanghai Municipality (12JC1408200), and the Scientific and Technological Support Program in Biological Medicine of Science and Technology Commission of Shanghai Municipality (13431900702).

Author Contributions

Conceived and designed the experiments: JP ZGL DLF. Performed the experiments: JP ZGL ZLF KH CH SX QJ ZQ WJS QND ZHB. Analyzed the data: JP DLF. Contributed reagents/materials/analysis tools: QND WJS. Contributed to the writing of the manuscript: JP DLF ZGL.

References

1. Kanis JA (1994) Assessment of fracture risk and its application to screening for postmenopausal osteoporosis: synopsis of a WHO report. WHO Study Group. Osteoporos Int 4: 368–381.
2. Qu B, Ma Y, Yan M, Wu HH, Fan L, et al. (2014) The economic burden of fracture patients with osteoporosis in western China. Osteoporos Int. 25: 1853–1860.
3. Brandi ML, Collin-Osdoby P (2006) Vascular biology and the skeleton. J Bone Miner Res 21: 183–192.
4. Mekraldi S, Lafage-Proust MH, Bloomfield S, Alexandre C, Vico L (2003) Changes in vasoactive factors associated with altered vessel morphology in the tibial metaphysis during ovariectomy-induced bone loss in rats. Bone 32: 630–641.
5. Ding WG, Wei ZX, Liu JB (2011) Reduced local blood supply to the tibial metaphysis is associated with ovariectomy-induced osteoporosis in mice. Connect Tissue Res 52: 25–29.
6. Vogt MT, Cauley JA, Kuller LH, Nevitt MC (1997) Bone mineral density and blood flow to the lower extremities: the study of osteoporotic fractures. J Bone Miner Res 12: 283–289.
7. Griffith JF, Wang YX, Zhou H, Kwong WH, Wong WT, et al. (2010) Reduced bone perfusion in osteoporosis: likely causes in an ovariectomy rat model. Radiology 254: 739–746.
8. Shih TT, Liu HC, Chang CJ, Wei SY, Shen LC, et al. (2004) Correlation of MR lumbar spine bone marrow perfusion with bone mineral density in female subjects. Radiology 233: 121–128.
9. Senel K, Baykal T, Seferoglu B, Altas EU, Baygutalp F, et al. (2013) Circulating vascular endothelial growth factor concentrations in patients with postmenopausal osteoporosis. Arch Med Sci 9: 709–712.
10. Mueller MD, Vigne JL, Minchenko A, Lebovic DI, Leitman DC, et al. (2000) Regulation of vascular endothelial growth factor (VEGF) gene transcription by estrogen receptors alpha and beta. Proc Natl Acad Sci U S A 97: 10972–10977.
11. Pufe T, Claassen H, Scholz-Ahrens KE, Varoga D, Drescher W, et al. (2007) Influence of estradiol on vascular endothelial growth factor expression in bone: a study in Gottingen miniature pigs and human osteoblasts. Calcif Tissue Int 80: 184–191.
12. Min JH, Yang H, Ivan M, Gertler F, Kaelin WG Jr, et al. (2002) Structure of an HIF-1alpha -pVHL complex: hydroxyproline recognition in signaling. Science 296: 1886–1889.
13. Maxwell PH, Wiesener MS, Chang GW, Clifford SC, Vaux EC, et al. (1999) The tumour suppressor protein VHL targets hypoxia-inducible factors for oxygen-dependent proteolysis. Nature 399: 271–275.
14. Jaakkola P, Mole DR, Tian YM, Wilson MI, Gielbert J, et al. (2001) Targeting of HIF-alpha to the von Hippel-Lindau ubiquitylation complex by O2-regulated prolyl hydroxylation. Science 292: 468–472.
15. Ohh M, Park CW, Ivan M, Hoffman MA, Kim TY, et al. (2000) Ubiquitination of hypoxia-inducible factor requires direct binding to the beta-domain of the von Hippel-Lindau protein. Nat Cell Biol 2: 423–427.
16. Shen X, Wan C, Ramaswamy G, Mavalli M, Wang Y, et al. (2009) Prolyl hydroxylase inhibitors increase neoangiogenesis and callus formation following femur fracture in mice. J Orthop Res 27: 1298–1305.
17. Wang Y, Wan C, Deng L, Liu X, Cao X, et al. (2007) The hypoxia-inducible factor alpha pathway couples angiogenesis to osteogenesis during skeletal development. J Clin Invest 117: 1616–1626.
18. Rankin EB, Wu C, Khatri R, Wilson TL, Andersen R, et al. (2012) The HIF signaling pathway in osteoblasts directly modulates erythropoiesis through the production of EPO. Cell 149: 63–74.
19. Weng T, Xie Y, Huang J, Luo F, Yi L, et al. (2014) Inactivation of Vhl in osteochondral progenitor cells causes high bone mass phenotype and protects against age-related bone loss in adult mice. J Bone Miner Res 29: 820–829.
20. Wan C, Gilbert SR, Wang Y, Cao X, Shen X, et al. (2008) Activation of the hypoxia-inducible factor-1alpha pathway accelerates bone regeneration. Proc Natl Acad Sci U S A 105: 686–691.
21. Wu C, Zhou Y, Chang J, Xiao Y (2013) Delivery of dimethyloxallyl glycine in mesoporous bioactive glass scaffolds to improve angiogenesis and osteogenesis of human bone marrow stromal cells. Acta Biomater 9: 9159–9168.
22. Fan W, Crawford R, Xiao Y (2010) Enhancing in vivo vascularized bone formation by cobalt chloride-treated bone marrow stromal cells in a tissue engineered periosteum model. Biomaterials 31: 3580–3589.
23. Wu C, Zhou Y, Fan W, Han P, Chang J, et al. (2012) Hypoxia-mimicking mesoporous bioactive glass scaffolds with controllable cobalt ion release for bone tissue engineering. Biomaterials 33: 2076–2085.
24. Zou D, Zhang Z, He J, Zhang K, Ye D, et al. (2012) Blood vessel formation in the tissue-engineered bone with the constitutively active form of HIF-1alpha mediated BMSCs. Biomaterials 33: 2097–2108.
25. Zou D, Zhang Z, He J, Zhu S, Wang S, et al. (2011) Repairing critical-sized calvarial defects with BMSCs modified by a constitutively active form of hypoxia-inducible factor-1alpha and a phosphate cement scaffold. Biomaterials 32: 9707–9718.
26. Donneys A, Weiss DM, Deshpande SS, Ahsan S, Tchanque-Fossuo CN, et al. (2013) Localized deferoxamine injection augments vascularity and improves bony union in pathologic fracture healing after radiotherapy. Bone 52: 318–325.
27. Farberg AS, Jing XL, Monson LA, Donneys A, Tchanque-Fossuo CN, et al. (2012) Deferoxamine reverses radiation induced hypovascularity during bone regeneration and repair in the murine mandible. Bone 50: 1184–1187.
28. Zhang W, Li G, Deng R, Deng L, Qiu S (2012) New bone formation in a true bone ceramic scaffold loaded with desferrioxamine in the treatment of segmental bone defect: a preliminary study. J Orthop Sci 17: 289–298.
29. Stewart R, Goldstein J, Eberhardt A, Chu GT, Gilbert S (2011) Increasing vascularity to improve healing of a segmental defect of the rat femur. J Orthop Trauma 25: 472–476.
30. Ding H, Gao YS, Wang Y, Hu C, Sun Y, et al. (2014) Dimethyloxaloylglycine Increases the Bone Healing Capacity of Adipose-Derived Stem Cells by Promoting Osteogenic Differentiation and Angiogenic Potential. Stem Cells Dev. 23: 990–1000.
31. Grewal BS, Keller B, Weinhold P, Dahners LE (2014) Evaluating effects of deferoxamine in a rat tibia critical bone defect model. J Orthop 11: 5–9.
32. Liu XD, Deng LF, Wang J, Qi J, Zhou Q, et al. (2007) [The regulation of hypoxia inducible factor-1alpha on osteoblast function in postmenopausal osteoporosis]. Zhonghua Wai Ke Za Zhi 45: 1274–1278.
33. Zhao Q, Shen X, Zhang W, Zhu G, Qi J, et al. (2012) Mice with increased angiogenesis and osteogenesis due to conditional activation of HIF pathway in osteoblasts are protected from ovariectomy induced bone loss. Bone 50: 763–770.
34. Yun SP, Lee MY, Ryu JM, Song CH, Han HJ (2009) Role of HIF-1alpha and VEGF in human mesenchymal stem cell proliferation by 17beta-estradiol: involvement of PKC, PI3K/Akt, and MAPKs. Am J Physiol Cell Physiol 296: C317–326.

35. Yen ML, Su JL, Chien CL, Tseng KW, Yang CY, et al. (2005) Diosgenin induces hypoxia-inducible factor-1 activation and angiogenesis through estrogen receptor-related phosphatidylinositol 3-kinase/Akt and p38 mitogen-activated protein kinase pathways in osteoblasts. Mol Pharmacol 68: 1061–1073.
36. Mazumdar J, O'Brien WT, Johnson RS, LaManna JC, Chavez JC, et al. (2010) O2 regulates stem cells through Wnt/beta-catenin signalling. Nat Cell Biol 12: 1007–1013.
37. Ren H, Cao Y, Zhao Q, Li J, Zhou C, et al. (2006) Proliferation and differentiation of bone marrow stromal cells under hypoxic conditions. Biochem Biophys Res Commun 347: 12–21.
38. Wagegg M, Gaber T, Lohanatha FL, Hahne M, Strehl C, et al. (2012) Hypoxia promotes osteogenesis but suppresses adipogenesis of human mesenchymal stromal cells in a hypoxia-inducible factor-1 dependent manner. PLoS One 7: e46483.
39. Zou D, Zhang Z, Ye D, Tang A, Deng L, et al. (2011) Repair of critical-sized rat calvarial defects using genetically engineered bone marrow-derived mesenchymal stem cells overexpressing hypoxia-inducible factor-1alpha. Stem Cells 29: 1380–1390.
40. Qu Z-H, Zhang X-L, Tang T-T, Dai K-R (2008) Promotion of osteogenesis through β-catenin signaling by desferrioxamine. Biochem Biophys Res Commun 370: 332–337.
41. Genetos DC, Toupadakis CA, Raheja LF, Wong A, Papanicolaou SE, et al. (2010) Hypoxia decreases sclerostin expression and increases Wnt signaling in osteoblasts. J Cell Biochem 110: 457–467.
42. Bidwell JP, Alvarez MB, Hood M Jr, Childress P (2013) Functional impairment of bone formation in the pathogenesis of osteoporosis: the bone marrow regenerative competence. Curr Osteoporos Rep 11: 117–125.
43. Li L, Yao XL, He XL, Liu XJ, Wu WC, et al. (2013) Role of mechanical strain and estrogen in modulating osteogenic differentiation of mesenchymal stem cells (MSCs) from normal and ovariectomized rats. Cell Mol Biol (Noisy-le-grand) Suppl 59: OL1889–1893.
44. Yang N, Wang G, Hu C, Shi Y, Liao L, et al. (2013) Tumor necrosis factor alpha suppresses the mesenchymal stem cell osteogenesis promoter miR-21 in estrogen deficiency-induced osteoporosis. J Bone Miner Res 28: 559–573.
45. Kusumbe AP, Ramasamy SK, Adams RH (2014) Coupling of angiogenesis and osteogenesis by a specific vessel subtype in bone. Nature 507: 323–328.
46. Jia P, Xu YJ, Zhang ZL, Li K, Li B, et al. (2012) Ferric ion could facilitate osteoclast differentiation and bone resorption through the production of reactive oxygen species. J Orthop Res 30: 1843–1852.
47. Ishii KA, Fumoto T, Iwai K, Takeshita S, Ito M, et al. (2009) Coordination of PGC-1beta and iron uptake in mitochondrial biogenesis and osteoclast activation. Nat Med 15: 259–266.
48. Zhao HX, Wang XL, Wang YH, Wu Y, Li XY, et al. (2010) Attenuation of myocardial injury by postconditioning: role of hypoxia inducible factor-1alpha. Basic Res Cardiol 105: 109–118.
49. Song YR, You SJ, Lee YM, Chin HJ, Chae DW, et al. (2010) Activation of hypoxia-inducible factor attenuates renal injury in rat remnant kidney. Nephrol Dial Transplant 25: 77–85.
50. Takaku M, Tomita S, Kurobe H, Kihira Y, Morimoto A, et al. (2012) Systemic preconditioning by a prolyl hydroxylase inhibitor promotes prevention of skin flap necrosis via HIF-1-induced bone marrow-derived cells. PLoS One 7: e42964.
51. Botusan IR, Sunkari VG, Savu O, Catrina AI, Grunler J, et al. (2008) Stabilization of HIF-1alpha is critical to improve wound healing in diabetic mice. Proc Natl Acad Sci U S A 105: 19426–19431.
52. Rey S, Lee K, Wang CJ, Gupta K, Chen S, et al. (2009) Synergistic effect of HIF-1alpha gene therapy and HIF-1-activated bone marrow-derived angiogenic cells in a mouse model of limb ischemia. Proc Natl Acad Sci U S A 106: 20399–20404.
53. Poynter JA, Manukyan MC, Wang Y, Brewster BD, Herrmann JL, et al. (2011) Systemic pretreatment with dimethyloxalylglycine increases myocardial HIF-1alpha and VEGF production and improves functional recovery after acute ischemia/reperfusion. Surgery 150: 278–283.
54. Patel TH, Kimura H, Weiss CR, Semenza GL, Hofmann LV (2005) Constitutively active HIF-1alpha improves perfusion and arterial remodeling in an endovascular model of limb ischemia. Cardiovasc Res 68: 144–154.
55. Sun Y, Li QF, Zhang Y, Hu R, Jiang H (2013) Isoflurane preconditioning increases survival of rat skin random-pattern flaps by induction of HIF-1alpha expression. Cell Physiol Biochem 31: 579–591.
56. Dempster DW, Compston JE, Drezner MK, Glorieux FH, Kanis JA, et al. (2013) Standardized nomenclature, symbols, and units for bone histomorphometry: a 2012 update of the report of the ASBMR Histomorphometry Nomenclature Committee. J Bone Miner Res 28: 2–17.
57. Zelzer E, Levy Y, Kahana C, Shilo BZ, Rubinstein M, et al. (1998) Insulin induces transcription of target genes through the hypoxia-inducible factor HIF-1alpha/ARNT. EMBO J 17: 5085–5094.
58. Fukuda R, Hirota K, Fan F, Jung YD, Ellis LM, et al. (2002) Insulin-like growth factor 1 induces hypoxia-inducible factor 1-mediated vascular endothelial growth factor expression, which is dependent on MAP kinase and phosphatidylinositol 3-kinase signaling in colon cancer cells. J Biol Chem 277: 38205–38211.
59. Botusan IR, Sunkari VG, Savu O, Catrina AI, Grunler J, et al. (2008) Stabilization of HIF-1 is critical to improve wound healing in diabetic mice. Proceedings of the National Academy of Sciences 105: 19426–19431.
60. Long F (2012) Building strong bones: molecular regulation of the osteoblast lineage. Nat Rev Mol Cell Biol 13: 27–38.
61. Rossini M, Gatti D, Adami S (2013) Involvement of WNT/beta-catenin signaling in the treatment of osteoporosis. Calcif Tissue Int 93: 121–132.
62. Xu XJ, Shen L, Yang YP, Zhu R, Shuai B, et al. (2013) Serum beta -Catenin Levels Associated with the Ratio of RANKL/OPG in Patients with Postmenopausal Osteoporosis. Int J Endocrinol 2013: 534352.
63. Shin DH, Kim JH, Jung YJ, Kim KE, Jeong JM, et al. (2007) Preclinical evaluation of YC-1, a HIF inhibitor, for the prevention of tumor spreading. Cancer Lett 255: 107–116.
64. Liu L, Yu Q, Lin J, Lai X, Cao W, et al. (2011) Hypoxia-inducible factor-1alpha is essential for hypoxia-induced mesenchymal stem cell mobilization into the peripheral blood. Stem Cells Dev 20: 1961–1971.
65. van de Wetering M, Cavallo R, Dooijes D, van Beest M, van Es J, et al. (1997) Armadillo coactivates transcription driven by the product of the Drosophila segment polarity gene dTCF. Cell 88: 789–799.
66. Reya T, Clevers H (2005) Wnt signalling in stem cells and cancer. Nature 434: 843–850.
67. Bouxsein ML, Boyd SK, Christiansen BA, Guldberg RE, Jepsen KJ, et al. (2010) Guidelines for assessment of bone microstructure in rodents using micro-computed tomography. J Bone Miner Res 25: 1468–1486.
68. Liu Y, Berendsen AD, Jia S, Lotinun S, Baron R, et al. (2012) Intracellular VEGF regulates the balance between osteoblast and adipocyte differentiation. J Clin Invest 122: 3101–3113.
69. Chapurlat RD, Delmas PD (2009) Bone microdamage: a clinical perspective. Osteoporos Int 20: 1299–1308.
70. Maes C, Goossens S, Bartunkova S, Drogat B, Coenegrachts L, et al. (2010) Increased skeletal VEGF enhances beta-catenin activity and results in excessively ossified bones. EMBO J 29: 424–441.
71. Henriksen K, Tanko LB, Qvist P, Delmas PD, Christiansen C, et al. (2007) Assessment of osteoclast number and function: application in the development of new and improved treatment modalities for bone diseases. Osteoporos Int 18: 681–685.
72. Spencer GJ, Utting JC, Etheridge SL, Arnett TR, Genever PG (2006) Wnt signalling in osteoblasts regulates expression of the receptor activator of NFkappaB ligand and inhibits osteoclastogenesis in vitro. J Cell Sci 119: 1283–1296.

CTXA Hip—An Extension of Classical DXA Measurements Using Quantitative CT

Christopher E. Cann[1,2], Judith E. Adams[3], J. Keenan Brown[1], Alan D. Brett[1]*

1 Mindways Software, Inc., Austin, Texas, United States of America, **2** Department of Radiology, University of California San Francisco, San Francisco, California, United States of America, **3** Department of Clinical Radiology, University of Manchester, Manchester, United Kingdom

Abstract

Bone mineral density (BMD) estimates for the proximal femur using Dual Energy X-ray Absorptiometry (DXA) are currently considered the standard for making a diagnosis of osteoporosis in an individual patient using BMD alone. We have compared BMD results from a commercial Quantitative CT (QCT) BMD analysis system, "CTXA Hip", which provides clinical data for the proximal femur, to results from DXA. We have also used CTXA Hip to determine cortical and trabecular contributions to total BMD. Sixty-nine patients were scanned using 3D QCT and DXA. CTXA Hip BMD measurements for Total Hip and Femoral Neck were compared to DXA results. Twenty-two women were scanned at 0,1,2 years and CTXA Hip and DXA results analyzed for long-term reproducibility. Long-term reproducibility calculated as root-mean-square averages of SDs *in vivo* was 0.012 g/cm^2 (CV = 1.8%) for CTXA Total Hip and 0.011 g/cm^2 (CV = 2.0%) for CTXA Femoral Neck compared to 0.014 g/cm^2 (CV = 2.0%) and 0.016 g/cm^2 (CV = 2.7%), respectively, for DXA. The correlation of Total Hip BMD CTXA vs. DXA was R = 0.97 and for Femoral Neck was R = 0.95 (SEE 0.044 g/cm^2 in both cases). Cortical bone comprised 62±5% (mean ± SD) of total hipbone mass in osteoporotic women. CTXA Hip provides substantially the same clinical information as conventional DXA and in addition provides estimates of BMD in separate cortical and trabecular bone compartments, which may be useful in evaluation of bone strength.

Editor: Hani A. Awad, University of Rochester, United States of America

Funding: The authors have no support or funding to report.

Competing Interests: Christopher Cann and Keenan Brown are stockholders of Mindways Software, Inc. Alan Brett and Keenan Brown are employees of Mindways Software, Inc.

* E-mail: alan@qct.com

Introduction

Osteoporosis is a major public health concern. It is estimated that up to 50% of women and 20% of men in the US are at risk for developing an osteoporosis-related fracture during their lifetime [1]. Bone mineral density (BMD) estimates may be used to test for osteoporotic fracture risk and to make decisions about the initiation of pharmacologic therapy. According to the official positions of the International Society for Clinical Densitometry (ISCD) [2] and the National Osteoporosis Foundation (NOF) [3], central DXA of the lumbar spine and proximal femur is the preferred method for bone mineral density (BMD) testing. Osteoporosis is diagnosed by central DXA in postmenopausal women and in men aged 50 years and older if the T-score of the lumbar spine or hip is −2.5 or less. Low bone mass or osteopenia is classified as a T-score of −1.0 or less [2].

Despite the fracture risk statistics, osteoporosis testing with dual-energy X-ray absorptiometry (DXA) remains underused [4]. However, BMD can also be assessed with other radiologic imaging tools, such as quantitative computed tomography (QCT) that may be available when access to DXA is restricted.

Historically, in spite of QCT having a number of advantages over DXA [5], the use of QCT was limited by a number of factors including the cost and availability of early CT scanners, and the time required for analysis using the first QCT systems. In addition, the original implementations of 2D QCT BMD measurement at the spine tended to show lower precision due to the operator dependence of 2D scan protocols based on tilting a CT gantry, and QCT is associated with a relatively high x-ray dose compared to DXA. However, modern MDCT machines are both fast and widely available, and have allowed the introduction of 3D QCT volumetric scan protocols, reducing operator dependence and enabling CV precision errors of 0.8% [6]. Contemporary low-dose CT techniques directed at focused regions of interest and utilizing Automatic Exposure Control (AEC) can minimize radiation exposure [7].

While DXA of the spine computes an "areal BMD" (aBMD) measurement by the projection of integral (cortical and trabecular) vertebral bone onto a 2D plane, QCT provides a volumetric BMD measure of the trabecular vertebral bone in isolation. This can have an advantage of superior sensitivity due to the higher metabolic rate of turnover of trabecular bone [5]; and can also avoid the confounding effects of joint-space narrowing, osteophytes, aortic calcification and other extra-osseous calcification that can artificially raise a DXA spine BMD measurement [8–11]. However, the measurement of isolated trabecular bone means that QCT vertebral T-scores are somewhat lower than DXA T-scores for the same age [12] and application of the established WHO classification of osteoporosis by DXA T-score is not appropriate. In order to facilitate the interpretation of QCT spine results, the American College of Radiology has in 2008 published guidelines for the performance of QCT [13]; based on these guidelines, volumetric trabecular BMD values from 120 to 80 mg/cm^3 are defined as osteopenic and BMD values below 80 mg/cm^3 as osteoporotic.

In addition to the spine, the hip is an important fracture risk site and therefore an important site for axial BMD measurement [14] and areal BMD measurement at the femoral neck is one of the clinical risk factors included in the WHO FRAX 10-year fracture risk calculation tool [15]. While 3D QCT systems for measurement at the hip have been proposed and developed for research [16], the volumetric BMD measurements from these tools lack the normal comparative data that exists for lumbar spine QCT.

CTXA Hip uses 3D QCT volume data sets to generate bone projection images that visually look like those generated by DXA. CTXA Hip exploits the anatomical detail in the 3D QCT data set to segment bone from surrounding tissues rather than relying on the dual-energy imaging method of DXA. While CTXA Hip and DXA use somewhat different technologies to generate bone projection images of the proximal femur, the projection images from both devices convey the same basic information—total bone mass per projected bone area. This leads to the hypothesis that CTXA Hip BMD estimates provide the same clinical utility as that afforded by DXA. Importantly, the areal BMD measurements and T-scores derived from CTXA Hip may be used with the WHO diagnostic classifications.

This kind of approach has been shown to have excellent correlation with DXA for areal BMD measurement for the Total Hip region [17]. In a previous study using CTXA Hip, Khoo et al compared it with DXA-derived areal bone mineral density and T-scores [18]. However, that study looked at a cohort of elderly patients aged 82.8+/−2.5 years (mean +/− SD) and did not utilize CTXA to derive separate measurement from cortical and trabecular compartments; CTXA Hip may provide more information than DXA from a study due to the greater anatomical detail accessible from the 3D QCT volume data set relative to the information present in the planar projection images intrinsic to DXA.

In this study, we compare CTXA Hip and DXA areal BMD measures at both the femoral neck and total hip regions in a cohort of women between the ages of 20–80 years. We also present cortical and trabecular BMD estimates from standard (DXA) hip ROIs derived using CTXA Hip as additional information available from this method.

Materials and Methods

QCT studies were performed using the QCT Pro calibration phantom and software system with the CTXA Hip analysis module (Mindways Software, Inc., Austin, TX). The Mindways liquid calibration phantom used in this study was based on the original QCT calibration system developed at University of California, San Francisco (UCSF) [19], and mineral density results are reported in terms of equivalent calibrated aqueous potassium phosphate density. The QCT Pro QA phantom included a reference tube that contains aqueous K_2HPO_4 with a concentration of 200.0±0.4 mg/cm^3, and was used within the software both as a cross-calibration reference and for monitoring scanner performance.

Quality assurance (QA) scans were performed once a month according to manufacturer's protocols. In brief, the QA phantom was placed above the calibration phantom and 8–10 axial slices were scanned using the same study protocol used for BMD studies as described below, see Figure 1.

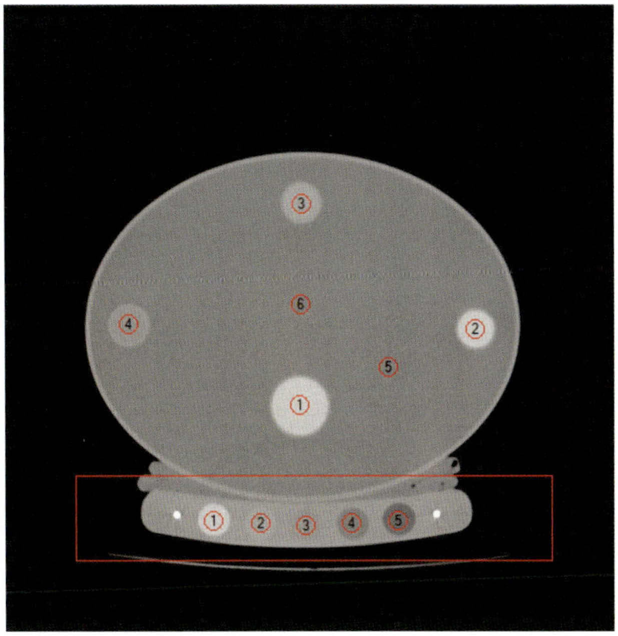

Figure 1. QA study axial image. Completed ROI placement in axial CT slice of quality assurance and CT calibration reference phantoms positioned for QA studies.

Subjects

Precision Study. A total of 22 subjects enrolled as placebo controls in an osteoporosis treatment study at the University of California, San Francisco (UCSF) comprised the precision study group. These "placebo" subjects were all postmenopausal osteoporotic women receiving hormone replacement therapy, calcium and vitamin D, and ranged in age from 55 to 72 years. All women were enrolled in that study by being identified as "osteoporotic" based on a spine or hip BMD T-score by DXA less than −2.5. Hip BMD was measured at yearly intervals for each subject using DXA and QCT. Ten of the 22 women received three hip BMD scans over a two year interval while 12 of the women received four hip BMD scans over a three year interval.

Interobserver Variability. The interobserver variability for BMD estimates using CTXA was estimated by comparing results obtained independently on the same in vivo data set by two trained operators. Data from a single clinical trial site were used for this analysis. Twenty eight studies were analyzed, and the results for estimated BMD of the femoral neck and total hip regions of interest were compared.

CTXA-DXA Comparison

A total of 69 patients having DXA exams for osteoporosis diagnostic testing were recruited from two clinical centers, the University of Manchester, UK, and Schenectady Radiology/Ellis Hospital, Schenectady, NY, for comparison of CTXA Hip and DXA results. Thirty patients were recruited at one center and 39 patients at the other. Seven patients were men and 62 were women. Ages ranged from 20–80 years, but the patients were predominantly postmenopausal women.

Ethics

All subjects involved in this study gave written informed consent, and all research protocols were approved by the Institutional Review Boards at the respective institutions: the

Institutional Review Board of Ellis Hospital, Schenectady, NY, USA; the Committee on Human Research (CHR), the UCSF Institutional Review Board holding Department of Health and Human Services Multiple Project Assurance #M-1169, University of California, San Francisco, USA; and the Ethics Committee of the University of Manchester, Manchester, UK.

Scanning Protocols

CTXA Examinations. CT image data analyzed for these studies using CTXA Hip were acquired using different CT scanner models at the three institutions. At UCSF, a GE9800 (GE Medical Systems, Waukesha, WI) was used, at the University of Manchester a Philips SR4000 (Philips Medical Systems, Best, Netherlands) was used, and at Schenectady Radiology a GE ProSpeed (GE Medical Systems, Waukesha, WI) was used. All CT scanners were maintained as specified by the manufacturers. In addition, all CT systems were further calibrated for QCT using the QCT Pro QA procedures.

Subjects were positioned supine on the CT scanner table, lying on top of a K_2HPO_4 CT calibration phantom and bolus bags so that the calibration phantom extended from the lumbar vertebrae to mid-thigh, to cover the pelvis and proximal femur region. Positioning was used so that the pelvis was as straight as possible and the knees were flat on the scanner table. Subjects were asked to put their feet together and remain still, but the feet were not restrained by a positioner. An anterior-posterior computed radiograph was obtained by the scanner from the iliac crest to mid-thigh, and the top of the femoral head to approximately 1 cm below the inferior extent of the lesser trochanter was defined graphically to define the scanning region. A contiguous series of scans was obtained, 3 mm thick every 3 mm, with a 40 cm display field-of-view (0.781 mm pixel size), and a standard abdomen reconstruction algorithm. Typically 40 images were obtained, with the time to acquire this image set approximately 3.5 minutes on the GE9800 and 1 minute on the Philips and ProSpeed scanners. Scanning parameters varied slightly depending on the capabilities of the CT scanner used and patient size, and were 80 kVp, 240 mAs for the GE9800, and 120 kVp, 100–200 mAs for the Philips and ProSpeed scanners. All subject and QA data were sent to Mindways where analysis was centralized.

DXA Examinations. DXA image data were acquired and analyzed at each site according to standard procedures used at those sites, including daily calibrations for quality control. A single individual at each site was responsible for all DXA analyses. At UCSF, DXA data were acquired using a Hologic QDR1000 (Hologic, Inc., Bedford, MA) scanner, while at the other two sites Hologic QDR4500 scanners were used. The DXA systems were calibrated and maintained in accordance with the manufacturer's specifications. The DXA data were acquired and analyzed according to the manufacturer's instructions.

Data Analysis

QA phantom data for each CT scanner were analyzed using the QCT Pro QA analysis module. Each QA study of 8–10 QA images acquired using the same technique as for subject scans was analyzed to determine CT scanner performance characteristics, and any deviations from expected performance were identified by the software. Any degradation of scanner performance identified by the QA software was resolved before subsequent subject data were analyzed. Subject results were referenced to the appropriate CT scanner QA results.

The QA phantom data is also used by the CTXA Hip software to detect and characterize differences in CT value response and make a correction to the CT calibration slope to compensate for "beam hardening" effects.

CT image data were analyzed in a standardized fashion with the CTXA Hip software, using the left proximal femur unless pathology prevented this. A square box region of interest was centered over the femoral neck as identified on the axial images, and a volumetric region of interest containing the proximal femur was extracted from the CT image data set for analysis. Segmentation of bone from surrounding non-bone tissue was performed using an adaptive algorithm controlled by three parameters. The first parameter defined a threshold below which a pixel could not be classified as bone (default: −250 mg/cm3). The second parameter defined the size of the neighborhood of pixels considered when adaptively modifying the local threshold. A default range corresponds to a neighborhood with a width of approximately five pixels. The third parameter was the initial threshold used to seed the adaptive algorithm, with pixels exceeding the initial threshold tentatively classified as "bone" and the remainder as "not bone" (default: 120 mg/cm3). The result of the segmentation process is a set of voxels identified as "bone" all contained within the outer cortex of the proximal femur. There was no further separation of voxels within this outer envelope as "marrow" vs. "bone" voxels. This 3D data set of bone voxels was then rotated such that the femoral shaft was vertical in the coronal and sagittal planes and the femoral neck was horizontal in the axial plane (Figure 2).

The CTXA Hip software generates a 2-dimensional image similar to a DXA image from the rotated 3D data set by summing all the bone voxels along lines perpendicular to the coronal plane. Each pixel of the resulting image represented the mass of mineral summed along that line, and was further characterized by a known pixel area, and a total volume of bone along the line. Regions of interest representing the common ROIs used for DXA analysis (Total Hip, Femoral Neck, Trochanter, Intertrochanter) were identified automatically on the projected image by the software (Figure 3). The lower extent of the Intertrochanter ROI was set at the lower junction of the lesser trochanter and the femoral shaft. The angle of the femoral neck axis, and the position and size of the femoral neck box ROI, were adjusted by the operator as required.

Results for areal BMD (g/cm^2), volumetric BMD (mg/cm^3), mass (g), area (cm^2) and volume (cm^3) for each of the ROIs were stored in the QCT Pro database and exported as text files for analysis.

In addition to the primary data analysis of total bone in the projected ROIs, the software also allows classification of bone voxels as "cortical" or "trabecular" based on a simple user-defined threshold. A threshold of 350 mg/cm^3 was used to separate "cortical" from "trabecular" bone in these ROIs. This value was chosen empirically as that which compartmentalized the major compressive and tensile trabecular bone groupings as "trabecular" bone. The choice of this threshold also identified higher density endocortical bone as "cortical" even though it was not part of the haversian cortex. The same measurements of area BMD, volumetric BMD, mass, area, and volume were given for each of these compartments. Compartmental analysis of the ROIs was performed for the group of 22 women recruited for the precision study as a homogeneous population of postmenopausal women identified as osteoporotic by DXA.

Statistical Analysis

The precision of area BMD (expressed in g/cm^2) measurements derived with the CTXA Hip was estimated by examining the dispersion of patient measurements acquired at approximately yearly intervals. The mean and standard deviation for the 3 or 4

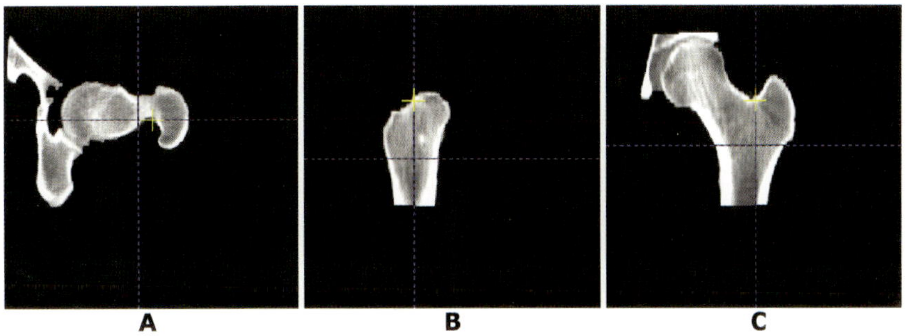

Figure 2. Proximal femur positioning. A) axial, B) sagittal and C) coronal images of segmented bone in proximal femur, rotated into a standard projection.

measurements for each patient were calculated without regard for the rate of bone change. Long-term precision was then estimated by calculating the root-mean-square average of the set of standard deviation estimates for the group of patients [20]. This method provides a conservative estimate of precision, and is justified because the women in this group on average were not losing bone (CTXA Hip Total Hip BMD mean and SEM for baseline, year 1 and year 2, 0.647±0.017, 0.644±0.018, 0.648±0.019 g/cm^2, $p>0.05$ for all comparisons by two tailed t-test).

For interobserver variability, significance of difference of means was tested using a two-tailed t-test.

The accuracy of the CTXA Hip BMD estimates relative to Hologic QDR DXA BMD estimates for the Total Hip and Femoral Neck ROIs was characterized by comparing CTXA Hip and DXA results from the same subject from the two sites using Hologic QDR4500 scanners. Results were first compared by individual site. Similarity of the distributions suggested pooling the results. Pooling of these results was objectively justified based on a two-sample t-test, assuming unequal variances, of the means of the bias distribution for each site. That is, the means of the distribution of patient-specific CTXA Hip minus DXA BMD results determined from paired subject measurements at each of the sites were compared by this method. No inconsistencies in the sample mean comparisons were found either for the total hip or femoral neck data at the 95% confidence level ($p<0.05$).

To ascertain the validity of t-tests, an Anderson-Darling test was used to detect significant deviations from normality in measurement distributions.

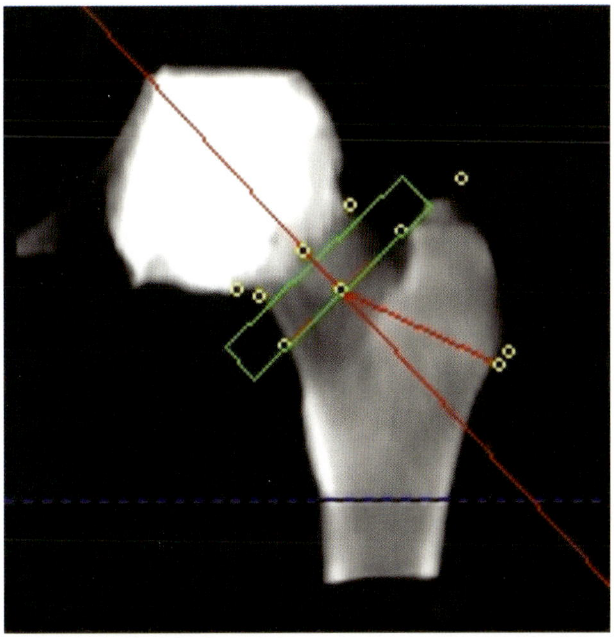

Figure 3. CTXA proximal femur ROI positions. CTXA projected image with standard regions of interest used for BMD calculations (femoral neck, trochanter, intertrochanter, and Total Hip as sum of these three regions). Position of femoral neck box and intertrochanter limit line at base of lesser trochanter, and rotation of femoral neck axis, are adjustable by user. Ward's Triangle ROI is displayed but not used in comparisons.

Results

The results of the long term in vivo precision studies are given in Table 1 (Table S1: "LongTerm In Vivo Precision CTXA vs DXA - Data"), both for precision in terms of the BMD value (g/cm^2) and as the coefficient of variation (CV,%), based on the distribution of the individual patient values. The mean BMD values by CTXA Hip and DXA are also given. There were no significant differences in precision between the CTXA Hip and the DXA results obtained in this study.

Interobserver variability results for CTXA Hip are given in Table 2 (Table S2: "Interobserver Comparison of CTXA BMD Estimates - Data"). The difference in total hip mean BMD estimates was not significant between the two observers at the 95% confidence level ($p = 0.055$), while the femoral neck difference was significant between the two observers at the 95% confidence level ($p = 0.026$). Even though statistically significant, the 1% difference between observers is similar to the 0.9–2.6% obtained using DXA (6,7).

No substantial evidence was found for rejecting the hypothesis that the data measurements are reasonably described by a normal sampling process using the Anderson-Darling test to detect

Table 1. Summary of Long-Term *In Vivo* Precision, CTXA vs. DXA, in Osteoporotic Subjects.

	Total Hip		Femoral Neck	
	CTXA	DXA	CTXA	DXA
Areal Density (g/cm^2)	0.645	0.700	0.551	0.598
Precision (g/cm^2)	0.012	0.014	0.011	0.016
CV (%)	1.8	2.0	2.0	2.7

Table 2. Interobserver Comparison of CTXA BMD Estimates (g/cm^2).

	Observer 1	Observer 2	Observer 2 - Observer 1	Observer 2 - Observer 1 (%)
Mean Total Hip BMD	0.668	0.675	0.007	1.0
SD Total Hip BMD	0.142	0.146	0.004	
Mean Femoral Neck BMD	0.585	0.578	−0.007	1.2
SD Femoral Neck BMD	0.121	0.118	−0.003	

significant deviations from normality in measurement distributions.

The correlation between BMD estimates made with CTXA Hip and DXA for total hip and femoral neck regions of interest are given in Table 3 (Table S3: "Correlation of CTXA Hip and DXA BMD results - Data"), for the two clinical sites independently and for pooled results. Figures 4 and 5 show the correlations for total hip and femoral neck graphically. Correlation coefficients of 0.92−0.97 were obtained for femoral neck and total hip ROIs, with Standard Error of the Estimates (SEE) of 0.043−0.047 g/cm^2.

The segmentation of total bone in the hip into compartments representing "cortical" and "trabecular" bone in DXA-like ROIs differentiates the measurement results of CTXA Hip analysis from DXA. For the study population, the total hip region of interest was found to contain 62.3%±4.8% (mean ± SD) "cortical" bone with the remaining 37.7%±4.8% bone belonging to the "trabecular" bone compartment defined by CTXA Hip. For the femoral neck the proportions were 57.7%±9.5% and 42.3%±9.5%, respectively.

Discussion

The focus on measurements of bone density at the proximal femur as a standard reference [14] has meant DXA has become the gold standard technology used to make these measurements. Theoretically QCT can produce a BMD estimate at the hip in two dimensions that has characteristics similar to DXA, and should give a BMD estimate that is highly correlated with a DXA result. The results of our study show that 2D projected BMD results obtained using the CTXA Hip software correlated highly with results obtained from a common DXA device (QDR4500), and these results are similar to those from other studies. Khoo et al, [18] showed correlation between DXA and CTXA of R = 0.89–0.93 in an older cohort, with a RMS errors of between 0.04–0.06 g/cm^2. In a comparison of a their own QCT aBMD projection algorithm for Total Hip region, Keyak et al [17] showed a correlation of R = 0.935 with an SEE of 0.046 g/cm^2.

The results obtained in our study are also similar to the relationship seen between DXA systems from Hologic and Lunar, where a correlation of R = 0.92 and SEE of 0.051 for the Femoral Neck ROI over the same BMD range in a similar population has been reported [21,22].

Long term in vivo precision is an important parameter for clinical practice, and we obtained results for CTXA Hip essentially identical to those from a Hologic QDR1000 system for osteoporotic patients studied under controlled conditions over a 2–3 year period. Our long-term precision in osteoporotic subjects is similar to short-term precision of 2.1–2.9% obtained by other researchers using DXA in similar populations [23,24], indicating that when properly performed QCT methods are just as precise as DXA. Our precision results are consistent with the observations of Khoo et al [18] where CTXA short-term precision estimates that were either non-inferior to or superior to DXA were reported. However, a limitation of the present study is that the results from only two observers where available for the reproducibility analysis.

We observed statistically significant differences in the slope and/or intercept of BMD results from CTXA Hip compared to Hologic DXA. In particular, CTXA Hip BMD estimates for the Total Hip ROI were found to be approximately 0.11 g/cm^2 lower than QDR 4500 results for the same population. This bias is well modeled by an additive (negative) bias term as shown in Figure 4 where the observed slope in the linear regression analysis was found to be not significantly different from unity. CTXA Hip BMD estimates for the Femoral Neck were also found to be less than the corresponding QDR 4500 results with an average bias of

Table 3. Correlation of CTXA Hip and DXA BMD Results (Site 1, Manchester; Site 2, Schenectady).

Total Hip						
	CTXA BMD	**DXA BMD**	**Slope**	**Intercept**	**R**	**SEE**
Site 1 (N = 30)	0.657±0.143	0.766±0.138	0.988	−0.100	0.95	0.046
Site 2 (N = 39)	0.755±0.175	0.851±0.170	0.999	−0.094	0.97	0.043
Site 1+2 (N = 69)	0.712±0.168	0.814±0.161	1.006	−0.106	0.97	0.044
Femoral Neck						
	CTXA BMD	**DXA BMD**	**Slope**	**Intercept**	**R**	**SEE**
Site 1 (N = 30)	0.564±0.117	0.645±0.123	0.876	−0.001	0.92	0.047
Site 2 (N = 34)	0.638±0.150	0.713±0.156	0.883	0.004	0.96	0.043
Site 1+2 (N = 64)	0.606±0.141	0.681±0.145	0.888	−0.004	0.95	0.044

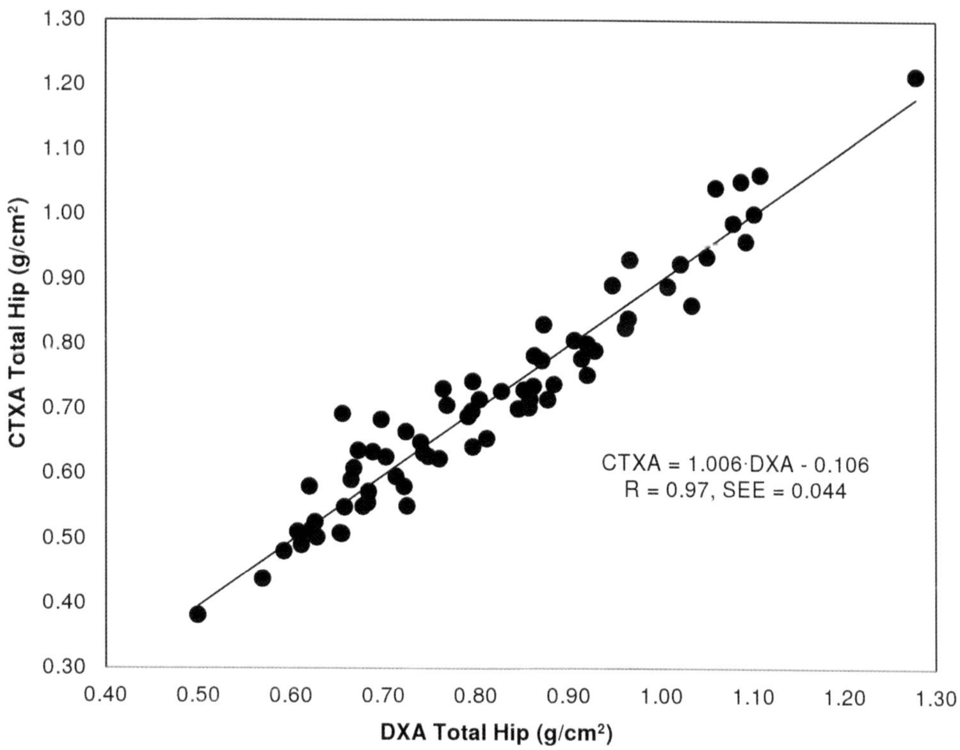

Figure 4. Correlation of area BMD for CTXA and DXA for total hip region of interest.

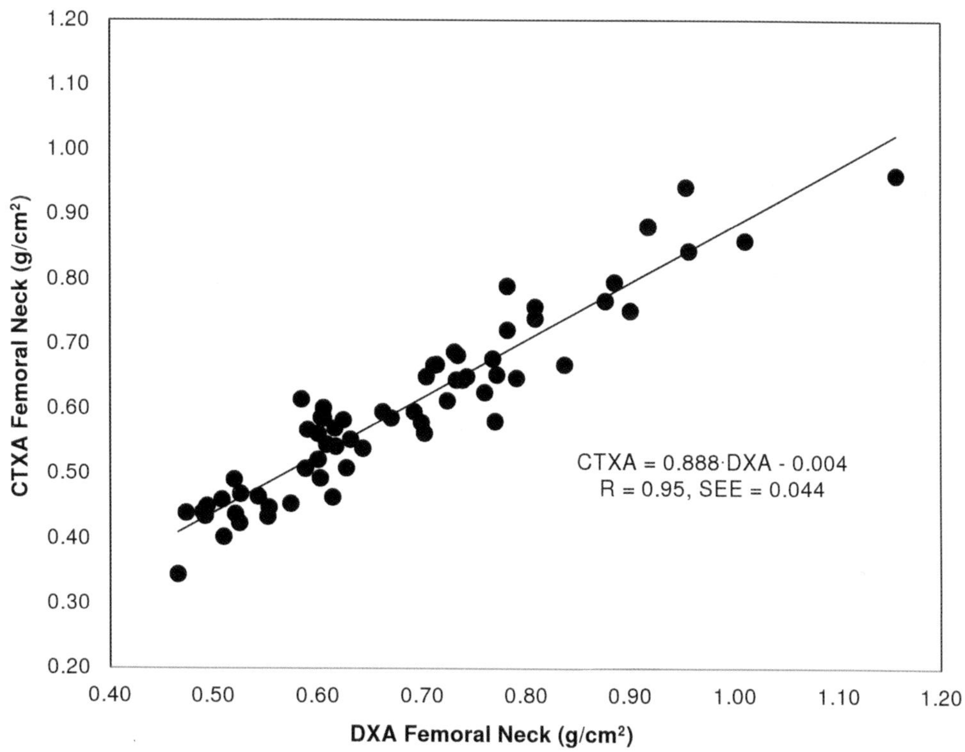

Figure 5. Correlation of area BMD for CTXA and DXA for femoral neck region of interest.

about 0.06 g/cm^2. In this case, however, linear regression analysis indicated the bias was better explained by a model slope significantly different than one with an additive offset not significantly different from zero. As can be seen in Table 1, we also observed statistically significant bias in CTXA Hip and QDR 1000 BMD estimates, with an average bias of about 0.05 g/cm2 at both measurement sites reported here for the osteoporotic patient population comprising our precision study group.

Biases in hip BMD estimates between bone densitometers from various manufacturers have been reported in numerous studies. Biases of the same magnitude we report here have been observed in comparison studies of DXA devices from Hologic, Lunar and Norland [21,22]. As noted by those authors, these differences may be due to technical differences in the way data are acquired and analyzed.

One cause of the differences between QCT (CTXA) aBMD and DXA-derived aBMD relates to the calibration phantoms used [25]. The Hologic DXA scanner uses solid calcium hydroxyapatite (CaHAP) standard for its calibration. QCT uses liquid potassium phosphate (K_2HPO_4) as a mineral standard. Although the mean CaHAP and K_2HPO_4 calibration standards are similar in the trabecular aBMD region, there are slight differences in the calibration slopes, with a propensity for K_2HPO_4 equivalent densities to be slightly lower than corresponding CaHAP equivalent densities. The difference is more pronounced when working at higher densities. Therefore, it is not surprising that QCT-derived mineral mass (BMC) at all corresponding sites of the proximal femur was significantly lower compared to DXA values (Table 1). In addition, the methods used for separating "soft tissue" components of the projection are also very different between QCT and DXA. DXA uses dual energy methods for this and in particular estimates the fat/lean ratio for tissue superimposed with the DXA bone signal. Essentially the soft-tissue component is subtracted in DXA. In CTXA, however, volumetric CT images are segmented into "bone" and "not bone" (mostly soft tissue, air and calibration phantom pixels) pixels using geometric, anatomical and physiological considerations. The "non-bone" pixels are completely removed from the image data prior to generating bone projections and so contribute essentially no signal (and no residual noise) component to the bone projection images and without dependencies on details of the nature and distribution of the surrounding tissue.

Next, DXA standardizes measurement positioning by controlling foot positioning during scanning. While the standard DXA foot positioning does result in turning the femoral neck axis outward such that the femoral neck axis is more nearly orthogonal to the x-ray projection direction, the orthogonality of the femoral neck axis to the projection direction is not what is controlled with DXA. This orthogonality is, however, what is being controlled within CTXA.

Another cause of differences is projection geometry. CTXA uses a parallel beam projection geometry. While older DXA units also use a parallel projection geometry, most DXA units today use fan beam projection geometries that include a depth-dependent magnification attribute. Depending upon DXA unit design, there can also be a residual magnification component related to how far a patient's bone sits above, say, the DXA device table top. In such a situation, DXA BMD estimates can be influenced by patient positioning, including factors that may be difficult to control between DXA scans–such as significant weight loss/gain resulting in an inability to position a patient in the same manner between two scans. All of these are on top of algorithmic variations in core image processing steps used to define various anatomical landmarks and reference lengths used to standardize BMD measurement on a particular device. For example, thresholds of 15% of the maximum BMD across a femoral neck profile to define the lateral margins of the femoral neck (and so the femoral neck width) are likely to be very different in a DXA image, that includes a non-zero, noisy background that is a residual of soft-tissue background subtraction, in comparison to a CTXA image that includes essentially no soft-tissue background and essentially no soft-tissue background noise.

Well-established biases in BMD estimates from different devices are currently handled in clinical densitometry practice by reporting normalized BMD estimates and interpreting normalized proximal-femur BMD scores from all DXA units using the same guidelines. The use of T-scores is the prevalent normalization method in use today [14], although alternative methods for generating "standardized" BMD estimates have been proposed [21,22]. When using the CTXA method, T-scores may be calculated by using conversion equations using the Hologic DXA-acquired NHANES III (National Health and Nutrition Examination Survey III) young normal data with conversion equations for the various anatomical regions [18]. This approach is similar to the adjustment made by DXA equipment manufacturers other than Hologic when using the NHANES III data to calculate T-scores [26]. Alternatively, young normal data may be gathered using the CTXA method in order to calculate T-scores. Although the normal subject data required for standardization of results by the computation of T-scores has been gathered for use with CTXA method and is in current clinical use that is not the subject of the study described here.

Osteoporosis represents a major public health issue, and there is a growing appreciation of the need for wider screening efforts. The recently revised and expanded recommendations by the U.S. Preventive Services Task Force (USPSTF) underscore the need for more screening [27]. The clinical utility of the CTXA hip method is in providing a BMD measurement where DXA may not be available due to space or financial constraints, but an underutilized CT scanner may be used such as in a rural healthcare facility. However, the disadvantage of a higher radiation dose must be considered in particular in younger individuals (e.g., peri-menopausal women).

The higher radiation exposure due to a dedicated QCT exam in comparison to a DXA study can be avoided by the re-use of a CT scan ordered for another reason. The use of QCT for BMD measurement at the lumber vertebrae and hip in conjunction with CT scans ordered for other reasons in the context of improving screening rates, has been explored in a number of studies [28–30] including for CT contrast-enhanced scans [31,32]. For patients undergoing screening CT colonography (CTC), a potential opportunity exists for concurrent BMD screening without the need for any additional imaging, radiation exposure, or patient time [30]. Such dual-use of CT images could increase screening rates or, alternatively, preclude the need for DXA screening in some individuals. Because standard CT colonography exams include the pelvis, CTXA femoral neck measurement rather than lumber spine measurement can be made which provides access to the diagnostic classification using WHO T-scores thresholds and the use of FRAX for fracture risk calculation. The ability of the CTXA method to produce areal BMD and T-scores at the femoral neck which may be used as input to the WHO FRAX tool is particularly important as the field moves away from relying solely on BMD measurement for fracture risk prediction [33].

We have compared a method of deriving DXA-like 2D projections of integral bone from volumetric CT scans to DXA measurements. In principle, there is a large amount of useful 3D information discarded by this approach. In this study, we have presented results from the use CTXA Hip analysis to segment "cortical" and "trabecular" bone compartments which exploits the 3D nature of the acquired 3D image data. In terms of fully 3D analysis of the proximal femur, several methods have been developed [34–39]. Within each anatomic subregion, the density, mass, and volume are computed for the cortical and trabecular components as well as for the integral bone envelope. For trabecular BMD measurements, the precision of these kinds of methods *in vivo* was found to range from 0.6% to 1.1% depending on the volume of interest assessed [34]. Several of these approaches also facilitate geometric and structural analyses of the minimum femoral neck cross section, computing cross-sectional area, estimates of cortical volume and thickness, and moments of inertia for strength estimation. There has also been comparison made of hip structural analysis (HSA) parameters derived by DXA and QCT [40]. However, as has been stated before, the lack of normal data for standardization and the prevailing use of DXA T-scores for diagnostic categorization currently limit these volumetric 3D hip analysis methods to research and clinical trials application.

Conclusion

We hypothesized that CTXA Hip BMD estimates could provide the same clinical utility as that afforded by DXA, and we believe our study results strongly support this hypothesis. High correlation of results from various combinations of DXA devices, along with consistency in measurement precision as characterized by SEE, interobserver variability, and assessment of long-term and short-term measurement precision have been accepted as a basis for using proximal femur results from all commercial DXA devices for clinical decision making within the context of any of numerous national and international clinical densitometry guidelines. Areal BMD and T-scores from CTXA Hip could provide standardized BMD measures from opportunistic osteoporosis screening using CT studies; or a method of osteoporosis screening in areas where DXA is unavailable. The 3D nature of QCT may also provide a more comprehensive estimate of bone strength parameters than similar analyses using DXA data.

Supporting Information

Table S1 Long Term In Vivo Precision CTXA vs DXA - Data.

Table S2 Interobserver Comparison of CTXA BMD Estimates - Data.

Table S3 Correlation of CTXA Hip and DXA BMD results - Data.

Author Contributions

Conceived and designed the experiments: CC JKB JA. Performed the experiments: CC JA. Analyzed the data: CC JKB ADB. Contributed reagents/materials/analysis tools: CC JKB. Wrote the paper: CC JKB JA ADB.

References

1. US Department of Health and Human Services (2004) Bone health and osteoporosis: a report of the Surgeon General. Rockville, MD. doi:10.2165/00002018-200932030-00004.
2. Lewiecki EM, Gordon CM, Baim S, Leonard MB, Bishop NJ, et al. (2008) International Society for Clinical Densitometry 2007 Adult and Pediatric Official Positions. Bone 43: 1115–1121. doi:10.1016/j.bone.2008.08.106.
3. National Osteoporosis Foundation (2013) Clinician's Guide to the Prevention and Treatment of Osteoporosis.
4. Curtis JR, Carbone LD, Cheng H, Hayes B, Laster A, et al. (2008) Longitudinal trends in use of bone mass measurement among older americans, 1999–2005. J Bone Miner Res 23: 1061–1067. doi:10.1359/jbmr.080232.
5. Adams JE (2009) Quantitative computed tomography. Eur J Radiol 71: 415–424. doi:10.1016/j.ejrad.2009.04.074.
6. Prior JC, Vigna YM, Wark JD, Eyre DR, Lentle BC, et al. (1997) Premenopausal ovariectomy-related bone loss: a randomized, double-blind, one-year trial of conjugated estrogen or medroxyprogesterone acetate. J Bone Miner Res 12: 1851–1863. doi:10.1359/jbmr.1997.12.11.1851.
7. Damilakis J, Adams JE, Guglielmi G, Link TM (2010) Radiation exposure in X-ray-based imaging techniques used in osteoporosis. Eur Radiol 20: 2707–2714. doi:10.1007/s00330-010-1845-0.
8. Yu EW, Thomas BJ, Brown JK, Finkelstein JS (2011) Simulated increases in body fat and errors in bone mineral density measurements by DXA and QCT. J Bone Miner Res 27: 119–124. doi:10.1002/jbmr.506.
9. Guglielmi G, Floriani I, Torri V, Li J, van Kuijk C, et al. (2005) Effect of Spinal Degenerative Changes on Volumetric Bone Mineral Density of the Central Skeleton as Measured by Quantitative Computed Tomography. Acta radiol 46: 269–275. doi:10.1080/02841850510012661.
10. Smith JA, Vento JA, Spencer RP, Tendler BE (1999) Aortic calcification contributing to bone densitometry measurement. J Clin Densitom 2: 181–183. doi:10.1385/JCD:2:2:181.
11. Liu G, Peacock M, Eilam O, Dorulla G, Braunstein E, et al. (1997) Effect of osteoarthritis in the lumbar spine and hip on bone mineral density and diagnosis of osteoporosis in elderly men and women. Osteoporos Int 7: 564–569.
12. Faulkner KG, von Stetten E, Miller P (1999) Discordance in patient classification using T-scores. J Clin Densitom 2: 343–350.
13. American College of Radiology (2008) ACR Practice Guideline for the Performance of Quantitative Computed Tomography (QCT) Bone Densitometry.
14. Kanis JA, McCloskey EV, Johansson H, Oden A, Melton LJ, et al. (2008) A reference standard for the description of osteoporosis. Bone 42: 467–475. doi:10.1016/j.bone.2007.11.001.
15. Kanis JA, Johnell O, Oden A, Johansson H, McCloskey E (2008) FRAX and the assessment of fracture probability in men and women from the UK. Osteoporos Int 19: 385–397. doi:10.1007/s00198-007-0543-5.
16. Genant HK, Engelke K, Prevrhal S (2008) Advanced CT bone imaging in osteoporosis. Rheumatology (Oxford) 47 Suppl 4: iv9–16. doi:10.1093/rheumatology/ken180.
17. Keyak JH, Sigurdsson S, Karlsdottir G, Oskarsdottir D, Sigmarsdottir A, et al. (2011) Male-female differences in the association between incident hip fracture and proximal femoral strength: a finite element analysis study. Bone 48: 1239–1245. doi:10.1016/j.bone.2011.03.682.
18. Khoo BCC, Brown JK, Cann CE, Zhu K, Henzell S, et al. (2009) Comparison of QCT-derived and DXA-derived areal bone mineral density and T scores. Osteoporos Int 20: 1539–1545. doi:10.1007/s00198-008-0820-y.
19. Cann CE, Genant HK (1980) Precise measurement of vertebral mineral content using computed tomography. J Comput Assist Tomogr 4: 493–500.
20. Glüer CC, Blake GM, Lu Y, Blunt BA, Jergas M, et al. (1995) Accurate assessment of precision errors: how to measure the reproducibility of bone densitometry techniques. Osteoporos Int 5: 262–270. doi:10.1007/BF01774016.
21. Genant HK, Grampp S, Glüer CC, Faulkner KG, Jergas M, et al. (1994) Universal standardization for dual x-ray absorptiometry: patient and phantom cross-calibration results. J Bone Miner Res 9: 1503–1514. doi:10.1002/jbmr.5650091002.
22. Hui SL, Gao S, Zhou XH, Johnston CC, Lu Y, et al. (1997) Universal standardization of bone density measurements: a method with optimal properties for calibration among several instruments. J Bone Miner Res 12: 1463–1470. doi:10.1359/jbmr.1997.12.9.1463.
23. Wahner HW, Looker A, Dunn WL, Walters LC, Hauser MF, et al. (1994) Quality control of bone densitometry in a national health survey (NHANES III) using three mobile examination centers. J Bone Miner Res 9: 951–960. doi:10.1002/jbmr.5650090621.
24. Slosman DO, Provvedini DM, Meunier PJ, Delmas PD, Sebert JL, et al. (1999) The use of different dual X-ray absorptiometry brands in a multicenter clinical trial: consequences and limits. J Clin Densitom 2: 37–44.
25. Goodsitt MM (1992) Conversion relations for quantitative CT bone mineral densities measured with solid and liquid calibration standards. J Bone Miner Res 19: 145–158.
26. Binkley N, Kiebzak GM, Lewiecki EM, Krueger D, Gangnon RE, et al. (2005) Recalculation of the NHANES database SD improves T-score agreement and reduces osteoporosis prevalence. J Bone Miner Res 20: 195–201. doi:10.1359/JBMR.041115.
27. Nelson H, Haney E, Dana T, Bougatsos C, Chou R (2010) Screening for Osteoporosis: An Update for the US Preventive Services Task Force. Ann Intern Med 153.

28. Papadakis AE, Karantanas AH, Papadokostakis G, Petinellis E, Damilakis J (2009) Can abdominal multi-detector CT diagnose spinal osteoporosis? Eur Radiol 19: 172–176. doi:10.1007/s00330-008-1099-2.
29. Link TM, Koppers BB, Licht T, Bauer JS, Lu Y, et al. (2004) In vitro and in vivo spiral CT to determine bone mineral density: initial experience in patients at risk for osteoporosis. Radiology 231: 805–811. doi:10.1148/radiol.2313030325.
30. Pickhardt PJ, Lee LJ, del Rio AM, Lauder T, Bruce RJ, et al. (2011) Simultaneous screening for osteoporosis at CT colonography: bone mineral density assessment using MDCT attenuation techniques compared with the DXA reference standard. J Bone Miner Res 26: 2194–2203. doi:10.1002/jbmr.428.
31. Bauer JS, Henning TD, Müeller D, Lu Y, Majumdar S, et al. (2007) Volumetric quantitative CT of the spine and hip derived from contrast-enhanced MDCT: conversion factors. AJR Am J Roentgenol 188: 1294–1301. doi:10.2214/AJR.06.1006.
32. Gruber M, Bauer JS, Dobritz M, Beer AJ, Wolf P, et al. (2013) Bone mineral density measurements of the proximal femur from routine contrast-enhanced MDCT data sets correlate with dual-energy X-ray absorptiometry. Eur Radiol 23: 505–512. doi:10.1007/s00330-012-2629-5.
33. Siris ES, Boonen S, Mitchell PJ, Bilezikian J, Silverman S (2012) What's in a name? What constitutes the clinical diagnosis of osteoporosis? Osteoporos Int 23: 2093–2097. doi:10.1007/s00198-012-1991-0.
34. Lang TF, Keyak JH, Heitz MW, Augat P, Lu Y, et al. (1997) Volumetric quantitative computed tomography of the proximal femur: precision and relation to bone strength. Bone 21: 101–108.
35. Kang Y, Engelke K, Kalender WA (2003) A new accurate and precise 3-D segmentation method for skeletal structures in volumetric CT data. IEEE Trans Med Imaging 22: 586–598. doi:10.1109/TMI.2003.812265.
36. Kang Y, Engelke K, Fuchs C, Kalender WA (2005) An anatomic coordinate system of the femoral neck for highly reproducible BMD measurements using 3D QCT. Comput Med Imaging Graph 29: 533–541. doi:10.1016/j.compmedimag.2005.05.002.
37. Camp JJ, Karwoski RA, Stacy MC, Atkinson EJ, Khosla S, et al. (2004) System for the analysis of whole-bone strength from helical CT images. In: Amini AA, Manduca A, Proc. SPIE 5369, Medical Imaging 2004: Physiology, Function, and Structure from Medical Images. pp. 74–88. doi:10.1117/12.535745.
38. Lang T, LeBlanc AD, Evans HJ, Lu Y, Genant HK, et al. (2004) Cortical and trabecular bone mineral loss from the spine and hip in long-duration spaceflight. J Bone Miner Res 19: 1006–1012. doi:10.1359/JBMR.040307.
39. Poole KES, Mayhew PM, Rose CM, Brown JK, Bearcroft PJ, et al. (2010) Changing structure of the femoral neck across the adult female lifespan. J Bone Miner Res 25: 482–491. doi:10.1359/jbmr.090734.
40. Khoo BCC, Brown K, Zhu K, Pollock M, Wilson KE, et al. (2012) Differences in structural geometrical outcomes at the neck of the proximal femur using two-dimensional DXA-derived projection (APEX) and three-dimensional QCT-derived (BIT QCT) techniques. Osteoporos Int 23: 1393–1398. doi:10.1007/s00198-011-1727-6.

Improved Anchorage of Ti6Al4V Orthopaedic Bone Implants through Oligonucleotide Mediated Immobilization of BMP-2 in Osteoporotic Rats

Julia V. Wölfle[1], Jörg Fiedler[2], Lutz Dürselen[3], Judith Reichert[4], Dieter Scharnweber[4], Anne Förster[5], Bernd Schwenzer[5], Heiko Reichel[1], Anita Ignatius[3], Rolf E. Brenner[2]*

1 Department of Orthopaedic Surgery, Centre of Musculoskeletal Research, University of Ulm, Ulm, Germany, **2** Division for Biochemistry of Joint and Connective Tissue Diseases, Department of Orthopaedic Surgery, Centre of Musculoskeletal Research, University of Ulm, Ulm, Germany, **3** Institute of Orthopaedic Research and Biomechanics, Centre of Musculoskeletal Research, University of Ulm, Ulm, Germany, **4** Max Bergmann Center of Biomaterials, TU Dresden, Dresden, Germany, **5** Institute of Biochemistry, TU Dresden, Dresden, Germany

Abstract

The aim of the present study was to test the biocompatibility and functionality of orthopaedic bone implants with immobilized oligonucleotides serving as anchor stands for rhBMP-2 and rhVEGF-A conjugated with complementary oligonucleotides in an osteoporotic rat model. Al_2O_3-blasted acid etched Ti6Al4V implants, carrying oligonucleotide anchor strands and hybridized with rhBMP-2 or rhVEGF-A through complementary 31-mer oligonucleotide stands were inserted into the proximal tibia of ovariectomized rats. At the time of surgery (15 weeks after ovariectomy) microCT analysis showed significantly lower bone mineral density compared to non-ovariectomized animals. Bone-implant contact (BIC) and pullout-force were not negatively affected by non-hybridized anchor strands. Twelve weeks after surgery, a significantly higher pullout force was found for BMP-2 hybridized to the anchor strands compared to non-hybridized anchor strands or native samples, and on histomorphometric analysis BIC was highest in the BMP group. Thus, we could show the biocompatibility and in vivo functionality of this modular, self-organizing system for immobilization and subsequent release of BMP-2 in vivo.

Editor: João Costa-Rodrigues, Faculdade de Medicina Dentária, Universidade do Porto, Portugal

Funding: This work has been funded by a grant from the German Federal Ministry of Education and Research (BMBF, FKZ 13N1006). The funders had no role in study design, data collection and analysis, decision to publish, or preparation of the manuscript.

Competing Interests: The authors have declared that no competing interests exist.

* E-mail: rolf.brenner@uni-ulm.de

Introduction

The coincidence of osteoarthritis and osteoporosis represents a major challenge to total joint replacement in orthopaedic surgery: Mäkkinen et al. found 74% osteopenic or osteoporotic patients in a subgroup of 53 female patients with advanced primary hip osteoarthritis scheduled for cement less total hip arthroplasty [1]. Whereas the relationship between osteoporosis and failure rate of dental implants is controversially discussed in literature [2–8], studies on the impact of osteoporosis on osseointegration of orthopaedic implants are less numerous and much less controversial. In an osteoporotic animal model impaired implant osseointegration into the tibia or femur has been repeatedly seen [6,9], most recently by Stadlinger et al. [10]. Alm et al. [11] found bone loss in Gruen zone 7 after cementless total hip arthroplasty in female patients with low bone mineral density, and Aro et al. [12] recently reported that low bone mineral density negatively affects initial stability and delays stem osseointegration after cementless hip joint replacement in women. Orthopaedic implant anchorage primarily depends on osteoconduction from periimplant bone tissue. Therefore, roughness and physico-chemical properties of implant surfaces have been optimized to increase osteoconductivity [13]. A further approach to improve osseointegration of titanium implants in osteoporotic bone is surface modification with bioactive molecules encouraging bone formation. In this context the method of binding and/or release of such factors is a crucial issue [13]. Promising results have been published by Michael et al. who achieved immobilization of bioactive molecules on the implant surface in a two-step procedure: First, short strands of nucleic acids – "anchor strands" – were entrapped into a titanium oxide layer on the implant surface [14,15]. Then, conjugates of bioactive molecules and complementary strands were hybridized to the surface modified with anchor strands [14,16]. It has been shown that bioactive molecules thus fixed on a titanium surface retain their bioactivity: Conjugates of RGD peptides and complementary strands hybridized to anodic immobilized anchor strands increased osteoblast attachment on the titanium surface compared to the control group [16].

Promising bioactive molecules for surface modification are bone morphogenetic protein 2 (BMP-2) and vascular endothelial growth factor A (VEGF-A): BMP-2 is probably one of the most important growth factors in bone formation which is currently used in a wide range of tissue-engineering products that allow complete regeneration of bone e.g. in long bone defects or pseudarthrosis [17–19]. VEGF-A induces angiogenesis, which is necessary for blood supply and may also provide osteoprogenitor cells derived from multipotent pericytes for implant integration [20]. Moreover, it exerts a chemoattractive effect on human mesenchymal progenitor

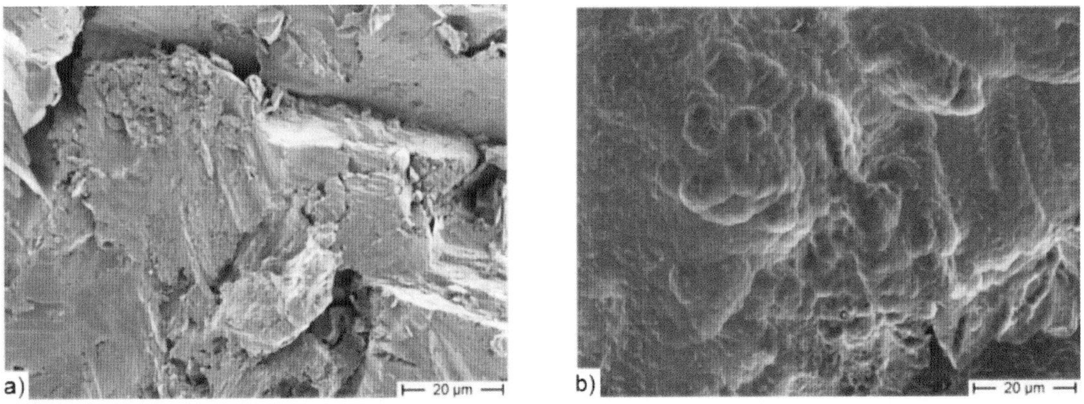

Figure 1. SEM-pictures of the orthopaedic implant surfaces a) before and b) after acid etching. Remaining Al_2O_3 particles were completely removed by etch process. In addition a gain in sub-µm structures was achieved.

cells [21–24]. Previous in vitro studies using the oligonucleotide-mediated immobilization technology indicated that BMP-2 and VEGF-A could be effectively bound to titanium surfaces. The growth factors were released over an extended time span and induced stimulatory effects on proliferation and osteogenic differentiation of mesenchymal stem cells as well as proliferative effects on endothelial cells in vitro [25,26]. Biological activity of released oligonucleotide conjugated BMP-2 and VEGF-A was preserved as indicated by the induction of alkaline phosphatase in C2C12 cells or van Willebrand Factor in mesenchymal stem cells in vitro [25,26].

Since in vivo responses and functionalities have not been tested so far, the aims of this study were (i) to investigate the biocompatibility of the above-mentioned surface modification and (ii) to explore the effects of BMP-2 and VEGF-A functionalization on orthopaedic implant osseointegration in the osteoporotic bone. Therefore, Al_2O_3-blasted acid etched titanium (AAT) implants, with anchor strands (ODN), and with rhBMP-2 modified with 31-mer Oligonucleotides (BMP-ODN) and rhVEGF-A modified with 31-mer Oligonucleotides (VEGF-ODN) hybridized to the anchor strands were inserted into the tibia metaphysis of female rats 15 weeks after ovariectomy.

Materials and Methods

Ethics Statement

The animal trial was conducted according to relevant national and international guidelines; the study was approved by the local governmental authorities (Regierungspräsidium Tübingen, registration number 982). All surgery was performed under adequate anaesthesia and analgesia, and all efforts were made to minimize suffering.

Animals

Sixty-four female ovariectomized WISTAR rats were supplied by Charles River Laboratories (Kißlegg, Germany). Ovariectomy had been performed at the age of 10 weeks. They were kept under climate-controlled conditions (21 +/− 1.5°C, 47.5 +/− 7.5% humidity, light-dark-cycle 12 hours/12 hours). Access to phytoestrogen-free diet and tap water was ad libitum. Mean body weight at the time of surgery was 397±32.2 grams.

Preparation of the orthopaedic bone implants

The orthopaedic implants consisted of an aluminium-oxide-blasted Ti6AlV4 cylindrical rod 5.2 mm in length with a diameter of 1.6 mm (kindly provided by Peter Brehm GmbH, Weisendorf, Germany). One end of the rod was threaded (length 1.2 mm) to enable biomechanical pullout testing. The samples were acid etched for 120 s in a mixture of 0.4 M HF and 1 M HNO_3 at room temperature and following cleaned two times 15 min in ultrapure water in a ultrasonic bath. Surface structure of the implants before and after acid etching is shown in Figure 1. Briefly, anodic polarization of the implants was performed in a custom electrochemical cell from acrylic glass with a gold wire acting as counter electrode and an Ag/AgCl reference electrode connected to the cell via a buffer-agarose salt bridge. Polarization was performed with the electrochemical system Voltalab 4.0 combined with a high-voltage booster HVB100 (Radiometer Analytical, Copenhagen). Ethanolic acetate buffer from 0.5 M acetate containing 5 M ethanol, pH 4.0 and phosphorylated 60mer single stranded oligonucleotides – briefly called anchor strand (AS) - at a concentration of 400 nM was used as electrolyte. Galvanostatic polarization at 7 mA/cm^2 was performed until a potential of 14.5 VAg/AgCl was reached. After several desorption steps (three times in the ethanolic acetate buffer, twice in sterilized ultrapure water; each for 30 s) to remove merely adsorbed and not entrapped anchor strands the implants were packed under dry argon atmosphere and sterilized by gamma irradiation with a standard dose of 25 kGy [14,16]. Conjugates of complementary strands of nucleic acid and recombinant human rhBMP-2 (Reliatech, Braunschweig, Germany) or recombinant human rhVEGF-A (VEGF165, Reliatech) respectively were hybridized to the surface modified with anchor strands directly before implantation under sterile conditions [25,26]. A final washing step was performed to eliminate unbound growth factors. Calculated from the density of single stranded oligonucleotides about 2 ng rhBMP2/mm^2 or 2 ng rhVEGF/mm^2 were immobilized on the orthopaedic implant surface.

Experimental design

The animals were randomly assigned 16 animals each to one of the following groups: (1) control group, (2) anchor strand group, (3) BMP-ODN group, or (4) VEGF-ODN group. According to which group they belonged to one of the following orthopaedic implants was inserted: (1) aluminium-oxide-blasted acid etched Ti6Al4V (AAT), (2) AAT with anchor strands (ODN), with (3) hybridized

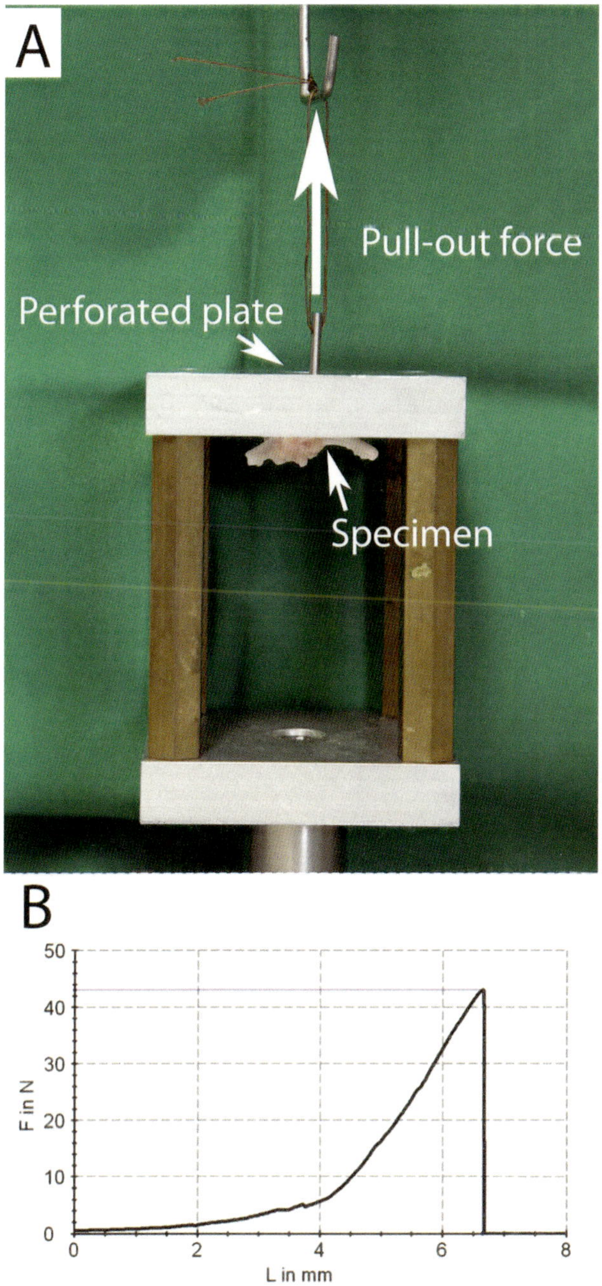

Figure 2. The threaded part of the orthopaedic implant was attached to a 200 N load cell (HBM, Darmstadt) of a standard testing machine (Zwick, Ulm, Figure 2A). A force-displacement diagram was recorded (Figure 2B), the load occurring before the first sudden drop of the tensile force was defined as maximum pullout force. F = force, L = length/displacement.

rhBMP-2 - modified with 31-mer Oligonucleotides (BMP-ODN) or (4) hybridized rhVEGF - modified with 31-mer Oligonucleotides (VEGF-ODN). Eight animals of each group were sacrificed after 4 weeks; the remaining animals 12 weeks after implant insertion. The left tibia was prepared for biomechanical testing, the right tibia for histomorphometric analysis, and the fourth vertebral body of the lumbar spine for analysis of bone mineral density.

To confirm reduced bone mineral density of the ovariectomized rat, four additional animals were sacrificed fifteen weeks after ovariectomy – i.e. at the time of surgery – and the bone mineral density of their fourth lumbar vertebral body was compared to the one of six otherwise identical animals who had not undergone ovariectomy.

Surgical Procedure

Fifteen weeks after ovariectomy the above-mentioned implants were inserted into the proximal tibia on both sides. Anaesthesia was administered by means of an inhalation device (Isoflurane 2%) and subcutaneous injection of analgesics (Tramadolor 20 mg/kg). The surgical technique was similar to the one described by Dayer et al. [27]: A 10 mm incision was made at the medial aspect of the proximal tibia, and the periosteum was incised ventrally to the medial collateral ligament. A 1.7 mm drill hole was made level with the insertion of the patella tendon just ventrally to the medial collateral ligament using hand-held drills held strictly perpendicular to the longitudinal axis of the tibia. The orthopaedic implant was then inserted into the bone. The threaded part remained outside and was covered by a 2 mm tube cut off from a venous catheter (fluorinated ethylene propylene, Vasofixx Braunüle® 18 G, Braun B., Melsungen, Germany) in order to prevent osseous overgrowth. Postoperative analgesia was ensured by adding Tramadolor to the drinking water (25 milligram per litre). Antibiotics (Clindamycine 45 mg/kg) were administered subcutaneously daily on the first three postoperative days.

Biomechanical Testing

For biomechanical testing a specifically designed cylindrical device with a matching internal thread was screwed onto the threaded part of the orthopaedic implant of the left tibia. To determine the pullout force of the implant the device was attached to a 200 N load cell (HBM, Darmstadt) of a standard testing machine (Z010, Zwick, Ulm, Germany; see Figure 2A). A force-displacement diagram (test speed 10 mm/s, preload 0.5 N) was recorded by the testing software (testXpert II, Zwick, Ulm, Germany) and the load occurring before the first sudden drop of the tensile force was defined as maximum pullout force (see Figure 2B).

Histomorphometric measurement

The right tibia including the inserted orthopaedic implant was embedded in Technovit VLC7200 (Kulzer, Germany) and ground down to sections of 100 μm along the longitudinal axis of the tibia. Masson-Goldner staining of the sections was used to visualize connective tissue surrounding the implant. The sections were inspected and scanned with a fully automated inverted light microscope (Leica DMI6000B, Wetzlar, Germany). To quantify the amount of bone surrounding the implant the following parameters were determined semi-automatically with the aid of an imaging analysis software (MetaMorph ®, Leica, Wetzlar, Germany): The bone-to-implant contact rate was calculated by dividing the total length of bone-to-implant contact by the total length around the orthopaedic implant within the tibia. The bone density within the medullar cavity was defined as the percentage of the area of osseous tissue within a 1 mm strip of medullar cavity just distal to the orthopaedic implant.

MicroCT scanning

The fourth vertebral body of the lumbar spine as well as two densitometric phantoms (250 mg/cm^3 and 750 mg/cm^3 hydroxyapatite bone-equivalent density) were scanned with a microCT

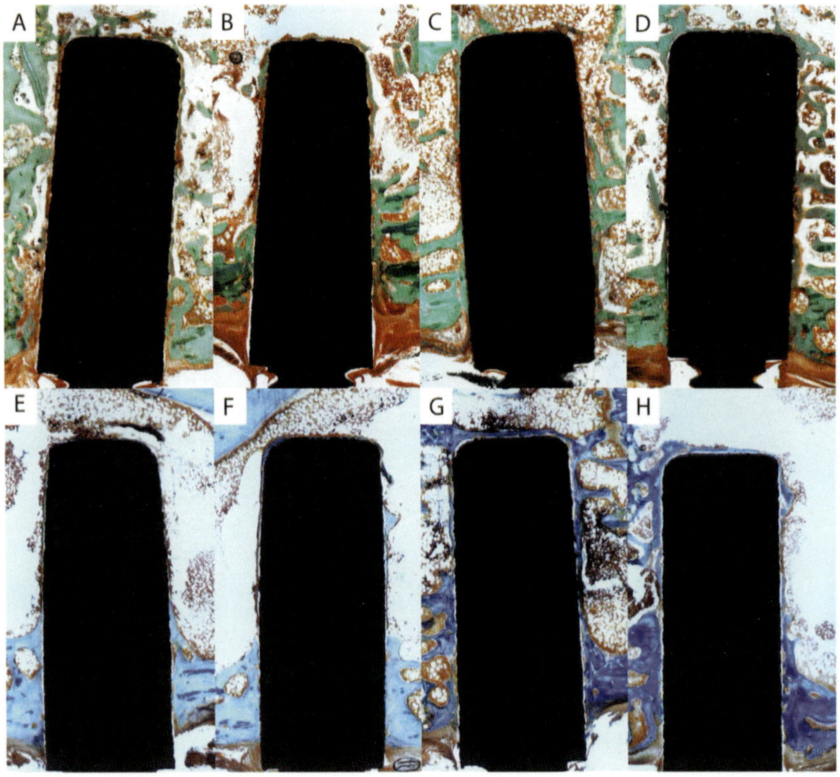

Figure 3. Photograph of trichrome-stains of 100 μm sections of the orthopaedic implant and surrounding osseous tissue (bone tissue in green/blue). Four weeks after surgery no relevant difference of bone-to-implant contact rate or bone density around implant is seen between AAT (A), ODN (B), BMP-ODN (C), and VEGF-ODN group (D). Twelve weeks after surgery bone-to-implant contact rate was increased within the BMP-ODN group (G) when compared to AAT (E) whereas the other groups (AAT (E), ODN (F), VEGF-ODN group (H)) showed no relevant differences. AAT: Al_2O_3-blasted acid etched titanium; ODN: anchor strands of oligonucleotides bound to titanium; BMP-ODN: rhBMP modified with 31-mer Oligonucleotides; VEGF-ODN: rhVEGF modified with 31-mer Oligonucleotides.

system (Skyscan 1172, Kontich, Belgium) with a resolution of 10 μm. As region of interest the trabecular bone starting ten slides below the upper endplate and ending ten slides above the lower endplate was then manually selected. After calibrating the image processing software (CT Analyser V1.11.4.2, Skyscan 1172, Kontich, Belgium) with the assistance of the two-densitometric phantoms the bone mineral density of the region of interest was determined. Then, the graylevel image was reduced to a binary image using Otsu's method of histogram shape-based image thresholding. Five bone structural parameters (bone volume fraction BV/TV, connectivity density Conn.D (measuring the degree of connectivity of trabeculae normalized by TV as explained in Bouxsein et al. [28]), trabecular number Tb.N, trabecular thickness Tb.Th, and trabecular separation Tb.Sp) were then automatically determined from the region of interest (CT Analyser V1.11.4.2, Skyscan 1172, Kontich, Belgium).

Statistical analysis

For statistical analysis the Statistical Package for Social Sciences (SPSS® Inc., IBM, version 19) was used. Due to the low number of animals per group non-parametric tests were used for statistical analysis. Mann-Whitney-U-Test was used to compare two groups (e.g. bone mineral density), Kruskal-Wallis-Test for more than two groups (e.g. pullout force). A probability value of less than 0.05 was considered to indicate statistical significance. Boxplots and median values were used to characterize the distribution of continuous variables.

Results

MicroCT scanning

MicroCT analysis of the four additional animals sacrificed 15 weeks after ovariectomy – i.e. at the time of the surgery – showed significantly lower bone mineral density when compared to six animals who had not undergone ovariectomy. More specific data is depicted in the supplement (Table S1).

Histomorphometric measurement

Within the sections of the orthopaedic bone implant inserted into the tibia a thin layer of osseous tissue covered large parts of the implant. The remaining surface of the orthopaedic implant was covered to a certain extent with a thin layer of non-mineralized connective tissue. This is exemplarily shown in Figure 3 by Masson-Goldner-Stains of non-decalcified 100 μm sections of the orthopaedic implants and the surrounding osseous tissue. Four weeks after surgery no significant difference of the bone-to-implant contact rate (BIC) of the orthopaedic implants of all four groups was measureable ($p = 0.927$, see Fig. 4). Twelve weeks after surgery bone-to-implant contact was highest in the BMP group (median 60.7%) though no significant difference between the groups could be found ($p = 0.927$).

In all ovariectomized animals cancellous bone was scarcely observed within the medullar cavity. Four weeks after surgery we did not see a significant difference between the four treatment groups ($p = 0.841$). With exception of the BMP-ODN group we found a further decrease of the bone density in the animals

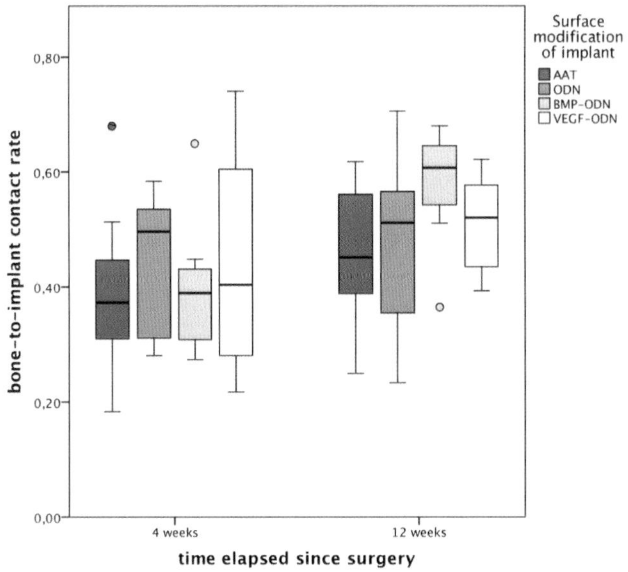

Figure 4. Bone-to-implant contact rate of animals sacrificed four and twelve weeks after implant insertion according to the surface modification of the orthopaedic implant. Bone-to-implant contact rate was highest in the BMP group (median 60.7%) 12 weeks after surgery though no significant difference could be found. AAT: Al_2O_3-blasted acid etched titanium; ODN: anchor strands of oligonucleotides bound to titanium; BMP-ODN: rhBMP modified with 31-mer Oligonucleotides; VEGF-ODN: rhVEGF modified with 31-mer Oligonucleotides.

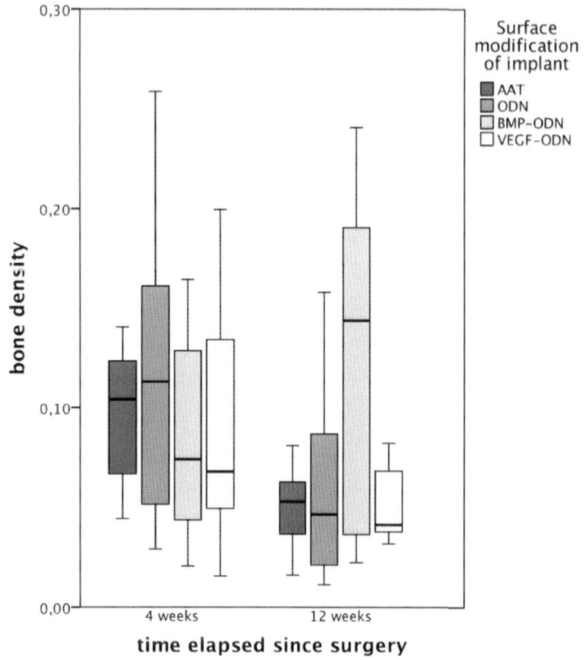

Figure 5. Bone density – i.e. percentage of area of osseous tissue within a 1 mm strip of medullar cavity just distal to the orthopaedic implant – of animals sacrificed four weeks and twelve weeks after implant insertion according to the surface modification of the implant. AAT: Al_2O_3-blasted acid etched titanium; ODN: anchor strands of oligonucleotides bound to titanium; BMP-ODN: rhBMP modified with 31-mer Oligonucleotides; VEGF-ODN: rhVEGF modified with 31-mer Oligonucleotides.

sacrificed after 12 weeks when compared to the animals sacrificed after 4 weeks. As shown in Fig. 5, 12 weeks after surgery bone density was highest in the BMP-ODN group (median BD 14.3%) though we did not find a significant difference between the four groups ($p = 0.488$).

Biomechanical testing

In the animals sacrificed after four weeks maximum pullout force was not significantly different between the treatment groups. As presented in Figure 6, we found a significant difference ($p = 0.034$) 12 weeks after surgery. Pullout force was significantly higher in the BMP-ODN group (median 81.8 N) in comparison with both the AAT group (median 57.0 N) as well as the ODN group (median 65.0 N).

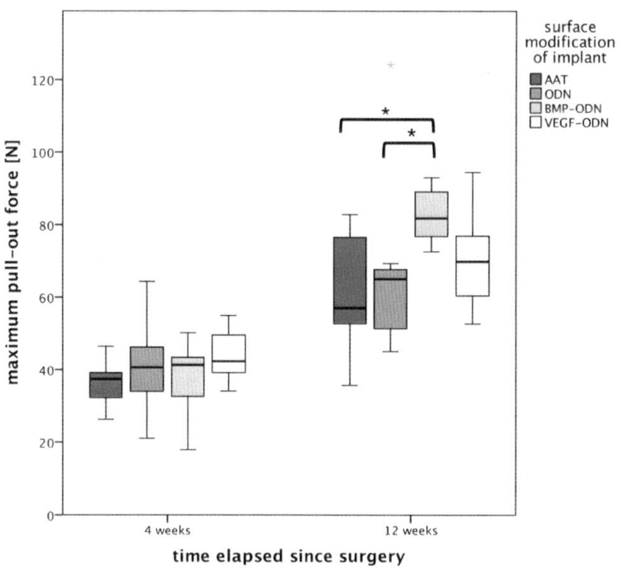

Figure 6. Boxplot of maximum pullout force according to surface modification four and 12 weeks after orthopaedic implant insertion. Asterisks represent significantly higher maximum pullout force in the BMP-ODN group 12 weeks after surgery (median 81.8 N) in comparison with both the AAT group (median 57.0 N) as well as the group (median 65.0 N) with $p<0.05$. AAT: Al_2O_3-blasted acid etched titanium; ODN: anchor strands of oligonucleotides bound to titanium; BMP-ODN: rhBMP modified with 31-mer Oligonucleotides; VEGF-ODN: rhVEGF modified with 31-mer Oligonucleotides.

Discussion

This animal study represents the first *in vivo* investigation of a new kind of orthopaedic implant surface functionalization, based on bioactive molecules immobilized through short complementary oligonucleotide anchor strands on a titanium surface using the specificity of nucleic acid hybridisation.

For reasons of clinical relevance ovariectomized rats were chosen for the study to simulate the compromised bone stock found in osteoporotic bone. The ovariectomized rat has been used as a model for osteoporosis in numerous studies [29-33]. It has been shown that after ovariectomy a biphasic pattern of cancellous bone loss occurs: During the first 100 days there is a rapid bone loss similar to high-turnover osteoporosis, which characterizes postmenopausal osteoporosis. Afterwards there is a relative stabilization at an osteopenic level with a slow bone loss resembling low-turnover osteoporosis, which is characteristic for senile osteoporosis [32,34]. Okamura et al. found that this difference of bone turnover in the ovariectomized rat affects the bone formation around a titanium implant: There was a significantly lower bone contact rate of the implant in the animals with low bone turnover (i. e. 15 weeks after ovariectomy) when compared to the high bone turnover group (i. e. 3 weeks after ovariectomy) [31]. Since we were focusing on senile osteoporosis, we performed the orthopaedic implant insertion 15 weeks after ovariectomy, i. e. in the phase of low-turnover osteoporosis. The decrease in bone density of the ovariectomized rats was confirmed by local histomorphometric and lumbar microCT analysis. This is in agreement with previous data from ovariectomized rats indicating the development of osteoporosis in both the spine and proximal tibia in the respective age and time span after ovariectomy [35].

Our results confirm the biocompatibility of the novel surface modification: no inflammatory response surrounding the orthopaedic titanium implants inserted into the tibia regardless of their surface modification was found. The thin layer of non-mineralized connective tissue partly covering the implant surface seen in our study was much thinner than the fibrous capsule consisting of up to 30 fibroblasts, which had been described by *van den* Beucken et al. [36] when examining the biocompatibility of transponders with multilayered DNA-coatings inserted subcutaneously in rats. The varying thickness of the connective tissue found in both our study and *van den* Beucken *et al.* corresponds to the amount of nucleic acid used in both cases (5 double layers of polyanionic DNA ±300 bp/molecule vs. a single layer of 60mer ODN). With respect to biocompatibility our findings correspond with their findings because they neither described any inflammatory cells surrounding the implant or differences of the tissue response between the coated and uncoated implants [36]. Moreover, we did not observe any case of infection indicating that the sterilization by gamma irradiation before the hybridisation step was effective.

Additionally, our data suggest that BMP-2 immobilized on the orthopaedic implant surface by hybridisation to short strands of nucleic acids preserved its bioactivity in vivo and exerted a biologic effect on the surrounding tissue. This corresponds to the recently published in vitro study by Schliephake et al. [26]. They found a retarded release of rhBMP-2 using this system of nanoanchoring compared to a simple adsorption based strategy. In the respective study only 20% of the hybridized conjugated BMP-2 had been released within 4 weeks and the released conjugated BMP-2 was biologically active as indicated by similar stimulation of alkaline phosphatase in C2C12 cells compared to native BMP-2 [26]. If the release kinetic was similar under in vivo conditions a sufficient amount of bioactive BMP-2 would have been locally available in the time span after surgery during which the benefit for orthopaedic implant anchorage was observed. This in vivo response also is concordant with previous in vitro results on stimulatory effects of titanium surfaces carrying identically immobilized BMP-2 on proliferation and osteogenic differentiation of human bone marrow stroma cells [26]. Accordingly, in the animals of the BMP-ODN group sacrificed after 12 weeks we found a significantly higher pullout force when compared to both the AAT and ODN group. Similarly, the median bone-to-implant contact rate and median periimplant bone density were highest in the BMP-ODN group 12 weeks after surgery. A number of previous animal studies using different species, dosages and immobilization/carrier systems have demonstrated positive effects of BMP-2 functionalization on primary stabilization of titanium implants [37]. In these approaches BMP-2 is released early after implantation and non-physiologically high concentrations have been used [38]. With the oligonucleotide mediated immobilization strategy we could observe positive effects on orthopaedic implant anchorage with rather low concentrations of BMP-2 after the primary phase of osseointegration. This may be explained by a favourable balance of growth factor bound on the surface and the amounts of BMP-2 available in diffusible form for an extended time span. To our knowledge, comparable studies in estrogen-deficient animal models of osteoporosis do not exist so far. In a rat bone defect model of the femur, however, a positive effect of BMP-2 loaded collagen carrier has previously been described which is consistent with our results [39]. Moreover, for statin coating of titanium implants with chitosan as a carrier positive effects on bone implant contact after 2 weeks in ovariectomized rats have recently been reported [10]. Statin induces the expression of BMP-2 in osteoblastic cells and also has positive early effects on osseointegration of implants in the non-compromised situation [40].

Since a reduction of local blood supply and VEGF-expression has been previously reported in ovariectomized mice [38] positive results of the VEGF-hybridisation could be expected at the start of our study. Nevertheless, we did not observe significant effects on both bone-implant contact and pullout force up to 12 weeks after implantation although an extended in vitro release of the growth factor and in vitro bioactivity of the released conjugated VEGF-A could previously be shown [25]. This may be partly explained by recent data of Lui et al. demonstrating that intracellular effects of VEGF-A but not the extracellular interaction with membrane-bound receptors are responsible for induction of osteogenic differentiation of mesenchymal stem cells [41]. Since the outcome parameters used in our study depend on the induction of mineralized bone tissue, we might have missed associated effects on vascularization or recruitment of undifferentiated mesenchymal stromal cells. We did not observe major differences in blood vessel density around the subcutaneous implants on a macroscopic level. Therefore, we cannot exclude that the local concentrations of released conjugated VEGF-A were too low to exert a biologic response. On all things considered, the question of a possible benefit of VEGF-A for orthopaedic implant integration in estrogen-deficient osteoporotic animals clearly deserves further investigation. Published in vivo studies addressing this issue are not available so far. If an effect on vascularisation could be achieved, a combined BMP2- and VEGF-hybridisation might have the potential for further optimization of orthopaedic implant anchorage in osteoporotic bone.

Conclusion

Our study is the first *in vivo* trial that shows the biocompatibility of an orthopaedic implant surface modification with short single strands of nucleic acids serving as anchor strands for complementary oligonucleotide conjugated bioactive molecules. Entrapped into a superficial titanium oxide layer of a Ti6Al4V implant the system is able to preserve the bioactivity of BMP-2 in vivo. Orthopaedic implant osseointegration in the compromised bone stock of estrogen-deficient osteoporotic rats was enhanced by hybridized conjugated BMP-2 molecules in a later phase of implant anchorage between 4 and 12 weeks after surgery compared with the native commercially used aluminium oxide-blasted and acid etched surface. This novel technique to functionalize biomaterial surfaces combines stable attachment of bioactive molecules and modifiable release kinetics with a high degree of flexibility in the production process. Therefore, its application for total joint replacement in osteoporotic patients seems promising.

Acknowledgments

The excellent technical assistance by Mr. Giovanni Ravalli is gratefully acknowledged.

Author Contributions

Conceived and designed the experiments: JVW JF LD DS BS HR AI REB. Performed the experiments: JVW JF JR AF REB. Analyzed the data: JVW JF LD REB. Contributed reagents/materials/analysis tools: JR DS AF BS AI. Wrote the paper: JVW JF AI REB. Contribution to drafting and revising the manuscript: LD JR DS AF BS HR.

References

1. Makinen TJ, Alm JJ, Laine H, Svedstrom E, Aro HT (2007) The incidence of osteopenia and osteoporosis in women with hip osteoarthritis scheduled for cementless total joint replacement. Bone 40: 1041–1047.
2. Alsaadi G, Quirynen M, Komarek A, van Steenberghe D (2007) Impact of local and systemic factors on the incidence of oral implant failures, up to abutment connection. J Clin Periodontol 34: 610–617.
3. Bornstein MM, Cionca N, Mombelli A (2009) Systemic conditions and treatments as risks for implant therapy. Int J Oral Maxillofac Implants 24 Suppl: 12–27.
4. Dao TT, Anderson JD, Zarb GA (1993) Is osteoporosis a risk factor for osseointegration of dental implants? Int J Oral Maxillofac Implants 8: 137–144.
5. Dvorak G, Arnhart C, Heuberer S, Huber CD, Watzek G, et al. (2011) Peri-implantitis and late implant failures in postmenopausal women: a cross-sectional study. J Clin Periodontol 38: 950–955.
6. Gaetti-Jardim EC, Santiago-Junior JF, Goiato MC, Pellizer EP, Magro-Filho O, et al. (2011) Dental implants in patients with osteoporosis: a clinical reality? J Craniofac Surg 22: 1111–1113.
7. Holahan CM, Koka S, Kennel KA, Weaver AL, Assad DA, et al. (2008) Effect of osteoporotic status on the survival of titanium dental implants. Int J Oral Maxillofac Implants 23: 905–910.
8. Moy PK, Medina D, Shetty V, Aghaloo TL (2005) Dental implant failure rates and associated risk factors. Int J Oral Maxillofac Implants 20: 569–577.
9. Yamazaki M, Shirota T, Tokugawa Y, Motohashi M, Ohno K, et al. (1999) Bone reactions to titanium screw implants in ovariectomized animals. Oral Surg Oral Med Oral Pathol Oral Radiol Endod 87: 411–418.
10. Stadlinger B, Korn P, Todtmann N, Eckelt U, Range U, et al. (2013) Osseointegration of biochemically modified implants in an osteoporosis rodent model. Eur Cell Mater 25: 326–340; discussion 339–340.
11. Alm JJ, Makinen TJ, Lankinen P, Moritz N, Vahlberg T, et al. (2009) Female patients with low systemic BMD are prone to bone loss in Gruen zone 7 after cementless total hip arthroplasty. Acta Orthop 80: 531–537.
12. Aro HT, Alm JJ, Moritz N, Makinen TJ, Lankinen P (2012) Low BMD affects initial stability and delays stem osseointegration in cementless total hip arthroplasty in women: a 2-year RSA study of 39 patients. Acta Orthop 83: 107–114.
13. Schliephake H, Scharnweber D (2008) Chemical and biological functionalization of titanium for dental implants. J Mater Chem: 2404–2414.
14. Michael J, Beutner R, Hempel U, Scharnweber D, Worch H, et al. (2007) Surface modification of titanium-based alloys with bioactive molecules using electrochemically fixed nucleic acids. J Biomed Mater Res B Appl Biomater 80: 146–155.
15. Beutner R, Michael J, Forster A, Schwenzer B, Scharnweber D (2009) Immobilization of oligonucleotides on titanium based materials by partial incorporation in anodic oxide layers. Biomaterials 30: 2774–2781.
16. Michael J, Schonzart L, Israel I, Beutner R, Scharnweber D, et al. (2009) Oligonucleotide-RGD peptide conjugates for surface modification of titanium implants and improvement of osteoblast adhesion. Bioconjug Chem 20: 710–718.
17. Bessa PC, Casal M, Reis RL (2008) Bone morphogenetic proteins in tissue engineering: the road from laboratory to clinic, part II (BMP delivery). J Tissue Eng Regen Med 2: 81–96.
18. Bessa PC, Casal M, Reis RL (2008) Bone morphogenetic proteins in tissue engineering: the road from the laboratory to the clinic, part I (basic concepts). J Tissue Eng Regen Med 2: 1–13.
19. Reddi AH (1998) Role of morphogenetic proteins in skeletal tissue engineering and regeneration. Nat Biotechnol 16: 247–252.
20. Modder UI, Khosla S (2008) Skeletal stem/osteoprogenitor cells: current concepts, alternate hypotheses, and relationship to the bone remodeling compartment. J Cell Biochem 103: 393–400.
21. Fiedler J, Leucht F, Waltenberger J, Dehio C, Brenner RE (2005) VEGF-A and PlGF-1 stimulate chemotactic migration of human mesenchymal progenitor cells. Biochem Biophys Res Commun 334: 561–568.
22. Deckers MM, Karperien M, van der Bent C, Yamashita T, Papapoulos SE, et al. (2000) Expression of vascular endothelial growth factors and their receptors during osteoblast differentiation. Endocrinology 141: 1667–1674.
23. Geiger F, Bertram H, Berger I, Lorenz H, Wall O, et al. (2005) Vascular endothelial growth factor gene-activated matrix (VEGF165-GAM) enhances osteogenesis and angiogenesis in large segmental bone defects. J Bone Miner Res 20: 2028–2035.
24. Mayr-Wohlfart U, Waltenberger J, Hausser H, Kessler S, Gunther KP, et al. (2002) Vascular endothelial growth factor stimulates chemotactic migration of primary human osteoblasts. Bone 30: 472–477.
25. Schliephake H, Strecker N, Forster A, Schwenzer B, Reichert J, et al. (2012) Angiogenic functionalisation of titanium surfaces using nano-anchored VEGF - an in vitro study. Eur Cell Mater 23: 161–169; discussion 169.
26. Schliephake H, Botel C, Forster A, Schwenzer B, Reichert J, et al. (2012) Effect of oligonucleotide mediated immobilization of bone morphogenic proteins on titanium surfaces. Biomaterials 33: 1315–1322.
27. Dayer R, Rizzoli R, Kaelin A, Ammann P (2006) Low protein intake is associated with impaired titanium implant osseointegration. J Bone Miner Res 21: 258–264.
28. Bouxsein ML, Boyd SK, Christiansen BA, Guldberg RE, Jepsen KJ, et al. (2010) Guidelines for assessment of bone microstructure in rodents using micro-computed tomography. J Bone Miner Res 25: 1468–1486.
29. Kalu DN (1991) The ovariectomized rat model of postmenopausal bone loss. Bone Miner 15: 175–191.
30. Kalu DN, Liu CC, Hardin RR, Hollis BW (1989) The aged rat model of ovarian hormone deficiency bone loss. Endocrinology 124: 7–16.
31. Okamura A, Ayukawa Y, Iyama S, Koyano K (2004) Effect of the difference of bone turnover on peri-titanium implant osteogenesis in ovariectomized rats. J Biomed Mater Res A 70: 497–505.
32. Wronski TJ, Dann LM, Scott KS, Cintron M (1989) Long-term effects of ovariectomy and aging on the rat skeleton. Calcif Tissue Int 45: 360–366.
33. Wronski TJ, Lowry PL, Walsh CC, Ignaszewski LA (1985) Skeletal alterations in ovariectomized rats. Calcif Tissue Int 37: 324–328.
34. Ozawa S, Ogawa T, Iida K, Sukotjo C, Hasegawa H, et al. (2002) Ovariectomy hinders the early stage of bone-implant integration: histomorphometric, biomechanical, and molecular analyses. Bone 30: 137–143.
35. Francisco JI, Yu Y, Oliver RA, Walsh WR (2011) Relationship between age, skeletal site, and time post-ovariectomy on bone mineral and trabecular microarchitecture in rats. J Orthop Res 29: 189–196.
36. van den Beucken JJ, Walboomers XF, Vos MR, Sommerdijk NA, Nolte RJ, et al. (2007) Biological responses to multilayered DNA-coatings. J Biomed Mater Res B Appl Biomater 81: 231–238.
37. Thorey F, Menzel H, Lorenz C, Gross G, Hoffmann A, et al. (2010) Enhancement of endoprosthesis anchoring using BMP-2. Technol Health Care 18: 217–229.
38. Ding WG, Wei ZX, Liu JB (2011) Reduced local blood supply to the tibial metaphysis is associated with ovariectomy-induced osteoporosis in mice. Connect Tissue Res 52: 25–29.
39. Sarban S, Senkoylu A, Isikan UE, Korkusuz P, Korkusuz F (2009) Can rhBMP-2 containing collagen sponges enhance bone repair in ovariectomized rats?: a preliminary study. Clin Orthop Relat Res 467: 3113–3120.
40. Moriyama Y, Ayukawa Y, Ogino Y, Atsuta I, Koyano K (2008) Topical application of statin affects bone healing around implants. Clin Oral Implants Res 19: 600–605.
41. Liu Y, Berendsen AD, Jia S, Lotinun S, Baron R, et al. (2012) Intracellular VEGF regulates the balance between osteoblast and adipocyte differentiation. J Clin Invest 122: 3101–3113.

24

Influence of Exercise on Bone Remodeling-Related Hormones and Cytokines in Ovariectomized Rats: A Model of Postmenopausal Osteoporosis

Lihui Li[1¶], Xi Chen[1,4¶], Shuang Lv[1], Miaomiao Dong[1], Li Zhang[1], Jiaheng Tu[1], Jie Yang[1], Lingli Zhang[1], Yinan Song[1], Leiting Xu[1,3]*, Jun Zou[2]*

1 School of Kinesiology, Shanghai University of Sport, Shanghai, China, **2** Scientific Research Department, Shanghai University of Sport, Shanghai, China, **3** Medical School of Ningbo University, Ningbo, China, **4** School of Sports Science, Wenzhou Medical University, Wenzhou, China

Abstract

This study aims to explore the effects of exercise on postmenopausal osteoporosis and the mechanisms by which exercise affects bone remodeling. Sixty-three Wistar female rats were randomly divided into five groups: (1) control group, (2) sham-operated group, (3) OVX (Ovariectomy) group, (4) DES-OVX (Diethylstilbestrol-OVX) group, and (5) Ex-OVX (Exercise-OVX) group. The rat osteoporosis model was established through ovariectomy. The Ex-OVX rats were made to run 251.2 meters every day, 6 d/wk for 3 months in a running wheel. Trabecular bone volume (TBV%), total resorption surface (TRS%), trabecular formation surface (TFS%), mineralization rate (MAR), bone cortex mineralization rate (mAR), and osteoid seam width (OSW) were determined by bone histomorphometry. The mRNA and protein levels of interleukin-1β (IL-1β_2), interleukin-6 (IL-6), and cyclooxygenase-2 (Cox-2) were determined by *in situ* hybridization and immunohistochemistry, respectively. Serum levels of estrogen estradiol (E_2), calcitonin (CT), osteocalcin (BGP), and parathyroid hormone (PTH) were determined by ELISA assays. The investigation revealed that compared to the control and the sham-operated groups, the OVX group showed significantly lower levels of TBV%, E_2, and CT, but much higher levels of TRS%, TFS%, MAR, OSW, BGP, and PTH. The Ex-OVX group showed increased TBV% and serum levels of E_2 and CT compared to the OVX group. Ovariectomy also led to a significant increase in IL-1β mRNA and protein levels in the bone marrow and IL-6 and Cox-2 protein levels in tibias. In addition, the Ex-OVX group showed lower levels of IL-1 mRNA and protein, IL-6 mRNA, and Cox-2 mRNA and protein than those in the OVX group. The upshot of the study suggests that exercise can significantly increase bone mass in postmenopausal osteoporosis rat models by inhibiting bone resorption and increasing bone formation, especially in trabecular bones.

Editor: Luc Malaval, Université de Lyon - Université Jean Monnet, France

Funding: This work was supported by Shanghai Key Lab of Human Sport Competence Development and Maintenance (Shanghai University of sport) (NO. 11DZ2261100), The National Natural Science Foundation of China (Grant No. 81170323). The funders had no role in study design, data collection and analysis, decision to publish, or preparation of the manuscript.

Competing Interests: The authors have declared that no competing interests exist.

* Email: zoujun777@126.com (JZ); xuleiting@nbu.edu.cn (LX)

¶ These authors are co-first authors on this work.

Background

Osteoporosis is a major health problem among the elderly and is characterized by low bone mineral density (T score for bone mineral density below 2.5) and microarchitectural deterioration of bone, leading to increased fracture risks [1]. Osteoporosis is prevalent among women, in particular postmenopausal women. Estrogen shortage/deficiency results in an increase in bone turnover, wherein the rate of osteoclastic resorption exceeds the rate of osteoblastic osteogenesis, leading to a net loss of bone mass. Many studies have indicated that hormone replacement therapies (HRT) can be used to prevent and/or treat postmenopausal osteoporosis. However, long-term estrogen supplementation poses several risks, e.g., endometrial cancer, breast cancer, ovarian cancer, and cardiovascular diseases, and is no longer recommended [2,3].

Previous studies suggest that estrogen may inhibit osteoclast activity through regulating the levels of serum CT and PTH [4]. Estrogen stimulates the synthesis of CT, which directly inhibits osteoclast differentiation and activity, and thus reduces the number of osteoclasts and serum concentration of Ca^{2+} [5]. PTH is one of the most important peptide hormones that regulate calcium and phosphorus homeostasis and bone remodeling [6]. Estrogen can decrease the expression of PTH and lead to a decrease in serum levels of PTH [7]. Estrogen also inhibits PTH-stimulated adenylate cyclase activity and thus PTH-stimulated bone resorption [8]. In addition, estrogen shortage has been found to increase serum levels of BGP (Bone Gla Protein) in postmenopausal women. BGP, also known as γ-carboxyglutamic acid protein, is a hormone-like peptide synthesized and secreted by osteoblasts [9]. BGP is not only an indicator of *in vivo* bone formation rate but also a positive regulator of bone mineralization.

In addition to these hormones, estrogen inhibits bone resorption by suppressing secretion of key osteolytic cytokines such as IL-1 and IL-6 by bone marrow stromal cells and osteoblasts. These cytokines are positive regulators of osteoclast activity and bone resorption [10,11]. Besides, these cytokines may crosstalk with each other to synergistically promote osteoclastogenesis and bone resorption. For example, IL-1, including both IL-1α and IL-1β subunits, can induce osteoblasts to secrete IL-6 to further promote bone resorption [11]. Estrogen, IL-1β, and IL-6 also regulate PGE production, which promotes proliferation and differentiation of osteoclast precursors. Previous studies have reported that PGE_2 could also stimulate bone resorption by increasing IL-6 transcription [12,13]. Furthermore, IL-1 was found to increase COX-2 expression at the mRNA and protein levels, leading to an increase in prostaglandin production. The stabilization of COX-2 mRNA is the most important basis of continued increase in COX-2 protein [14].

Previous studies have shown that increased physical activity is effective in maintaining or even increasing bone and muscle mass in postmenopausal women [15]. Appropriate long-term exercise helps to prevent the development of postmenopausal osteoporosis [16]. Exercise is also effective in maintaining BMD in early postmenopausal women. Kemmler et al. reported that exercises that can improve muscle function might improve overall fitness, maintain bone health, and reduce fall risk [17]. Thus, exercise has been proposed as a preventative measure for osteoporosis. However, the exact mechanisms by which exercise regulates bone remodeling and improves bone quality remain unclear. In animal studies, exercise is generally considered to increase the peak bone mass. Joo et al. showed that treadmill running improves trabecular bone microarchitecture, bone density, and cortical geometry in young growing female rats [18]. Tromp et al. showed that mechanical loading has beneficial effects on bone mineral content (BMC) and bone mineral density of ovariectomized rats [19]. Sakakura et al. showed that exercise has a beneficial effect on tibia and the neck of the condyloid process in ovariectomized rats, probably by increasing serum levels of progesterone [20]. However, how exercise exerts its beneficial effects on bone is not well understood.

We hypothesize that exercise executes its positive influence on bone mass and quality by regulating the synthesis of hormones and cytokines that are involved in bone remodeling. We found that exercise escalates the levels of estrogen in OVX rats, which may suppress the expression of bone resorption stimulators such as CT, IL-1, and IL-6, to inhibit bone resorption. Moreover, we found that exercise also increases bone formation in ovariectomized rats although the mechanisms need further investigation. The results demonstrate that exercise assists in preventing bone loss in rat model of postmenopausal osteoporosis.

Materials and Methods

Animals

This study was carried out in strict accordance with the recommendations from the Ethical Committee of Shanghai University of Sports on the Care and Use of Animal Subjects in Research (Permit Number: [2008](2)), following the protocols approved by the committee. All animals were housed in a temperature- and humidity-controlled environment with a 12 h light/12 h dark cycle with free access to food (standard laboratory chow) and water *ad libitum*. All surgery was performed under sodium pentobarbital anesthesia, and all possible efforts were made to minimize suffering.

Surgical Procedures

A total of 63 female Wistar rats (200 g to 220 g) were obtained from the Laboratory Animal Center of the Academy of Military

Table 1. The mRNA sequence of IL-1β target genes.

Group	The mRNA sequence of IL-1β target genes							
No.1	5′	ACAAA	ATACC	TGTGG	CCTTG	GGCCT	CAAGG	3′
No.2	5′	GAAGA	AGATG	GAAAA	GCGAT	TTGTC	TTCAA	3′
No.3	5′	CAACT	GGTAC	ATCAG	CACCT	CTCAA	GCAGA	3′

Table 2. The mRNA sequence of IL-6 target genes.

Group	The mRNA sequence of IL-6 target genes							
No.1	5′	CTCCG	CAAGA	GACTT	CCAGC	CAGCT	GCCTT	3′
No.2	5′	CTTCC	AAACT	GGATA	TAACC	AGGAA	ATTTG	3′
No.3	5′	ATTTC	TAAAG	GTCAC	TATGA	GGTCT	ACTCG	3′

Table 3. The mRNA sequence of COX-2 target genes.

Group	The mRNA sequence of COX-2 target genes							
No.1	5′	ATGTA	TGAGT	GTGGG	ATTTG	ACCAG	TATAA	3′
No.2	5′	GAACG	TTGTG	AATAA	CATTC	CCTTC	CTTCG	3′
No.3	5′	TGCCT	CAATT	CAGTC	TCTCA	TCTGC	AATAA	3′

Medical Sciences, PCLA (License No. SCXK-(military) 2002-001) and maintained in the Laboratory Animal Rooms (License No. SYK11-00-0039) of the Institute of Basic Theory, Chinese Academy of Chinese Medical Sciences. The rats were randomly divided into five groups: control group (n = 13), sham-operated group (n = 13), OVX group (n = 13), DES-OVX group (n = 13), and Ex-OVX group (n = 11). Rats in the OVX group, the DES-OVX group, and the Ex-OVX group were ovariectomized. To remove the ovaries, rats were anesthetized using an intraperitoneal injection of pentobarbital sodium (48 mg/kg) while in prone position. They were shaved along the midaxillary line, 0.5 cm away from the lateral border of the spine below the last rib, exposing the surgical field. An incision on the skin was made on one side through the musculature and peritoneum, and the ovary was subsequently retracted and removed. Tubal ligation was performed, and then the wound was closed. The same procedure was repeated on the other side. The procedure was also performed on rats belonging to the sham-operated group, except that the ovaries of these rats were retracted and put back into their abdomen and some adipose tissues around their ovaries were removed.

Physical exercise protocol for animals

Two and a half months after surgery, a two-week acclimation period of wheel running training was conducted. Rats in the Ex-OVX group were given access to a running wheel (40 cm diameter, homemade) for 10 min on d 1, with an increase of 10 min/d thereafter until 1 h/d was reached. Wheel revolutions and running distance were counted and automatically recorded using a counter. Three months after surgery, rats in the Ex-OVX group were made to run 200 revolutions (251.2 meters) in the running wheel every day, 6 d/wk for 3 months. Rats belonging to the DES-OVX group were intragastrically administered with Diethylstilbestrol (0.045 mg/kg; concentration, 0.0045 mg/ml; Beijing Yimin Pharmaceutical Co., Ltd., Batch No. H11020899). The control, OVX, and sham-operated groups were given distilled water every day, 6 d/wk for 3 months.

Animal tissue preparation

Rats in all groups were given two intraperitoneal injections of tetracycline hydrochloride (30 mg/kg; Aozehui Technology and Trade Company, US22105) 3 and 16 d before exercising. Five and a half months after surgery, all rats were anesthetized using an intraperitoneal injection of pentobarbital sodium (45 mg/kg; Beijing Tongxian Yucai Fine Chemical Works, Batch No. 950427). When rats appeared to clamping as judged by independent animal care personnel with no knowledge of the protocol design, they were euthanized by Carbon monoxide in a box. Then rats' blood samples were collected from the femoral arteries. The tibias were harvested, with the right tibias being used for undecalcified bone sections to determine bone morphometric indices and the left ones being used for decalcified bone frozen sections for in situ hybridization to detect IL-1β, IL-6, and COX-2 mRNA levels. The blood obtained from the femoral arteries was centrifuged (2000 r/min) and the supernatant was collected. The serum was transferred to an Eppendorf tube and preserved at −20°C for future detection of E2, calcitonin, osteocalcin, and parathyroid hormone.

Bone histomorphometry

The proximal one-third of the right tibias of the rats were obtained and the soft tissues, along with some cortex at both ends, were removed. The samples were dehydrated in increasing concentrations of ethanol (twice at each concentration, each time for 24 h), and xylene was used as a transparency agent (50% ethanol + 50% xylene 30 min, and xylene 30 min twice). The next step was resination of the samples by immersing them in the solutions described below: Solution I: 75 ml methyl methacrylate (Beijing Yili Fine Chemical Co. Ltd., Batch No. 960523), 25 ml dibutyl phthalate (DBP; Beijing Chemical Reagent Company, Batch No. 970628); Solution II: 1 g benzoyl peroxide (Beijing Jinlong Chemical Reagent Co. Ltd., Batch No. 20000420) added to Solution I; Solution III: 2.5 g benzoyl peroxide added to Solution I. Each of these solutions was mixed using a magnetic stirrer. The specimens were sequentially immersed in Solutions I, II, and III, for 36 hrs each. Afterwards, 5 ml of Solution III was injected into a small bottle containing penicillin. The specimens were placed in the bottle. The closed bottle was then placed in an incubator. Polymerization was performed at 40°C for 3 d to 4 d. A hard, colorless, transparent block with embedded samples was formed. The block was taken out and shaped using a file. The resulting undecalcified bone sections were cut at a thickness of 5 or 10 μm on a microtome (Autocut 2040, Reichert-Jung, Heidelberg, Germany) with a tungsten steel blade. The 5 μm-thick undecalcified bone sections were placed in methyl methacrylate for 2 h and then twice in xylene, each time for 1 h. After deresination, the sections were again dehydrated with increasing concentrations of ethanol and stained with toluidine blue. The 10 μm-thick undecalcified bone sections were directly subjected to fluorescence observation.

Leica QWin image analysis software was used to determine the morphometric indices of the undecalcified bone sections using the method reported by Liu [21]. The morphometric indices of trabecular bone, including trabecular bone volume (TBV%), total

Table 4. TBV, TRS, and TFS percentages in the five groups.

Group	TBV%	TRS%	TFS%
control group	31.75 ± 6.23	3.65 ± 1.32	4.07 ± 1.21
sham-operated group	31.05 ± 5.88	3.76 ± 1.37	3.91 ± 1.29
OVX group	$13.21 \pm 3.91^{\square\square **}$	$9.48 \pm 2.63^{\square\square **}$	$7.92 \pm 1.76^{\square\square **}$
DES-OVX group	$25.81 \pm 4.79^{\square * \triangle\triangle}$	$5.09 \pm 1.79^{\square * \triangle\triangle}$	$5.31 \pm 1.37^{\square * \triangle\triangle}$
Ex-OVX group	$16.90 \pm 4.52^{\square\square ** \triangle \blacktriangle\blacktriangle}$	$8.59 \pm 1.65^{\square\square ** \blacktriangle\blacktriangle}$	$9.58 \pm 1.56^{\square\square ** \triangle \blacktriangle\blacktriangle}$

compared with the control group: $^{\square}p<0.05$, $^{\square\square}p<0.01$;
compared with the sham-operated: $^{*}p<0.05$, $^{**}p<0.01$;
compared with the OVX group: $^{\triangle}p<0.05$, $^{\triangle\triangle}p<0.01$;
compared with the DES-OVX group: $^{\blacktriangle\blacktriangle}p<0.01$.

Table 5. The levels of MAR, mAR, and OSW in the five groups.

Group	MAR (μm/d)	mAR (μm/d)	OSW (μm)
control group	1.31 ± 0.25	1.98 ± 0.38	10.17 ± 1.90
sham-operated group	1.49 ± 0.27	2.11 ± 0.32	9.77 ± 1.90
OVX group	$2.52\pm0.40^{\square\square**}$	$3.31\pm0.56^{\square\square**}$	$16.79\pm3.85^{\square\square**}$
DES-OVX group	$1.73\pm0.33^{\triangle\triangle}$	$2.06\pm0.31^{\triangle\triangle}$	$10.32\pm2.63^{\triangle\triangle}$
Ex-OVX group	$2.22\pm0.33^{\square\square**\blacktriangle\blacktriangle}$	$2.62\pm0.36^{\square\square**\triangle\triangle\blacktriangle\blacktriangle}$	$14.85\pm2.25^{\square\square**\blacktriangle\blacktriangle}$

compared with the control group: $^{\square\square}p<0.01$;
compared with the sham-operated: $^{**}p<0.01$;
compared with the OVX group: $^{\triangle\triangle}p<0.01$;
compared with the DES-OVX group: $^{\blacktriangle\blacktriangle}p<0.01$.

resorption surface (TRS%), trabecular formation surface (TFS%), and mineralization rate (MAR), as well as those of the inner surface of the cortex bone, including osteoid seam width (OSW) and bone cortex mineralization rate (mAR), were calculated.

Quantitation of IL-1β, IL-6, and COX-2

The proximal one-third of the left tibias of the rats was harvested with the soft tissues removed. The tibias were then fixed in 4% paraformaldehyde for 24 h, fully rinsed using PBS, and decalcified for 3 wk at 4°C using 10% EDTA/PBS. The decalcification solution was changed every other day. The decalcified bones were rinsed with PBS and then dehydrated in 15% sucrose solution/PBS for 24 h. Frozen sections were later cut at 10 μm on a refrigerated microtome (BRIGHT–5030, UK).

Immunohistochemical staining was used to detect IL-1β, IL-6, and COX-2 protein levels. IL-1β, IL-6, and COX-2 mRNA levels in the rat tibias were determined using in situ hybridization kits (Wuhan Boster Biological Technology, Ltd.). Oligonucleotide probes for IL-1β, IL-6, and COX-2 were labeled with digoxin. The mRNA sequences transcribed from the human IL-1β genes are shown in **Table 1**. The only difference among the sequences of rat, mouse, and human lies on 1 bp/90 bp. The mRNA sequences transcribed from the rat and mouse IL-6 genes are shown in **Table 2**. The mRNA sequences transcribed from the human COX-2 target genes are shown in **Table 3**. The only difference among the sequences of rat, mouse, and human lies on 5 bp/90 bp. In the morphometric analysis that used the Leica Q Win image analysis software, a positive reaction was indicated by brown coloration of the cytoplasm. More than five high-power fields (×400) below the epiphyseal plate within the medullary cavity were randomly picked and analyzed. The mRNA and protein level of IL-6 and COX-2 in osteoblasts was determined by the ratio of positive cells area per trabecular area in high-power field, and the mRNA and protein level of IL-1β in bone marrow was determined by the ratio of positive cells area per high-power field (without trabecular area), the mean was calculated and recorded as the percentage of positively reacting cells (%).

Measurement of serum CT, BGP, PTH, and E_2

ELISA assays were adapted to determine the levels of serum CT, BGP, PTH, and E_2. ELISA kits for rat BGP, CT, and PTH were purchased from Market Company (Batch Nos. RE030, IR108, and IR067) and the E_2 kit was purchased from Tianjing Jiuding Biomedical Engineering Ltd. (Batch No. ESBL4287).

Statistical analysis

Data are presented as mean ± standard deviation. Statistical evaluation was performed using one-way ANOVA. Data were compared between groups, and a Q-test was performed.

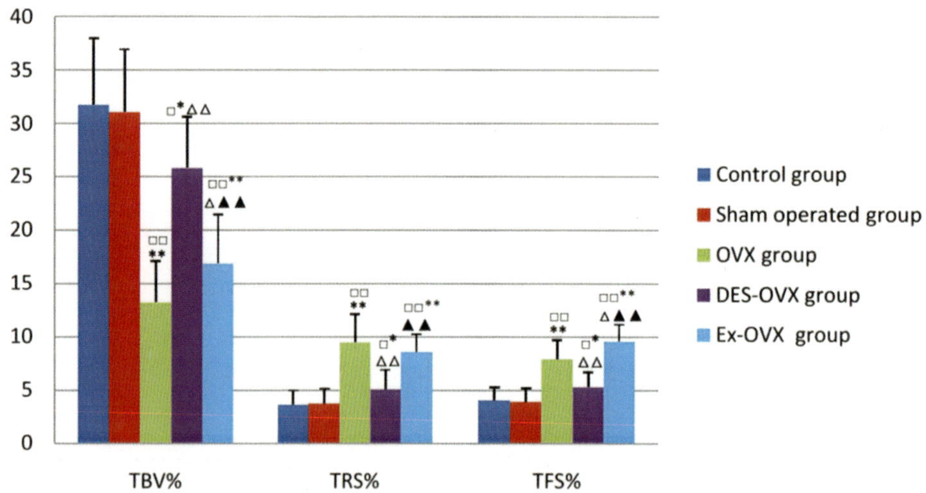

Figure 1. TBV, TRS, and TFS percentages in the five groups. compared with the control group: $^{\square}p<0.05$, $^{\square\square}p<0.01$; compared with the sham-operated: $^{*}p<0.05$, $^{**}p<0.01$; compared with the OVX group: $^{\triangle}p<0.05$, $^{\triangle\triangle}p<0.01$; compared with the DES-OVX group: $^{\blacktriangle\blacktriangle}p<0.01$.

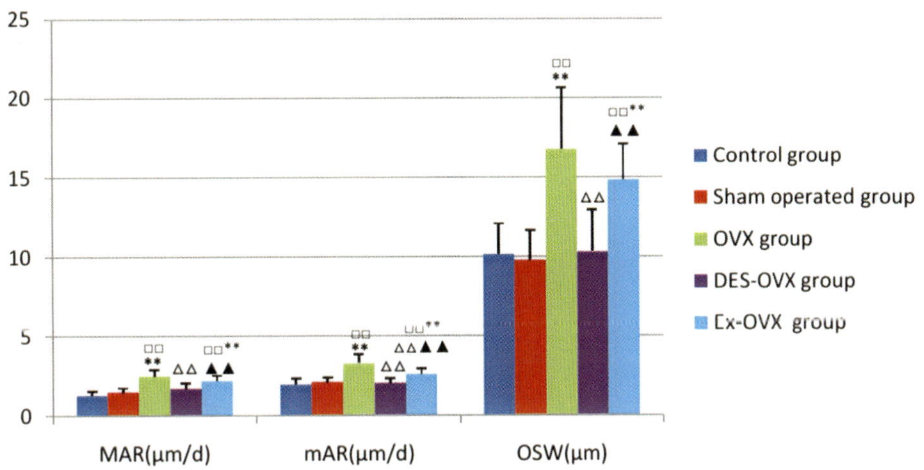

Figure 2. MAR, mAR, and OSW in the five groups. compared with the control group: □□$p<0.01$; compared with the sham-operated: **$p<0.01$; compared with the OVX group: △△$p<0.01$; compared with the DES-OVX group: ▲▲$p<0.01$.

Significant differences were considered at $p<0.05$ and highly significant differences at $p<0.01$.

Results

In this study, we studied the effects of exercise on bone remodeling parameters of ovariectomized rats by histomorphometry and explored whether bone remodeling-related hormones and cytokines are involved.

Effect of exercise on bone histomorphometric parameters

As shown in **Table 4 and Figure 1**, the TBV% of the OVX group was significantly lower than the control and the sham-operated groups, which was accompanied by increased TRS, confirming that ovariectomy led to increased bone resorption and bone loss in rats. Moreover, the OVX group rats also showed higher levels of TFS%, MAR, mAR, and OSW than the control and sham-operated group rats (**Table 5 and Figure 2**), suggesting that these rats also displayed increased bone formation, which is likely caused by the coupling between bone resorption and formation. Thus, ovariectomized rats showed high bone turnover rate, with the increase in bone resorption being greater than that in bone formation. These findings are in accordance with previous studies and suggest that the surgery was successful in this study. To confirm these findings, we also treated ovariectomized rats with DES and found that DES almost completely reversed the bone loss and restored the bone parameters. In addition, none of the parameters was significantly different between the sham-operated group and the normal control group, which excludes the impact of surgical factors.

More importantly, exercise significantly increased the bone mass in the Ex-OVX group rats, which could be attributable to a decrease in bone resorption and an increase in bone formation, as TRS% was decreased whereas TFS% was increased compared to the OVX group. These bone histomorphometric parameters were measured in trabecular bones. On the other hand, the cortical bone parameters including MAR, mAR, and OSW were slightly decreased in the EX-OVX rats compared to OVX rats. These results suggest exercise can inhibit bone resorption and increase trabecular bone formation, which helps to prevent further bone loss in ovariectomized rats.

Effect of exercise on serum levels of CT, BGP, PTH, and E_2

We then analyzed some of the hormones that are involved in bone remodeling, especially the hormones whose levels are altered in post-menopausal osteoporotic patients and animal models. As shown in **Table 6 and Figure 3**, rats in the OVX group had much lower E_2 whereas DES-OVX rats showed E2 levels that were comparable to the control rats. Interestingly, exercise significantly increased serum levels of E2, which might be

Table 6. The levels of CT, BGP, PTH, and E_2 in the five groups.

Group	CT (pg/ml)	BGP (ng/ml)	PTH (pg/ml)	E2 (pg/ml)
control group	9.98±1.33	4.76±0.90	41.72±9.14	40.36±15.91
sham-operated group	10.13±1.24	4.94±1.03	42.30±12.52	40.87±19.61
OVX group	5.88±1.02□□**	10.14±1.06□□**	54.03±10.27□□*	5.09±1.07□□**
DES-OVX group	8.78±1.09□**△△	3.09±1.06□□**△△	44.13±6.60△△	37.38±12.78△△
Ex-OVX group	7.30±1.61□□**△▲	8.85±1.81□□**△▲▲	51.65±11.83□	6.98±1.46□□**△△▲▲

compared with the control group: □$p<0.05$, □□$p<0.01$;
compared with the sham-operated: *$p<0.05$, **$p<0.01$;
compared with the OVX group: △$p<0.05$, △△$p<0.01$;
compared with the DES-OVX group: ▲$p<0.05$, ▲▲$p<0.01$.

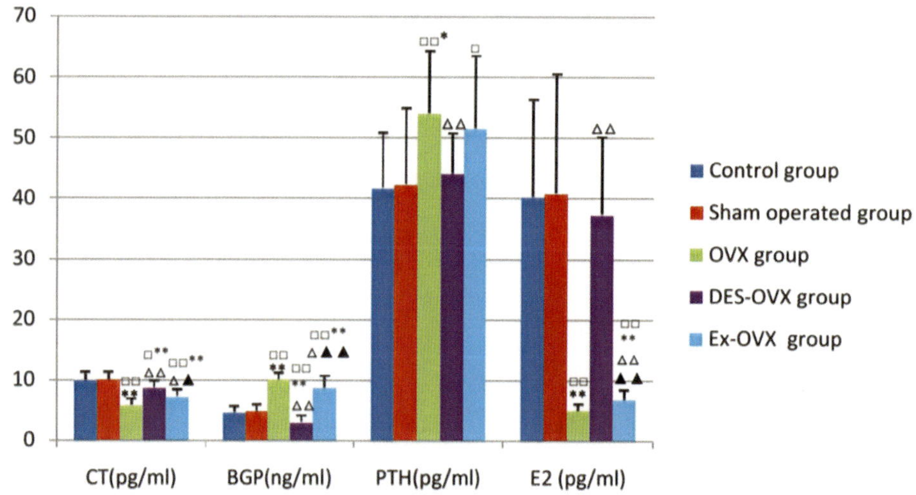

Figure 3. CT, BGP, PTH, and E_2 in the five groups. compared with the control group: □$p<0.05$, □□$p<0.01$; compared with the sham-operated: *$p<0.05$, **$p<0.01$; compared with the OVX group: △$p<0.05$, △△$p<0.01$; compared with the DES-OVX group: ▲$p<0.05$, ▲▲$p<0.01$.

synthesized and secreted by organs other than the ovary [22]. The increase in E2 levels was expected to inhibit bone resorption.

Moreover, the levels of CT, a negative regulator of osteoclast differentiation and activity, were decreased in OVX rats. On the other hand, the levels of PTH, a positive regulator of bone resorption, were increased in the OVX group compared to the control and the sham-operated groups. Additionally, the change in these two hormones was restored to close to normal levels in the DES-OVX group. These results suggest that estrogen deficiency led to a decrease in CT but an increase in PTH in ovariectomized rat. Furthermore, the levels of BGP, an osteoblast-produced hormone that promotes bone mineralization and acts as an indicator of in vivo bone formation rate, was also increased in ovariectomized rats. These results are consistent with our finding that estrogen deficiency leads to enhanced bone formation, in which BGP might play a positive role.

We also found that rats in the Ex-OVX group showed higher levels of CT and lower levels of BGP than the OVX rats, without significantly changing the levels of PTH. Note that the Ex-OVX group still showed lower levels of CT and E2, as well as higher levels of BGP and PTH, than the control and the sham-operated groups. These findings suggest that exercise may inhibit bone loss and prevent osteoporosis by regulating the serum levels of CT, PTH, and BGP.

Alteration of protein levels of IL-1β in the bone marrow and IL-6 and COX-2 in tibias

As shown in **Table 7 and Figure 4**, the OVX rats showed an increase in the protein levels of IL-1β, IL-6, and COX-2 compared to the control and the sham-operated groups, which were all restored to normal levels in the DES-OVX group, suggesting that estrogen deficiency is the reason behind the alteration of the expression of these proteins. Moreover, we found that the Ex-OVX group had much lower levels of IL-1β, IL-6, and COX-2 than the OVX group. These results suggest that exercise could partially inhibit the expression of IL-1β, IL-6, and COX-2, which helps to suppress bone resorption.

Alteration of mRNA levels of IL-1β in the bone marrow and IL-6 and COX-2 in tibias

To validate the above finding, we also analyzed the mRNA levels of these proteins on bone sections by in situ hybridization. As shown in **Table 8 and Figure 5**, the OVX rats showed much higher levels of IL-1β, IL-6, and COX-2 mRNA than the control and the sham-operated groups, which were restored to normal levels in the DES-OVX group. Moreover, the Ex-OVX group rats showed much lower levels of IL-1β, IL-6, and COX-2 mRNA than the OVX group. These results suggest that exercise could inhibit the expression of these cytokines at the mRNA level.

Table 7. IL-1β, IL-6, and COX-2 protein levels in the five groups.

Group	IL-1βprotein expression (%)	IL-6protein expression (%)	COX-2protein expression (%)
control group	4.84±1.17	5.32±0.92	5.04±0.94
sham-operated group	5.30±1.24	5.41±1.07	5.26±1.08
OVX group	10.76±1.80□□**	8.64±1.65□□**	11.36±2.14□□**
DES-OVX group	5.18±1.05△△	6.03±1.25△△	5.69±0.99△△
Ex-OVX group	7.48±1.37□□**△△▲▲	7.65±1.20□□**▲▲	7.99±1.50□□**△△▲▲

compared with the control group: □□$p<0.01$;
compared with the sham-operated: **$p<0.01$;
compared with the OVX group: △△$p<0.01$;
compared with the DES-OVX group: ▲▲$p<0.01$.

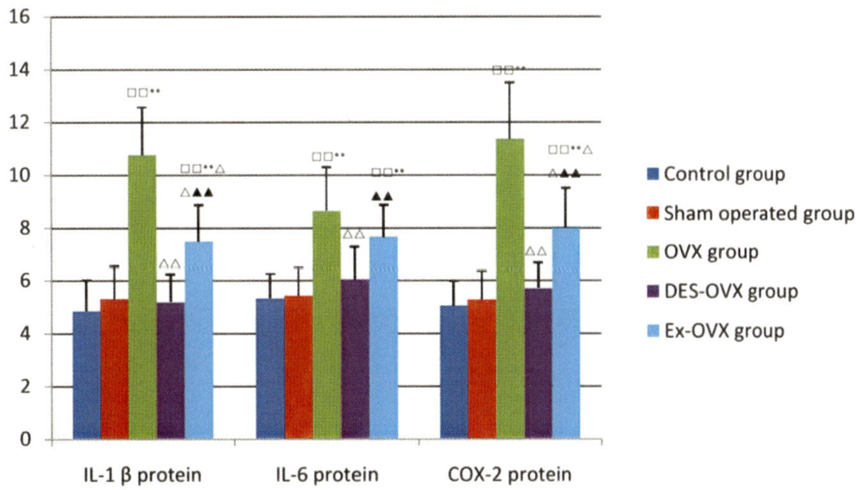

Figure 4. IL-1β, IL-6, and COX-2 protein expression in the five groups. compared with the control group: $^{\square\square}p<0.01$; compared with the sham-operated: $^{**}p<0.01$; compared with the OVX group: $^{\triangle\triangle}p<0.01$; compared with the DES-OVX group: $^{\blacktriangle\blacktriangle}p<0.01$.

Discussion

Ovariectomized rats and mice are well-established models for the study of the pathogenesis of postmenopausal osteoporosis and are widely used for evaluation and development of new drugs for treatment of postmenopausal osteoporosis [23–25]. Here we used the rat model to study the possible effect of exercise on bone remodeling. Consistent with the previous results, we found that ovariectomized rats exhibited a significant decrease in bone mass, whereas bone resorption indexes TRS%, PTH, and bone formation markers TFS%, MAR, OSW, mAR, and BGP, were all significantly increased. This finding indicates that ovariectomy increases bone turnover rate, wherein bone resorption outpaces bone formation, leading to the development of osteoporosis. Moreover, DES was found to reverse all these changes in ovariectomized rats.

Previous studies have shown that osteoporosis-related bone loss in postmenopausal rat was partially prevented by moderate exercise [26–28]. Our findings support this concept and provide more histomorphometric evidence. Rats in the EX-OVX group showed higher TBV% than those in the OVX group, indicating that running wheel improves cancellous bone in ovariectomized rats. Compared to the OVX group, the EX-OVX group rats showed a modest decrease in bone resorption rate, which is correlated with an increase in serum levels of estrogen and CT. On the other hand, exercise increased bone formation, especially of trabecular bones, which is reflected by an increase in TFS%. However, bone formation rate at the endosteal surface of cortical bones in the EX-OVX group was lower than that in the OVX group, suggesting that exercise may differentially regulate bone formation in trabecular and cortical bones. It seems that exercise can partially prevent estrogen deficiency-induced bone loss by suppressing bone resorption and increasing bone formation. While it is still debated whether decreased bone resorption or increased bone formation is the main reason behind exercise-induced bone mass elevation [29,30], our results support the involvement of both events.

Estrogen exerts its anti-osteoporotic activity by directly or indirectly regulating bone resorption [31,32]. While there is convincing evidence that estrogen, acting via estrogen receptor α, stimulates osteoclast apoptosis and suppresses osteoblasts apoptosis [33], estrogen has been shown to act on MSCs and osteoblasts to regulate the expression of cytokines and growth factors that control osteoclast differentiation and activity. Since long-term HRT has adverse effects, caution is expected in choosing HRT for prevention and treatment of osteoporosis in women [34,35]. On the other hand, a number of studies have shown that appropriate intensities of exercise can increase serum levels of estradiol and testosterone, which helps to improve osteoblast proliferation and activity, leading to an increase in bone mass and density [36,37].

Table 8. IL-1β, IL-6, and COX-2 mRNA levels in the five groups.

Group	IL-1βmRNA expression (%)	IL-6mRNA expression (%)	COX-2mRNA expression (%)
control group	6.17±0.99	5.48±1.08	5.28±1.01
sham-operated group	6.14±1.10	5.68±1.13	5.14±1.13
OVX group	11.20±2.02$^{\square\square**}$	9.07±1.33$^{\square\square**}$	10.49±1.36$^{\square\square**}$
DES-OVX group	6.59±1.23$^{\triangle\triangle}$	5.53±1.10$^{\triangle\triangle}$	5.52±1.00$^{\triangle\triangle}$
Ex-OVX group	9.45±1.53$^{\square\square**\triangle\blacktriangle\blacktriangle}$	7.90±1.05$^{\square\square**\triangle\blacktriangle\blacktriangle}$	7.81±1.38$^{\square\square**\triangle\triangle\blacktriangle\blacktriangle}$

compared with the control group: $^{\square\square}p<0.01$;
compared with the sham-operated: $^{**}p<0.01$;
compared with the OVX group: $^{\triangle}p<0.05$, $^{\triangle\triangle}p<0.01$;
compared with the DES-OVX group: $^{\blacktriangle\blacktriangle}p<0.01$.

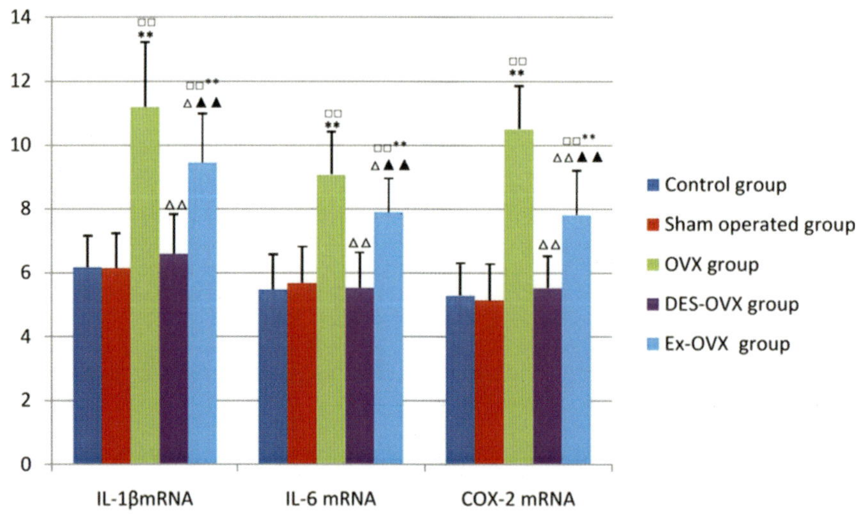

Figure 5. IL-1β, IL-6, and COX-2 mRNA expression in the five groups. compared with the control group: □□*p*<0.01; compared with the sham-operated: ***p*<0.01; compared with the OVX group: △*p*<0.05, △△*p*<0.01; compared with the DES-OVX group: ▲▲*p*<0.01.

However, some clinical studies showed that the estrogen levels were unchanged in response to exercise [38]. This discrepancy could be caused by the difference in the intensities of exercise, the age and ethnicity of the patients, or both. Nevertheless, this study shows that wheel running increases serum E_2 in ovariectomized rats, which can slow down bone loss induced by ovariectomy. In addition, the levels of CT, an inhibitor of osteoclast differentiation and activity [5], are also decreased after ovariectomy, likely due to estrogen shortage. Indeed, previous studies have shown that estrogen stimulates the synthesis of CT [4]. We found that exercise also increases the levels of CT in ovariectomized rats, which might be a result of increased estrogen.

We found that the OVX group rats showed higher levels of BGP and PTH than the control group. BGP is a hormone-like peptide synthesized and secreted by osteoblasts and is significantly increased in the serum of postmenopausal women [9]. It has pro-minerilization function and is an indicator of in vivo bone formation rate. Thus, it is possible that estrogen regulates bone formation and bone resorption thorugh these two hormones as well. The observation that supplementation with diethylstilbestrol reversed the alteration in BGP and PTH expression in ovariectomized rats suggests that estrogen deficiency is the underlying cause for the change in BGP and PTH levels. In addition, we found that exercise decreases the levels of BGP in ovariectomized rats, which might be due to the increase in the E2 levels.

Our study further showed that the protein and mRNA levels of the bone marrow IL-1β and osteoblastic IL-6 and COX-2 were increased in ovariectomized rats. The change in the levels of these proteins was highly related to E_2, as there is no significant difference between the DES-OVX group and the sham-operated group. Charatcharoenwitthaya et al. demonstrated that in humans, like in rodents, part of the effects of estrogen deficiency on increased bone resorption is mediated by IL-1 [39]. Moreover, IL-6 can enhance osteoclastogenesis in vivo and in vitro, which could be prevented by 17 beta-estradiol or an antibody against IL-6. Thus, IL-1 and IL-6 play critical roles in estrogen-regulated osteoclastogenesis. Moreover, IL-1 and IL-6 regulate the expression of Cox-2 and therefore the production of PGE_2, which also increases osteoclast activity and bone resorption [40]. Our study revealed that exercise could effectively decrease the mRNA and protein levels of IL-1, IL-6, and Cox-2 in ovariectomized rats. These results, taken together, suggest that exercise may regulate serum levels of the hormones and cytokines via E2, to inhibit bone resorption and to prevent further bone loss in estrogen deficiency-induced osteoporosis models.

While therapeutic HRT inhibits both osteogenesis and bone resorption, with inhibition of bone resorption being the dominant effect, we found that exercise inhibits bone resorption but increases osteogenesis. The dual beneficial effects of exercise may have positive impact on bone geometry in addition to bone mass and density. As such, an increasing number of researchers are considering using exercise or combination of exercise with drugs such as bisphosphonates to treat osteoporosis [41,42].

Conclusions

Overall, our study revealed that exercise acts on both bone formation and bone resorption to slow down bone loss in ovariectomized rat models. Exercise not only increases the serum levels of E2 but also affects the expression of hormones that play critical roles in bone remodeling, such as CT, BGP and PTH. Moreover, exercise also inhibits the expression of IL-1, IL-6, and Cox-2 to negatively regulate osteoclastogenesis and bone resorption. However, the interaction between these cytokines and hormones needs further investigation.

Author Contributions

Conceived and designed the experiments: JZ. Performed the experiments: SL MD. Analyzed the data: LZ JY. Contributed reagents/materials/analysis tools: LZ JT. Wrote the paper: LL LX YS XC. Provided suggestions and wrote most of the revised version: XC LX.

References

1. Nih Consensus Development Panel on Osteoporosis Prevention D, Therapy (2001) Osteoporosis prevention, diagnosis, and therapy. JAMA 285: 785–795.
2. Lacey JV, Jr., Mink PJ, Lubin JH, Sherman ME, Troisi R, et al. (2002) Menopausal hormone replacement therapy and risk of ovarian cancer. JAMA 288: 334–341.
3. Nelson HD, Humphrey LL, Nygren P, Teutsch SM, Allan JD (2002) Postmenopausal hormone replacement therapy: scientific review. JAMA 288: 872–881.
4. Doggrell SA (2004) Recent important clinical trials of drugs in osteoporosis. Expert Opin Pharmacother 5: 1635–1638.
5. Karsdal MA, Henriksen K, Arnold M, Christiansen C (2008) Calcitonin: a drug of the past or for the future? Physiologic inhibition of bone resorption while sustaining osteoclast numbers improves bone quality. BioDrugs 22: 137–144.
6. Gesty-Palmer D, Luttrell LM (2011) 'Biasing' the parathyroid hormone receptor: a novel anabolic approach to increasing bone mass? Br J Pharmacol 164: 59–67.
7. Carrillo-Lopez N, Roman-Garcia P, Rodriguez-Rebollar A, Fernandez-Martin JL, Naves-Diaz M, et al. (2009) Indirect regulation of PTH by estrogens may require FGF23. J Am Soc Nephrol 20: 2009–2017.
8. Nakamura M, Udagawa N, Matsuura S, Mogi M, Nakamura H, et al. (2003) Osteoprotegerin regulates bone formation through a coupling mechanism with bone resorption. Endocrinology 144: 5441–5449.
9. Price PA, Parthemore JG, Deftos LJ (1980) New biochemical marker for bone metabolism. Measurement by radioimmunoassay of bone GLA protein in the plasma of normal subjects and patients with bone disease. J Clin Invest 66: 878–883.
10. Edwards CJ, Williams E (2010) The role of interleukin-6 in rheumatoid arthritis-associated osteoporosis. Osteoporos Int 21: 1287–1293.
11. Kwan Tat S, Padrines M, Theoleyre S, Heymann D, Fortun Y (2004) IL-6, RANKL, TNF-alpha/IL-1: interrelations in bone resorption pathophysiology. Cytokine Growth Factor Rev 15: 49–60.
12. Subbaramaiah K, Marmo TP, Dixon DA, Dannenberg AJ (2003) Regulation of cyclooxgenase-2 mRNA stability by taxanes: evidence for involvement of p38, MAPKAPK-2, and HuR. J Biol Chem 278: 37637–37647.
13. Denkert C, Weichert W, Winzer KJ, Muller BM, Noske A, et al. (2004) Expression of the ELAV-like protein HuR is associated with higher tumor grade and increased cyclooxygenase-2 expression in human breast carcinoma. Clin Cancer Res 10: 5580–5586.
14. de Araujo Junior RF, Souza TO, de Medeiros CA, de Souza LB, Freitas Mde L, et al. (2013) Carvedilol decrease IL-1beta and TNF-alpha, inhibits MMP-2, MMP-9, COX-2, and RANKL expression, and up-regulates OPG in a rat model of periodontitis. PLoS One 8: e66391.
15. Going S, Lohman T, Houtkooper L, Metcalfe L, Flint-Wagner H, et al. (2003) Effects of exercise on bone mineral density in calcium-replete postmenopausal women with and without hormone replacement therapy. Osteoporos Int 14: 637–643.
16. Evans EM, Racette SB, Van Pelt RE, Peterson LR, Villareal DT (2007) Effects of soy protein isolate and moderate exercise on bone turnover and bone mineral density in postmenopausal women. Menopause 14: 481–488.
17. Kemmler W, von Stengel S, Engelke K, Haberle L, Kalender WA (2010) Exercise effects on bone mineral density, falls, coronary risk factors, and health care costs in older women: the randomized controlled senior fitness and prevention (SEFIP) study. Arch Intern Med 170: 179–185.
18. Joo YI, Sone T, Fukunaga M, Lim SG, Onodera S (2003) Effects of endurance exercise on three-dimensional trabecular bone microarchitecture in young growing rats. Bone 33: 485–493.
19. Tromp AM, Bravenboer N, Tanck E, Oostlander A, Holzmann PJ, et al. (2006) Additional weight bearing during exercise and estrogen in the rat: the effect on bone mass, turnover, and structure. Calcif Tissue Int 79: 404–415.
20. Sakakura Y, Shide N, Tsuruga E, Irie K, Yajima T (2001) Effects of running exercise on the mandible and tibia of ovariectomized rats. J Bone Miner Metab 19: 159–167.
21. Liu SQ (1996) Plastic-embedded undecalcified bone tissue glasscutter slicing technology. Chinese Journal of Pathology 25: 49.
22. Wood CE, Stavisky RC, Nowak J, Kaplan JR (2012) Stimulatory adrenocortical effects of a selective estrogen receptor modulator in ovariectomized female macaques. Toxicol Pathol 40: 55–61.
23. Saville PD (1969) Changes in skeletal mass and fragility with castration in the rat; a model of osteoporosis. J Am Geriatr Soc 17: 155–166.
24. Inada M, Matsumoto C, Miyaura C (2011) [Animal models for bone and joint disease. Ovariectomized and orchidectomized animals]. Clin Calcium 21: 164–170.
25. Chachra D, Lee JM, Kasra M, Grynpas MD (2000) Differential effects of ovariectomy on the mechanical properties of cortical and cancellous bone in rat femora and vertebrae. Biomed Sci Instrum 36: 123–128.
26. Barengolts EI, Curry DJ, Bapna MS, Kukreja SC (1993) Effects of endurance exercise on bone mass and mechanical properties in intact and ovariectomized rats. J Bone Miner Res 8: 937–942.
27. Chen Y, Wang S, Bu S, Wang Y, Duan Y, et al. (2011) Treadmill training prevents bone loss by inhibition of PPARgamma expression but not promoting of Runx2 expression in ovariectomized rats. Eur J Appl Physiol 111: 1759–1767.
28. Winters-Stone KM, Dobek J, Nail LM, Bennett JA, Leo MC, et al. (2013) Impact + resistance training improves bone health and body composition in prematurely menopausal breast cancer survivors: a randomized controlled trial. Osteoporos Int 24: 1637–1646.
29. Iwamoto J, Takeda T, Ichimura S (1998) Effects of moderate intensity exercise on tibial bone mass in mature ovariectomized rats: bone histomorphometry study. Keio J Med 47: 162–167.
30. Barengolts EI, Lathon PV, Curry DJ, Kukreja SC (1994) Effects of endurance exercise on bone histomorphometric parameters in intact and ovariectomized rats. Bone Miner 26: 133–140.
31. Gong YS, Chen J, Zhang QZ, Zhang JT (2006) Effect of 17beta-oestradiol and ginsenoside on osteoporosis in ovariectomised rats. J Asian Nat Prod Res 8: 649–656.
32. Zhao X, Wu ZX, Zhang Y, Yan YB, He Q, et al. (2011) Anti-osteoporosis activity of Cibotium barometz extract on ovariectomy-induced bone loss in rats. J Ethnopharmacol 137: 1083–1088.
33. Nakamura T, Imai Y, Matsumoto T, Sato S, Takeuchi K, et al. (2007) Estrogen prevents bone loss via estrogen receptor alpha and induction of Fas ligand in osteoclasts. Cell 130: 811–823.
34. Cummings SR, Ensrud K, Delmas PD, LaCroix AZ, Vukicevic S, et al. (2010) Lasofoxifene in postmenopausal women with osteoporosis. N Engl J Med 362: 686–696.
35. Prestwood KM, Kenny AM, Kleppinger A, Kulldorff M (2003) Ultralow-dose micronized 17beta-estradiol and bone density and bone metabolism in older women: a randomized controlled trial. JAMA 290: 1042–1048.
36. Scott JP, Sale C, Greeves JP, Casey A, Dutton J, et al. (2014) Treadmill running reduces parathyroid hormone concentrations during recovery compared with a nonexercising control group. J Clin Endocrinol Metab 99: 1774–1782.
37. Wallace BA, Cumming RG (2000) Systematic review of randomized trials of the effect of exercise on bone mass in pre- and postmenopausal women. Calcif Tissue Int 67: 10–18.
38. Campbell KL, Westerlind KC, Harber VJ, Bell GJ, Mackey JR, et al. (2007) Effects of aerobic exercise training on estrogen metabolism in premenopausal women: a randomized controlled trial. Cancer Epidemiol Biomarkers Prev 16: 731–739.
39. Charatcharoenwitthaya N, Khosla S, Atkinson EJ, McCready LK, Riggs BL (2007) Effect of blockade of TNF-alpha and interleukin-1 action on bone resorption in early postmenopausal women. J Bone Miner Res 22: 724–729.
40. Yuk TH, Kang JH, Lee SR, Yuk SW, Lee KG, et al. (2002) Inhibitory effect of Carthamus tinctorius L. seed extracts on bone resorption mediated by tyrosine kinase, COX-2 (cyclooxygenase) and PG (prostaglandin) E2. Am J Chin Med 30: 95–108.
41. Leblanc A, Matsumoto T, Jones J, Shapiro J, Lang T, et al. (2013) Bisphosphonates as a supplement to exercise to protect bone during long-duration spaceflight. Osteoporos Int 24: 2105–2114.
42. Liu M, Zhong C, He RX, Chen LF (2012) Icariin associated with exercise therapy is an effective treatment for postmenopausal osteoporosis. Chin Med J (Engl) 125: 1784–1789.

Seven Day Insertion Rest in Whole Body Vibration Improves Multi-Level Bone Quality in Tail Suspension Rats

Rui Zhang[1], He Gong[1]*, Dong Zhu[2]*, Jiazi Gao[1], Juan Fang[1], Yubo Fan[3]

1 Department of Engineering Mechanics, Jilin University, Changchun, Jilin, People's Republic of China, **2** Department of Orthopedic Surgery, No. 1 Hospital of Jilin University, Changchun, Jilin, People's Republic of China, **3** School of Biological Science and Medical Engineering, Beihang University, Beijing, People's Republic of China

Abstract

Objective: This study aimed to investigate the effects of low-magnitude, high-frequency vibration with rest days on bone quality at multiple levels.

Methods: Forty-nine three-month-old male Wistar rats were randomly divided into seven groups, namely, vibrational loading for *X* day followed by *X* day rest (VLXR, *X* = 1, 3, 5, 7), vibrational loading every day (VLNR), tail suspension (SPD), and baseline control (BCL). One week after tail suspension, rats were loaded by vibrational loading (35 Hz, 0.25 g, 15 min/day) except SPD and BCL. Fluorescence markers were used in all rats. Eight weeks later, femora were harvested to investigate macromechanical properties, and micro-computed tomography scanning and fluorescence test were used to evaluate microarchitecture and bone growth rate. Atomic force microscopy analyses and nanoindentation test were used to analyze the nanostructure and mechanical properties of bone material, respectively. Inductively coupled plasma optical emission spectroscopy was used for quantitative chemical analyses.

Results: Microarchitecture, mineral apposition rate and bone formation rate and macromechanical properties were improved in VL7R. Grain size and roughness were significantly different among all groups. No statistical difference was found for the mechanical properties of the bone material, and the chemical composition of all groups was almost similar.

Conclusions: Low-magnitude, high-frequency vibration with rest days altered bone microarchitecture and macro-biomechanical properties, and VL7R was more efficacious in improving bone loss caused by mechanical disuse, which provided theoretical basis and explored the mechanisms of vibration for improving bone quality in clinics.

Editor: João Costa-Rodrigues, Faculdade de Medicina Dentária, Universidade do Porto, Portugal

Funding: This work is supported by the National Natural Science Foundation of China (Nos. 11322223 and 11272134), the 973 Program (No. 2012CB821202), and the Program for New Century Excellent Talents in University (NCET-12-0024). The funders had no role in study design, data collection and analysis, decision to publish, or preparation of the manuscript.

Competing Interests: The authors have declared that no competing interests exist.

* E-mail: gonghe1976@yahoo.com (HG); swyxgc@126.com (DZ)

Introduction

Bone tissue is a complex composite biological material with the ability for functional adaptation. Mechanical environment is an important factor in controlling and influencing bone structure. Osteoporosis is a systemic skeletal disease characterized by low bone mass and microarchitecture deterioration of bone tissue, with a consequent increase in bone fragility and susceptibility to fracture [1]. Many factors contribute to onset of bone loss. In addition to hormone deficiency, microgravity can also lead to bone loss. For astronauts staying four to six months in space, the mineral content of lower limb bones decreases remarkably, and the rate of loss of bone mineral density (BMD) is almost 1.6% per month [2,3]. In a gravitational environment for the duration of space travel, deterioration of some bone structures is irreversible though the bone mass has started to increase [4].

Pharmacologic treatment is the most popular intervention to prevent osteoporosis, but is unsuitable for all patients because of potential side effects [5]. Thus, non-invasive and non-pharmacologic therapy is a focus of current research in osteoporosis treatment [6,7]. Low-level mechanical stimuli can improve both quantity and quality of trabecular bone in 6 to 8 years old female sheep, which (if applicable in humans) may serve as an effective intervention for osteoporosis [8]. After daily mechanical stimulation of the hindlimbs of adult sheep for a year with 20 min bursts of very-low-magnitude, high-frequency vibration, the density of trabecular bone in the proximal femur significantly increases (by 34.2%) than those in controls [6]. A pilot randomized controlled trial in disabled children demonstrated that low-magnitude, high-frequency mechanical stimuli are anabolic to trabecular bone, and may provide a non-pharmacologic treatment for bone fragility [9]. In addition, clinical studies of bone responses to exercise, bed rest, and microgravity confirmed the sensitivity of bone to physical and environmental stimuli [10]. The beneficial effects on bone mass and strength can be attributed to the sensitivity of bone cells to mechanical stimuli. However, bone cells lose mechanical sensitivity soon after stimulation, and a rest interval between each low-magnitude load cycle can create a potent anabolic stimulus [11–13]. Compared with daily loading, Ma et al. found that low-magnitude, high-frequency mechanical vibration is more effective in improving bone microarchitecture and biomechanical properties in ovariectomised rodents if the long-duration mechanical stimulus is separated by several rest days [14]. However, the influence of vibration with rest days on osteoporosis caused by mechanical disuse remains unknown. Long-term limb disuse may disorder normal bone metabolism. Bone tissue is below or next to the threshold of bone remodeling, and the amount of bone resorption in remodeling process is greater than bone formation, which results in decreased bone mass. However, this is different from osteoporosis caused by the decline of ovarian function in women after menopause, which may increase the mechanical set point of mechanostat [15]. Because of the different nature between disuse osteoporosis and estrogen-deficient osteoporosis, the bone qualities in response to this new type of low-magnitude, high-frequency intermittent mechanical intervention strategy proposed by Ma et al. [14] need to be further investigated through mechanical disuse model for the osteoporosis caused by weightlessness.

The mechanical properties of bone are determined by not only the structure and geometry, but also the tissue properties of bone material itself [16]. Considerable evidence demonstrated that bone mass and microarchitecture are sensitive to mechanical stimuli, and a feedback regulatory mechanism between external load and metabolism must exist [17]. This mechanism needs to be explored thoroughly using multi-level investigations, i.e. mechanical testing or micro-computed tomography (micro-CT) for bone qualities (e.g., elastic modulus or BMD) [18]. Atomic force microscopy (AFM) was recently used to improve our knowledge of the nanostructure of bone material because the dimensions of many microarchitecture features of interest in bone tissue are several micrometers or less [19–25]. In addition, elastic properties of bone microarchitecture components differ from the macroscopic values, and nanoindentation is a mechanical microprobe method that allows the direct simultaneous measurement of elastic modulus and hardness of the material [26–29].

The previous studies on the effects of low-magnitude, high-frequency vibration on bone quality mainly concerned one or several aspects of bone property (e.g., mechanical property, mineral content, or microarchitecture) [6–10], [14], [30], but little is known about macro-micro-nano multi-level bone quality in response to the low-magnitude, high-frequency vibration with rest days, which was essential for better understanding the underlying mechanism for this mechanical intervention strategy. Accordingly, this study aimed to explore the effects of low-magnitude, high-frequency mechanical vibration on bone quality at multiple levels when the long-duration mechanical stimulus was separated by several rest days rather than daily loading. Macro- and micro-mechanical and morphological investigations were performed in this study to determine the bone mechanical properties, nanostructure of bone material, and material properties of femora with mechanical methods separated by 1, 3, 5, and 7 d rests in the loading cycle compared with daily loading in tail suspension rodents.

Materials and Methods

Materials

This study was performed in strict accordance with the recommendations of the Laboratory Animal Standardization Committee. The protocol was approved by the Medical Ethics Committee of No. 1 Hospital of Jilin University (2013-145). All efforts were made to minimize suffering of animals.

A total of 49 three-month-old male Wistar rats were purchased from the Experimental Animal Center of Jilin University. These rats were housed as singletons, and provided with a standard rodent diet (autoclaved NIH-31 with 6% fat; 18% protein; Ca:P, 1:1; and fortified with vitamins and minerals) and tap water during the experimental period. The environmental temperature was 24±2°C in natural light condition. All rats were randomly divided into seven groups, namely, vibrational loading for X day followed by X day rest (VLXR, $X = 1, 3, 5, 7$), vibrational loading every day (VLNR), tail suspension (SPD), and baseline control (BCL). The temporal schematic was shown in Fig. 1A. Non-invasive tail suspension was applied on all rats except those used for baseline control (BCL, n = 7), which were fed without any treatment. One week after tail suspension, high-frequency, low-magnitude whole body vibration was performed for eight weeks, which was similar with the study of Ma et al. [14]. The animals that were loaded by whole body vibration stimuli (35 Hz, 0.25 g, 15 min/day) on the first day were given one rest day, that is, vibrational loading with 1 d rest (VL1R, n = 7). Further groups were similarly created as follows: vibrational loading for 3 d followed by 3 d rest (VL3R, n = 7), vibrational loading for 5 d followed by 5 d rest (VL5R, n = 7), vibrational loading for 7 d followed by 7 d rest (VL7R, n = 7), and no rest day or vibrational loading every day (VLNR, n = 7). The rats in the tail suspension group (SPD, n = 7) were suspended without mechanical loading during the eight-week experimental period. The equipment for vibrational loading was assembled manually with a vibrational platform and a controller whose frequency and acceleration were adjustable (Fig. 1B). The weights of rats were measured before the experiment, one week after the suspension, and per week during the experiment. At day 42 and day 43 of the experimental protocol, all rats were treated with subcutaneous injection of calcein (dose: weight, 5 mg:1 kg) and tetracycline (dose: weight, 30 mg:1 kg), respectively. At day 52 and day 53 of the experimental protocol, calcein and tetracycline were re-injected to create a fluorescence maker [31,32]. All the rats were sacrificed at eight weeks, and the femurs were prepared for tests following removal of skin, muscle, and tendons.

Micro-CT Scanning

Left femurs were initially fixed with 80% ethanol (EtOH). Then, quantitative analysis of microarchitecture of trabecular bone in the femoral head was performed with micro-CT scanning (Skyscan 1076, Skyscan, Belgium). The spatial resolution for specimen scanning was set to 18 μm. The microarchitecture parameters of trabecular bone in the femoral head, such as bone volume fraction (BV/TV), trabecular thickness (Tb.Th), trabecular number (Tb.N), trabecular separation (Tb.Sp), and BMD were calculated by CTAn (CTAn, Skyscan, Belgium) [33].

Three-point Bending Mechanical Test

After micro-CT scanning, left femurs were cleaned in normal saline and a three-point bending mechanical test was performed on each left femur using an electronic universal testing machine (AG-X plus, Shimadzu, Kyoto, Japan). The test was performed with a fulcrum span of 20 mm and an actuator speed of 1 mm/min. Failure load was recorded, and energy absorption was determined as the area under the force-deflection curve until the point of failure. The elastic modulus was calculated using the following equation:

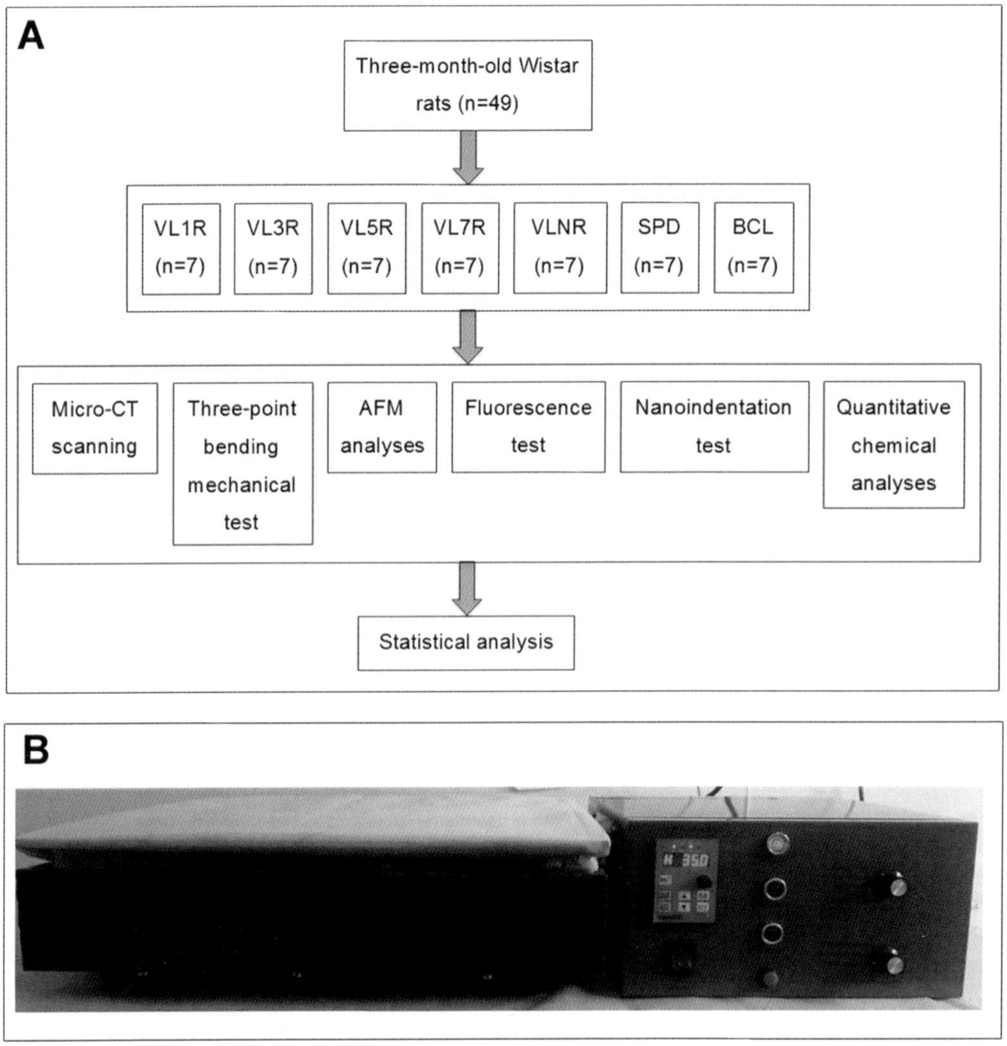

Figure 1. Temporal schematic of experiment and equipment for vibrational loading. (A) The temporal schematic; (B) The equipment for vibrational loading, which was assembled manually with a vibrational platform and a controller.

$$E = \frac{L^3}{48I}\left(\frac{\Delta F}{\Delta f}\right) \quad (1)$$

where L is the fulcrum span, $\frac{\Delta F}{\Delta f}$ is the slope of force-deflection curve, and I is the moment of inertia of an area. The cortical thickness of the fracture position was measured for calculating the elastic modulus.

AFM Analyses

After three-point bending mechanical test, sections of the left proximal femurs were cleaned in normal saline and dehydrated in increasing EtOH concentration from 85% to 100%. Longitudinal cortical bone specimens with a thickness of 2 mm were cut along the femoral shaft axis from femur shafts with a low-speed diamond saw under constant deionized water irrigation. Longitudinal trabecular bone specimens with a thickness of 1 mm to 2 mm were similarly cut from femur heads along the femoral neck axis.

Each bone sample (after 5 min of washing in ultrasonic bath, and natural drying) was placed horizontally onto the sample disk and imaged by a Multimode quadrex SPM with a Nanoscope IIIe controller (Veeco Instruments, USA). Imaging was operated under ambient conditions in standard AFM tapping mode using a commercial Silicon AFM probe (Tap300AI-G, BudgetSensors Instruments, Bulgaria) with a 125 μm cantilever length, a 40 Nm^{-1} constant force, a 300 kHz resonant frequency, and a tip radius lower than 10 nm. The size of mineral grains, i.e. the collagen bundles and the hydroxyapatite crystals, was measured using NanoScope Analysis version 1.4.0, as described by Milovanovic et al. [25].

Fluorescence Test

Right femurs were initially fixed with 80% EtOH, and dehydrated similar to left proximal femurs. Then, right femurs were embedded separately in polymethylmethacrylate (PMMA), ensuring that all bones were not demineralized. Each embedded right femur was sectioned into proximal femur and femur shaft. The right proximal femurs were cut along the coronal plane with a low-speed diamond saw under constant deionized water irrigation, which exposed the cancellous bone. Right femur shafts were then cut along the horizontal plane using a similar method, which exposed the cortical bone. Slices for fluorescence test were cut from right femur shafts. Then, the remaining parts were used for nanoindentation test. The mineral apposition rate (MAR) and bone formation rate (BFR/Tb.Ar) were calculated under fluorescence microscopy [34]. Laser scanning confocal microscopy (FV500, Olympus Corporation, Japan) was used to take pictures of analyzed fields, and one picture per right femur was obtained, and a total of 49 fluorescence images were obtained. MAR and BFR/Tb.Ar were measured by Image-Pro Plus software.

Nanoindentation Test

In this study, elastic modulus (E) and hardness (H) of longitudinal and transverse trabecular bone material, as well as those of longitudinal cortical bone material, were measured. Longitudinal trabecular bones with a thickness of 2 mm cut from left femoral heads were used for nanoindentation test in the longitudinal direction, and were also embedded separately in PMMA. Longitudinal cortical bones with a thickness of 2 mm cut from right femur shafts were used for nanoindentation test in the longitudinal direction, and transverse cancellous bones with a thickness of 2 mm of right femur heads were tested in the transverse direction. All the embedded samples were metallographically polished using silicon carbide abrasive papers of decreasing grit size (600, 800, 1500, and 2000 grit), and finally on microcloths with finer grades of diamond suspensions to the finest, 0.05 μm grit, to produce smooth surfaces for nanoindentation test. Specimens were washed in deionized water between each polishing step to remove debris. Nanoindentation tests were performed using Nano Indenter G200 (Agilent Technologies, Ltd., Santa Clara, CA, USA). A sharp Berkovich diamond indenter, a three-sided pyramid with the angle of 76°54′ between two edges, was used for all measurements. The specimens to be examined were located in the microscope and positioned beneath the indenter using the x–y table. The indenter was then slowly driven toward the surface at a constant displacement rate of 10 nm/s until surface contact was detected by the changes in the load and displacement signals. After contact, a permanent hardness impression was made by driving the indenter into the specimen to a depth of 1000 nm at a constant loading rate of 750 μN/s, holding at this load for a period of 10 s and then unloading to 15% of the peak load at a rate equal to half that used during loading. At the end of the unloading cycle, the indenter was held on the surface for a period of 100 s to establish the rate of thermal drift in the machine and specimen for correction of the data, and then completely withdrawn [35].

All indents were conducted at the similar site based on the optical microscopy observation to eliminate any local effects (Fig. 2A). Three indented areas (Fig. 2B) were selected for each trabecular specimen, and five indentations were made in each target area and 15 indentations were made in every sample, and the areas for each cortical specimen were similarly selected. A total of 2205 indentations were made. E and H were determined using the method of Oliver and Pharr [36]. The quantities of concern include the peak load (P_{max}), the contact area (A), and the contact stiffness (S). The equations used to calculate hardness (H) and effective indentation modulus (E_{ef}) from the measured quantities are:

$$H = \frac{P_{\max}}{A} \tag{2}$$

and

$$S = \frac{2}{\sqrt{\pi}}\beta E_{ef}\sqrt{A} \tag{3}$$

The effective modulus (E_{ef}) for the indentor-specimen combination can be derived from

$$\frac{1}{E_{ef}} = \frac{1-\nu_b^2}{E_b} + \frac{1-\nu_i^2}{E_i} \tag{4}$$

Where $\nu_b = 0.3$ and E_b are Poisson's ratio and elastic modulus for the bone material, respectively; $\nu_i = 0.07$ and $E_i = 1140$ GPa are the same quantities for the indenter, and the factor $\beta = 1.034$ is a constant for the Berkovich indenter. The basic assumption involved in this method is that the sample behaves purely elastically during unloading. Any indentation close to the mounting PMMA was removed to minimize the effects of embedding on the measurements.

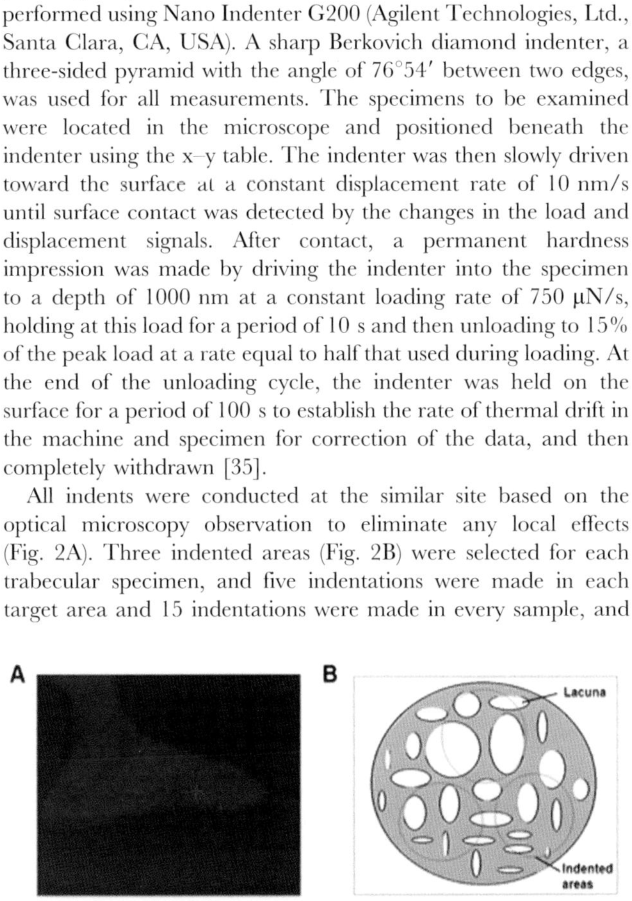

Figure 2. Indentation sites for nanoindentation test. Sample thickness is 2 mm. (A) Actual indented sites marked by red cross under optical microscopy; (B) Sketch map of indented areas marked by red circle.

Quantitative Chemical Analyses

Trabecular bones in each group were powdered to micron-sized particles using an electric grinder (Bosch Mkm 6000), and seven samples were prepared. Inductively coupled plasma optical emission spectroscopy (ICP-OES; 1.15 kW, 27 MHz; IRIS Intrepid, Thermo Electron Corporation, USA) was used for quantitative chemical analyses [37]. The user-friendly Quick Quant scan-based procedure was used to compare the intensities for measured elements in the samples with the intensities measured for standards with known concentrations. Calibration curves were calculated, and the concentrations of the measured elements in the samples were determined.

Statistical Analysis

Differences of all groups in the macro- and micromechanical and morphological properties of femurs were analyzed using Kruskal-Wallis H test of K independent sample nonparametric test. After that, Nemenyi test of two independent samples was used to determine differences of all mechanical and morphological parameters between every two groups. Data analysis was performed with SPSS 16.0 software, and the significance level was 0.05.

Results

Microarchitecture of Proximal Femurs Evaluated by Micro-CT Scanning

The region of interest (ROI) in the micro-CT image was selected one by one manually. The trabecular bones of femoral heads were included in the ROI as much as possible, and the 3D

Table 1. Microarchitecture parameters evaluated by micro-CT scanning.

	VL1R	VL3R	VL5R	VL7R	VLNR	SPD	BCL
BMD (g/cm^3)	$0.70\pm0.02^{a,b,c,d,e,f}$	$0.74\pm0.03^{a,b,c,e}$	$0.65\pm0.01^{a,b,c,d}$	$0.79\pm0.11^{a,b,c}$	$0.61\pm0.10^{a,b}$	$0.58\pm0.07^{b,c}$	$0.91\pm0.14^{a,c}$
BV/TV (%)	$72.06\pm1.26^{a,b,c,d,e,f}$	$77.41\pm1.47^{a,b,c,d,e}$	$83.87\pm2.35^{a,b,c}$	$87.04\pm2.84^{a,b,c}$	$62.87\pm1.86^{a,b}$	$50.43\pm2.31^{b,c}$	$89.62\pm2.17^{a,c}$
Tb.Th (mm)	$0.21\pm0.01^{a,b,c,e}$	$0.22\pm0.03^{a,b,c,e}$	$0.19\pm0.01^{a,b,c,d}$	$0.22\pm0.01^{a,b,c}$	$0.15\pm0.11^{a,b}$	$0.13\pm0.00^{b,c}$	$0.26\pm0.05^{a,c}$
Tb.N (mm^{-1})	$3.22\pm0.14^{a,b,c,d,f}$	$4.18\pm0.82^{a,b,c,d,e}$	$3.48\pm0.24^{a,b,c,d}$	$4.92\pm0.41^{a,b,c}$	$3.27\pm0.08^{a,b}$	$2.20\pm0.11^{b,c}$	$5.43\pm0.21^{a,c}$
Tb.Sp (mm)	$0.15\pm0.01^{a,b,c,d,f}$	$0.12\pm0.02^{a,b,c,e}$	$0.14\pm0.01^{a,b,c,d}$	$0.11\pm0.01^{a,b,c}$	$0.18\pm0.03^{a,b}$	$0.20\pm0.02^{b,c}$	$0.09\pm0.04^{a,c}$

n = 7 values per group. Values are shown as the median±SE. BMD - bone mineral density; BV/TV - bone volume fraction; Tb.Th - trabecular thickness; Tb.N - trabecular number; Tb.Sp - trabecular separation.
[a]Statistically different from SPD ($P<0.05$).
[b]Statistically different from BCL ($P<0.05$).
[c]Statistically different from VLNR ($P<0.05$).
[d]Statistically different from VL7R ($P<0.05$).
[e]Statistically different from VL5R ($P<0.05$).
[f]Statistically different from VL3R ($P<0.05$).

microarchitecture parameters calculated from CTAn are shown in Table 1. The three-dimensional (3D) reconstruction of micro-CT images of the trabecular bone in the femoral head is shown in Fig. 3. Compared with SPD, the trabeculae in the BCL are much denser, thicker and inseparable, whereas VL7R created a major improvement of trabecular microarchitecture compared with SPD, in which trabecular density, thickness and continuity were improved after eight weeks mechanical interventions. Table 1 shows variances in microarchitecture parameters of the different groups. BMD and BV/TV in all experimental groups were statistically higher than those in SPD ($P<0.05$), and VL7R exhibited significantly higher values than VLNR ($P<0.05$) and other vibrational loading groups ($P<0.05$), and there were statistical difference between VL1R, VL3R and VL5R ($P<0.05$). Furthermore, all these mechanical interventions with rest days displayed greater Tb.Th than daily loading ($P<0.05$), whereas VL7R showed the most obvious increase ($P = 0.006$). Dramatic increases in Tb.N of the femoral head were observed in all mechanical interventions, and the maximum was observed in VL7R than that in VLNR ($P = 0.001$). A statistically lower Tb.Sp was detected in the mechanical interventions with rest days than that in daily loading ($P<0.05$). There were improvements in all above microarchitecture parameters in VL1R, VL3R and VL5R than VLNR ($P<0.05$), but the statistical results between VL1R, VL3R and VL5R were not the same.

Failure Load, Elastic Modulus, and Energy Absorption Measured by Three-point Bending Test

The macro-biomechanical parameters measured by three-point bending test are shown in Fig. 4. BCL had the maximum failure load, elastic modulus, and energy absorption ($P<0.05$), whereas SPD had the minimum values ($P<0.05$). For failure load, a significant enhancement was observed in all experimental groups than that in SPD, and a significant increase was exclusively observed in VL7R than that in VLNR ($P = 0.006$) and other vibrational loading groups ($P<0.05$) (Fig. 4A). Dramatic increases in elastic modulus and energy absorption were observed in all experimental groups than those in SPD. Among all the vibration groups with rest days, elastic modulus and energy absorption were significantly higher in VL7R than those in VLNR ($P<0.05$) and other vibrational loading groups ($P<0.05$) (Figs. 4B and 4C), and there were no statistical difference between VL1R, VL3R and VL5R (Fig. 4).

Nanostructure of Bone Material Tested by AMF

Typical AFM topographic images and phase images of the nanostructure of trabecular bone material in the femoral head are shown in Fig. 5. Figs. 5-(T) show topographic images of VL1R, VL3R, VL5R, VL7R, VLNR, SPD and BCL. Scanning electron microscopy (SEM) (Figs. 5-(S)) revealed that bone minerals are fused together and form a sheet-like structure in a coherent manner [38]. The AFM phase Figs. 5-(P) obtained in our study show that the observed nanostructure of trabecular bone material exhibited a continuous phase, which is consistent with the SEM; nevertheless, the granular organization of the phase was evident in our sample (Figs. 5-(P)). The grain sizes of trabecular bone and cortical bone are listed in Table 2. Significant increases in grain sizes were observed in Figs. 5-(T)-SPD than those in Figs. 5-(T)-BCL, which showed a minimum grain size and a significantly narrower range (77 nm to 113 nm, Table 2). By contrast, the maximum values were detected in Figs. 5-(T)-SPD ($P<0.05$). Grain size was significantly smaller in Figs. 5-(T)-VL7R than that in Figs. 5-(T)-SPD among all the vibration groups with rest days ($P<0.05$). Grain size of Figs. 5-(T)-VL7R, Figs. 5-(T)-VL7R and

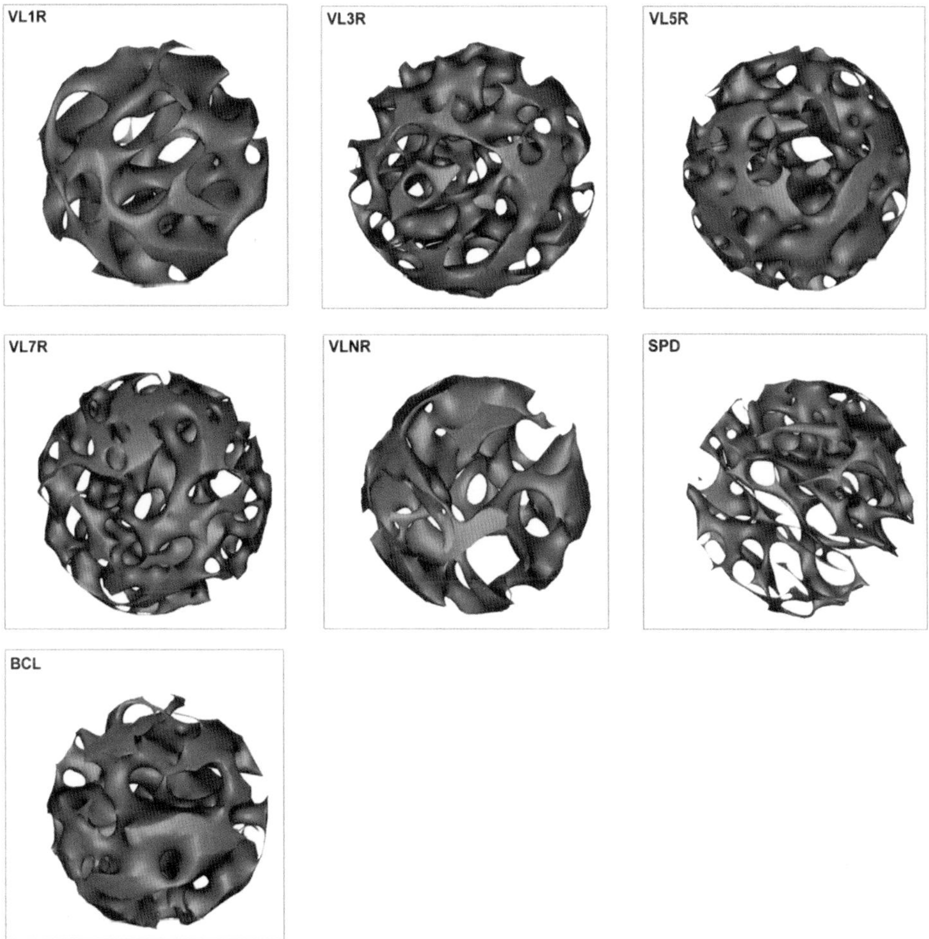

Figure 3. 3D reconstruction of micro-CT images of trabecular bone in femoral heads. VL1R: vibrational loading for 1 d followed by 1 d rest group; VL3R: vibrational loading for 3 d followed by 3 d rest group; VL5R: vibrational loading for 5 d followed by 5 d rest group; VL7R: vibrational loading for 7 d followed by 7 d rest group; VLNR: vibrational loading for no rest day or vibrational loading every day; SPD: tail suspension group; BCL: baseline control group.

Figs. 5-(T)-VL7R were improved than Figs. 5-(T)-VLNR ($P<0.05$), and statistical difference was detected between VL1R, VL3R and VL5R ($P<0.05$). The nanostructure of cortical bone material was similar to that of trabecular bone, and the size of grains differed among all experimental groups. Moreover, Figs. 5-(T)-SPD showed an unexpectedly low mean saturation roughness of the trabecula (approximately 70 nm, $P<0.05$), which showed that larger grains were flattened. By contrast, the mean saturation roughness values in Figs. 5-(T)-BCL and Figs. 5-(T)-VL7R were significantly higher (approximately 110 nm to 130 nm, $P<0.05$).

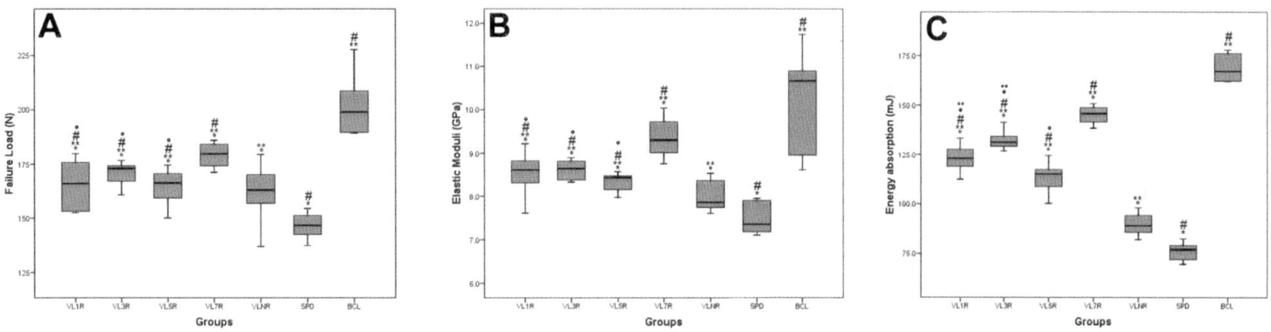

Figure 4. Macro-biomechanical parameters measured by three-point bending test. (A) Failure load; (B) Elastic modulus; (C) Energy absorption. *Statistically different from BCL ($P<0.05$). **Statistically different from SPD ($P<0.05$). #Statistically different from VLNR ($P<0.05$). ˙Statistically different from VL7R ($P<0.05$). ¨Statistically different from VL5R ($P<0.05$).

Table 2. Grain size of trabecular bone and cortical bone.

	VL1R	VL3R	VL5R	VL7R	VLNR	SPD	BCL
Tb.(nm)	$294\pm43^{a,b,c,d,e,f}$	$347\pm31^{a,b,c,d,e}$	$415\pm39^{a,b,c,d}$	$220\pm21^{a,b,c}$	$493\pm38^{a,b}$	$684\pm57^{b,c}$	$95\pm18^{a,c}$
Ct.(nm)	$316\pm23^{a,b,c,d,e,f}$	$359\pm34^{a,b,c,d,e}$	$413\pm37^{a,b,c,d}$	$197\pm16^{a,b,c}$	$521\pm43^{a,b}$	$659\pm49^{b,c}$	$110\pm13^{a,c}$

n = 7 values per group. Sample thickness is 2 mm. Values are shown as the median±SE. Tb. - trabecular bone; Ct. - cortical bone.
[a]Statistically different from SPD ($P<0.05$).
[b]Statistically different from BCL ($P<0.05$).
[c]Statistically different from VLNR ($P<0.05$).
[d]Statistically different from VL7R ($P<0.05$).
[e]Statistically different from VL5R ($P<0.05$).
[f]Statistically different from VL3R ($P<0.05$).

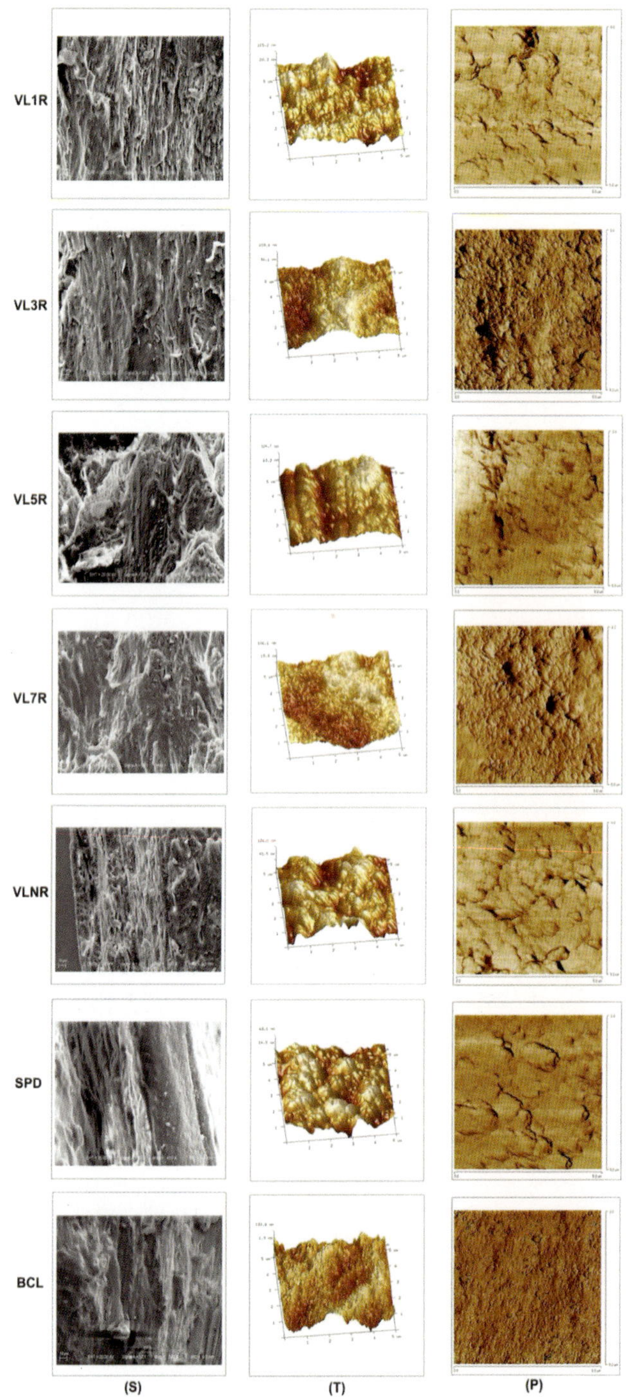

Figure 5. Scanning electron microscopy (SEM) images (Mag = 500X), AFM topographic images (5 μm×5 μm) and phase images (5 μm×5 μm) of the trabecular bone in femoral head. Sample thickness is 2 mm. Column (S): scanning electron microscopy; Column (T): AFM topographic images; Column (P): AFM phase images. Row VL1R: vibrational loading for 1 d followed by 1 d rest group; Row VL3R: vibrational loading for 3 d followed by 3 d rest group; Row VL5R: vibrational loading for 5 d followed by 5 d rest group; Row VL7R: vibrational loading for 7 d followed by 7 d rest group; Row VLNR: vibrational loading for no rest day or vibrational loading every day; Row SPD: tail suspension group; Row BCL: baseline control group.

Bone Growth Measured by Fluorescence Test

Fluorescence marker lines were clearly observed in the fluorescence graph in Fig. 6. The MAR and BFR/Tb.Ar are shown in Fig. 7. Maximum values were detected in BCL ($P<0.05$), whereas minimum values were detected in SPD ($P<0.05$). A significant increase was exclusively found in VL7R than that in VLNR ($P=0.001$) and other vibration groups with rest days ($P<0.05$). The MAR and BFR/Tb.Ar were increased in VL1R, VL3R and VL5R than VLNR ($P<0.05$), and there were statistical difference between VL1R, VL3R and VL5R ($P<0.05$).

E and H of Bone Material Evaluated by Nanoindentation Test

A summary of E, H, and E/H ratio of the trabecular and cortical bone sites as determined by nanoindentation is shown in Table 3. All data were obtained at an indentation depth of approximately 1000 nm [35]. E, H, and E/H ratio of longitudinal cortical bone (Ct.L) were greater than those of longitudinal trabecular bone (Tb.L), followed by transverse trabecular bone (Tb.T). No statistical difference was found in E, H, and E/H ratio for all groups ($P_{Tb.T}=0.845$, $P_{Tb.L}=0.172$, and $P_{Ct.L}=0.100$ for E; $P_{Tb.T}=0.707$, $P_{Tb.L}=0.414$, and $P_{Ct.L}=0.179$ for H; $P_{Tb.T}=0.898$, $P_{Tb.L}=0.540$, and $P_{Ct.L}=0.231$ for E/H ratio).

Bone Composition Evaluated by Quantitative Chemical Analyses

Results of quantitative chemical analyses (Table 4) show unchanged levels of calcium and phosphorus in all groups ($P=0.983$), and no significant difference was found in the Ca/P ratio ($P=0.991$).

Discussion

BMD decreased when hindlimbs were suspended and high-frequency, and low-magnitude mechanical stimuli could improve the biomechanical properties and microarchitecture in various sites, including cancellous and shaft cortical bones [39–42]. Whole-body vibration mitigated the reduction of bone strength in long-term hindlimb unloading rats and the complexity of trabecular bone could be preserved [43–45]. Low-magnitude, high-frequency mechanical stimuli may provide a non-pharmacologic treatment for bone loss. But bone cells lose mechanical sensitivity soon after stimulation, and a rest interval between each low-magnitude load cycle may create a potent anabolic stimulus [11–13]. Therefore, high-frequency, low-magnitude whole body vibration with rest days was put forward. However, the most effective number of rest days for treating bone loss was still

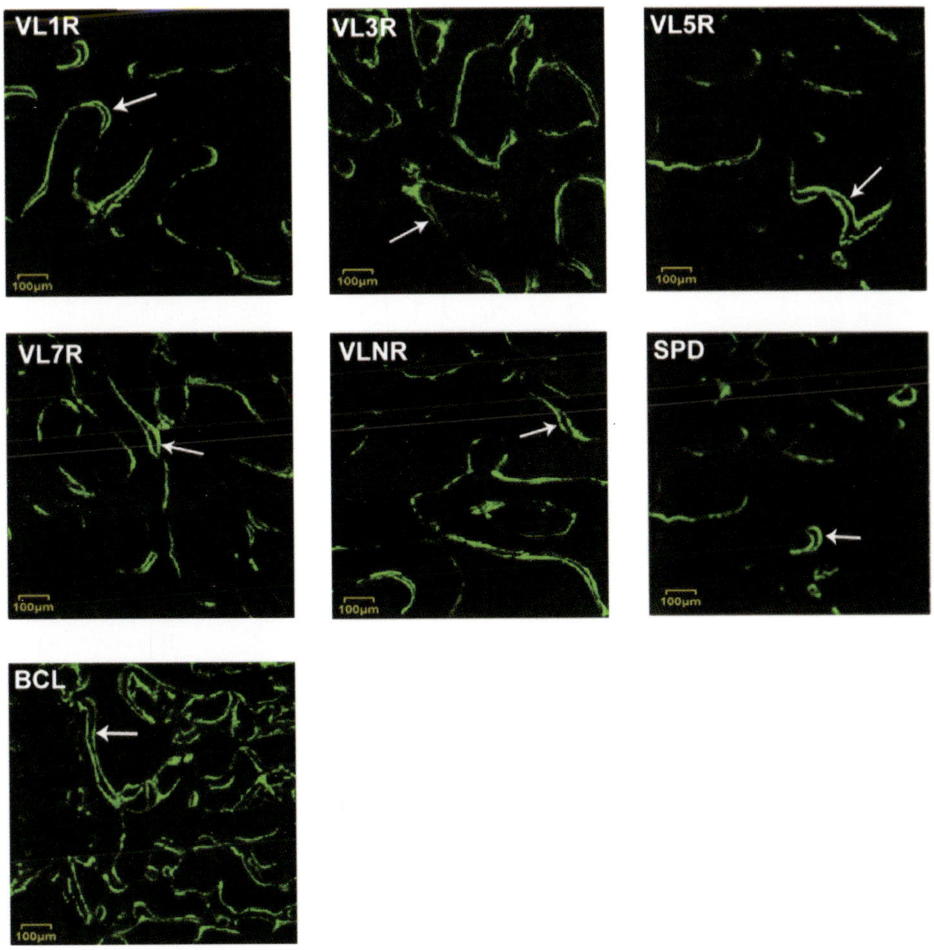

Figure 6. Fluorescence graphs of cancellous bones in proximal femurs. Arrows show the areas where the mineral apposition rate and bone formation rate were measured. VL1R: Vibrational loading for 1 d followed by 1 d rest group; VL3R: Vibrational loading for 3 d followed by 3 d rest group; VL5R: Vibrational loading for 5 d followed by 5 d rest group; VL7R: Vibrational loading for 7 d followed by 7 d rest group; VLNR: Vibrational loading for no rest day or vibrational loading every day; SPD: Tail suspension group; BCL: Baseline control group.

Table 3. *E*, *H*, and *E/H* ratio of the trabecular and cortical bone sites as determined by nanoindentation.

		VL1R	VL3R	VL5R	VL7R	VLNR	SPD	BCL
Tb.T	*E* (GPa)	14.90±1.02	15.00±1.11	15.00±1.23	15.00±0.89	14.90±0.74	14.90±1.35	15.00±1.41
	H (GPa)	0.20±0.01	0.20±0.01	0.19±0.03	0.20±0.02	0.19±0.03	0.20±0.02	0.20±0.01
	E/H	74.50±3.41	75.00±4.29	77.90±2.79	74.00±2.76	77.90±4.73	75.00±1.96	75.00±2.47
Tb.L	*E* (GPa)	23.72±2.11	23.50±2.64	23.58±1.89	23.16±2.13	23.20±2.29	23.65±3.01	23.15±1.74
	H (GPa)	1.24±0.03	1.23±0.11	1.20±0.10	1.13±0.09	1.15±0.03	1.19±0.10	1.21±0.06
	E/H	19.37±2.12	19.15±1.71	19.72±1.22	20.39±1.59	20.05±2.85	19.87±1.97	19.40±2.18
Ct.L	*E* (GPa)	30.20±2.94	30.20±3.15	30.20±2.76	30.40±2.18	30.60±3.31	30.10±2.87	30.80±2.09
	H (GPa)	1.49±0.12	1.49±0.09	1.49±0.04	1.49±0.01	1.49±0.01	1.49±0.04	1.50±0.10
	E/H	20.34±1.86	20.20±1.43	20.34±0.98	20.54±1.03	20.54±2.10	20.20±1.74	20.53±1.35

n = 7 values per group. Sample thickness is 2 mm. Values are shown as the median±SE. Tb.T - transverse trabecular bone; Tb.L - longitudinal trabecular bone; Ct.L - longitudinal cortical bone; *E* - elastic modulus; *H* - hardness; *E/H* - ratio of elastic modulus and hardness.

Table 4. Chemical composition of trabecular bone in femoral head (ICP-OES).

	VL1R	VL3R	VL5R	VL7R	VLNR	SPD	BCL
Ca [%]	24.34±2.51	24.92±1.91	24.59±2.55	24.72±3.02	24.82±2.37	24.51±2.62	24.59±2.29
P [%]	11.32±0.42	11.40±0.23	11.44±0.21	11.56±0.32	11.43±0.24	11.39±0.40	11.38±0.25
Ca/P ratio	2.15±0.19	2.19±0.21	2.15±0.23	2.14±0.17	2.18±0.21	2.15±0.19	2.16±0.23
Mg [%]	0.46±0.04	0.47±0.02	0.50±0.01	0.50±0.01	0.50±0.03	0.46±0.02	0.48±0.01
Sr [%]	0.0070±0.00	0.0069±0.00	0.0066±0.00	0.0069±0.00	0.0069±0.00	0.0067±0.00	0.0070±0.00
Fe [%]	0.015±0.00	0.016±0.00	0.013±0.00	0.015±0.00	0.012±0.00	0.013±0.00	0.023±0.00
Ba [%]	<0.005±0.00	<0.005±0.00	<0.005±0.00	<0.005±0.00	<0.005±0.00	<0.005±0.00	<0.005±0.00
K [%]	0.093±0.01	0.092±0.01	0.11±0.02	0.10±0.01	0.10±0.01	0.087±0.01	0.098±0.01
Na [%]	0.61±0.03	0.67±0.02	0.78±0.01	0.70±0.01	0.72±0.02	0.61±0.01	0.70±0.02

n = 7 values per group. Values are shown as the median±SE. ICP-OES - inductively coupled plasma optical emission spectroscopy.

unknown. Based on the 5 working days, VL5R was established in this study, and two smaller groups, i.e. VL1R and VL3R and one bigger group, i.e. VL7R were created. Groups of vibrational loading every day (VLNR), tail suspension (SPD), and baseline control (BCL) were also included for comparison to investigate multi-level mechanical properties, morphology, and chemical composition of bone to explore the effects of high-frequency, low-magnitude whole body vibration with different rest days.

In this study, macromechanical properties (i.e., failure load, elastic modulus, and energy absorption) increased in all experimental groups than those in SPD, and VL7R was significantly higher than VLNR (P<0.05) and other vibration groups with rest days (P<0.05). Similar results were detected in microarchitecture parameters, including increased BV/TV, BMD, Tb.Th, Tb.N, and lower Tb.Sp, of VL7R than those of VLNR (P<0.05) and other vibration groups with rest days (P<0.05). A 3D reconstruction of micro-CT images (Fig. 3) and fluorescence graphs (Fig. 7) showed that the trabeculae of BCL were significantly denser and thicker than SPD or vibrational loading groups, and bone growth in BCL was significantly greater than that in other groups. By contrast, significant trabecular deterioration was observed in rodents after tail suspension without mechanical intervention. Stimuli with rest days resulted in a major improvement of trabecular microarchitecture than SPD such that trabecular density, thickness, and continuity improved and bone growth rate was higher, and VL7R was more effective than VL1R, VL3R or VL5R. Whole-body vibration mitigated the reduction of bone strength in long-term hindlimb unloading rats, and mechanical stimulation in the form of whole-body vibration limited reduction of bone density when it was applied during the unloading [43,45], which was similar to the results of this study. However, our study showed that the vibrational loading for 7 d followed by 7 d rest appeared to be the optimal loading strategy for the bone loss caused by mechanical disuse, since significant differences were found in all above parameters.

The AFM phase images obtained in this study show that the observed nanostructure of the bone material exhibited a continuous phase and evident granular structure, which was consistent with the observation of Milovanovic et al. [25]. Compared with BCL, the grain sizes in all experimental groups were larger. In addition to crystal growth, two additional processes can increase mineral size, namely, crystal secondary nucleation leading to crystal proliferation and aggregation of preformed crystals [46]. Increased grain size in SPD cannot be explained by the increase in amount of minerals because our quantitative chemical analyses revealed unchanged calcium and phosphorus levels, as well as Ca/P ratio, in all experimental groups. Our findings indicate that in SPD, the existing mineral was reorganized by aggregation to larger grains, similar to the suggestion for turkey-leg tendon maturation [47,48]. Lower roughness in SPD, despite its larger grains, also supported the reorganization hypothesis, in which fused grains formed a larger flattened structure. Small mineral grain size of vibrational groups in this study was attributed to new bone formed in the remodeling process [49], and in all vibration groups with rest days, mineral grain size of VL7R was significantly smaller than VLNR (P<0.05) and other vibration groups with rest days (P<0.05), which showed that VL7R was more efficacious in improving bone loss and promoting bone formation. By contrast, large grains were possibly located in sites that have not undergone the bone remodeling process for a considerable amount of time. However, further experimental studies are needed for direct investigation of the mechanisms of grain enlargement. Nanoindentation test was used in this study to investigate the material properties of trabecular and cortical bones. Nanoindentation, which is a different method from conventional microhardness techniques, measures relatively smaller areas of bone material and provides estimates for both E and H. In this study, E and H of trabeculae and cortical bones were measured, and the average E and H of trabecular bone were considerably smaller than those of cortical bone (P<0.05). The E/H ratio, which represents the overall behavior of bone during the indentation process with respect to fracture toughness, was useful to describe material deformation during indentation and determine the brittleness of a material (ductile materials with higher E/H value) [50]. However, no significant difference in bone material properties was observed among all groups (P>0.05). Thus, the effect of disuse on the collagen bone matrix should be investigated. Other studies found that E and H of lamellae are unrelated to age, gender, and body mass index, and reductions in the mechanical integrity of whole bone must be caused by other factors, such as changes in tissue mass and organization [51,52]. Many of these changes are possibly caused by structural and histological features rather than

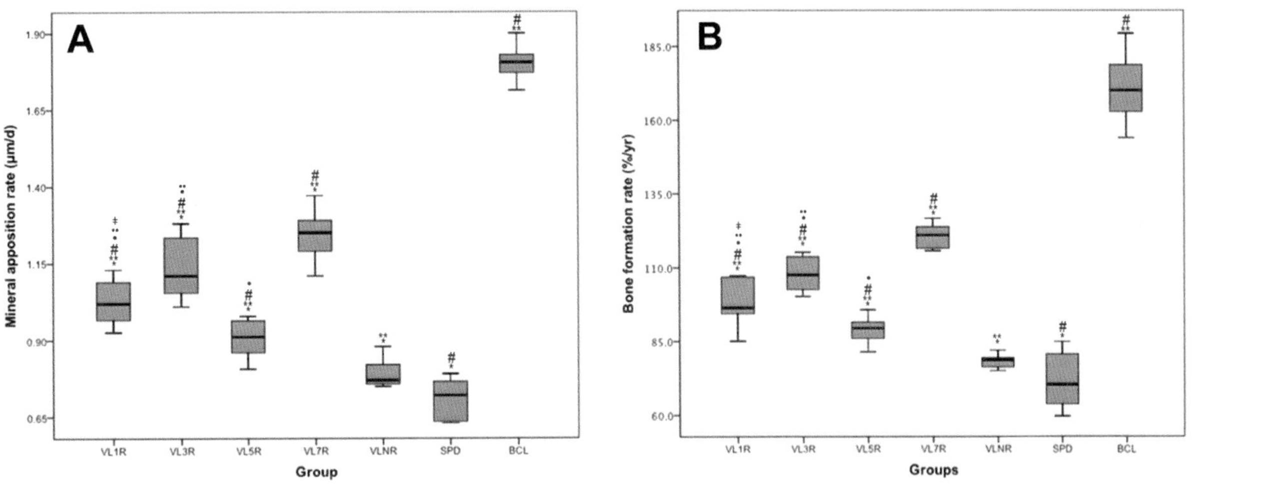

Figure 7. Mineral apposition rate and bone formation rate. *Statistically different from BCL (P<0.05). **Statistically different from SPD (P<0.05). #Statistically different from VLNR (P<0.05). ˙Statistically different from VL7R (P<0.05). ¨Statistically different from VL5R (P<0.05). ‡Statistically different from VL3R (P<0.05).

alterations in the bone matrix itself, and these changes warrant further investigation [53,54].

Some investigations suggested that high-frequency and low-magnitude mechanical signal may suppress adipose, non-esterified free fatty acid, and triglyceride contents in the liver or reduce a downstream challenge to liver morphology and function in rodents fed with a high-fat diet [55,56]. This mechanical efficacy to inhibit adipogenesis may increase with additional loading bouts if a refractory period is incorporated [57]. In this study, weights of animals sustained in tail suspension showed a similar ascending trend over seven weeks of vibration. However, animals loaded with mechanical stimuli appeared to lose weight in the last week ($P < 0.05$). The variation in weight was similar to that reported by Ma et al. [14]. At the same time, hindlimb-unloading induced loss of mass in muscles, but the response of BMD to altered loading conditions did not necessarily depend on the response of muscle mass [39]. Further studies will be performed to understand the mechanism of weight loss and the response of BMD to muscle mass affected by vibration stimuli.

This study had several limitations. First, three-month-old male rats were selected to exclude the influence of hormones with respect to osteoporosis of ovariectomised rats caused by estrogen deficiency [14]. In future studies, female rats with the same age will be investigated to determine the effect of gender. Second, though three-month-old male rats have been carefully limited in this study, body mass or size of all rats was not measured daily, which could have been responsible for the differences between individuals. Likewise, the behavioral monitoring may have been able to recognize any potential differences in activity levels between animals (those that were not undergoing tail suspension), and this study did not establish a group of tail suspension with 15 min of free activities instead of vibration stimuli, but the experimental groups only had different vibration cycles, and statistical results were unaffected by free activities during the vibration period. Further studies will record body mass or size and perform the behavioral monitoring daily, which would help eliminate those from being variables that potentially cloud the results, and an experimental group with tail suspension rodents and free activities will be included to determine the influence of free activities on bone quality. Third, bilateral femurs were used because the rat femoral heads were too small to collect all necessary specimens. In relation to the investigation on Caucasian women, which showed no significant difference in BMD of bilateral femoral necks, trochanters, and hips [58], bilateral differences were ignored in this study. Fourth, the bone turnover markers P1NP and CTX-I on rat serum were not studied to quantify the difference of bone formation and bone resorption between different groups, and this will be quantified in further studies. The number of days that rats underwent vibrational loading and rest is smaller than seven. However, vibrational loading for X day followed by X day rest (VLXR, $X = 1, 3, 5, 7$) were studied in contrast with vibrational loading every day (VLNR), and this study showed that high-frequency, low-magnitude whole body vibration with rest days was efficacious in improving bone quality than daily loading. In future studies, the days of vibrational loading and rest will be diversified. Fifth, the samples were dehydrated before the experiment, which were different from fresh samples. Because the quantity of samples was limited, and the same sample was used for a variety of experimental study. Thus, considering the different experimental needs, all the samples were dehydrated in the same condition, which would not affect the statistical significance. The mechanical experiments on fresh samples will be carried out in the later study to make it closer to the reality.

This study showed that bone mineral reorganization and spatial arrangement were modified by high-frequency, low-magnitude whole body vibration with different rest days, which resulted in the recombination of mineral grains into different sizes and changes in mineral apposition rate and bone formation rate. The micro-architecture of bone was affected, which resulted in statistical differences in macromechanical properties. However, the mechanical properties of the bone material were not altered. This study investigated the influence of high-frequency, low-magnitude whole body vibration on bone loss caused by mechanical disuse in multiple levels, and showed that high-frequency, low-magnitude whole body vibration with 7 d rests was more efficacious in improving macro-biomechanical properties and microarchitecture than daily loading, which provided a theoretical basis for improving bone quality using this mechanical intervention in clinics.

Author Contributions

Conceived and designed the experiments: RZ HG DZ. Performed the experiments: RZ. Analyzed the data: RZ JZG JF. Contributed reagents/materials/analysis tools: HG DZ YF. Wrote the paper: RZ HG.

References

1. Lane NE (2006) Epidemiology, etiology, and diagnosis of osteoporosis. Am J Obstet Gynecol 194: S3–S11.
2. LeBlanc A, Shackelford L, Schneider V (1998) Future human bone research in space. Bone 22: S113–S6.
3. Ruff C, Beck T, Newman D, Oden M, Shaffner G, et al. (1999) Skeletal consequences of reduced gravity environments. 1st Biennial Space Biomed. Inv. Workshop 1: 86–7.
4. Lafage V, Dubousset J, Lavaste F, Skalli W (2002) Finite element simulation of various strategies for CD correction. Stud Health Technol Inform 91: 428–32.
5. Rahmani P, Morin S (2009) Prevention of osteoporosis-related fractures among postmenopausal women and older men. CMAJ 181: 815–20.
6. Rubin C, Turner AS, Bain S, Mallinckrodt C, McLeod K, et al. (2001) Low mechanical signals strengthen long bones. Nature 412: 603–4.
7. Tezval M, Biblis M, Sehmisch S, Schmelz U, Kolios L, et al. (2011) Improvement of femoral bone quality after low-magnitude, high-frequency mechanical stimulation in the ovariectomized rat as an osteopenia model. Calcif Tissue Int 88: 33–40.
8. Rubin C, Turner AS, Müller R, Mittra E, McLeod K, et al. (2002) Quantity and quality of trabecular bone in the femur are enhanced by a strongly anabolic, noninvasive mechanical intervention. J Bone Miner Res 17: 349–57.
9. Ward K, Alsop C, Caulton J, Rubin C, Adams J, et al. (2004) Low magnitude mechanical loading is osteogenic in children with disabling conditions. J Bone Miner Res 19: 360–9.
10. Rubin C, Recker R, Cullen D, Ryaby J, McCabe J, et al. (2004) Prevention of postmenopausal bone loss by a low-magnitude, high-frequency mechanical stimuli: a clinical trial assessing compliance, efficacy, and safety. J Bone Miner Res 19: 343–51.
11. Robling AG, Hinant FM, Burr DB, Turner CH (2002) Shorter, more frequent mechanical loading sessions enhance bone mass. Med Sci Sports Exerc 34: 196–202.
12. Saxon LK, Robling AG, Alam I, Turner CH (2005) Mechanosensitivity of the rat skeleton decreases after a long period of loading, but is improved with time off. Bone 36: 454–64.
13. Srinivasan S, Weimer DA, Agans SC, Bain SD, Gross TS (2002) Low-magnitude mechanical loading becomes osteogenic when rest is inserted between each load cycle. J Bone Miner Res 17: 1613–20.
14. Ma RS, Zhu D, Gong H, Gu GS, Huang X, et al. (2012) High-frequency and low-magnitude whole body vibration with rest days is more effective in improving skeletal micro-morphology and biomechanical properties in ovariectomised rodents. Hip Int 22: 218–26.
15. Gong H, Zhang M, Zhang H, Zhu D, Yang L (2006) Theoretical analysis of contributions of disuse, basic multicellular unit activation threshold, and osteoblastic formation threshold to changes in bone mineral density at menopause. J Bone Miner Metab 24: 386–94.
16. Feng L, Jasiuk I (2011) Multi-scale characterization of swine femoral cortical bone. J Biomech 44: 313–20.

17. Ruimerman R, Huiskes R, Lenthe GH, Janssen JD (2001) A computer simulation model relating bone-cell metabolism to mechanical adaptation of trabecular architecture. COMPUT METHOD BIOMEC 4: 433–448.
18. Wang LZ, Cheung JT, Pu F, Li DY, Zhang M, et al. (2011) Why do woodpeckers resist head impact injury: A Biomechanical Investigation. PLoS ONE 6(10): e26490.
19. Thurner PJ, Müller R, Kindt JH, Schitter G, Fantner GE, et al. (2005) Novel techniques for high-resolution functional imaging of trabecular bone. In: Proceedings of the SPIE, p. 515–26.
20. Thurner PJ, Oroudjev E, Jungmann R, Kreutz C, Kindt JH, et al. (2007) Imaging of bone ultrastructure using atomic force microscopy. In: Méndez-Vilas A, Díaz J, editors. Modern research and educational topics in microscopy. Badajoz: Formatex, p. 37–48.
21. Hassenkam T, Fantner GE, Cutroni JA, Weaver JC, Morse DE, et al. (2004) Highresolution AFM imaging of intact and fractured trabecular bone. Bone 35: 4–10.
22. Hassenkam T, Jøgensen HL, Lauritzen JB (2006) Mapping the imprint of bone remodeling by atomic force microscopy. Anat Rec A 288: 1087–94.
23. Hassenkam T, Jøgensen HL, Pedersen MB, Kourakis AH, Simonsen L, et al. (2005) Atomic force microscopy on human trabecular bone from an old woman with osteoporotic fractures. Micron 36: 681–7.
24. Chappard D, Legrand E, Baslé MF, Audran M (2011) New laboratory tools in the assessment of bone quality. Osteoporos Int 22: 2225–40.
25. Milovanovic P, Potocnik J, Stoiljkovic M, Djonic D, Nikolic S, et al. (2011) Nanostructure and mineral composition of trabecular bone in the lateral femoral neck: Implications for bone fragility in elderly women. Acta Biomater 7: 3446–51.
26. Pharr GM, Oliver WC (1992) Measurement of thin film mechanical properties using nanoindentation. MRS Bull 17: 28–33.
27. Doerner MF, Nix WD (1986) A method for determining the data from depth-sensing indentation instruments. J Mater Res 1: 601.
28. Ascenzi A, Baschieri P, Benvenuti A (1990) The bending properties of a single osteon. J Biomech 23, 763–71.
29. Lotz JC, Gerhart TN, Hayes WC (1991) Mechanical properties of metaphyseal bone in the proximal femur. J Biomech 24: 317–29.
30. Manske SL, Good CA, Zernicke RF, Boyd SK (2012) High-Frequency, Low-Magnitude Vibration Does Not Prevent Bone Loss Resulting from Muscle Disuse in Mice following Botulinum Toxin Injection. PLoS ONE 7(5): e36486.
31. Hembree M, Buschang PH, Carrillo R, Rossouw PE (2009) Effects of intentional damage to the roots and surrounding structures with miniscrew implants. Am J Orthod Dentofacial Orthop, 135(3): 280.e1–9.
32. Brisceno CE, Rossouw PE, Carrillo R, Spears R, Buschang H (2009) Healing of the roots and surrounding structures after intentional damage with miniscrew implants. Am J Orthod Dentofacial Orthop, 135(3). 292–301.
33. Dempster DW, Compston JE, Drezner MK, Glorieux FH, Kanis JA, et al. (2013) Standardized nomenclature, symbols, and units for bone histomorphometry: a 2012 update of the report of the ASBMR histomorphometry nomenclature committee. J Bone Miner Res 28: 1–16.
34. Li XJ, Jee WS, Chow SY, Woodbury DM (1990) Adaptation of cancellous bone to aging and immobilization in the rat: a single photon absorptiometry and histomorphometry study. The Anatomical Record 227: 12–24.
35. Rho JY, Ting Y, Tsui TY, Pharr GM (1997) Elastic properties of human corticaland trabecular lamellar bone measured by nanoindentation. Biomaterials 18: 1325–30.
36. Oliver WC, Pharr GM (1992) An improved technique for determining hardness and elastic modulus using load and displacement sensing indentation experiments. J Mater Res 7: 1564–83.
37. Rankovic D, Kuzmanovic M, Savovic J, Pavlovic M, Stoiljkovic M, et al. (2010) The effect of potassium addition on plasma parameters in argon dc plasma arc. J Phys D: Appl Phys 43: 335202.
38. Chen PY, Toroian D, Price PA, McKittrick J (2011) Minerals Form a Continuum Phase in Mature Cancellous Bone. Calcif Tissue Int 88: 351–361.
39. Yamauchi H, Mashiko S, Kimura M, Miyano S, Yonemoto K (2003) Responses of bone mineral density to isometric resistance exercise during hindlimb unloading and subsequent recovery. J Sport Med Phys Fit 52: 119–130.
40. Rubin CT, Sommerfeldt DW, Judex S, Qin YX (2001) Inhibition of osteopenia by low magnitude, high-frequency mechanical stimuli. Drug Discov Today 6: 848–58.
41. Gilsanz V, Wren TA, Sanchez M, Dorey F, Judex S, et al. (2006) Low-level, high-frequency mechanical signals enhance musculoskeletal development of young women with low BMD. J Bone Miner Res 21: 1464–74.
42. Flieger J, Karachalios T, Khaldi L, Raptou P, Lyritis G (1998) Mechanical stimulation in the form of vibration prevents postmenopausal bone loss in ovariectomized rats. Calcif Tissue Int 63: 510–4.
43. Li ZL, Tan C, Wu YH, Ding Y, Wang HJ, et al. (2012) Whole-body vibration and resistance exercise prevent long-term hindlimb unloading-induced bone loss: independent and interactive effects. Eur J Appl Physiol 112: 3743–53.
44. Matsuda J, Kurata K, Hara T, Higaki H (2009) Mechanical Vibration Applied in the Absence of Weight Bearing Suggest Improved Fragile Bone. 13th International Conference on Biomedical Engineering IFMBE Proceedings 23: 1766–8.
45. Yang PF, Jia B, Ding C, Wang Z, Qian AR, et al. (2009) Whole-Body Vibration Effects on Bone Before and After Hind-Limb Unloading in Rats. ASEM 80: 88–93.
46. Boskey AL (2001) Bone mineralization. In: Cowin SC, editor. Bone mechanics handbook. Boca Raton, FL: CRC Press: 5/1–5/33.
47. Landis WJ, Hodgens KJ, Song MJ, Arena J, Kiyonaga S, et al. (1996) Mineralization of collagen may occur on fibril surfaces: evidence from conventional and high-voltage electron microscopy and three-dimensional imaging. J Struct Biol 117: 24–35.
48. Landis WJ, Song MJ, Leith A, McEwen L, McEwen BF (1993) Mineral and organic matrix interaction in normally calcifying tendon visualized in three dimensions by high-voltage electron microscopic tomography and graphic image reconstruction. J Struct Biol 110: 39–54.
49. Su X, Sun K, Cui FZ, Landis WJ (2003) Organization of apatite crystals in human woven bone. Bone 32: 150–62.
50. Fan ZF, Smith P, Rauch F, Harris GF (2007) Nanoindentation as a means for distinguishing clinical type of osteogenesis imperfecta. Compos Part B 38: 411–5.
51. Hoffler CE, Moore KE, Kozloff K, Zysset PK, Goldstein SA (2000) Age, gender and bone lamellae elastic moduli. J Orthop Res 18: 432–7.
52. Hoffler CE, Moore KE, Kozloff K, Zysset PK, Brown MB, et al. (2000) Heterogeneity of bone lamellar-level elastic moduli. Bone 26: 603–9.
53. Rho JY, Zioupos P, Curry JD, Pharr GM (2002) Microstructural elasticity and regional heterogeneity in human femoral bone of various ages examined by nano-indentation. J Biomech 35: 189–98.
54. Sun LW, Fan YB, Li DY, Zhao F, Xie T, et al. (2009) Evaluation of the mechanical properties of rat bone under simulated microgravity using nanoindentation. Acta Biomater 5: 3506–11.
55. Rubin CT, Capilla E, Luu YK, Busa B, Crawford H, et al. (2007) Adipogenesis is inhibited by brief, daily exposure to high-frequency, extremely low magnitude mechanical signals. PNAS 104: 17879–84.
56. Luu YK, Ozcivici E, Capilla E, Adler B, Chan E, et al. (2010) Development of diet induced fatty liver disease in the aging mouse is suppressed by brief daily exposure to low-magnitude mechanical signals. Int J Obes (Lond) 34: 401–5.
57. Sen B, Xie ZH, Case N, Styner M, Rubin CT, et al. (2011) Mechanical signal influence on mesenchymal stem cell fate is enhanced by incorporation of refractory periods into the loading regimen. J Biomech 44: 593–9.
58. Faulkner KG, Genant HK, McClung M (1995) Bilateral comparison of femoral bone density and hip axis length from single and fan beam DXA scans. Calcif Tissue Int 56: 26–31.

Variation in the *MC4R* Gene Is Associated with Bone Phenotypes in Elderly Swedish Women

Gaurav Garg[1], Jitender Kumar[2], Fiona E. McGuigan[1], Martin Ridderstråle[3], Paul Gerdhem[4], Holger Luthman[5], Kristina Åkesson[1]*

1 Clinical and Molecular Osteoporosis Research Unit, Department of Clinical Sciences, Lund University and Department of Orthopaedics, Skåne University Hospital, Malmö, Sweden, **2** Department of Medical Sciences, Molecular Epidemiology and Science for Life Laboratory, Uppsala University, Uppsala, Sweden, **3** Clinical Obesity Research, Department of Endocrinology, Skåne University Hospital, Malmö, Sweden, **4** Department of Clinical Science, Intervention and Technology, Karolinska Institutet, Department of Orthopaedics, Karolinska University Hospital, Stockholm, Sweden, **5** Medical Genetics Unit, Department of Clinical Sciences, Lund University, Malmö, Sweden

Abstract

Osteoporosis is characterized by reduced bone mineral density (BMD) and increased fracture risk. Fat mass is a determinant of bone strength and both phenotypes have a strong genetic component. In this study, we examined the association between obesity associated polymorphisms (SNPs) with body composition, BMD, Ultrasound (QUS), fracture and biomarkers (Homocysteine (Hcy), folate, Vitamin D and Vitamin B12) for obesity and osteoporosis. Five common variants: rs17782313 and rs1770633 (melanocortin 4 receptor *(MC4R)*; rs7566605 (insulin induced gene 2 (*INSIG2*); rs9939609 and rs1121980 (fat mass and obesity associated *(FTO)* were genotyped in 2 cohorts of Swedish women: PEAK-25 (age 25, n = 1061) and OPRA (age 75, n = 1044). Body mass index (BMI), total body fat and lean mass were strongly positively correlated with QUS and BMD in both cohorts (r^2 = 0.2–0.6). *MC4R* rs17782313 was associated with QUS in the OPRA cohort and individuals with the minor C-allele had higher values compared to T-allele homozygotes (TT vs. CT vs. CC: BUA: 100 vs. 103 vs. 103; p = 0.002); (SOS: 1521 vs. 1526 vs. 1524; p = 0.008); (Stiffness index: 69 vs. 73 vs. 74; p = 0.0006) after adjustment for confounders. They also had low folate (18 vs. 17 vs. 16; p = 0.03) and vitamin D (93 vs. 91 vs. 90; p = 0.03) and high Hcy levels (13.7 vs 14.4 vs. 14.5; p = 0.06). Fracture incidence was lower among women with the C-allele, (52% vs. 58%; p = 0.067). Variation in *MC4R* was not associated with BMD or body composition in either OPRA or PEAK-25. SNPs close to *FTO* and *INSIG2* were not associated with any bone phenotypes in either cohort and *FTO* SNPs were only associated with body composition in PEAK-25 ($p \leq 0.001$). Our results suggest that genetic variation close to *MC4R* is associated with quantitative ultrasound and risk of fracture.

Editor: Joseph Devaney, Children's National Medical Center, Washington, United States of America

Funding: The funders had no role in study design, data collection and analysis, decision to publish, or preparation of the manuscript. Financial support for the study was received from the Swedish Research Council (Grant K2009-53X-14691-07-3)(www.vr.se), Greta and Johan Kock Foundation, A Påhlsson Foundation, A Österlund Foundation, Herman Järnhardt Foundation, King Gustav V and Queen Victoria Foundation, Malmö University Hospital Research Foundation, Research and Development Council of Region Skåne, Sweden and the Swedish Medical Society.

Competing Interests: The authors have declared that no competing interests exist.

* E-mail: Kristina.Akesson@med.lu.se

These authors contributed equally to this work.

Introduction

Osteoporosis and obesity are both multifactorial disorders that in recent years have become major public health problems. At one time considered to be mutually exclusive, it is now recognized that these conditions share many genetic and environmental risk factors and are linked to each other through a number of complex regulatory pathways [1,2]. Epidemiological studies have shown that increased body weight is positively associated with bone mass, while low body weight is a risk factor for bone loss and osteoporosis [3]. The positive effect of body weight on bone mass may be attributable to a number of factors: increased mechanical load which has an anabolic effect on bone [4]; conversion of steroid precursors to estrogen in peripheral adipose tissue [5] or through the secretion of bone active hormones from β-cells in the pancreas and adipocytes themselves [6]. Homocysteine (Hcy), vitamin B12, vitamin D and folate are biomarkers for a number of pathologies including cardiovascular disease and diabetes and a strong correlation between these biomarkers with BMI has been reported [7–10]. Elevated levels of Hcy and low levels of vitamin D are strong and independent risk factors for osteoporotic fracture risk [11,12].

Studies have shown that variation in diet and life style modulate Hcy, folate and vitamin B12 [13,14], all of which are important components in intermediary metabolism. Elevated Hcy levels have been associated with detrimental effects on bone metabolism, however, whether Hcy and other biochemical parameters play a causal role or act as markers for other mechanisms underlying these pathologies is unclear [15].

The complex relationship between fat cells and bone has been under intense scrutiny. Adipocytes and osteoblasts share a common progenitor, the pluripotent mesenchymal stem cell, and there is a degree of plasticity between the two cell types [16–19]. Differentiation to a particular lineage is regulated by numerous transcription factors and with increasing age there is a shift away from osteoblast towards adipocyte production [19] which in conjunction with increased osteoclast function may lead to osteoporosis [20].

At the genetic level a number of association studies have identified single nucleotide polymorphisms (SNPs) close to genes contributing to both osteoporosis and body composition [21–30]. To date, few bivariate genome-wide association studies (GWAS) for osteoporosis and obesity have been performed [31] although GWAS for obesity and its associated pathological outcomes have identified a number of SNPs close to genes expected to also play an important role in bone metabolism [31]. In the current study, we selected five SNPs identified through GWAS: rs17782313_*MC4R*; rs1770633_*MC4R*; rs7566605_*INSIG2*; rs9939609_*FTO* and rs1121980_*FTO*.

The *FTO* gene is highly expressed in the hypothalamus and is involved in energy homeostasis through the control of energy expenditure [32]. Located on chromosome 16, the *FTO* gene has nine exons and spans more than 400 kb. The SNPs associated with BMI in the GWAS lie in the first intron that harbors a region highly conserved across different species [33]. Individuals with the rs9939609 variant allele were shown to have a 31% increased risk per variant allele, of developing obesity [34,35]. Variation in the *FTO* gene has been analyzed for association with BMD in a number of populations including children and adults [36] and in a mouse knockout model, BMD was lower in the *FTO* knockout compared to controls [37].

The *MC4R* gene on chromosome 18 encodes the MC4 protein, a G-protein coupled receptor that plays a major role in the central regulation of body weight through maintaining energy homeostasis and the suppression of food intake [38]. Genetic variation in the *MC4R* gene has been identified as responsible for monogenic forms of obesity [39]. In a GWAS by Loos et al., SNPs present in the intergenic region upstream of *MC4R* were associated with BMI [33]. Patients deficient in *MC4R* have been reported to have increased BMD and decreased bone resorption [40], while genetic variation has been evaluated for association with bone mass, but only in children [41].

The *INSIG2* gene has been reported to be associated with increased risk of obesity [42]. SNP rs7566605, located 10 kb upstream of the *INSIG2* gene transcription start site, was associated with fat mass. *INSIG2* is a candidate gene for increased BMI; it binds to the sterol regulatory element-binding protein complex (*SREBP*) and reduces the activity of cholesterol and fatty acid synthesis in the endoplasmic reticulum [43]. Although variation in the *INSIG2* gene has recently identified in a GWAS for BMD [44], it has not been yet fully explored.

The rationale for our study was to comprehensively evaluate the association between selected obesity associated polymorphisms and aspects of bone strength, a complex trait not captured by BMD alone. Since the skeletal fragility associated with osteoporosis reflects reduced bone quality as well as quantity, we have assessed micro-architectural properties of bone, bone geometry and long-term fracture risk in addition to BMD and body composition. Furthermore, in order to understand the mechanisms underlying these associations, we have also evaluated the association between these polymorphisms and biomarkers for obesity and bone mass. By studying two differently aged cohorts we have evaluated age-related differences in the contribution of obesity associated polymorphisms with bone phenotypes.

Materials and Methods

Subjects

Two population based cohorts of Swedish women were studied; the OPRA cohort consisting of 1044 elderly women all aged exactly 75 and prospectively followed for 10 years and the PEAK-25 cohort consisting of 1061 women all aged exactly 25. Details of the two cohorts have been published [45,46]. Participants gave written informed consent and the study was approved by the Regional Ethical Review Board in Lund according to the Helsinki agreement.

Measurement of Bone Phenotypes and Body Composition Using DXA

Bone mineral density (g/cm^2) at the femoral neck (FN), lumbar spine (LS) and total body (TB) was measured using dual-energy x-ray absorptiometry (Lunar Prodigy: PEAK-25; Lunar DPX-L: OPRA (Lunar Corporation, Madison, WI, USA)). Fat and lean mass for total body (TB) and trunk were also measured using the same instrument. Calibrations were performed daily using a phantom supplied by the manufacturer. Precision error (coefficient of variation) for DXA scanning was 0.94%, 1.45%, 4.01% for TB, LS and FN respectively in the OPRA cohort [47] and 0.90% and 0.65% for FN and LS respectively in PEAK-25 [48]. For the OPRA cohort, all measurements at baseline were performed using the same instrument, while analyses of scans were made with software versions 1.33 and 1.35.

Hip geometry was assessed only in the OPRA cohort by employing the software provided by Lunar® (Lunar Corporation, WI, USA) for the DPX-L scanner. The following phenotypes were analyzed: Hip Axis Length (mm); femoral neck width (mm); Cross Sectional Moment of Inertia [CSMI] (Cm^4) and Section Modulus [SM] (Cm^3). To minimize variability, all variables were analyzed by a single operator. The coefficient of variation for these measurements was between 0.6 and 3.7% [49].

Ultrasound measurements (Speed of Sound (SOS) (m/s)), Broadband Ultrasound Attenuation ((BUA) (dB/MHz)) and Stiffness Index (SI)) were performed on the right calcaneus using the Lunar Achilles (R) system (Lunar Corporation Madison, WI, USA) to assess bone quality in both cohorts. The precision was 1.5% for derivatives of BUA and SOS [50]. Daily calibrations were made to control the long-term stability of the apparatus.

Fracture Ascertainment

In the PEAK-25 cohort the fracture incidence is low, therefore fracture data was analyzed only in the OPRA cohort. Self-reported fractures sustained between age 20 and 75 were recorded and verified from the radiological files [51]. The majority of fractures (>99%) occurring in the elderly women were attributable to low energy trauma.

Blood Sample Collection and Biochemical Phenotypes Measurements

Non-fasting blood samples were collected before noon for DNA isolation (PEAK-25 and OPRA) and to assay serum concentration of biochemical markers (OPRA). Samples were stored at −80°C until analysis. Assays were performed at the Department of Clinical Chemistry, Malmö, Skåne University Hospital according to accredited methods. Biochemical phenotypes, available only in the OPRA cohort, were assayed using standardized analytical protocols. Total serum Hcy (µmol/L) was measured using HPLC. Serum vitamin B12 (pmol/L) and folate (nmol/L) were measured using Elecsys assays (Roche Diagnostics, Mannheim, Germany) and serum 25-hydroxy vitamin D (25OHD) (nmol/L) was assessed by liquid chromatography mass spectrophotometry (LC-MS) [52].

Genotyping and Statistical Analysis

Five obesity associated SNPs from three genes were genotyped in both cohorts (Table S1) [33,42]. Sequenom's iPlex Gold system (Sequenom, San Diego, CA) was employed to score the genotypes. A total of 993 women from the OPRA and 1001 women from the PEAK-25 cohort were genotyped successfully. Approximately 3% of the samples from each cohort were genotyped in duplicate with 100% concordance. Departures from Hardy-Weinberg equilibrium were tested using the χ^2 test with one degree of freedom (HWE Program, Jurg Ott and Rockefeller University, New York). Linkage disequilibrium (LD) between SNPs from the same gene was tested using Haploview (http://www.broad.mit.edu/mpg/haploview/). Statistical analysis was performed using SPSS (version 20.0, SPSS Inc., Chicago, IL).

Using a co-dominant model (comparing the three genotypes, under the assumption that neither of the alleles is dominant), genotype specific differences between the phenotypes were analyzed with the Kruskal-Wallis test and to determine association adjusting for confounding factors (height, and smoking) regression analysis was performed. Gene interaction with Hcy was analyzed comparing the lowest and highest quartiles of serum Hcy levels, where quartile 1 was considered 'Normal' (<11.6 µmol/L) and quartile 4 'High' (>17.5 µmol/L). The $\chi 2$ test was used to analyze association between genotypes and categorical variables. Multiple statistical tests were performed, however since most of the phenotypes are dependent, we report uncorrected p-values (two-tailed) and associations were considered nominally significant at the level $p<0.05$.

Results

The general and clinical characteristics of the women from the two differently aged cohorts are reported in **Table 1**. Genotype and allele frequencies did not differ between cohorts (**Table 2**). All SNPs conformed to HWE ($p>0.05$). Both SNPs from the *FTO* gene were in strong LD (OPRA, $D' = 0.98$, $r^2 = 0.84$; PEAK-25, $D' = 0.99$, $r^2 = 0.87$) therefore only rs9939609 was used for further analysis. No LD was observed for the *MC4R* SNPs ($D' = 0.45$, $r^2 = 0.13$).

The PEAK-25 participants had lower BMI and fat mass and higher lean mass compared to the elderly individuals from OPRA (**Table 1**). As previously reported, fat and lean mass were strongly positively associated with BMD [26,53], with lean mass making a greater contribution than fat mass to BMD in young women (data not shown). For QUS phenotypes, the positive association with fat and lean mass was very similar in the elderly women, while in the young women the contribution from lean mass was stronger (**Table 3**).

Table 1. Cohort Baseline Details.

Variable	PEAK-25	OPRA
Age (years)	25.5 (25.3–25.7)	75.2 (75.1–75.3)
Weight (kg)	63.0 (57.1–70.0)	67 (60–75)
Height (cm)	168 (163–172)	160 (157–164)
BMI (kg/m^2)	22.4 (20.5–24.6)	26.0 (23.4–28.7)
Smokers#	440 (44%)	354 (34%)
Adult Fracture*	–	534 (51.1%)
Body Composition		
Total Body Fat mass (kg)	19.6 (15.2–25.1)	26.0 (20.8–31.3)
Trunk Fat mass (kg)	9.3 (6.9–12.2)	12.7 (9.8–15.4)
% Fat mass- Total Body	31.7 (26.5–36.4)	39.2 (34.1–43.1)
% Fat mass- Trunk	32.5 (26.2–38.9)	40.1 (35.3–44.1)
BMD (g/cm^2)		
Total Body	1.17 (1.12–1.22)	1.00 (0.94–1.07)
Femoral Neck	1.04 (0.97–1.13)	0.75 (0.66–0.85)
Lumbar Spine	1.05 (0.99–1.13)	0.97 (0.86–1.10)
Quantitative Ultrasound		
BUA (dB/MHz)	116 (110–124)	102 (96–109)
SOS (m/s)	1571 (1551–1595)	1522 (1505–1540)
Stiffness Index	98 (88–109)	71 (62–80)
Hip Geometry		
Hip Axis Length (mm)	–	105 (102–109)
Femoral Neck Width (mm)	–	34 (32–36)
Cross-Sectional Area (cm^2)	–	131 (114–155)
CSMI (cm^4)	–	10281 (8253–13188)
Femoral Neck Shaft Angle (°)	–	129 (126–131)
Biochemistry		
Homocysteine (µmol/L)	–	14.1 (11.6–17.5)
Vitamin B12 (pmol/L)	–	308 (238–409)
Folate (nmol/L)	–	18.0 (14.0–27.0)
Vitamin D (nmol/L)	–	92.1 (74.3–112.2)

Median (Interquartile Range) reported for continuous variables; Number (%) for discrete variables. #Current or former smokers; BUA- Broadband Ultrasound Attenuation; SOS- Speed of Sound; CSMI- Cross Sectional Moment of Inertia; *Fracture of any type sustained after age 20 and before baseline.

Association between Obesity Associated Polymorphisms and Body Composition

SNP rs9939609_*FTO* was associated with a number of body composition measurements including weight, BMI, and fat mass in PEAK-25 (**Table 4**). Individuals carrying the minor allele had higher BMI, fat mass (TB and trunk) but no association was found with lean mass (**Table 4**). The association with rs9939609_*FTO* remained after adjusting for smoking status and height ($p = 0.001$ to $p<0.0001$) (**Table 4**). We observed trends for BMI, TB fat mass and percentage trunk-fat in the same direction in the OPRA cohort, but these did not reach statistical significance. After adjustment for height and smoking status an association with percentage of trunk-fat was observed with rs9939609_*FTO* ($p = 0.007$). No association between *MC4R* or *INSIG2* polymorphisms and body composition were observed in the OPRA and PEAK-25 cohorts (data not shown).

Obesity Associated Polymorphisms and Association with BMD, QUS and Geometry

SNP rs1121980 from the *FTO* gene was excluded from analysis. The remaining four SNPs were analyzed for association with bone density, but no significant genotype related differences in BMD at any skeletal site were observed in either cohort (data not shown).

Polymorphisms were also analyzed for association with bone quantitative ultrasound in both cohorts. The rs17782313_*MC4R* showed association with BUA, SOS and SI in OPRA ($p = 0.007$–0.001) (**Table 5**) and individuals carrying the minor C-allele had higher values compared to homozygotes for the common allele. The association remained even after adjustment for height and smoking ($p = 0.02$–0.0004) (**Table 5**) and additional adjustment

Table 2. Genotype and Allele Frequencies.

	OPRA				PEAK-25			
SNP_Gene Symbol	**Major Allele Homozygotes No. (%)**	**Heterozygotes No. (%)**	**Minor Allele Homozygotes No. (%)**	**MAF**	**Major Allele Homozygotes No. (%)**	**Heterozygotes No. (%)**	**Minor Allele Homozygotes No. (%)**	**MAF**
rs9939609_FTO	354 (36)	499 (50)	139 (14)	0.39	319 (32)	499 (50)	182 (18)	0.43
rs1121980_FTO	312 (32)	500 (51)	170 (17)	0.43	282 (29)	492 (50)	211 (21)	0.47
rs7566605_INSIG2	448 (46)	424 (43)	111 (11)	0.33	449 (45)	421 (43)	116 (12)	0.33
rs17782313_MC4R	550 (57)	362 (38)	53 (5)	0.24	564 (57)	363 (37)	59 (6)	0.24
rs17700633_MC4R	456 (46)	439 (44)	98 (10)	0.32	482 (48)	414 (42)	98 (10)	0.31

MAF- Minor allele frequency.

Table 3. Effect Sizes of Lean and Fat Mass on Bone Quantitative Ultrasound (QUS) Phenotypes.

		QUS Variable	
OPRA	**BUA**	**SOS**	**Stiffness**
Total Body Fat mass	0.30	0.21	0.28
Total Body Lean mass	0.32	0.22	0.28
Trunk Fat mass	0.32	0.23	0.31
Trunk Lean mass	0.31	0.21	0.30
PEAK-25			
Total Body Fat mass	0.14	−0.03[a]	0.05[a]
Total Body Lean mass	0.34	0.20	0.28
Trunk Fat mass	0.14	−0.02[a]	0.06[a]
Trunk Lean mass	0.27	0.14	0.22

Reported values are standardized β-coefficients; covariates are adjusted for height and smoking status.
All coefficients are significant at $p<0.01$ except for those marked [a] which are non-significant.

for weight ($p = 0.015$ to 0.007). Similar trends were observed in the PEAK-25 cohort but were not statistically significant. Polymorphisms close to *FTO* and *INSIG2* were not associated with ultrasound phenotypes in either cohort.

Femoral neck geometry is an important component of hip fracture risk and we evaluated SNP-phenotype associations in the OPRA cohort. The rs7566605_*INSIG2* showed association with FN width ($p = 0.03$), with individuals carrying the minor allele having a lower mean value compared to subjects homozygous for the major allele (34.1 vs. 34.5 mm), but this did not withstand adjustment for height and weight. Polymorphisms from *FTO* and *MC4R* did not show any association with bone geometry (data not shown).

Obesity Associated Polymorphisms and Association with Biomarkers and Fracture

The association between obesity associated polymorphisms, biochemical risk factors and fracture was evaluated in the OPRA cohort. Carriers of rs17782313_*MC4R* C-allele had high Hcy ($p = 0.06$), low serum folate ($p = 0.03$) and low vitamin D ($p = 0.03$) (**Table 5**). After adjustment for smoking and height, the association remained for folate ($p = 0.01$) and vitamin D ($p = 0.02$).

We wanted to determine whether the association between *MC4R* SNPs and QUS was influenced in relation to normal (<11.6 μmol/L) and high (>17.5 μmol/L) levels of Hcy. Only in the high Hcy group was rs17782313_*MC4R* associated with QUS ($p = 0.03$ to $p = 0.005$) and this association remained even after adjustment for height and smoking ($p = 0.007$ to $p = 0.001$) (**Table 6**) and additionally adjusted for weight the association remained significant ($p = 0.01$ to 0.002). Interestingly, in the high Hcy group, vitamin D levels decreased with number of C-alleles, in direct contrast with the observation in the normal Hcy group (**Table 6**). As expected, proportionally fewer women fractured prior to baseline in the lowest (BMI<23.4; 63.9%) compared to the highest BMI quartile (BMI >28.7; 52.3%); $p = 0.009$).

Variation in *FTO* and *INSIG2* did not appear to make an important contribution to fracture risk, even when smoking, TB-BMD and any one of body weight, BMI or fat mass were

Table 4. Association of rs9939609_*FTO* with Bone and Body Composition Phenotypes in the PEAK-25 Cohort.

Phenotypes	TT (n = 319)	TA (n = 499)	AA (n = 182)	β-Value (Adjusted) Co-Dominant#	P-value[a]	P- value[b]
Weight	61.5 (57.0–68.7)	63.0 (57.0–69.2)	64.3 (58.0–72.3)	1.57 (0.69 to 2.44)	0.038	0.0004
BMI	22.1 (20.2–24.2)	22.2 (20.5–24.5)	23.0 (21.1–25.4)	0.550 (0.24 to 0.86)	0.004	0.001
Total Body Fat mass	19.0 (14.5–23.9)	19.4 (15.2–24.8)	21.1 (16.5–26.9)	1.36 (0.67 to 2.05)	0.004	0.0001
Total Body Lean mass	40.3 (37.4–43.3)	40.0 (37.1–43.1)	40.1 (37.1–43.5)	0.15 (−0.17 to 0.46)	0.63	0.36
% Fat mass - Total Body	30.5 (25.7–35.2)	31.7 (26.3–36.4)	32.9 (28.0–38.4)	1.17 (0.56 to 1.78)	0.002	0.0001
Trunk Fat mass	8.9 (6.6–11.6)	9.3 (6.9–12.1)	10.3 (7.7–13.5)	0.764 (0.39 to 1.14)	0.004	0.00007
% Fat mass - Trunk	31.2 (25.3–37.9)	32.5 (26.1–38.4)	34.12 (28.1–41.0)	1.36 (0.78 to 1.85)	0.002	0.0001
Total Body BMD	1.16 (1.12–1.22)	1.17 (1.12–1.23)	1.18 (1.13–1.22)	0.003 (−0.003 to 0.009)	0.52	0.38
Femoral neck BMD	1.04 (0.97–1.12)	1.04 (0.97–1.14)	1.06 (0.97–1.12)	0.003 (−0.007 to 0.014)	0.86	0.53
Lumbar Spine BMD	1.23 (1.15–1.31)	1.24 (1.14–1.33)	1.24 (1.14–1.33)	−0.001 (−0.012 to 0.010)	0.93	0.85
BUA	116 (109–124)	117 (117–123)	117 (110–124)	−0.015 (−0.977 to 0.946)	0.87	0.97
SOS	1569 (1552–1594)	1573 (1551–1596)	1572 (1550–1593)	−0.881 (−3.871 to 2.109)	0.60	0.56
Stiffness Index	96.5 (87.3–108.0)	98.0 (88.9–109.6)	99.0 (87.6–107.4)	−0.254 (−1.604 to 1.096)	0.65	0.71

Reported values are median (interquartile range); #(TT vs. TA vs. AA) [a]Kruskal-Wallis; [b]Linear regression - after adjustment for height and smoking.

included in the regression model. Women carrying the *MC4R*_rs17782313 C-allele showed a non-significant trend towards fewer fractures although there was no allele dose effect (52.1% vs. 58.5%). As expected, compared to women without a baseline fracture, QUS values were lower in those with a fracture regardless of genotype (data not shown), however, within the fracture category women with the rs17782313_*MC4R* C-allele had higher QUS values ((BUA: 97 vs. 100 vs. 103; p = 0.04); (SOS: 1516 vs. 1517 vs. 1517; p = 0.18); (SI: 67 vs. 70 vs. 72; p = 0.021)) consistent with a lower fracture incidence.

Discussion

Obesity is an established risk factor for a number of complex disorders including cardiovascular complications, diabetes mellitus and hypertension, but it has been suggested to be protective against osteoporosis [54]. A complex, differential influence from lean and fat mass on bone strength is suggested [54,55] and the current study supports the supposition that lean mass makes a larger contribution to BMD during young age while fat mass plays a major role for BMD in later stages of life [54,55].

Table 5. Association of rs17782313_*MC4R* with Body Composition, Bone and Biochemistry phenotypes in the OPRA Cohort.

Phenotypes	TT (n = 550)	TC (n = 362)	CC (n = 53)	β-value (Adjusted) Co-Dominant#	P-value[a]	P-value[b]
Weight	66 (60–75)	68 (59–76)	67 (62–75)	0.419 (−0.703 to 1.542)	0.65	0.46
BMI	26.0 (23.3–28.4)	26.0 (23.5–29.1)	26.2 (23.4–27.8)	0.157 (−0.283 to 0.596)	0.58	0.49
Total Body Fat mass	25.8 (20.5–31.1)	26.0 (20.9–31.9)	27.1 (22.4–30.4)	0.431 (−0.419 to 1.281)	0.70	0.32
% Fat mass Total Body	38.5 (34.0–42.7)	39.1 (34.4–42.2)	40.0 (35.4–41.7)	0.485 (−0.276 to 1.247)	0.72	0.21
Trunk Fat mass	12.5 (9.8–15.3)	13.0 (9.7–15.7)	13.0 (10.4–14.8)	0.144 (−.280 to 0.568)	0.69	0.50
% Fat mass- Trunk	39.1 (34.2–42.7)	39.6 (34.5–43.0)	39.4 (35.8–41.9)	0.52 (−0.266 to 1.237)	0.55	0.26
Total Body BMD	0.997 (0.941–1.061)	1.011 (0.944–1.073)	1.003 (0.934–1.062)	0.004 (−0.006 to 0.015)	0.52	0.44
Femoral Neck BMD	0.752 (0.660–0.848)	0.751 (0.680–0.846)	0.724 (0.628–0.825)	−0.005 (−0.019 to 0.009)	0.33	0.52
Lumbar Spine BMD	0.97 (0.86–1.10)	0.98 (0.87–1.09)	0.95 (0.84–1.12)	0.009 (−0.044 to 0.061)	0.83	0.75
BUA	100 (95–108)	103 (97–109)	103 (95–108)	1.72 (0.606 to 2.833)	0.007	0.002
SOS	1521 (1504–1539)	1526 (1509–1544)	1524 (1506–1540)	4.227 (1.119 to 7.335)	0.024	0.008
Stiffness Index	69.0 (61.0–79.0)	73.4 (65.0–82.5)	74.0 (61.0–81.3)	2.59 (1.11 to 4.07)	0.001	0.0006
Homocysteine	13.7 (11.6–16.9)	14.4 (11.6–17.7)	14.5 (11.6–18.3)	0.337 (−0.355 to 1.028)	0.06	0.34
Folate	18.0 (15.0–28.0)	17.0 (14.0–24.0)	16.0 (14.0–22.0)	−1.544 (−2.734 to −0.353)	0.028	0.013
Vitamin D	92.6 (76.7–115.5)	91.1 (72.5–109.2)	90.2 (70.3–110.5)	−3.744 (−6.914 to −0.573)	0.027	0.018

Values are median (Interquartile Range); #(TT vs. TC vs. CC); [a]Kruskal-Wallis; [b]Linear regression after adjustment for height and smoking; Units: folate and vitamin D (nmol/L), homocysteine (μmol/L).

Table 6. SNP *rs17782313_MC4R* Interacts with Homocysteine to Influence Bone Quality.

'Normal' homocysteine levels (<11.6 μmol/L) (n = 237)						
Phenotype	**TT**	**TC**	**CC**	**β-Value (Adjusted)**	**p value[a]**	**p value[b]**
	(130)	**(79)**	**(13)**	**Co-Dominant[#]**		
Total Body Fatmass	24.3 (18.7–29.2)	25.9 (21.1–30.4)	22.6 (19.4–28.7)	0.749 (−0.809 to 2.309)	0.35	0.35
Folate	32 (19–44)	29 (20–44)	32 (20–35)	−0.931 (−3.547 to 1.686)	0.76	0.48
Vitamin D	91.8 (77.2–115.5)	96.8 (73.7–111.0)	104 (72.3–134.0)	4.421 (−2.398 to 11.24)	0.46	0.21
BUA	101.4 (95.1–108.7	102 (98–109.7)	104.3 (93.0–108.7)	1.504 (−0.5546 to 3.563)	0.34	0.15
SOS	1522 (1505–1541)	1529 (1510–1547)	1538 (1508–1554)	3.893 (−2.348 to 10.13)	0.26	0.22
Stiffness Index	71 (62–80.6)	74 (65.5–83)	79 (57.6–84.7)	2.791 (−0.1968 to 5.779)	0.16	0.06
'High' homocysteine levels (>17.5 μmol/L) (n = 246)						
Phenotype	**TT**	**TC**	**CC**	**β-Value (Adjusted)**	**p value[a]**	**p value[b]**
	(111)	**(90)**	**(16)**	**Co-Dominant[#]**		
Total Body Fatmass	26.1 (19.6–31.4)	24.5 (19.2–33.2)	28.8 (24.9–30.7)	0.759 (−1.319 to 2.838)	0.49	0.48
Folate	14 (12–17)	14 (12–16)	14 (12–15)	−0.201 (−1.44 to 1.038)	0.87	0.75
Vitamin D	93.6 (75.6–116.9)	85.7 (68.9–106.7)	80.3 (64.2–104.3)	−7.394 (−13.9 to −0.8903)	0.08	0.026
BUA	98.7 (93.0–107.7)	103.5 (97–109)	106 (95.1–107.7)	4.356 (1.732 to 6.979)	0.006	0.001
SOS	1510 (1502–1535.9)	1519 (1508.2–1543)	1524 (1501–1539.9)	9.316 (2.572 to 16.06)	0.028	0.007
Stiffness Index	67 (59.9–77.9)	72 (64–82.5)	77 (64–76.8)	5.445 (2.188 to 8.702)	0.005	0.001

Values are median (Interquartile Range);
[#](TT vs. TC vs. CC);
[a]Kruskal-Wallis;
[b]Linear regression after adjustment for height and smoking.

FTO has been well described in relation to body composition and obesity phenotypes [33,34,36,37]. In our study, we observed higher BMI and fat mass in relation to the rs9939609_*FTO* C-allele; however it is interesting that the association was only seen in the young women. This is consistent with suggestions that the effect size of obesity susceptibility genes varies with age [56]. Although the underlying mechanisms are unclear, data from a mouse model has shown that mRNA expression of *FTO* is regulated by nutritional intake and expression levels vary according to feeding and fasting behavior [32] and we might speculate that food intake patterns differ between young and elderly individuals. We did not find any association with BMD or other bone phenotypes in either the young or elderly cohort of women. An age-specific effect has been reported in at least one study alongside suggestions that *FTO* could be a genetic marker for peak bone mass [36] due to the potential role of *FTO* in postnatal growth [37]. Our results do not support this however since the women in the PEAK-25 cohort are at an age where peak bone mass is assumed to have been reached. Nonetheless this does not rule out the possibility that *FTO* variants could be associated with skeletal growth trajectory in childhood and adolescence. Although we found no direct association between variations in the vicinity of *FTO* and BMD or QUS parameters, it is likely that any effect of the gene on bone is indirect, through BMI and fat mass.

MC4R is crucial in the regulation of body weight and monogenic forms of obesity commonly result from mutations in its gene. Although we observed a trend for higher BMI and fat mass in both cohorts with the C-allele, the association with *MC4R* did not reach significance, which contrasts with the findings reported in GWAS [33] and other association studies [57]. In the current study, we have shown for the first time that variation in the *MC4R* gene is associated with QUS phenotypes. A trend towards better bone quality with carriage of the variant *MC4R* rs17782313 C-allele was observed in the young women, but was more pronounced in the elderly women. Furthermore this association appeared to be mediated by both direct and indirect mechanisms which may explain in part the age specific effect observed, since a higher BMI, as displayed by the older women, is positively associated with bone strength. Although a genetic association between *MC4R* gene polymorphism and bone mass has been reported, albeit in children [41], we found no association with BMD or bone structural traits (femoral neck geometry) in our study.

One of the novel findings of our study is that *MC4R* is associated with altered vitamin D, folate and Hcy levels, which are associated with obesity. Vitamin D deficiency associated with obesity has been shown at all ages and independent of sex in a recent meta-analysis [58]. The results from our study indicates that a gene environment interaction has the potential to improve bone quality through increased fat mass in elderly women, demonstrated by the fact that the strongest association between *MC4R* and QUS was in the elevated Hcy group. This finding is in keeping with what is known about *MC4R* expression, i.e. that it is altered in response to environmental stimuli through hypothalamic neuronal networks, and recent studies suggest this has an important role in bone homeostasis [59].

Although in a meta-analysis of GWAS [39] variation in *INSIG2* was associated with femoral neck BMD, in our cohorts *INSIG2* was not associated with BMD, body composition or bone quality, although this is unsurprising since we have analyzed a BMI associated SNP which is not in LD ($r^2 = 0.01$; $D' = 0.39$) with the SNP identified in the BMD GWAS. In our study, although width at the femoral neck was narrower in elderly women with the variant allele, the association was attenuated after adjustment for height and weight and furthermore indices of bone strength and hip fracture rates were not different. To date, none of the GWAS for bone geometry have shown evidence of association within or near the *INSIG2* gene [60–63].

The strengths of this study include the extensive data collected on body composition, bone related phenotypes and biochemical risk factors for obesity and osteoporosis. By including two differently aged cohorts we have the possibility to distinguish age related effects of genetic variation on these phenotypes. The cohorts studied are well-characterized, large, of identical age within each cohort and the majority of women were of Swedish origin. Whether the findings are applicable to other ethnic groups requires replication in other populations. A limitation of the study is that biomarker data was not available in the PEAK-25 cohort, which would have enabled us to identify if there are age related effects associated with the homocysteine-*MC4R*-obesity relationship.

In summary, our data provides novel evidence that variation in the obesity associated gene *MC4R* is associated with improved quantitative ultrasound phenotypes, an important component of bone strength.

Acknowledgments

The authors acknowledge the participants of the study. Thanks are also extended to Dr Mattias Callréus for data collection, Åsa Almgren, Siv Braun and Lisa Quensell for data management, Jan-Åke Nilsson for statistical advice, Lisa Jansson for genotyping and the research nurses at the Clinical and Molecular Osteoporosis Research Unit.

Author Contributions

Conceived and designed the experiments: KÅ PG FM JK HL. Performed the experiments: GG JK. Analyzed the data: GG JK. Contributed reagents/materials/analysis tools: KÅ FM HL GG JK. Wrote the paper: GG JK FM. Revising and Approving manuscript: GG JK FM HL PG MR KÅ.

References

1. Deng FY, Lei SF, Li MX, Jiang C, Dvornyk V, et al. (2006) Genetic determination and correlation of body mass index and bone mineral density at the spine and hip in Chinese Han ethnicity. Osteoporos Int 17: 119–124.
2. Sun X, Lei SF, Deng FY, Wu S, Papacian C, et al. (2006) Genetic and environmental correlations between bone geometric parameters and body compositions. Calcif Tissue Int 79: 43–49.
3. Wardlaw GM (1996) Putting body weight and osteoporosis into perspective. Am J Clin Nutr 63: 433S–436S.
4. Skerry TM, Suva LJ (2003) Investigation of the regulation of bone mass by mechanical loading: from quantitative cytochemistry to gene array. Cell Biochem Funct 21: 223–229.
5. Horowitz MC (1993) Cytokines and estrogen in bone: anti-osteoporotic effects. Science 260: 626–627.
6. Reid IR (2002) Relationships among body mass, its components, and bone. Bone 31: 547–555.
7. Nakazato M, Maeda T, Takamura N, Wada M, Yamasaki H, et al. (2011) Relation of body mass index to blood folate and total homocysteine concentrations in Japanese adults. Eur J Nutr 50: 581–585.
8. Vaya A, Ejarque I, Tembl J, Corella D, Laiz B (2011) Hyperhomocysteinemia, obesity and cryptogenic stroke. Clin Hemorheol Microcirc 47: 53–58.
9. Vaya A, Rivera L, Hernandez-Mijares A, de la Fuente M, Sola E, et al. (2012) Homocysteine levels in morbidly obese patients: its association with waist circumference and insulin resistance. Clin Hemorheol Microcirc 52: 49–56.
10. Jungert A, Roth HJ, Neuhauser-Berthold M (2012) Serum 25-hydroxyvitamin D3 and body composition in an elderly cohort from Germany: a cross-sectional study. Nutr Metab (Lond) 9: 42.
11. Ensrud KE, Ewing SK, Fredman L, Hochberg MC, Cauley JA, et al. (2010) Circulating 25-hydroxyvitamin D levels and frailty status in older women. J Clin Endocrinol Metab 95: 5266–5273.
12. van Meurs JB, Dhonukshe-Rutten RA, Pluijm SM, van der Klift M, de Jonge R, et al. (2004) Homocysteine levels and the risk of osteoporotic fracture. N Engl J Med 350: 2033–2041.
13. McLean RR, Jacques PF, Selhub J, Tucker KL, Samelson EJ, et al. (2004) Homocysteine as a predictive factor for hip fracture in older persons. N Engl J Med 350: 2042–2049.
14. Morris MS, Jacques PF, Selhub J (2005) Relation between homocysteine and B-vitamin status indicators and bone mineral density in older Americans. Bone 37: 234–242.
15. Vacek TP, Kalani A, Voor MJ, Tyagi SC, Tyagi N (2013) The role of homocysteine in bone remodeling. Clin Chem Lab Med 51: 579–590.
16. Bellows CG, Heersche JN (2001) The frequency of common progenitors for adipocytes and osteoblasts and of committed and restricted adipocyte and osteoblast progenitors in fetal rat calvaria cell populations. J Bone Miner Res 16: 1983–1993.
17. Beresford JN, Bennett JH, Devlin C, Leboy PS, Owen ME (1992) Evidence for an inverse relationship between the differentiation of adipocytic and osteogenic cells in rat marrow stromal cell cultures. J Cell Sci 102 (Pt 2): 341–351.
18. Carnevale V, Romagnoli E, Del Fiacco R, Pepe J, Cipriani C, et al. (2010) Relationship between bone metabolism and adipogenesis. J Endocrinol Invest 33: 4–8.
19. Gimble JM, Robinson CE, Wu X, Kelly KA (1996) The function of adipocytes in the bone marrow stroma: an update. Bone 19: 421–428.
20. Rosen CJ, Bouxsein ML (2006) Mechanisms of disease: is osteoporosis the obesity of bone? Nat Clin Pract Rheumatol 2: 35–43.
21. Ackert-Bicknell CL, Demissie S, Marin de Evsikova C, Hsu YH, DeMambro VE, et al. (2008) PPARG by dietary fat interaction influences bone mass in mice and humans. J Bone Miner Res 23: 1398–1408.
22. Bustamante M, Nogues X, Mellibovsky L, Agueda L, Jurado S, et al. (2007) Polymorphisms in the interleukin-6 receptor gene are associated with bone mineral density and body mass index in Spanish postmenopausal women. Eur J Endocrinol 157: 677–684.
23. Cha S, Yu H, Kim JY (2012) Bone mineral density-associated polymorphisms are associated with obesity-related traits in Korean adults in a sex-dependent manner. PLoS One 7: e53013.
24. Fairbrother UL, Tanko LB, Walley AJ, Christiansen C, Froguel P, et al. (2007) Leptin receptor genotype at Gln223Arg is associated with body composition, BMD, and vertebral fracture in postmenopausal Danish women. J Bone Miner Res 22: 544–550.
25. McGuigan F, Larzenius E, Callreus M, Gerdhem P, Luthman H, et al. (2008) Variation in the bone morphogenetic protein-2 gene: effects on fat and lean body mass in young and elderly women. Eur J Endocrinol 158: 661–668.
26. McGuigan FE, Larzenius E, Callreus M, Gerdhem P, Luthman H, et al. (2007) Variation in the BMP2 gene: bone mineral density and ultrasound in young adult and elderly women. Calcif Tissue Int 81: 254–262.
27. Piters E, de Freitas F, Nielsen TL, Andersen M, Brixen K, et al. (2012) Association study of polymorphisms in the SOST gene region and parameters of bone strength and body composition in both young and elderly men: data from the Odense Androgen Study. Calcif Tissue Int 90: 30–39.
28. Xiao WJ, He JW, Zhang H, Hu WW, Gu JM, et al. (2011) ALOX12 polymorphisms are associated with fat mass but not peak bone mineral density in Chinese nuclear families. Int J Obes (Lond) 35: 378–386.
29. Zhao J, Bradfield JP, Li M, Zhang H, Mentch FD, et al. (2011) BMD-associated variation at the Osterix locus is correlated with childhood obesity in females. Obesity (Silver Spring) 19: 1311–1314.
30. Zhao LJ, Guo YF, Xiong DH, Xiao P, Recker RR, et al. (2006) Is a gene important for bone resorption a candidate for obesity? An association and linkage study on the RANK (receptor activator of nuclear factor-kappaB) gene in a large Caucasian sample. Hum Genet 120: 561–570.
31. Liu YZ, Pei YF, Liu JF, Yang F, Guo Y, et al. (2009) Powerful bivariate genome-wide association analyses suggest the SOX6 gene influencing both obesity and osteoporosis phenotypes in males. PLoS One 4: e6827.
32. Gerken T, Girard CA, Tung YC, Webby CJ, Saudek V, et al. (2007) The obesity-associated FTO gene encodes a 2-oxoglutarate-dependent nucleic acid demethylase. Science 318: 1469–1472.

33. Loos RJ, Lindgren CM, Li S, Wheeler E, Zhao JH, et al. (2008) Common variants near MC4R are associated with fat mass, weight and risk of obesity. Nat Genet 40: 768–775.
34. Frayling TM, Timpson NJ, Weedon MN, Zeggini E, Freathy RM, et al. (2007) A common variant in the FTO gene is associated with body mass index and predisposes to childhood and adult obesity. Science 316: 889–894.
35. Rouskas K, Kouvatsi A, Paletas K, Papazoglou D, Tsapas A, et al. (2012) Common variants in FTO, MC4R, TMEM18, PRL, AIF1, and PCSK1 show evidence of association with adult obesity in the Greek population. Obesity (Silver Spring) 20: 389–395.
36. Guo Y, Liu H, Yang TL, Li SM, Li SK, et al. (2011) The fat mass and obesity associated gene, FTO, is also associated with osteoporosis phenotypes. PLoS One 6: e27312.
37. Gao X, Shin YH, Li M, Wang F, Tong Q, et al. (2010) The fat mass and obesity associated gene FTO functions in the brain to regulate postnatal growth in mice. PLoS One 5: e14005.
38. Tao YX (2010) The melanocortin-4 receptor: physiology, pharmacology, and pathophysiology. Endocr Rev 31: 506–543.
39. Willer CJ, Speliotes EK, Loos RJ, Li S, Lindgren CM, et al. (2009) Six new loci associated with body mass index highlight a neuronal influence on body weight regulation. Nat Genet 41: 25–34.
40. Ahn JD, Dubern B, Lubrano-Berthelier C, Clement K, Karsenty G (2006) Cart overexpression is the only identifiable cause of high bone mass in melanocortin 4 receptor deficiency. Endocrinology 147: 3196–3202.
41. Timpson NJ, Sayers A, Davey-Smith G, Tobias JH (2009) How does body fat influence bone mass in childhood? A Mendelian randomization approach. J Bone Miner Res 24: 522–533.
42. Herbert A, Gerry NP, McQueen MB, Heid IM, Pfeufer A, et al. (2006) A common genetic variant is associated with adult and childhood obesity. Science 312: 279–283.
43. Gong Y, Lee JN, Brown MS, Goldstein JL, Ye J (2006) Juxtamembranous aspartic acid in Insig-1 and Insig-2 is required for cholesterol homeostasis. Proc Natl Acad Sci U S A 103: 6154–6159.
44. Estrada K, Styrkarsdottir U, Evangelou E, Hsu YH, Duncan EL, et al. (2012) Genome-wide meta-analysis identifies 56 bone mineral density loci and reveals 14 loci associated with risk of fracture. Nat Genet 44: 491–501.
45. Gerdhem P, Brandstrom H, Stiger F, Obrant K, Melhus H, et al. (2004) Association of the collagen type 1 (COL1A 1) Sp1 binding site polymorphism to femoral neck bone mineral density and wrist fracture in 1044 elderly Swedish women. Calcif Tissue Int 74: 264–269.
46. Kumar J, Swanberg M, McGuigan F, Callreus M, Gerdhem P, et al. (2011) LRP4 association to bone properties and fracture and interaction with genes in the Wnt- and BMP signaling pathways. Bone 49: 343–348.
47. Lenora J, Akesson K, Gerdhem P (2010) Effect of precision on longitudinal follow-up of bone mineral density measurements in elderly women and men. J Clin Densitom 13: 407–412.
48. Callreus M, McGuigan F, Ringsberg K, Akesson K (2012) Self-reported recreational exercise combining regularity and impact is necessary to maximize bone mineral density in young adult women: a population-based study of 1,061 women 25 years of age. Osteoporos Int 23: 2517–2526.
49. Tenne M, McGuigan FE, Ahlborg H, Gerdhem P, Akesson K (2010) Variation in the PTH gene, hip fracture, and femoral neck geometry in elderly women. Calcif Tissue Int 86: 359–366.
50. Karlsson MK, Obrant KJ, Nilsson BE, Johnell O (1998) Bone mineral density assessed by quantitative ultrasound and dual energy X-ray absorptiometry. Normative data in Malmo, Sweden. Acta Orthop Scand 69: 189–193.
51. Gerdhem P, Akesson K (2007) Rates of fracture in participants and non-participants in the Osteoporosis Prospective Risk Assessment study. J Bone Joint Surg Br 89: 1627–1631.
52. Gerdhem P, Ivaska KK, Isaksson A, Pettersson K, Vaananen HK, et al. (2007) Associations between homocysteine, bone turnover, BMD, mortality, and fracture risk in elderly women. J Bone Miner Res 22: 127–134.
53. Gerdhem P, Ringsberg KA, Akesson K, Obrant KJ (2003) Influence of muscle strength, physical activity and weight on bone mass in a population-based sample of 1004 elderly women. Osteoporos Int 14: 768–772.
54. Namwongprom S, Rojanasthien S, Mangklabruks A, Soontrapa S, Wongboontan C, et al. (2013) Effect of fat mass and lean mass on bone mineral density in postmenopausal and perimenopausal Thai women. Int J Womens Health 5: 87–92.
55. Hawamdeh ZM, Sheikh-Ali RF, Alsharif A, Otom AH, Ibrahim AI, et al. (2013) The Influence of Aging on the Association Between Adiposity and Bone Mineral Density in Jordanian Postmenopausal Women. J Clin Densitom. [Epub ahead of print].
56. Kvaloy K, Kulle B, Romundstad P, Holmen TL (2013) Sex-specific effects of weight-affecting gene variants in a life course perspective-The HUNT Study, Norway. Int J Obes (Lond) 9: 1221–9.
57. Liem ET, Vonk JM, Sauer PJ, van der Steege G, Oosterom E, et al. (2010) Influence of common variants near INSIG2, in FTO, and near MC4R genes on overweight and the metabolic profile in adolescence: the TRAILS (TRacking Adolescents' Individual Lives Survey) Study. Am J Clin Nutr 91: 321–328.
58. Vimaleswaran KS, Berry DJ, Lu C, Tikkanen E, Pilz S, et al. (2013) Causal relationship between obesity and vitamin D status: bi-directional Mendelian randomization analysis of multiple cohorts. PLoS Med 10: e1001383.
59. Patel MS, Elefteriou F (2007) The new field of neuroskeletal biology. Calcif Tissue Int 80: 337–347.
60. Chen Y, Xiong DH, Guo YF, Pan F, Zhou Q, et al. (2010) Pathway-based genome-wide association analysis identified the importance of EphrinA-EphR pathway for femoral neck bone geometry. Bone 46: 129–136.
61. Hsu YH, Zillikens MC, Wilson SG, Farber CR, Demissie S, et al. (2010) An integration of genome-wide association study and gene expression profiling to prioritize the discovery of novel susceptibility Loci for osteoporosis-related traits. PLoS Genet 6: e1000977.
62. Liu YZ, Wilson SG, Wang L, Liu XG, Guo YF, et al. (2008) Identification of PLCL1 gene for hip bone size variation in females in a genome-wide association study. PLoS One 3: e3160.
63. Zhao LJ, Liu XG, Liu YZ, Liu YJ, Papasian CJ, et al. (2010) Genome-wide association study for femoral neck bone geometry. J Bone Miner Res 25: 320–329.

Permissions

All chapters in this book were first published in PLOS ONE, by The Public Library of Science; hereby published with permission under the Creative Commons Attribution License or equivalent. Every chapter published in this book has been scrutinized by our experts. Their significance has been extensively debated. The topics covered herein carry significant findings which will fuel the growth of the discipline. They may even be implemented as practical applications or may be referred to as a beginning point for another development.

The contributors of this book come from diverse backgrounds, making this book a truly international effort. This book will bring forth new frontiers with its revolutionizing research information and detailed analysis of the nascent developments around the world.

We would like to thank all the contributing authors for lending their expertise to make the book truly unique. They have played a crucial role in the development of this book. Without their invaluable contributions this book wouldn't have been possible. They have made vital efforts to compile up to date information on the varied aspects of this subject to make this book a valuable addition to the collection of many professionals and students.

This book was conceptualized with the vision of imparting up-to-date information and advanced data in this field. To ensure the same, a matchless editorial board was set up. Every individual on the board went through rigorous rounds of assessment to prove their worth. After which they invested a large part of their time researching and compiling the most relevant data for our readers.

The editorial board has been involved in producing this book since its inception. They have spent rigorous hours researching and exploring the diverse topics which have resulted in the successful publishing of this book. They have passed on their knowledge of decades through this book. To expedite this challenging task, the publisher supported the team at every step. A small team of assistant editors was also appointed to further simplify the editing procedure and attain best results for the readers.

Apart from the editorial board, the designing team has also invested a significant amount of their time in understanding the subject and creating the most relevant covers. They scrutinized every image to scout for the most suitable representation of the subject and create an appropriate cover for the book.

The publishing team has been an ardent support to the editorial, designing and production team. Their endless efforts to recruit the best for this project, has resulted in the accomplishment of this book. They are a veteran in the field of academics and their pool of knowledge is as vast as their experience in printing. Their expertise and guidance has proved useful at every step. Their uncompromising quality standards have made this book an exceptional effort. Their encouragement from time to time has been an inspiration for everyone.

The publisher and the editorial board hope that this book will prove to be a valuable piece of knowledge for researchers, students, practitioners and scholars across the globe.

List of Contributors

Hossam M. Abdallah and Ali M. El-halawany
Department of Natural Products, Faculty of Pharmacy, King Abdulaziz University, Jeddah, Saudi Arabia
Department of Pharmacognosy, Faculty of Pharmacy, Cairo University, Cairo, Egypt

Ahmed M. Al-Abd
Pharmacology Department, Medical Division, National Research Center, Giza, Egypt
Department of Pharmacology and Toxicology, Faculty of Pharmacy, King Abdulaziz University, Jeddah, Saudi Arabia

Gihan F. Asaad
Pharmacology Department, Medical Division, National Research Center, Giza, Egypt
Pharmacology Department, Faculty of Pharmacy, Jazan University, Jazan, Saudia Arabia

Ashraf B. Abdel-Naim
Department of Pharmacology and Toxicology, Faculty of Pharmacy, King Abdulaziz University, Jeddah, Saudi Arabia

Guoqing Qian, Kathy Xue1, Lili Tang, Franklin Wang and Jia-Sheng Wang
Department of Environmental Health Science, University of Georgia, Athens, Georgia, United States of America

Xiao Song
Department of Epidemiology and Biostatistics, University of Georgia, Athens, Georgia, United States of America

Ming-Chien Chyu
Department of Mechanical Engineering, Texas Tech University, Lubbock, Texas, United States of America

Barbara C. Pence
Laboratory Science and Primary Care, Texas Tech University Health Sciences Center, Lubbock, Texas, United States of America

Chwan-Li Shen
Laboratory Science and Primary Care, Texas Tech University Health Sciences Center, Lubbock, Texas, United States of America
Department of Pathology, Texas Tech University Health Sciences Center, Lubbock, Texas, United States of America
Laura W. Bush Institute for Women's Health, Texas Tech University Health Sciences Center, Lubbock, Texas, United States of America

Yongzheng He, Shi Chen, Xiaohua Wu, Jin Yuan, Xianlin Yang, Li Jiang, Mingjiang Xu and Feng-Chun Yang
Department of Pediatrics, Indiana University School of Medicine, Indianapolis, Indiana, United States of America

Steven D. Rhodes
Department of Anatomy and Cell Biology, Indiana University School of Medicine, Indianapolis, Indiana, United States of America

Xianqi Li and Naoyuki Takahashi
Division of Hard Tissue Research, Matsumoto Dental University, Shiojiri, Nagano, Japan

Khalid S. Mohammad and Theresa A. Guise
Department of Medicine, Indiana University School of Medicine, Indianapolis, Indiana, United States of America

Yang Wang, Ling Li, Benjamin T. Moore, Xian-Hao Peng, Joan M. Lappe, Robert R. Recker and Peng Xiao
Osteoporosis Research Center, School of Medicine, Creighton University, Omaha, Nebraska, United States of America

Xiang Fang
Biostatistical Core, Office of Research and Compliance, Creighton University, Omaha, Nebraska, United States of America

Minoru Sugiura, Kazunori Ogawa, Yoshinori Ikoma and Masamichi Yano
Citrus Research Division, National Institute of Fruit Tree Science, Shizuoka City, Shizuoka, Japan

Mieko Nakamura
Department of Community Health and Preventive Medicine, Hamamatsu University School of Medicine, Hamamatsu City, Shizuoka, Japan

Eugenia Negredo, Anna Bonjoch Carla Estany and Jordi Puig
Lluita contra la SIDA Foundation, Hospital Universitari Germans Trias i Pujol, Universitat Autónoma de Barcelona, Barcelona, Spain

Nuria Perez- Alvarez
Lluita contra la SIDA Foundation, Hospital Universitari Germans Trias i Pujol, Universitat Auto`noma de Barcelona, Barcelona, Spain
Statistics and Operations Research Department, Universitat Politècnica de Catalunya, Barcelona, Spain

Bonaventura Clotet
Lluita contra la SIDA Foundation, Hospital Universitari Germans Trias i Pujol, Universitat Auto`noma de Barcelona, Barcelona, Spain
Irsicaixa Foundation, Barcelona, Spain

Moisés Gómez-Mateu and Guadalupe Gómez
Statistics and Operations Research Department, Universitat Politècnica de Catalunya, Barcelona, Spain

Joaquin Rosales, Silvana di Gregorio and Luis del Rio
CETIR Centre Mè dic, Barcelona, Spain

Bo Ma, Qi Zhang, Yonglu Wang, Jing Li and Yinhui Liu
School of Pharmaceutical Sciences, Nanjing University of Technology, Nanjing, People's Republic of China

Jiannan Liu
Department of Respiration, Jiangsu Geriatric Hospital, Nanjing, People's Republic of China

Hanjie Ying
School of Life Science and Pharmaceutical Engineering, Nanjing University of Technology, Nanjing, People's Republic of China

Jiye A and Jianguo Sun
Key Laboratory of Drug Metabolism and Pharmacokinetics, China Pharmaceutical University, Nanjing, People's Republic of China

Di Wu
Laboratory for Systems Biology, Division of Clinical Pharmacology and Therapeutics, The Children's Hospital of Philadelphia, Philadelphia, Pennsylvania, United States of America
Kinetic Modeling and Simulation (KMAS) Core, Institute of Translational Medicine and Therapeutics, University of Pennsylvania, Philadelphia, Pennsylvania, United States of America

Ying-Hsien Chen., Wei-Shiung Yang, Yen-Hung Lin, Mao-Shin Lin, Yi-Lwun Ho and Ming-Fong Chen
National Taiwan University College of Medicine, Taipei, Taiwan
Department of Internal Medicine, National Taiwan University Hospital, Taipei, Taiwan

Yen-Wen Wu
National Taiwan University College of Medicine, Taipei, Taiwan
Department of Internal Medicine, National Taiwan University Hospital, Taipei, Taiwan
Department of Nuclear Medicine, National Taiwan University Hospital, Taipei, Taiwan
Department of Nuclear Medicine, Far Eastern Memorial Hospital, New Taipei City, Taiwan

Chi-Ming Lee
National Taiwan University College of Medicine, Taipei, Taiwan
Department of Internal Medicine, National Taiwan University Hospital, Taipei, Taiwan
Cardiovascular Center, National Taiwan University Hospital Yun-Lin Branch, Dou-Liu City, Taiwan

Shoei-Shen Wang, Nai- Kuan Chou and Ron-Bin Hsu
National Taiwan University College of Medicine, Taipei, Taiwan
Department of Surgery, National Taiwan University Hospital, Taipei, Taiwan

Cristina Eller-Vainicher, Iacopo Chiodini, Elisa Cairoli and Paolo Beck-Peccoz
Endocrinology and Diabetology Unit, Medical Sciences Department, Fondazione Istituto di Ricovero e Cura a Carattere Scientifico Cà Granda Ospedale Maggiore Policlinico, Milan, Italy

Ivana Santi
Istituto Geriatrico Azienda di Servizi alla Persona Istituti Milanesi Martinitt e Stelline e Pio Albergo Trivulzio, Milan, Italy

Marco Massarotti
Istituto di Ricovero e Cura a Carattere Scientifico Humanitas, Rozzano, Milan, Italy

Luca Pietrogrande
Orthopedic Clinic, Dipartimento di Medicina, Chirurgia e Odontoiatria San Paolo, University of Milan, Milan, Italy

Matteo Longhi
Unit of Reumathology, Istituto di Ricovero e Cura a Carattere Scientifico Istituto Ortopedico Galeazzi, Milan, Italy

Valter Galmarini
Azienda Ospedaliera Fatebenefratelli e Oftalmico, Milan, Italy

Giorgio Gandolini
Istituto di Ricovero e Cura a Carattere Scientifico Don Gnocchi, Milan, Italy

Maurizio Bevilacqua
Endocrinology and Diabetes Unit, Luigi Sacco Hospital (Vialba), University of Milan, Milan, Italy

Enzo Grossi
Bracco Medical Department, San Donato Milanese, Milan, Italy
Semeion Research Centre, Rome, Italy

Yong-Jun Liu, Qing Tian, Hui Shen and Inderpal S. Thethi
School of Public Health and Tropical Medicine, Tulane University, New Orleans, Louisiana, United States of America

Hong-Wen Deng
School of Public Health and Tropical Medicine, Tulane University, New Orleans, Louisiana, United States of America
Center of System Biomedical Sciences, School of Medical Instrument and Food Engineering, University of Shanghai for Science and Technology, Shanghai, P. R. China

Shu Ran, Yu-Fang Pei, Lei Zhang, Ying-Ying Han, Yong Lin and Xue-Zhen Zhu
Center of System Biomedical Sciences, School of Medical Instrument and Food Engineering, University of Shanghai for Science and Technology, Shanghai, P. R. China

Rong Hai
Inner Mongolia People's Hospital, Hohhot, P. R. China

Tie-Lin Yang
School of Life Science and Technology, Xi'an Jiaotong University, Xi'an, Shanxi, P. R. China

Yan-Fang Guo
School of Basic Medical Science, Institute of Bioinformatics, Southern Medical University, Guangzhou, Guangdong, P. R. China

Peggy Benisch, Tatjana Schilling, Lothar Seefried, Nadja Raaijmakers, Melanie Krug, Martina Regensburger, Sabine Zeck, Regina Ebert and Franz Jakob
Orthopedic Center for Musculoskeletal Research, University of Wuerzburg, Wuerzburg, Germany

Ludger Klein-Hitpass
Institute of Cell Biology (Tumor Research), University Hospital Essen, Essen, Germany

Sönke P. Frey
Department of Trauma, Hand-, Plastic- and Reconstructive Surgery, University Hospital of Wuerzburg, Wuerzburg, Germany

Thorsten Schinke and Michael Amling
Department of Osteology and Biomechanics, University Medical Center Hamburg Eppendorf, Hamburg, Germany

Clive Henry Buckle., Evy De Leenheer and Michelle Anne Lawson
Department of Human Metabolism, University of Sheffield Faculty of Medicine, Dentistry and Health, Sheffield, United Kingdom

Peter Ian Croucher
Department of Human Metabolism, University of Sheffield Faculty of Medicine, Dentistry and Health, Sheffield, United Kingdom
Garvan Institute for Medical Research, Sydney, Australia

Kwee Yong and Neil Rabin
Department of Haematology, University College London, London, United Kingdom

Mark Perry
Department of Anatomy, University of Bristol, Bristol, United Kingdom

Karen Vanderkerken
Department of Haematology and Immunology, Vrije Universiteit Brussel, Brussels, Belgium

Ellen Wright, Peter T. Schofield, Paul Seed and Mariam Molokhia
Department of Primary Care and Public Health Sciences, King's College London, London, United Kingdom

Hongbao Cao
Department of Biomedical Engineering, Tulane University, New Orleans, Louisiana, United States of America

Yu-Ping Wang
Department of Biomedical Engineering, Tulane University, New Orleans, Louisiana, United States of America
Department of Biostatistics and Bioinformatics, Tulane University, New Orleans, Louisiana, United States of America

Shufeng Lei
Center for Genetic Epidemiology and Genomics, School of Public Health, Medical College of Soochow University, Suzhou, P. R. China

Hong-Wen Deng
Department of Biostatistics and Bioinformatics, Tulane University, New Orleans, Louisiana, United States of America

M. Mofizul Islam, Laurann Yen, Paresh Dawda, Tanisha Jowsey and Ian S. McRae
Australian Primary Health Care Research Institute, Australian National University, Canberra, Australian Capital Territory, Australia

Jose M. Valderas
Health Services and Policy Research, University of Exeter Medical School, Exeter, England, United Kingdom

Marilyn L. Kwan, Joan C. Lo, Cecile A. Laurent, Janise M. Roh, Malini Chandra, Charles P. Quesenberry Jr. and Lawrence H. Kushi
Division of Research, Kaiser Permanente Northern California, Oakland, California, United States of America

Li Tang, Theresa E. Hahn, Chi-Chen Hong, Lara Sucheston-Campbell, Christine B. Ambrosone and Song Yao
Department of Cancer Prevention and Control, Roswell Park Cancer Institute, Buffalo, New York, United States of America

Dawn L. Hershman
Department of Medicine and the Herbert Irving Comprehensive Cancer Center, Columbia University, New York, New York, United States of America

Philippe Ravaud
U1153, Institut National de la Santé et de la Recherche Mé dicale, Paris, France,
Centre d'E´pid é miologie Clinique, H ôpital Hôtel Dieu AP-HP, Paris, France
Université Paris Descartes, PRES Sorbonne Paris Cité, Paris, France

Clémence Palazzo
U1153, Institut National de la Santé et de la Recherche Mé dicale, Paris, France
Centre d'E´pid é miologie Clinique, H ôpital Hôtel Dieu AP-HP, Paris, France
Université Paris Descartes, PRES Sorbonne Paris Cité, Paris, France
Service de rééducation et réadaptation de l'appareil locomoteur et des pathologies du rachis, Hôpital Cochin AP-HP, Paris, France

Serge Poiraudeau
U1153, Institut National de la Santé et de la Recherche Mé dicale, Paris, France
Université Paris Descartes, PRES Sorbonne Paris Cité, Paris, France
Service de rééducation et réadaptation de l'appareil locomoteur et des pathologies du rachis, Hôpital Cochin AP-HP, Paris, France
Institut fédératif de recherche sur le handicap, Institut National de la Sante´ et de la Recherche Mé dicale, Paris, France

Agathe Papelard
Service de rééducation et réadaptation de l'appareil locomoteur et des pathologies du rachis, Hôpital Cochin AP-HP, Paris, France
Institut fe´de´ ratif de recherche sur le handicap, Institut National de la Sante´ et de la Recherche Mé dicale, Paris, France

Jean-François Ravaud
Institut fédé ratif de recherche sur le handicap, Institut National de la Santé et de la Recherche Mé dicale, Paris, France
U988, Institut National de la Santé et de la Recherche Médicale, Villejuif, France
UMR 8211, Centre national de la recherche scientifique, Villejuif, France

Shuai Zheng, Zhao-Ming Zhong, Xiu-Hua Wu, Zhi-Ping Huang, Wei Li1, Ruo-Ting Ding, Hui Yu and Jian-Ting Chen
Department of Orthopedic Spinal Surgery, Nanfang Hospital, Southern Medical University, Guangdong Province, Guangzhou, China

Guo-Xian Chen
Department of Orthopedic Spinal Surgery, Nanfang Hospital, Southern Medical University, Guangdong Province, Guangzhou, China
Department of Orthopedic, the First Hospital of Putian City, Fujian Province, Putian City, China

Shuai Qin
Department of ophthalmology, The People's Hospital of Zhuhai, Zhuhai, China

Miyuki Takasu, Takuji Yamagami, Yuko Nakamura, Daisuke Komoto, Yoko Kaichi, Chihiro Tani, Shuji Date, Masao Kiguchi and Kazuo Awai
Department of Diagnostic Radiology, Graduate School of Biomedical Sciences, Hiroshima University, Hiroshima, Japan

Jun Wu, Dengshun Miao and Wen Sun
The Research Center for Bone and Stem Cells, Department of Anatomy, Histology and Embryology, Nanjing Medical University, Nanjing, P.R. of China

Hua Wang and Ying Yin
The Research Center for Bone and Stem Cells, Department of Anatomy, Histology and Embryology, Nanjing Medical University, Nanjing, P.R. of China
Institute of Dental Research, Stomatological College, Nanjing Medical University, Nanjing, P.R. of China

Jingning Liu
Department of Geriatrics, The Second Affiliated Hospital of Nanjing Medical University, Nanjing, P.R. of China

Zilu Wang
Institute of Dental Research, Stomatological College, Nanjing Medical University, Nanjing, P.R. of China

Yoshiteru Miyauchi, Hiroya Kanagawa, Eri Katsuyama, Atsuhiro Fujie, Wu Hao, Toshimi Tando, Ryuichi Watanabe, Kana Miyamoto, Hideo Morioka, Morio Matsumoto and Yoshiaki Toyama
Department of Orthopedic Surgery, Keio University School of Medicine, Shinjuku-ku, Tokyo, Japan

Yuiko Sato
Department of Orthopedic Surgery, Keio University School of Medicine, Shinjuku-ku, Tokyo, Japan
Department of Musculoskeletal Reconstruction and Regeneration Surgery, Keio University School of Medicine, Shinjuku-ku, Tokyo, Japan

Tami Kobayashi and Takeshi Miyamoto
Department of Orthopedic Surgery, Keio University School of Medicine, Shinjuku-ku, Tokyo, Japan
Department of Integrated Bone Metabolism and Immunology, Keio University School of Medicine, Shinjuku-ku, Tokyo, Japan

Shigeyuki Yoshida and Mayu Morita
Department of Dentistry and Oral Surgery, Keio University School of Medicine, Shinjuku-ku, Tokyo, Japan

Meng Wei and Stephen C. Deutsch
Cedars-Sinai Medical Care Foundation, Beverly Hills, California, United States of America

Run Yu
Division of Endocrinology, Cedars-Sinai Medical Center, Los Angeles, California, United States of America

Jia Peng, Shen Xing, Kang Hui, Chen Hao, Qi Jin, Zhou Qi, Wang Jin Shen, Qian Nian Dong, Zhou Han Bing and Deng Lian Fu
Shanghai Institute of Traumatology and Orthopaedics, Shanghai Key Laboratory for Prevention and Treatment of Bone and Joint Diseases with Integrated Chinese- Western Medicine, Ruijin Hospital, Jiao Tong University School of Medicine, Shanghai, China

Zuo Gui Lai
Shanghai Institute of Traumatology and Orthopaedics, Shanghai Key Laboratory for Prevention and Treatment of Bone and Joint Diseases with Integrated Chinese- Western Medicine, Ruijin Hospital, Jiao Tong University School of Medicine, Shanghai, China
Department of Orthopaedics, Qian Fo Shan Hospital, Shang Dong University, Ji Nan, China

Zhang Lian Fang
Shanghai Institute of Traumatology and Orthopaedics, Shanghai Key Laboratory for Prevention and Treatment of Bone and Joint Diseases with Integrated Chinese- Western Medicine, Ruijin Hospital, Jiao Tong University School of Medicine, Shanghai, China
Department of Orthopaedics, The First Affiliated Hospital of Soochow University, Suzhou, China

J. Keenan Brown and Alan D. Brett
Mindways Software, Inc., Austin, Texas, United States of America

Christopher E. Cann
Mindways Software, Inc., Austin, Texas, United States of America
Department of Radiology, University of California San Francisco, San Francisco, California, UnitedStates of America

Judith E. Adams
Department of Clinical Radiology, University of Manchester, Manchester, United Kingdom

Julia V. Wö lfle and Heiko Reichel
Department of Orthopaedic Surgery, Centre of Musculoskeletal Research, University of Ulm, Ulm, Germany

Jörg Fiedler and Rolf E. Brenner
Division for Biochemistry of Joint and Connective Tissue Diseases, Department of Orthopaedic Surgery, Centre of Musculoskeletal Research, University of Ulm, Ulm, Germany

Lutz Dürselen and Anita Ignatius
Institute of Orthopaedic Research and Biomechanics, Centre of Musculoskeletal Research, University of Ulm, Ulm, Germany

Judith Reichert and Dieter Scharnweber
Max Bergmann Center of Biomaterials, TU Dresden, Dresden, Germany

Anne Förster and Bernd Schwenzer
Institute of Biochemistry, TU Dresden, Dresden, Germany

Lihui Li, Shuang Lv, Miaomiao Dong, Li Zhang, Jiaheng Tu, Jie Yang, Lingli Zhang and Yinan Song
School of Kinesiology, Shanghai University of Sport, Shanghai, China

Jun Zou
Scientific Research Department, Shanghai University of Sport, Shanghai, China

Leiting Xu
School of Kinesiology, Shanghai University of Sport, Shanghai, China
Medical School of Ningbo University, Ningbo, China

Xi Chen
School of Kinesiology, Shanghai University of Sport, Shanghai, China
School of Sports Science, Wenzhou Medical University, Wenzhou, China

Rui Zhang, He Gong, Jiazi Gao and Juan Fang
Department of Engineering Mechanics, Jilin University, Changchun, Jilin, People's Republic of China

Dong Zhu
Department of Orthopedic Surgery, No. 1 Hospital of Jilin University, Changchun, Jilin, People's Republic of China

Yubo Fan
School of Biological Science and Medical Engineering, Beihang University, Beijing, People's Republic of China

Jitender Kumar
Department of Medical Sciences, Molecular Epidemiology and Science for Life Laboratory, Uppsala University, Uppsala, Sweden

Martin Ridderstråle
Clinical Obesity Research, Department of Endocrinology, Ska°ne University Hospital, Malmö, Sweden

Paul Gerdhem
Department of Clinical Science, Intervention and Technology, Karolinska Institutet, Department of Orthopaedics, Karolinska University Hospital, Stockholm, Sweden

Holger Luthman
Medical Genetics Unit, Department of Clinical Sciences, Lund University, Malmö, Sweden

Gaurav Garg, Fiona E. McGuigan and Kristina Åkesson
Clinical and Molecular Osteoporosis Research Unit, Department of Clinical Sciences, Lund University and Department of Orthopaedics, Skåne University Hospital, Malmö, Sweden

Index